a LANGE medical book

Introduction to
Clinical Psychiatry

first edition

a LANGE medical book

Introduction to
Clinical Psychiatry

first edition

Edited by

G. David Elkin, MD
Attending Psychiatrist
San Francisco General Hospital
Associate Clinical Professor
Department of Psychiatry
University of California, San Francisco

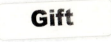

APPLETON & LANGE
Stamford, Connecticut

Notice: The authors and the publisher of this volume have taken care to
make certain that the doses of drugs and schedules of treatment are correct
and compatible with the standards generally accepted at the time of
publication. Nevertheless, as new information becomes available, changes in
treatment and in the use of drugs become necessary. The reader is advised to
carefully consult the instruction and information material included in the
package insert of each drug or therapeutic agent before administration.
This advice is especially important when using, administering, or recommending
new or infrequently used drugs. The authors and publisher disclaim all responsibility
for any liability, loss, injury, or damage incurred as a consequence, directly
or indirectly, of the use and application of any of the contents of this volume.

Prentice Hall International (UK) Limited, *London*
Prentice Hall of Australia Pty. Limited, *Sydney*
Prentice Hall Canada, Inc., *Toronto*
Prentice Hall Hispanoamericana, S.A., *Mexico*
Prentice Hall of India Private Limited, *New Delhi*
Prentice Hall of Japan, Inc., *Tokyo*
Simon & Schuster Asia Pte. Ltd., *Singapore*
Editora Prentice Hall do Brasil Ltda., *Rio de Janeiro*
Prentice Hall, *Upper Saddle River, New Jersey*

ISSN: 1098–7029
ISBN: 0–8385–4333–2

Acquisitions Editor: David A. Barnes
Senior Development Editor: Amanda M. Suver
Development Editor: Amy R. Marks
Production Editor: Jeanmarie Roche
Art Coordinator: Eve Siegel
Illustrator: Wendy Jackelow

ISBN 0-8385-4333-2

90000

9 780838 543337

PRINTED IN THE UNITED STATES OF AMERICA

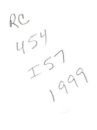

Contents

19. Cross-cultural Issues in Psychiatry

David Elkin, MD, Elizabeth Lee, MD, Arthur Sorrell, MD,
JoEllen Brainin-Rodriguez, MD,
Heather Clague, MPH, & Robert Harvey, MD

20. Psychiatric Issues in the Homeless

Kyra Minninger, MD, & David Elkin, MD

Authors

JoEllen Brainin-Rodriguez, MD
Attending Psychiatrist, San Francisco General Hospital, and Associate Clinical Professor, Department of Psychiatry, University of California, San Francisco

Louann Brizendine, MD
Associate Professor, Langley Porter Psychiatric Institute, Department of Psychiatry, University of California, San Francisco

Robert P. Cabaj, MD
Chief, Department of Psychiatry, San Mateo County Medical Center, San Mateo, California, and Assistant Clinical Professor, Department of Psychiatry, University of California, San Francisco

Cameron S. Carter, MD
Associate Professor of Psychiatry, Western Psychiatric Institute and Center, Department of Psychiatry, University of Pittsburgh

Heather Clague, MPH
Class of 1999, University of California, San Francisco School of Medicine

John DiMartini, PhD
Private Practice, Oakland, California

David Elkin, MD
Attending Psychiatrist, San Francisco General Hospital, and Associate Clinical Professor, Department of Psychiatry, University of California, San Francisco

Adriana Feder, MD
Psychiatry Attending, Columbia–Presbyterian Medical Center and Assistant Professor, Department of Psychiatry, Columbia University, New York

Francisco Gonzalez, MD
Assistant Clinical Professor, Department of Psychiatry, University of California, San Francisco

Robert Harvey, MD
Attending Psychiatrist, San Francisco General Hospital, and Assistant Clinical Professor, Depart-

ment of Psychiatry, University of California, San Francisco

Elizabeth Lee, MD
Attending Psychiatrist, Department of Psychiatry, San Mateo County Medical Center, San Mateo, California

Kyra Minninger, MD
Private Practice, San Francisco, and Assistant Clinical Professor, Department of Psychiatry, University of California, San Francisco

James M. Mol, PhD
Clinical Manager, Department of Psychology, McAuley Behavioral Health Services, Saint Mary's Hospital, San Francisco

Kalpana I. Nathan, MD
Attending Psychiatrist, Veterans Administration Palo Alto Health Care System, and Assistant Clinical Professor, Department of Psychiatry, Stanford University, California

Emily Newman, MD
Attending Psychiatrist, San Francisco General Hospital, and Assistant Clinical Professor, Department of Psychiatry, University of California, San Francisco

Sudha Prathikanti, MD
Attending Psychiatrist, San Francisco General Hospital, and Assistant Clinical Professor, Department of Psychiatry, University of California, San Francisco

Susan Scheidt, PhD
Attending Psychologist, San Francisco General Hospital, and Assistant Clinical Professor, Department of Psychiatry, University of California, San Francisco

Arthur Sorrel, MD
Psychiatry Resident, University of California, San Francisco

Claudia E. Toomey, PhD
Private practice, Oakland, California

Sophia Vinogradov, MD
Director, Psychiatric Outpatient Clinic, San Francisco Veterans Administration Medical Center, and Assistant Professor in Residence, Department of Psychiatry, University of California, San Francisco

Sheldon Vile, MD
Private practice, San Rafael, California

Amelia J. Wilcox, PhD
Attending Psychologist, San Francisco General Hospital, and Assistant Clinical Professor, Department of Psychiatry, University of California, San Francisco

Kristin Yaffe, MD
Director, Memory Disorders Clinic, San Francisco Veterans Administration Medical Center, and Assistant Clinical Professor, Department of Psychiatry, University of California, San Francisco

Mark Zaslav, PhD
Director of Training, Psychology Department, San Francisco Veterans Administration Medical Center and Assistant Clinical Professor, Department of Psychiatry, University of California, San Francisco

Preface

Students frequently have many questions about mental illness and its treatment. This book begins with the premise that psychiatric disorders are widespread and are commonly encountered in medical settings. Estimates have shown that during any given year over 20% of the US population suffers from at lease one psychiatric disorder. Patients in general medical clinics, specialty clinics, and hospitals exhibit high rates of depression, anxiety, and substance use disorders, as well as other mental health problems. The costs of psychiatric disorders are enormous in terms of health care service dollars, loss of productivity, and human suffering by both patients and their families. The social stigma associated with mental illness often prevents patients from seeking help. Many do not seek treatment because of a lack of knowledge or feelings of shame or hopelessness. However, when patients do ask for help, they turn most often to their general physician or another nonpsychiatric medical provider. Moreover, because of changes in the health care system, primary care providers are increasingly expected to assess, diagnose, and sometimes treat psychiatric disorders. Treatment of many of these disorders by the nonpsychiatric physician can be highly efficacious thanks to advances in psychopharmacology, psychotherapy, and other disciplines.

This textbook is designed for the nonpsychiatric medical practiner. Its primary objective is to introduce students to a wide range of psychiatric diagnoses and the basic features of major psychiatric disorders. It also emphasizes interviewing techniques and diagnostic skills. Approximately one quarter of the text consists of case studies that illustrate key principles and underscore the human dimension of these disorders. Less emphasis is placed on treatment, the principles of which are often more advanced and are likely to be discussed with supervising residents and attending physicians.

Beginning with a review of patient assessment and the mental status exam, this textbook introduces and defines key terms that are the basis of a vocabulary of psychiatric descriptors and conditions. Chapters on major psychiatric disorders follow. The last quarter of the book is devoted to special topics in psychiatric care including special populations, patients affected by HIV, systems-based approaches, cross-cultural care, women's issues, and homelessness.

Working with psychiatric patients typically evokes strong and confusing emotional reactions among clinicians. These responses provide important information about patients that can contribute to more accurate diagnosis and effective treatment. Accordingly each chapter includes a section on emotional reactions to patients and the implications of these responses. The legal and ethical issues related to each disorder are also considered. Students are usually taught about ethics in a separate course in their preclinical or clinical years. However, ethical considerations arise frequently in patient care and it is my belief that sensitivity to and competence in dealing with these issues are essential to future clinicians.

The references at the end of each chapter depict a key sampling of psychiatric literature, including Internet and World Wide Web sites that, along with their linked sites, provide current information about related disorders and issues. In addition to the canonical references, many chapters offer a sampling of first-hand patient accounts of their experiences wrestling with different disorders.

These accounts, along with the case studies given in every chapter, address an important, but sometimes overlooked, facet of medicine and psychiatry: the patient. DSM-IV categories and differential diagnosis skills are important but should not become an end in themselves. To maintain a focus on the patient, the cases (which have been changed or combined to protect the confidentiality of actual patients) and the references to personal accounts are intended to remind readers of the human "face" of often-devastating mental illnesses.

Another important goal of this textbook is to stimulate students to use their clinical experiences to learn about themselves as well as their patients, to recognize the universality of suffering, to be aware of the tendencies to distance oneself from or to dehumanize patients, and to ponder some of the difficult questions posed by a career in medicine. I hope that students will be encouraged to ask themselves, Who am I?; What are my limitations, biases, and strengths?; How can I help the patients for whom I am responsible?; and How do these experiences relate to my own professional and personal growth and development? Considering these questions is part of the challenge and promise of this profession, which is by turns so consuming, difficult, rewarding, and inspiring.

ACKNOWLEDGMENTS

I would like to extend my thanks to the numerous colleagues who made this book possible. At Appleton & Lange, John Dolan and Gregory Huth played key roles in formulating the project, and Amanda Suver and John Butler saw the book through its development and completion, providing invaluable assistance and guidance. The development editor, Amy Marks, patiently helped to polish chapters into their final form. The input and constructive feedback of colleagues and contributors at San Francisco General Hospital and at the University of California, San Francisco, Medical Center is reflected in the quality of this text as it goes to print. Friends, family, and especially my wife and son provided much-appreciated input, support, and encouragement.

The materials in this textbook have vastly benefitted over the years from constructive feedback from students and residents in many departments at the University of California, San Francisco, and from students and faculty at the University of California, Davis. Although they are too numerous to thank individually, I would like to express my appreciation to the many students, colleagues, and instructors who have helped to shape my own vision of this fascinating and complex field. I am also grateful to the many patients who have taught me more than they could often realize and whose suffering, humor, strength, and courage have left me with lasting lessons and insights about medicine and humanity.

David Elkin
San Francisco
June, 1998

Introduction to Psychiatric Diagnosis & Patient Evaluation

1

David Elkin, MD

Most medical students will enter nonpsychiatric fields such as general medicine, primary care, or family practice, or specialty fields such as dermatology, surgery, or neurology. Nevertheless, all physicians must have a basic understanding of mental illness and its treatment. Changes in the health-care system have resulted in nonpsychiatric physicians becoming increasingly responsible for the diagnosis and treatment of mental illness. Psychiatry is therefore becoming increasingly relevant to the practice of medicine. Psychiatric disorders are now known to be common in both inpatient and outpatient settings, and studies in the past decade have demonstrated significant increases in morbidity, mortality, and costs related to untreated psychiatric disorders in medically ill patients.

INCIDENCE OF PSYCHIATRIC DISORDERS

In any given year in the United States, over 50 million people—or over 20% of the population—has a diagnosable mental disorder that interferes with their ability to function at work or in relationships. Thirty million people suffer from anxiety disorders such as panic disorder and post-traumatic stress disorder. Between 8 and 12 million people experience an episode of depression annually, and up to one in five individuals has a depressive episode in their lifetime. Dementia affects as many as 10 million people per year, and its incidence is increasing rapidly as the post–World War II baby boomers are aging. One percent of the population has schizophrenia, and a similar proportion has bipolar disorder, which is characterized by mood swings from depression to mania. There are 30,000 completed suicides each year, and tens of thousands of others are left disabled by suicide attempts. Suicide is now the third leading cause of death for young people aged 15–24.

The cost of mental illness is staggering, with $55.4 billion expended annually in direct costs for mental illness, and $11.4 billion spent per year in direct costs for substance use. Indirect costs for mental illness and substance use based on absenteeism, lost work productivity, accidents, and premature deaths have been estimated at $273 billion per year. Compared to the costs of chronic physical illnesses, mental illness is slightly less costly than heart disease but is more expensive than diabetes, pulmonary disease, and other widely recognized physical ailments. These statistics fail to capture the degree to which patients and their families suffer as a result of these illnesses.

In spite of the huge emotional and financial burden of mental illness, psychiatric disorders remain grossly underrecognized and undertreated. Only one in five people who have mental illness ever seek treatment. Of those affected, many fear the stigma of mental illness and do not come to mental health professionals for help. Instead, many are seen in medical outpatient clinics and medical emergency rooms.

In numerous studies a high percentage of patients in primary care clinics have been found to experience mental illness. Among the top 10% of patients accessing the health care system for physical complaints, almost two–thirds have either an anxiety or mood disorder.

At any given time in a typical group of 100 medical outpatients, 40 will be suffering significant psychosocial distress. Twenty-five people will meet the full criteria for a psychiatric disorder, although in some urban public health clinics that number may rise to one-half or even two-thirds of all patients. Despite the availability of additional training and public health campaigns, physicians will make an accurate psychiatric diagnosis only half the time. Physicians will prescribe treatment for fewer than one in five of those individuals who have a psychiatric disorder. In some cases the treatment prescribed will be inappropriate and ineffective, for example, as when tranquilizers are prescribed for symptoms of depression.

Patients may also have psychiatric symptoms that are caused by medical illness. These patients may be mistakenly diagnosed as having depression, anxiety,

1

or psychosis, in which case their underlying medical problems go undetected and untreated.

There are several reasons why physicians so often fail to diagnose mental illness. First, patients themselves may lack the insight needed to realize that they have a psychiatric disorder and instead may present in a medical clinic with numerous somatic (physical) complaints. Many factors that contribute to the failure to diagnose these patients are believed to be associated with physicians themselves. Primary care providers may be ignorant about mental illness or may lack basic psychiatric training; some are not convinced that psychiatric disorders are as "real" as medical illnesses and focus only on physical complaints. Others may view psychiatric problems as moral problems and echo the widespread belief that psychiatric illness is the result of a personal failing. The brief time allotted for most patient visits—now at an average of less than 10 minutes per patient—may cause the physician to focus on physical symptoms to the exclusion of discussing psychosocial illness.

Psychiatric consultation may not be readily available in some clinical settings, or the cost of referral may be prohibitive in cost-conscious clinics. Under many managed care health plans, primary care providers are often expected to diagnose and treat patients who have psychiatric illnesses. An increasing body of research shows that the ultimate cost of not treating psychiatric disorders may be very expensive indeed, with far more inappropriate visits and tests in medical settings, decreased satisfaction with physicians, and increased morbidity and mortality from medical conditions due to diminished adherence and other factors. The emotional suffering that psychiatric disorders cause patients and their families is less visible or easily understood by observers and is an important reason to provide prompt evaluation and treatment for mental illness.

ETIOLOGY OF PSYCHIATRIC DISORDERS

Dramatic advances in understanding the etiology of psychiatric disorders have occurred in the past several decades. However, our understanding of the confluence of biological, psychological, and social factors remains incomplete. The contribution of genetics to disease and behavior of illness derive from twin studies and other probes of hereditary influences. Other biological explanations are derived from pharmacologic actions of medications that implicate different neurotransmitter imbalances in psychiatric illness. Structural abnormalities can be detected with computed tomography (CT) and magnetic resonance imaging (MRI) scans of the head, whereas PET (positron emission tomography) and real-time MRI provide a window into brain function.

Despite the abundant evidence for biological factors as the cause of psychiatric disorders, this is only part of the picture. Psychological causes for psychiatric illness are also well documented, including the aberrant developmental process in patients who have personality disorders, the effects of poor self-esteem on judgment and decision making in depression, psychological factors that initiate and maintain substance use, and the fears and avoidance seen in anxiety disorders. A consideration of the patient's style of coping with stress and anxiety is also important in the understanding and treatment of mental illness. Patients use many different psychological defense mechanisms to manage anxiety, but they are sometimes unaware of their use of these coping strategies. The unconscious nature of selected aspects of mental functioning is explored in subsequent chapters.

Social and environmental factors have also been causally linked to psychiatric disorders. Major life stressors often precede psychiatric disorders, and mental illness may precipitate disruption in an individual's family life, workplace, and social support. Family background and current social and work relationships should be characterized. The patient's cultural background is another important social factor that often greatly affects the formation of symptoms and the patient's and his or her family's understanding of psychiatric disorders.

Of course, etiologic factors do not determine illness independently as they are presented above. A sophisticated view of mental illness recognizes the interplay of biological, psychological, and environmental factors.

THE *DSM-IV* & MAJOR PSYCHIATRIC DISORDERS

Psychiatric disorders have been classified using the *Diagnostic Statistical Manual* (4th edition) or *DSM-IV*. Successive editions of the *DSM* have updated diagnostic categories based on clinical research. The *DSM-IV* divides psychiatric disorders into the following major groupings (see listed chapters for coverage of each grouping):

- **dementia and delirium** (see Chapter 3)
- **psychotic disorders** (eg, schizophrenia; see Chapter 4)
- **affective disorders** (eg, major depression [see Chapter 5] and bipolar [affective] disorder, formerly known as manic-depressive illness [see Chapter 6])
- **anxiety disorders** (eg, panic disorder, social phobia, simple phobia, generalized anxiety disorders, obsessive-compulsive disorder, and post-traumatic stress disorder; see Chapters 7 and 8)

- **somatoform disorders** (eg, conversion disorder, pain disorder, hypochondriasis, somatization disorder, and body dysmorphic disorder; see Chapter 9)
- **dissociative disorders** (see Chapter 10)
- **substance use disorders** (eg, abuse of alcohol, cocaine, heroin, or other drugs; see Chapter 11)
- **personality disorders** (see Chapter 12)

Disorders are specified on the following axes of the *DSM-IV:*

- **Axis I:** major psychiatric disorders, including dementia, delirium, depression, mania, substance dependence/abuse, anxiety disorders; also includes psychosis, depression, mania, anxiety, or personality change due to a medical condition
- **Axis II:** personality disorders, disorders of development, including childhood disorders such as mental retardation
- **Axis III:** medical conditions
- **Axis IV:** psychosocial stressors in the patient's life
- **Axis V:** global assessment on a scale of 0–100 of how well the patient is able to function in an overall sense (eg, psychological, social, and occupational function)

The *DSM-IV* helps to standardize the diagnosis of psychiatric disorders by using objective criteria for categories of illness that have been validated clinically. Thus a major strength of the *DSM-IV* is that it provides a common ground and language for clinicians to describe, report, and discuss psychiatric disorders. However, differences often exist (eg, in history, symptomatology, illness expression, and other key issues) between two patients who have the same disorder. Thus these disease classifications are not a substitute for a thorough understanding of individual patients and their experiences.

THE PSYCHIATRIC EVALUATION

The evaluation of the psychiatric patient should follow a stepwise process (see Figure 1–1). This includes a review of the patient's chart and collateral sources of information. The patient should be interviewed with particular attention to the history of the present illness, the patient's past psychiatric and medical histories, and the mental status examination, including relevant physical findings. The clinician then constructs a differential diagnosis of likely psychiatric disorders that could account for symptoms. Students will probably develop a formulation about a

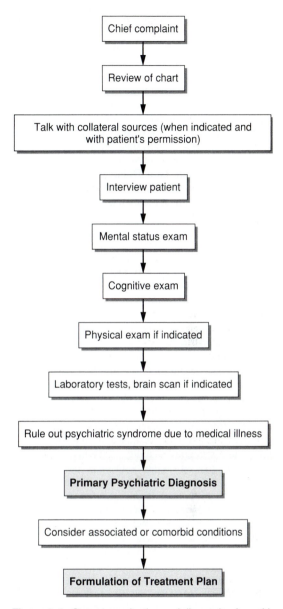

Figure 1–1. Steps to evaluation and diagnosis of psychiatric symptoms.

patient's condition and a treatment plan in consultation with the resident and attending physician. The clinician's emotional reactions to the patient may provide a rich source of information. Legal and ethical issues should also be considered.

THE INTERVIEW PROCESS

Establish the Purpose and the Context of the Interview. Students may take for granted that their patients are familiar with the goals and circumstances of the interview. But many patients need to be oriented. An example might be, "Good morning Mr. Smith. Thank you for agreeing to be interviewed. I'm Gweneth Jones, a third-year medical student, and these are my classmates. I'd like to ask you a series of questions about what has been happening to you so that the attending doctor and I can determine how we can best help you. I also have a brief set of questions to check your concentration and memory that should take 5 minutes or so. I have an hour, until 3 PM, and would like to leave some time for you to ask questions. Do you have any questions before we begin?"

Be Clear About Your Role. Students should explain their role within the team structure, stating explicitly that they are students who work and communicate with residents and attending physicians. Students should explain the limitations of their role when relevant, such as needing back-up to make significant clinical decisions, countersigning orders, and so on. Students can identify themselves as a part of the treating team and explain their capacity to function as a patient advocate. It is unethical, illegal, and inadvisable for a student to introduce or indirectly refer to himself or herself as a physician.

Put Yourself & the Patient at Ease. If a patient appears anxious, the student can ask the patient if anything is bothering him or her, and if anything can be done to improve the situation. Before beginning to interact with the patient, the student should check his or her own emotions. Many students find that they are concerned and preoccupied with forgetting key points in the interview or questions intended to test the patient's cognitive ability. Students may find it useful to carry an outline with these points written down and that patients will tolerate the student's use of memory prompts, particularly if the student states explicitly the purpose of these reminders as a means for ensuring a complete interview.

Build Rapport. Students should seek to form an alliance with patients. Demonstrating understanding and empathy for the patient's circumstances may make many patients feel that the student is truly interested and capable of helping them. It also helps ensure communication and has been shown to be therapeutic in many instances.

Follow-up on Issues That Elicit Strong Emotions. Patients sometimes become sad, angry, or happy, or they display other strong emotional responses. Many interviewers simply continue asking questions. Instead, it is advisable to pause and explore the patient's response by asking questions such as, "It looks like you're feeling sad. Could you tell me what you are thinking about?" or "You seemed to become very angry when I asked about your boss. What was happening there?" Attending to the patient's emotional states often yields valuable information and also helps strengthen the therapeutic alliance between the interviewer and the patient by acknowledging the importance of the patient's subjective experiences.

Adjust the Interviewing Style. Students can use a range of open- and closed-ended questions depending on the patient and the situation. Closed-ended questions are designed to elicit a brief response, for example, "What is your date of birth?" Open-ended questions are less specific and invite a broader range of patient responses, for example, "Can you tell me what brought you to the clinic today?" Closed-ended questions produce accurate responses but provide so much structure to the interview that they may deprive the interviewer of a better sense of the patient's style of thinking, by masking a patient's disorganized or psychotic thoughts or causing a patient to "close down."

Open-ended questions help to illuminate the patient's thoughts, emotions, and style of organizing information but are disadvantageous with patients who are garrulous and need the student's help in organizing their thoughts. It is often useful to begin an interview with an open-ended question in order to develop a sense of the patient's spontaneous thoughts. A student could begin the interview by asking, "What brought you to the clinic today?" and then allowing the patient to explain for 5 minutes.

Make Smooth Transitions. When shifting areas of inquiry, many clinicians forget to explain the reasons for pursuing these areas of information, or they fail to introduce the new topics. For example, a student can say, "It's been helpful to review your history. Now I'd like to switch gears and ask about some of the medications that you have been taking."

Clarify Confusing Points. The interviewer is encouraged to ask the patient about responses that are unclear. This can be done with genuine interest and respect, by stating, "I'm not clear on what you just said about the stress that you are under. Let me restate what I think you said, and you can tell me if I understood correctly."

Avoid Making Assumptions. It is important to understand the patient's perspective on his or her own life and illness. Interviewers may apply their own reasoning, values, and judgments on patients without being aware that they are doing so. For example, many medical professionals assume that patients who are dependent on drugs or alcohol recognize that substance use is a problem and want to receive treatment. This assumption may reflect the interviewer's own hypothetic response if he or she were dependent on drugs, but many patients may minimize a substance use problem and deny a need to change at all.

Use "Here and Now" Interventions. This powerful technique focuses on what is happening during the interview. If a patient says that he or she becomes uncomfortable when talking to other people, the interviewer can ask "What about in here—are you uncomfortable talking to me?" Another worthwhile intervention that can be used during or at the end of the interview is to ask the patient, "How has this interview been for you?"

Be Aware of Emotional Reactions. Interviewers should try to be aware of their own thoughts and feelings, which may affect their behavior toward a patient or may indicate the patient's emotional state.

Leave 5 Minutes to Fill in Missing Clinical Data. Interviews often work best if 5 minutes are left at the end of the interview to review psychiatric symptoms, clarify confusing areas, or give the patient an opportunity to ask questions without feeling rushed. Remember to help identify areas of relative strength for patients. For some patients, reviewing the psychiatric history may highlight problem areas or engender a sense of shame. It is therefore advisable to inquire about the patient's personal strengths and positive attributes toward the end of the interview.

Solicit Feedback. Students may finish an interview wondering how they performed. They may ruminate about a mistake they feel they made, an error they missed, or an omission. It is helpful to ask for feedback from patients, for example, "How did this interview go for you?"

Make the Acquisition of Interviewing Skills a Lifelong Goal. Although interviewing skills are essential for almost any clinician, students are often expected to learn about interviewing in a much less stringent manner than their other clinical skills. Students are encouraged to actively solicit observation and feedback from peers and supervisors. Finally, students should watch and learn from other professionals but strive to develop their own style.

Be Prepared to Handle Special Problems. Problems that may occur during the interview may seem particularly troublesome if the student is not prepared to handle them. This section covers some of the more common problematic situations encountered during the interview.

- **The patient asks the interviewer to leave.** Patients may refuse to cooperate with the interview, particularly in inpatient psychiatric settings where patients are hospitalized against their will or have more severe psychiatric disturbances. Suggested strategies include exploring why the patient does not want to talk, and if he or she has any specific fears about the interview. Otherwise, it may be worth trying to engage the patient in a discussion of nonpsychiatric or medical issues, such as asking about the television show currently on or about the book the patient is reading. If the patient still refuses to be interviewed, the student should indicate what time he or she will return to attempt the interview again, and why the information the patient furnishes will be of mutual benefit.
- **The patient seeks assurances about his or her diagnosis or treatment.** Some patients will ask about their diagnosis. It may be helpful to review the diagnoses being considered, but if the condition is unclear it may be best to explain that the team does not know the diagnosis yet, that the assessment process is continuing, and that the patient will receive updates on his or her condition and proposed treatment on a daily basis.
- **The patient offers information only if the student promises not to reveal it.** Students should always maintain free communication with their resident and attending supervisors and should never agree to keep information from them. Withholding important clinical information could easily render the diagnosis and treatment plan less accurate and effective. Or students will have to break the agreement in the event that critical information is disclosed, such as suicidal thoughts, which can lower a patient's trust in the treating team. Patients who try to divide team members often have personality disorders associated with impulsive and suicidal behavior.
- **The patient wants to continue to work with the student after the end of the rotation.** Students should be clear that their relationship with the patient will finish with the end of their rotation.
- **The patient asks the student on a date.** Students should always maintain professional attitudes and behavior toward patients. Friendship or romantic relationships with patients at best endanger the treatment and at worst can cause significant distress or worsening of psychiatric disorders.
- **The patient makes sexual advances or is verbally, sexually, or physically abusive toward the student.** Any form of abuse should be reported to a supervisor immediately. Most medical schools have a zero-tolerance policy toward sexual harassment by staff members as well.

THE PSYCHIATRIC HISTORY & MENTAL STATUS EXAMINATION

Psychiatry differs from other medical specialties in the lack of reliable laboratory tests available to help identify specific disorders. Psychiatric diagnosis is based primarily on the patient's history and mental status examination.

1. HISTORY

Chief Complaint. Ask the patient why he or she came to the outpatient clinic or hospital. If the psychiatric consultation was requested by another physician, ask the reason for the referral. Characterize the current illness by asking the patient how long he or she has experienced symptoms, whether any stressors were associated with the onset of the illness, and how the patient understands his or her illness.

Psychiatric Review of Symptoms. Ask the patient briefly about core symptoms of the major psychiatric disorders listed above if these symptoms were not included in the history of the current illness. Table 1–1 reviews questions to ask to screen for features of most major psychiatric disorders. Primary screening questions should be part of every initial evaluation. If a patient's response to a primary question is positive, ask follow-up questions.

Substance Use. Ask the patient about substance use patterns, including intake of alcohol and use of illicit drugs such as marijuana, cocaine, heroin, and hallucinogens. It may be helpful to have the patient estimate his or her use of drugs and alcohol over the preceding week to avoid vague or inaccurate responses.

Past Psychiatric History. Ask the patient about previous psychiatric illnesses, including contact with mental health professionals, psychiatric hospitalizations, and medications prescribed.

Social & Developmental History. Ideally the interviewer should compile a thorough biography of the patient, including details about his or her birth, developmental milestones, childhood (including relationships with parents, siblings, and friends), school experiences, and work or military experience (if any).

Medical History. Note all current and past medical problems.

Medications. Ask the patient to list all prescription and over-the-counter medications currently being taking, and whether he or she is adhering to the prescription instructions. If the patient is hospitalized, medications taken before and during hospitalization should be listed. Students should determine how often medications listed as prn (meaning "as needed for . . . ") are actually taken.

Family History. Ask the patient about the incidence of psychiatric and medical illness in his or her family members.

2. MENTAL STATUS EXAMINATION

Appearance & Behavior. Note key features of the patient's appearance and behavior, including grooming, hygiene, and dress; whether the patient's apparent age matches his or her chronologic age; eye contact and attitude toward the examiner; gait and bearing; mannerisms; and psychomotor slowing or agitation.

Language. Consider the patient's use of language, with particular attention to rhythm, rate, and loudness. Note any difficulties with language such as garbled or slurred speech or difficulties with word-finding.

Emotions. Note the patient's emotional state (eg, depressed, happy, anxious), usually based on the patient's self-report. **Affect** refers to the objective assessment of the patient's emotional state and can be divided into several dimensions:

- The **objective description** of the patient's mood, as seen by the interviewer.
- **Range of affect,** or the spectrum of moods displayed by the patient. Common descriptions of affective range include (a) **full** (ie, normal), since most people have shifts in mood, either up or down, throughout a conversation, depending on what is being discussed; (b) **restricted,** which applies to depressed patients, who show mostly sadness, or manic patients, who have an elevated mood; or (c) **flat,** which describes patients who show very little emotion, most commonly seen in patients who have schizophrenia.
- **Lability** describes the quickness with which the patient's moods shift. A patient who has a labile mood might, for example, shift from tearfulness to extreme anger within seconds.
- **Appropriateness** refers to how well the patient's emotional tone matches the subject he or she is discussing. If a patient is describing a suicide attempt and becomes tearful and sad, the patient's affect will appear appropriate to the examiner. However, if the same patient were to laugh and start joking with the examiner while relating the details of the suicide attempt, a mismatch of mood and content would be readily apparent to the interviewer, who probably would feel quite uncomfortable. Thus the interviewer's emotional response to the patient will provide a gauge of the appropriateness of the patient's emotions.

Thought Process. **Thought process** describes the flow of the patient's thoughts. Several categories are used to characterize a patient's though processes:

- **Goal-oriented (linear):** The patient will answer in a straightforward manner that is easily followed by the interviewer. For example,
  Student: What brought you to the hospital?
  Patient: I was feeling more depressed than ever—as soon as the doctors saw me they told me I'd need to stay for a week or more.
- **Circumstantiality:** The patient gives a roundabout answer with unnecessary information but does return to the original question.
  Student: What brought you to the hospital?
  Patient: It's a long story, I've been feeling pretty depressed for a long time. My childhood was pretty rough. . . . You're asking about this time, though. I started to feel like I couldn't go on like this any more. That's when I made an appointment here, and they admitted me right away because I was feeling so depressed.
- **Tangentiality:** The patient's thoughts veer off into unrelated areas without reference to the original idea or question. This may occur when the pa-

Table 1–1. Topics for screening questions for core psychiatric disorders.[1]

Core Symptoms	Primary (Initial) Screening Questions	Follow-up Questions
Dementia	Memory problems	Problems with concentration, abstract thinking, judgment, behavior
Delirium	Disorientation	Disturbed sleep cycles, illusions, problems with memory or concentration
Schizophrenia	Hallucinations, delusions, paranoia	Disorganized thoughts; magical powers, telepathy, precognition
Depression	Depressed mood, suicidal thoughts, sleep disturbance, loss of pleasure, change in appetite and weight	Fatigue; feelings of hopelessness; decreased sexual drive; feelings of worthlessness or guilt; trouble with decision-making, concentration
Bipolar disorder	Elevated mood, decreased need for sleep	Speaking or thinking faster than usual; grandiose feelings; increased spending, pleasurable activities
Anxiety disorders	Episodes of anxiety, panic; obsessive thoughts, compulsive behaviors; phobias or avoidant behavior	Generalized restlessness, irritability, or nervousness; intrusive thoughts about contamination, harming others, symmetry; compulsive handwashing, checking, hoarding, rituals
PTSD	Exposure to traumatic event(s); flashbacks, nightmares	Hypervigilance, arousal symptoms; survivor guilt
Somatoform Disorders	Unexplained physical symptoms	Chronic health concerns, pain despite negative exams and tests; conviction of malformed body part
Dissociative disorders	Feelings of depersonalization, derealization; loss of time, blackouts	Sensing another person existing inside and taking control, no memory of childhood
Substance use	History of alcohol and drug use, legal, relationship, or work problems due to substance use; last drink	"CAGE" questions (see Chapter 11)
Personality disorders (cluster B)	Emotional lability and reactivity; impulsive behavior; suicidal behavior, self-mutilation; arrests, legal problems	
Eating disorders	Subjective sense of being overweight; bingeing, purging (inducing vomiting)	Restrictive or ritualistic behaviors around food; laxative abuse, excessive exercising
AIDS (risk factors)	High-risk behavior (not using condoms, sterilizing needles)	

[1]Primary screening questions should be part of every initial evaluation. If any responses to primary topics are positive, further topics from follow-up column should be addressed.

tient is anxious, is being evasive or defensive, or has dementia or a mild case of delirium.

Student: What brought you to the hospital?

Patient: I've never been in a hospital like this before. All of the people working here, it's hard to know what everybody does. Me, I've been an auto mechanic since I was 16 years old. Cars have gotten a lot more complicated since 1970, let me tell you. When I started working at Sam's Garage we didn't have the modern equipment you see now . . .

- **Flight of ideas:** The patient races from one thought to the next. Thought processes often speed along faster than the patient's speech can keep up. This is most commonly seen in mania.

Student: What brought you to the hospital?

Patient: Hospitals are incredible collections of social forces and high technology . . . do you realize that technology is increasing exponentially, with computer speed doubling every 6 months? I have a plan to help people tap into their own natural growth potential using the Internet, we could double the collective intelligence of the planet. The whole planet, from here to Tibet . . . do you know about the oppression in Tibet . . .

Student: Umm, I was asking about how you . . .

Patient (interrupting): . . . the mountains there are incredibly challenging, but I've figured out a new system that will allow anyone to climb them. I've got another idea to combine a global positioning technology with climbing equipment, if you have $100,000 to invest I can guarantee you won't miss out . . .

- **Loose associations:** The patient exhibits a loss of connectedness between ideas, as far as the examiner can discern. This is most common in psychosis or delirium.
  Student: What brought you to the hospital?
  Patient: There are these worms . . . you expect the spolisisms, the . . .
  Student: What's a "spolisism?"
  Patient: My mother annihilated it. . . a car vaccine wouldn't make it. Lung disease cancels discordance, sometimes . . .
- **Thought blocking:** The patient's thoughts will cease in midstream, without a discernible cause for the interruption. This is sometimes seen in psychosis.
  Student: What brought you to the hospital?
  Patient: I couldn't get down to it anymore, my mother—(stops, continues to look ahead)
  Student: What about your mother?
  Patient: (continues to look vacant)
- **Concrete thinking:** The patient lacks the ability to think in abstract categories; therefore, the patient's responses are extremely literal. This is seen in dementia, in patients with low intelligence, and sometimes in psychosis.
  Student: What brought you to the hospital?
  Patient: A car.
  Student: No, I mean why did you decide to come to the hospital today?
  Patient: I don't know. My wife said I should come here and she drove me.
- **Perseveration:** This term refers to repeated behaviors, mannerisms, or patterns of speech. Perseveration is often a sign of central nervous system dysfunction.
  Student: What brought you to the hospital?
  Patient: I don't know, it's a global thing. You would have to understand the global issues. It just seems very global when you think about it.

Thought Content. During the interview, the clinician should note any of the following types of thought content:

- **Delusions** are fixed, false beliefs that are not shared by the patient's cultural group and are resistant to being disproved by a rational approach. Commonly encountered delusions can be characterized as paranoid, grandiose, somatic, or shared.
- **Paranoid delusions** involve a conviction that the patient is being plotted against, stalked, or pursued by a person or group of persons.
- **Grandiose delusions (delusions of grandeur)** involve the belief that the patient is more talented, accomplished, or famous than he or she actually is.

- **Somatic delusions** are marked by a conviction that something is wrong with the patient's body, as in the case of a patient who is certain that he or she has cancer despite lack of physical evidence.
- **Shared delusions** (*folie á deux*) occur when the patient and another person (usually a family member) both believe in the same delusion.
- **Paranoia** is a general sense of suspiciousness, hypervigilance, and a tendency to overreact and misinterpret environmental clues as dangerous.
- **Suicidal ideation** refers to thoughts of suicide. These may range from fleeting thoughts of passive death (eg, "Maybe it would be easier if I were to just die.") to more active rumination (constant, detailed thoughts of killing oneself, including a specific plan and fantasies of how friends, family, and coworkers would react).
- **Homicidal ideation** involves thoughts of killing other people.
- **Ideas of reference** occur when patients misinterpret commonplace events and feel that they are receiving special messages, usually through modern communication media, such as a patient thinking that a television news anchor is touching her hair to send the patient a special signal.
- **Hallucinations** are false sensory impressions that originate within the patient, such as hearing voices (**auditory hallucinations**) or seeing imaginary people who do not exist (**visual hallucinations**). Hallucinations can exist in any sensory modality (eg, auditory, visual, tactile, olfactory, and gustatory). Auditory and visual hallucinations are more common than the other forms and may be seen in patients who have schizophrenia, delirium, and severe depression or mania. Olfactory hallucinations may be a feature of seizure activity centered in the temporal lobes, near the olfactory nerve. Tactile hallucinations, such as feeling bugs running over one's body, are often seen in delirium due to alcohol withdrawal. Unilateral findings such as monoaural hallucinations (ie, hearing sounds in one ear) may indicate a CNS disturbance.
- **Illusions** are sensory misimpressions based on actual sensory input. They are found most commonly in delirium. For example, a delirious patient may mistake a white handle for a cigarette, or a hospital laundry cart for a fruit stand.

Judgment, Insight, & Impulse Control. Judgment is a global assessment of the patient's ability to gather and process information, anticipate problems, evaluate alternatives, and plan for future difficulties. Generally, judgment is graded as good, fair, or poor. An example of a patient who has poor judgment is one who is brought to the hospital after trying to leap into traffic at the urging of an auditory hallucination. If the patient is asked how things will be different after being discharged from the hospital and he or she responds, "I need to kill myself. It's the only way out," judgment would be said to be poor. An example of a patient who has fair judgment is one who, when asked the same question, would answer, "I guess that I could call the psychiatry clinic if I feel that way again," but would have no back-up plan.

Insight refers to the patient's awareness of his or her mental illness and the ability to connect this disturbance to other problems. Like judgment, insight can be said to good, fair, or poor. A patient who is aware that hallucinations and paranoia are features of a relapse of schizophrenia has good insight. If the same patient was unsure if these symptoms were a feature of the illness, or was not sure they were really happening, insight would be said to be fair or poor. The patient who insists that these phenomena are real and that the doctors are part of a conspiracy to confuse him has poor insight.

Impulse control can be assessed by observing the patient during the interview. Examples of poor impulse control include the patient who becomes angry and throws his food tray into the hall, or the manic patient who on admiring the student's watch attempts to pull the jewelry from the student's wrist.

Cognitive Examination. The **cognitive examination** tests higher cognitive functioning. This examination (unlike the rest of the mental status examination) involves discrete questions and is best performed halfway or two-thirds through the initial interview. Students should mention the cognitive examination early in the interview and try to make a smooth transition to this portion of the interview. For example, the student might say, "You mentioned that you've been having difficulty concentrating recently. I'd like to spend 5 minutes asking you some questions to test your concentration and memory." The basic components of the cognitive examination include the following areas:

- **Level of consciousness**
- **Orientation** to person, place, and time
- **Concentration:** ask the patient to subtract sevens serially from 100 or to name the months of the year backward
- **Memory:** give the patient four words and then have the patient repeat the words. Five minutes later ask the patient to repeat the words again. Give category prompts and then offer a list of three choices if the patient cannot recall one or more words.
- **Visuospatial skills:** ask the patient to copy a complex figure (usually two overlapping geometric figures such as a square and pentagon)
- General **fund of knowledge:** ask the patient to name the current president of the United States or to name five major cities
- **Abstracting ability:** ask the patient about the similarities between two objects in the same class, such as an apple and an orange
- **Language ability:** ask the patient to identify several common objects on sight and to perform commands written on paper (but not spoken)
- **Ability to follow two-or three-step commands:** ask the patient to execute a series of two- or three-step actions (eg, "Please touch your nose and then clap your hands.")

DIFFERENTIAL DIAGNOSIS

After establishing the clinical database for the patient, the differential diagnosis—a list of possible psychiatric disorders that could account for the patient's symptoms—should be considered.

The first step in differential diagnosis is to consider and rule out a medical illness that could be causing the psychiatric problems. Medical diseases can produce psychiatric symptoms that suggest a primary mental disorder; in some cases, these are the first or only symptoms. For example, hypothyroidism may be present with symptoms of depression, including sadness, low energy, weight gain, and increased sleep. Pulmonary emboli (clots in the blood vessels of the lungs) can manifest with no other symptoms than anxiety.

Since medical illness can perfectly mimic psychiatric symptoms, it is not possible for physicians to tell whether a given patient has an underlying medical problem without a thorough physical examination and appropriate laboratory tests, such as an MRI head scan, thyroid function tests, or a lumbar puncture to examine cerebrospinal fluid. This step in differential diagnosis, along with a review of medical diseases that can mimic psychiatric disorders, is considered in detail in Chapter 2.

A principal diagnosis should then be selected. Students should list factors in the patient's history, mental status examination, and laboratory results that do or do not support this diagnosis. Whenever possible, students should seek a single diagnosis that can account for the patient's symptoms (this is known as Occam's principle). When more than one diagnosis is cited (such as a psychiatric disorder and substance use), the interplay of these conditions should be considered.

At least three other diagnostic possibilities should be listed along with a consideration of features from the patient's case that make these diagnoses less likely. Frequently associated psychiatric diagnoses should be considered. For example, when a diagnosis of post-traumatic stress disorder is made, students should question whether substance use or depression is also present.

FORMULATION & ASSESSMENT

At this point, the patient's history is reviewed, along with chief pertinent negative and positive findings in the mental status examination. Biological, psychological, and social factors are then considered. Biological variables include genetic predisposition toward illness based on family history, medications, any relevant medical illness, and any structural abnormalities indicated by head scans or suggested by a past history of head trauma.

Psychological factors vary depending on the patient's history and illness, as well as the psychological framework in which the patient's difficulties are considered. The **psychodynamic model** focuses on difficulties in the patient's childhood development, and how hidden conflict, usually involving sexuality or aggression, continues to affect the patient's life through feelings, thoughts, and behavior. Self-psychology shifts the focus to the patient's realization in childhood of limitations, and difficulties in adulthood adjusting to those limitations while maintaining a stable internal image of one's physical and emotional self.

The **control mastery perspective** examines irrational ideas, with particular emphasis on guilt, that develop in childhood and shape the patient's expectations and relationships in adulthood. Existential issues may be particularly relevant in patients facing life-threatening illness or trauma, with concerns about the meaning of life, the nature of death, the difficulties inherent in forging relationships, and the individual's conflict between freedom and responsibility. **Cognitive-behavioral approaches** link the thoughts and behaviors that patients report, while deemphasizing the role of development and unconscious mental functioning. This approach often features homework assignments and an active approach to changing the patient's thinking and behaviors.

Social factors include any relevant problems or supports in the patient's environment, at home, at work, or in a hospital setting for medical inpatients. Psychosocial stressors that may have precipitated or exacerbated a patient's condition should be listed. Examples include a breakup in a relationship, the death of a friend or family member, unemployment, or physical trauma. The patient's support system, including family and social contacts, should be considered.

Based on the information gleaned from the patient and available collateral sources of information, such as family members, a previous therapist, or medical records, students should develop a formulation of the patient's case that links psychological, biological, and social factors in understanding the patient's current state. Suggested parameters include major themes or conflicts in the patient's life; links between present and past difficulties; areas of impairment in psychological functioning and anticipated problems in the treatment plan; and personal strengths, skills, or attributes.

TREATMENT

MEDICATION

Medication may be warranted for treatment of many psychiatric conditions. Major classifications of psychiatric medications include antidepressants, antipsychotics, and sedative-hypnotics. Patients should always be fully informed about the medications they have been prescribed, including any side effects. Adherence to medication is a significant problem in psychiatry.

Antidepressants

The antidepressants include the older tricyclic antidepressants (TCAs), which increase the neurotransmitter norepinephrine. Major anticholinergic side effects include dry mouth, blurry vision, constipation, and sedation. Serotonin-specific re-uptake inhibitors (SSRIs) increase levels of serotonin. They cause nausea, headaches, and occasional agitation or insomnia initially but may have more chronic effects on sex drive and function.

TCAs and SSRIs are effective for depression and anxiety disorders. SSRIs also reduce obsessive-compulsive symptoms. TCAs are the only antidepressants that also relieve chronic pain. They are lower in cost but generally have more side effects than do SSRIs and are toxic at lower levels, a particularly important consideration when treating patients who have expressed suicidal thoughts.

Monoamine oxidase inhibitors (MAOIs) have fallen into disuse because patients must maintain a strict tyramine-free diet in order to avoid a hypertensive crisis. Newer antidepressants include nefazodone (Serzone), which increases serotonin both pre- and post-synaptically; venlafaxine (Effexor), a mixed serotonin and norepinephrine agent; and buproprion (Wellbutrin), which appears to act on dopamine receptors.

Antipsychotics

The antipsychotic class of medications consists of older medications, such as chlorpromazine (Thorazine), thioridazine (Mellaril), and haloperidol (Haldol), which block dopamine receptors, and newer antipsychotic agents such as clozapine (Clozaril), risperidone (Risperdal), and olanzapine (Zyprexa). These agents are effective for psychotic conditions such as schizophrenia, or depression or mania with psychotic features (ie, those with symptoms of hallucinations, paranoia, and disorganized thinking).

Sedative-hypnotics

Benzodiazepines affect the GABA neurotransmitter system and relieve anxiety. Their side effects include sedation, reduced reflexes, tolerance, and the potential for addiction. They are generally used for the short-term treatment of anxiety and sometimes as a sleep aid.

PSYCHOTHERAPY

Medications are often not necessary for milder psychiatric conditions. Studies have shown that even when medications are helpful, the combination of psychotherapy and medication ensures a full recovery with the smallest chance for relapse. **Interpersonal psychotherapy** uses the relationship between the therapist and the patient as the curative agent. Therapy may be supportive in nature, for example, helping the patient to re-identify strengths and to increase self-confidence. **Cognitive-behavioral psychotherapy** focuses on controlling negative thinking and attempts cognitive restructuring so that the patient can look at situations more positively. **Psychodynamic psychotherapy** in particular focuses on past events and internal conflicts that may interfere with the patient's ability to achieve his or her full potential.

Brief psychotherapy is defined as a course of treatment limited to 6–20 sessions. **Group psychotherapy** allows patients to receive support from others who can understand their disorder and helps patients achieve more effective relationships with friends, significant others, and coworkers. Group psychotherapy is less expensive than other forms and is extremely effective. It may be used more frequently in the face of an increased emphasis on cost control and managed care.

OTHER TREATMENT MODALITIES

Social services address the patient's housing, eligibility for benefits, and disposition planning. **Case management** refers to active engagement with recidivistic patients, not only in the medical setting but in the patient's home or neighborhood.

EMOTIONAL REACTIONS TO PATIENTS

Emotional reactions to patients are an inevitable and natural component of clinical encounters. The theoretic term used to describe these reactions is **countertransference;** the patient's reactions to the clinician are called **transference.** Countertransference may have roots in a number of factors related to the patient and the clinician.

Physicians and trainees have their own areas of comfort and discomfort with different kinds of patients and different psychiatric disorders, based on their previous experiences, backgrounds, and personal and societal values. The stigma of mental illness can affect the physician's clinical judgments.

Factors related to the patient may stimulate emotional reactions in the clinician. This form of emotional resonance has been compared to the acoustic resonance of two tuning forks, or the strings of two musical instruments. Specific psychiatric illnesses may stimulate somewhat predictable emotional responses in physicians. For example, interviewing a depressed patient may leave the interviewer feeling tired, powerless, or sad; similarly, a disorganized, psychotic patient may generate feelings of confusion or fear.

Students should realize that interactions between any two people represent a dynamic process and can be thought of an interpersonal "field" in which the interplay of transference and countertransference between the patient and the student creates changing patterns of communication and emotions. For example, working with a depressed patient who is feeling needy and dependent may initially cause a student to feel helpful and important, but these positive feelings may give way to resentment and frustration if the patient talks continuously and causes the interview to run over time limits.

Emotional reactions are therefore an important phenomenon for several reasons. Increased awareness of one's own reaction to a patient leads to a more rapid and sensitive response to the patient's emotional state. A student who feels angry while interviewing a patient might consider whether he or she is picking up on the patient's anger or rage, even if the patient appears pleasant and exhibits no overt signs of hostility. With increased clinical experience, students may come to correlate particular emotional reactions with different psychiatric diagnoses, enabling them to consider specific diagnoses at an early stage.

Clinicians need to be aware of their emotional responses to patients so that patient care is not compromised. For example, a physician who is uncomfortable with self-destructive patients might fail to ask appropriate or adequate questions to identify patients at risk for suicide. Studies suggest that increased familiarity with one's own dynamic inner emotional life is consistent with increased self-knowledge and personal growth of the physician at any level of training. Trainees and physicians who are aware of their own emotional "blind spots" are less likely to miss important information, are able to work more effectively with a broad range of patients, and can provide leadership to other members of their medical team when working with difficult patients.

LEGAL & ETHICAL ISSUES

A complete review of the principles of bioethics is beyond the scope of this book. Each chapter reviews some of the more salient ethical issues raised in the treatment of specific psychiatric disorders. However, a basic familiarity with the principles of medical ethics is vital. Ethical issues frequently arise in the care of patients in medical settings and even more so in the care of patients who have psychiatric illnesses.

Although physicians can rely on scientific research, accepted standards of clinical care, and laws and legal guidelines in making decisions about clinical care, each ethical dilemma is often unique to the patient and his or her own physical, emotional, and cultural circumstances. Generally physicians follow a professional code that provides guidelines to work with patients and families. This code is derived from the tradition of Hippocrates and modified somewhat by case law and state and federal laws. However, technical advancements in medicine and increasingly complex systems of health-care delivery have created situations in which professional, legal, and ethical principles lead to different conclusions.

PRINCIPLE-BASED MODEL OF ETHICS

Basic principles of ethics include considerations of **autonomy, beneficence, non-malfeasance,** and **justice.** Additional concerns include **cultural values,** health-care providers' countertransference, and other factors. The application of these principles to the treatment of patients who have specific psychiatric illnesses is discussed at the conclusion of each chapter. The following sections discuss these principles in general terms.

Autonomy

Autonomy refers to the principle of self-determination that is particularly prominent in Western cultures. It is essential to know what the patient's wishes are with respect to his or her illness. In general, every effort should be made to respect a patient's personal autonomy. However, autonomy may be compromised if the patient has diminished a **decision-making capability.** Psychiatric illness can interfere with a patient's ability to make rational decisions.

To function with maximum autonomy, a patient is also entitled to **informed consent.** A patient must receive a thorough explanation of his or her illness and be fully informed about possible benefits and risks of different proposed treatments, including the option to refuse treatment. The capacity to give informed consent for a medical intervention rests on the patient's ability to understand the illness, the prognosis and proposed treatment, and alternatives, as well as the ability to weigh the risks and benefits of having medical treatment. Patients who are able to meet the criteria for informed consent may refuse medical interventions. Note that the diagnosis of a psychiatric illness does not automatically mean that a patient cannot give informed consent. Autonomy also extends to the patient's right to privacy and **confidentiality.** Physicians are sometimes permitted to break confidentiality in the event of emergencies such as suicidal or homicidal intent or in cases involving minors.

Beneficence

Beneficence refers to the physician's responsibility to do the most good for the patient. It is sometimes invoked as a reason to limit the autonomy of a patient whose ability to make decisions or to care for himself or herself has been compromised.

Non-malfeasance

Non-malfeasance is based on the time-honored Hippocratic principle *primum non nocere* ("first do no harm"). Usually this involves the physician and the patient weighing the risks and benefits of a given procedure. Physicians must be certain that they are offering care that carries the least chance of illness or death. When risk of injury or death is unavoidable, physicians must make certain that benefits truly outweigh possible harm. This issue may also arise in research studies.

Justice

Justice is a complex ethical issue that demands consideration of the fairness of a proposed treatment or intervention. Here justice refers not only to the patient but the cost to society and how these principles are weighed together.

Countertransference

Countertransference, or the physician's emotional reaction to patients, should also be considered. Likable patients often receive more care, perhaps leading to an improved prognosis; and hostile, difficult, and personality-disordered patients are more commonly ignored or given poorer quality care. Physicians should strive to treat patients equally, regardless of their own feelings toward individual patients.

Other Factors

Cross-cultural factors may become highly relevant since ethical issues involve the patient's background and values. Physicians need to be sensitive to the patient's views, which may involve a different understanding of illness, involvement of family, attitudes toward medication, the stigma of mental illness, and mistrust of Western medicine. **Third-party issues** arise frequently in the funding of health care, and the intrusion of insurance companies or other agencies in the clinical care decisions and the doctor-patient relationship. Physicians working for health-care organizations may find a conflict of interest between responsibilities to their patients and to their employers.

Other factors include the influence of the **group dynamics** on the medical team's decision-making. The phenomenon of **group-think** occurs when health-care members reinforce, rather than challenge, their own clinical reasoning and are unaware of their communal "blind spots" that lead to erroneous decision-making.

OTHER ETHICAL CONSIDERATIONS

The strengths of the principle-based model of ethics outlined above are a case-based approach firmly grounded in moral philosophy and a reproducible methodology that can be applied in a scientific manner. But this model is only one approach to bioethics. Further, it has been criticized on the grounds that it conveys only a superficial understanding of how these principles should be applied and that it favors consideration of objective principles at the expense of the patient's subjective experience of his or her illness. The **narrative approach** is an alternative method to bioethics that emphasizes the patient's experience of illness within the unique context of the patient's life, culture, and individual psychology. This approach is less influenced by the values inherent in modern medical systems.

Concern for ethical issues is important in maintaining the highest standards of patient care. These issues are also essential to the growth and development of students and residents. Medical trainees are sometimes confronted by clinical situations in which the so-called right course of action is unclear. Trainees are exposed to situations in which they may feel that their residents and attending physicians did not act in the best interests of a patient. Such experiences may be upsetting to students as real-world events clash with cherished internal values, principles, and ideals about how physicians should think, feel, and behave. Ide-

ally, students will find a forum to discuss these issues and experiences and will grow professionally and personally as they come to appreciate the strengths and weaknesses of the medical system in which they train. Most medical centers have ethics committees that offer confidential case-based consultation that students may find helpful. The alternative may be a gradual diminution of moral sense and interest, and a growing cynicism about the practice of medicine.

CONCLUSION

Psychiatric disorders are commonly encountered by all clinicians, yet they remain underdiagnosed and undertreated. The current era of a rapidly evolving system of health care and the economic and psychological cost of mental disorders to patients, their families, and society makes it essential for every physician to have a working knowledge of psychiatric disorders. Physicians should be able to perform an initial evaluation for these disorders, develop a differential diagnosis, formulate an assessment of the patient's condition, and in some clinical settings design a treatment plan. At the same time, clinicians should strive to develop their interviewing skills, to become aware of their own emotional reactions to patients, and gain familiarity with the legal and ethical issues that are often encountered in working with patients who have mental illness.

REFERENCES

American Association of Bioethics. http://www.med.umn.edu/aab/

American Psychiatric Association: *Diagnostic and Statistical Manual of Mental Disorders, 4th edition (DSM-IV).* American Psychiatric Press, 1994.

American Psychiatric Association: American Psychiatric Association practice guidelines for psychiatric evaluation of adults. Am J Psychiatr 1995;152:11(Suppl):65.

Basch MF: *Understanding Psychotherapy: The Science Behind the Art.* Basic Books, 1988.

Gabbard GO: Psychodynamic psychiatry in clinical practice: the DSM-IV edition. American Psychiatric Press, 1994.

Goldman LS: Psychiatry in primary care: possible roles for organized medicine. Psychiatr Ann 1997;27(6):425.

Hebert P: *Doing Right: A Practical Guide to Ethics for Medical Trainees and Professionals.* Oxford University Press, 1996.

Hughes CC: Culture in clinical psychiatry. Page 41 in: *Culture, Ethnicity and Mental Illness.* Gaw A (editor). American Psychiatric Press, 1993.

Internet Mental Health. Http://www.mentalhealth.com/

Jecker NS, Jonsen AR, Pearlman RA. *Bioethics: An Introduction to the History, Methods, and Practice.* Jones & Bartlett Publishers, 1997.

Kessler RC et al: Lifetime and 12-month prevalence of DSM-III-R psychiatric disorders in the United States: results from the National Comorbidity Survey. Arch Gen Psychiatr 1994;51:8.

Lo B: *Resolving Ethical Dilemmas: A Guide for Clinicians.* Williams & Wilkins, 1996.

Mental Illness in America (National Institute of Health). http://mentalhealth.com/book/p45-mhus.html

Othmer E, Othmer S: *The Clinical Interview Using DSM-IV. Vol 1: Fundamentals.* American Psychiatric Press, 1994.

Shea SC: *Psychiatric Interviewing: The Art of Understanding.* Saunders, 1988.

Sims A: *Symptoms in the Mind: An Introduction to Descriptive Psychopathology,* 2nd ed. Bailliere Tindall, 1996.

Sperry L, Gudeman JE, Faulkner LR: *Psychiatric Case Formulation.* American Psychiatric Association Press, 1992.

Stahl SM: *Essential Psychopharmacology: Neuroscientific*

Basis and Practical Applications. Cambridge University Press, 1996.

Strub RL, Black EW: *The Mental Status Examination in Neurology.* FA Davis Company, 1977.

Trzepacz PT, Baker RW: *The Psychiatric Mental Status Examination.* Oxford University Press, 1993.

Zaubler TS, Viederman M, Fins JJ: Ethical, legal and psychiatric issues in capacity, competency and informed consent: an annotated bibliography. Gen Hosp Psychiatr 1996;18:155.

Medical Mimics of Psychiatric Disorders

2

David Elkin, MD

Many medical conditions can cause symptoms that mimic primary psychiatric disorders, including mood disorders (mania or depression), psychosis (with symptoms similar to schizophrenia), anxiety, or personality disorders. The incidence of these **medical mimics** of psychiatric disorders is high, and certain patients are particularly vulnerable. Mental status changes associated with these conditions may include cognitive dysfunction such as short-term memory or concentration problems. Clinicians should rule out these medical (previously termed organic) conditions before making a purely psychiatric diagnosis. Legal and ethical issues may arise in caring for patients who have medical illnesses that mimic psychiatric disorders.

INCIDENCE

The incidence of medical illness that causes or exacerbates psychiatric symptoms is remarkably high. Undiagnosed medical problems are also common in patients who do have psychiatric disorders, and these problems lead to unnecessary suffering and thousands of deaths annually as a result of delays in diagnosis and treatment.

The risk is probably highest in patients who have severe, chronic mental illness such as schizophrenia and schizoaffective disorder. These patients are unlikely to have access to or the skills needed to obtain regular medical attention, and their mental illness may interfere with their ability to give a coherent medical history. Studies show that although 20–50% of patients who have psychotic disorders also have a serious medical illness; less than half will receive the appropriate workup, diagnosis, and treatment for these medical conditions. In many cases medical illnesses cause or aggravate psychotic symptoms. Drug and alcohol use may further complicate the clinical presentation of patients who have these disorders.

Other patient populations at increased risk of having medical illnesses that aggravate or mimic psychiatric conditions include the elderly, patients who are HIV positive, or those who have dementia. As many as one-half of patients who are diagnosed with a **conversion disorder,** in which physical symptoms are believed to be the result of a psychological disorder, will later be shown to have an undiagnosed medical problem.

DIAGNOSTIC ASSESSMENT

Many physicians erroneously assume they can easily distinguish symptoms caused by primary psychiatric disorders from those caused by an underlying medical problem.. This is not the case; psychiatric symptoms often look identical, whether they are caused by medical or psychological factors. Sometimes medical illnesses produce psychiatric symptoms as well as cognitive dysfunction, including problems with short-term memory, concentration, or visuospatial skills such as drawing. Although anxiety, depression, and psychosis can cause mild problems with these cognitive tasks, the presence of moderate to severe cognitive dysfunction almost invariably indicates the presence of an underlying medical disorder.

In most cases, medical illnesses that cause or exacerbate psychiatric symptoms do not produce cognitive problems. The clinical presentation of these medical illnesses will closely mimic that seen in depression, mania, psychosis, anxiety, or personality disorders. The clinician will not be able to determine whether a medical condition exists without performing a thorough workup, including a complete history, physical examination, and laboratory tests. Family histories and collaborative information from families or friends may be very helpful. Thus the first step in working up a patient with psychiatric symptoms should be to rule out an underlying medical disease process. Table 2–1 summarizes factors that increase the likelihood of an underlying medical problem.

The language used to distinguish between medical

Table 2–1. Factors that increase the likelihood of a medical cause for psychiatric symptoms.

Older age of onset
Lack of prior psychiatric history
Negative family psychiatric history
Cognitive dysfunction or decline
Atypical presentation (history, symptoms, course)
Unilateral hallucinations
Alteration in level of consciousness, orientation
Failed response to prior treatment, or sudden unexplained or new symptoms

and psychiatric phenomena reflects and creates tremendous gaps in our knowledge of psychiatric conditions. The *DSM-IV* uses the terms "medical" and "psychiatric" instead of the older terminology of "organic" and "functional," respectively, but this division is based more on the semantics and philosophy of the Western construct that divides "mind" and "body" than on the existence of two absolutely discreet, mutually exclusive categories. Consider, for example, that strong evidence indicates that depression, mania, psychosis, and other psychiatric disorders result from imbalances of neurotransmitters in the CNS. Or that schizophrenia is likely the result of a defect in the development of deeper brain structures. Or that reduced functioning is observed in the dominant prefrontal areas of the brains of depressed patients, and that depressed patients who improve in psychotherapy without medication have probably experienced a return of neurotransmitter levels to normal. Is psychotherapy then a biological therapy modality? The categories used to cleave medical from psychiatric illness are useful in a practical sense, but the theoretical gaps reflect a philosophical dilemma that continues to perplex Western medicine.

Einstein warned that "your theory will determine your observations," and the medical corollary is that physicians will tend to pursue only the observations and diagnoses they have considered. Many healthcare workers will unwittingly neglect physical findings, or fail to order appropriate tests, because they assume that a patient's problems are based on a psychiatric disorder rather than a medical illness.

The mental status examination is useful in diagnosing psychiatric disorders due to medical conditions. Detailed information regarding the duration and severity of abnormal affect and thought processes, hallucinations, and delusions should be sought. These characterizations should be augmented by historical data obtained from family members and health-care workers. The cognitive examination is especially important. Patients who have psychiatric symptoms caused by medical illness sometimes exhibit cognitive dysfunction, that is, disturbances of concentration, short-term memory, abstracting ability, or visuospatial ability. The presence of cognitive dysfunction should increase the physician's suspicion

that an underlying medical disorder may be causing a patient's psychiatric symptoms.

The converse is not true: Since cognitive dysfunction is not always present in medical conditions that mimic psychiatric disorders, a normal cognitive examination does not eliminate the possibility of a medical condition. The case examples in the next section illustrate this variability.

Another potential oversight involves medical illnesses in patients who have a known psychiatric history. Patients who have depression, bipolar disorder, and schizophrenia get sick too, and any change in the baseline of these patients should trigger a review of their medical status.

Robert A, a patient with a 20-year history of schizophrenia who had been stable on antipsychotic medications for many years, began to exhibit increasingly bizarre behavior in the psychiatric outpatient clinic, including pulling off his pants in front of other patients. The mental health team assumed that Mr. A was noncompliant with his medication (despite protests to the contrary from the family). His antipsychotic medication dosage was increased, with little or no effect on his behavior. After taking increasing dosages of his medication for several months, Mr. A had a seizure. A computed tomography (CT) scan revealed a brain tumor, presumably the cause of his altered behavior. Resection of the tumor was deemed impossible, and Mr. A died shortly thereafter.

To accurately diagnose psychiatric disorders due to medical conditions, physicians must follow five basic principles:

1. A psychiatric diagnosis (eg, schizophrenia or major depression) should be made only after a medical condition has been ruled out as the cause of psychiatric symptoms.
2. A thorough history should always be obtained from the patient. The history should include the onset and course of symptoms, previous psychiatric and medical history, a review of all prescription and over-the-counter medications taken by the patient, and a family history that includes medical as well as psychiatric illness.
3. A thorough physical examination should be conducted and appropriate laboratory tests performed.
4. Extra diligence may be required to detect a medical disorder, especially in cases involving patients who have atypical presentations, those who are well-known to the mental health system, or those who are particularly unlikable.
5. Physicians should still consider the possibility of a missed medical diagnosis at a later time.

SPECIFIC MEDICAL CAUSES
OF PSYCHIATRIC CONDITIONS

This section describes some of the disease processes that can mimic psychiatric illnesses. Table 2–2 lists various medical problems that can cause psychiatric symptoms.

Intracranial Lesions & Masses

Brain tumors can cause mania, depression, psychosis, and personality change, either by displacing brain tissue or as a side effect of treatment (eg, surgery, radiation therapy, or chemotherapy). Symptoms are often accompanied by cognitive dysfunction such as short-term memory loss and problems with concentration.

Victor B, a 49-year-old male, was seen by the psychiatry resident on call after Mr. B had told the emergency room's internal medicine resident that he was planning to kill himself. Mr. B appeared tired, depressed, and irritable. He exhibited psychomotor slowing, with slow speech, gait, and mannerisms. He was angry to be receiving a psychiatric consultation, saying, "I didn't say I would kill myself, I said I would kill myself if someone didn't figure out what's wrong with me—it was just an expression!"

Mr. B explained that his symptoms had begun 6 months earlier and had worsened gradually. He was depressed, had less energy and initiative, was sleeping poorly, and felt anxious throughout the day. His marriage to his second wife 1 year earlier had started out well, but he felt that he couldn't "keep up with her." He also described decreased sex drive and an inability to enjoy usually pleasurable activities.

Mr. B was also disturbed by other problems with his concentration and memory. He would forget numbers on the way to use a telephone. He worked in a bar and was having trouble making change for customers. He also noted that he was having trouble using the bar's drink dispenser: "I used to know those buttons by heart, but now I have to stop and look at which one I'm pushing or I'll get it wrong." Because Mr. B worked in a bar, the psychiatry resident asked him whether he'd had any problems with alcohol. "I did," he said, "but I stopped cold turkey a year ago when I got married because my wife insisted." Mr. B's wife confirmed this statement.

Cognitive testing was remarkable for slowed concentration—Mr. B could perform serial sevens and name the months of the year backward, but at a speed that seemed slow both to him and to the interviewer. His short-term memory may have been affected: He learned four items on the first try but could recall only three items at 5 minutes, even when given category or list prompts. His visuospatial skills also seemed impaired, as evidenced by the trouble he experienced while drawing a clock. There were no abnormalities of language or speech. The neurologic examination was unremarkable. Laboratory tests also were normal, including liver function tests, which made current alcohol dependence seem less likely.

The psychiatric team felt that Mr. B's cognitive dysfunction was mild and could be easily explained by a diagnosis of major depression. But the resident was impressed by Mr. B's visuospatial and memory problems. The psychiatry resident was also struck by the fact that Mr. B experienced increasing cognitive problems after stopping alcohol, when his memory and concentration problems should have improved.

An electroencephalogram (EEG) was abnormal, and a magnetic resonance imaging (MRI) scan of the patient's head revealed a very small tumor at the out-flow of the fourth ventricle, resulting in the equivalent of normal pressure hydrocephalus. Removal of the tumor led to rapid correction of the patient's depression and all cognitive deficits. The tumor was an adenocarcinoma, believed to be a metastasis from lung cancer, diagnosed some time later.

Mr. B regained his energy and noted improvement in his marriage. He lived several years, without recurrence of his depression.

Diagnosis. Major depression due to a medical disorder (metastatic cancer) (Axis I); adenocarcinoma with intracranial metastasis (Axis III).

Strokes (cerebrovascular accidents) can also cause a number of conditions, including any of the psychiatric syndromes described above, as well as dementia or delirium. Depending on their size and location, strokes may not manifest with sensory, motor, or speech problems but with psychiatric symptoms instead. Patients who have fluent aphasia produce nonsensical, disjointed speech, which may be mistaken for the loose associations and disorganized thoughts seen in patients who have schizophrenia. A diagnosis of stroke should always be considered, especially with increasing age and other risk factors (eg, obesity, high cholesterol, smoking, family history). MRI scans provides more resolution than do CT scans.

Cardiopulmonary Conditions

Cardiopulmonary problems are extremely common in the United States. Congestive heart failure, and other conditions that result in reduced blood flow to the brain (eg, arrhythmias or atherosclerotic blockage of the carotid arteries), may produce symptoms of depression. Nearly a million pulmonary emboli occur in the United States population each year, but

Table 2–2. Medical conditions causing psychiatric symptoms.

Medical Illness	Examples	Psychosis	Depression	Mania	Anxiety	Dementia	Delirium
Intracranial lesions/ masses	CNS tumors and metastases	x	x	x	x	x	
	Stroke	x	x		x	x	x
Cardiopulmonary problems	Congestive heart failure		x		x		x
	Pulmonary emboli				x		
	Cardiac arrythmias				x		x
Reduced CNS bloodflow	Anemia		x		x		
Electrolyte abnormalities	Hypercalcemia	x	x				
Temporal lobe epilepsy	Temporal lobe epilepsy	x			x		
Endocrine disorders	Hypothyroidism	x	x			x	
	Hyperthyroidism	x		x	x		
	Cushing's syndrome	x	x	x			
	Addison's disease		x				
Connective tissue disorders	Multiple sclerosis		x				
	Systemic lupus erythema- tosus	x	x	x	x		
Cancer	Pancreatic carcinoma		x				
	Pheochromocytoma				x		
Infections (CNS or systemic)	Neurosyphilis	x				x	
	Meningitis						x
	HIV	x	x	x		x	
	Lyme disease		x			x	
Medication	Corticosteroids	x	x	x			
	Birth control pills		x		x		
	Beta blockers		+				
Vitamin deficiencies	Thiamine deficiency	x	x		x		x
Substance use	Alcohol use		x		x	x	x
	Alcohol withdrawal	x			x		x
	Cocaine/methamphetamines	x		x	x		
Sleep abnormalities	Sleep apnea		x			x	
	Shift work		x				
Rare conditions	Wilson's disease	x					
	Porphyria			x	x		

only 10% of these incidents will produce symptoms (or health-related behaviors) that result in contact with a physician and a laboratory test to confirm the diagnosis. The other 90% will not be diagnosed. Individuals experiencing these incidents may have few or no symptoms, but some will report a need to hyperventilate, a subjective sense of doom, or other symptoms of anxiety.

Hypoxemia

Decreased oxygen delivery to the brain (**hypoxemia**)—regardless of the cause—can result in depression, anxiety, personality change, dementia, or delirium. For example, congenital heart failure or anemia frequently cause fatigue and other symptoms seen in depression.

Electrolyte Abnormalities

Electrolyte abnormalities are extremely common in hospitalized patients. Abnormalities can result from many conditions, including renal disease, dehydration, and increased output of urine (**diuresis**). These disturbances are measured in blood but are distributed uniformly throughout the body, including the cerebrospinal fluid. When the brain is exposed to abnormal levels of electrolytes, delirium, depression, anxiety, psychosis, or personality change can occur.

Claude D, a 59 year-old male, had been diagnosed recently with lung cancer. His behavior became troublesome over the 3 days since his admission, especially after he had been told that his cancer had spread to his bones. The nurses noted that he was increasingly agitated, hostile, and paranoid. His paranoia took the form of questioning what the nurses and doctors were writing in his chart, thinking, and saying. He began lurking around the nurses' station, spying on them, taking notes on their conversations, and trying to steal his chart.

None of the hospital staff knew Mr. D prior to his admission, but it was widely believed that he had a "difficult" personality as a baseline. He denied a history of alcohol abuse. Although he appeared anxious and paranoid, he had no noticeable cognitive deficits. He refused formal testing but his short-term memory and concentration appeared intact. His vital signs were normal, and he showed no fluctuation of consciousness or disorientation, making delirium unlikely. His anger and irrational thinking were most prominent whenever he was confronted about the inappropriateness of his reactions to medical personnel.

Routine laboratory analysis showed an elevated level of serum calcium, over 14 mg/dl (normal is ~8 mg/dl). Presumably the increase in osteoclastic activity caused by the metastasis led to elevated calcium levels. Mr. D received an intravenous infusion of medication that brought his calcium down to normal levels by the next day.

Mr. D's personality had also undergone a remarkable transformation by the next day. Instead of being hostile and paranoid, he seemed concerned about his treatment and prognosis. He stopped spying on the nurses and was appropriate in every interaction with the medical staff.

Over the next several days however, Mr. D's behavior and attitude slowly reverted to his previous state, as his calcium levels increased slowly above 13 mg/dl. He became paranoid and irrational and threatened to refuse all treatment. Over the next several weeks, while he received daily radiation therapy for his bone metastases, this pattern repeated itself several times. When his calcium level was normal, his behavior was appropriate; as his calcium level increased, his paranoia returned.

Diagnosis. Personality change due to a medical condition (hypercalcemia) (Axis I); metastatic lung cancer, hypercalcemia (Axis III).

Discussion. Mr. D's paranoia and agitation were not investigated immediately because the medical team assumed that he was at or near his personality baseline and that any exacerbation of the baseline was the result of purely psychological causes (ie, a reaction to a terminal illness and the stress of treatment).

This case further illustrates the connection between "mind" and "body," between a medical condition and a psychiatric set of symptoms, specifically the issue of personality change. Changes in personality should always be investigated thoroughly, both by thorough history-gathering as well as physical and laboratory examination.

Temporal Lobe Epilepsy

Temporal lobe epilepsy (TLE) (also known as complex partial seizure disorder or psychomotor seizures) differs considerably from grand mal seizures. Rather than occurring in a motor strip and resulting in muscle contractions, TLE involves synchronized discharge of cells in the temporal lobes. Electrical activity here may produce a variety of effects: "fear" attacks, which may resemble the symptoms of panic attacks; hallucinations, either visual, auditory, or olfactory; or dissociative phenomena in which the patient feels his or her surroundings are "unreal" or "dreamlike." Between seizures, patients may have symptoms of depression, anxiety, or psychosis. Between 7 and 23% of patients who have TLE exhibit psychiatric symptoms that mimic schizophrenia.

Some important distinguishing characteristics of TLE include olfactory hallucinations, extensive and compulsive writing (hypergraphia), periods of diminished consciousness, and a history of head trauma. Other symptoms such as extreme religious beliefs and decreased sex drive may also be found in schizophrenia and do not aid in differential diagnosis. Misdiagnosis of TLE as schizophrenia leads to the prescription of antipsychotic medication, which will lower the seizure threshold and may worsen the patient's condition. Also, even sleep-deprived EEGs with nasopharyngeal leads positioned near the temporal lobes will fail to reveal TLE in half of all cases, so the physician needs to be mindful of the diagnosis.

Stefan K, a 45-year-old man, was enrolled in group therapy for panic attacks. His attacks were consistent with panic disorder: 20–30 minute episodes of fear, knotting in his stomach, palpitations, numbness in his fingertips, and a feeling of dread. Mr. K worked as a prison guard, but the panic attacks, which occurred several times a week, caused so much emotional distress, shame, and embarrassment that he left his job with a medical disability.

A brief attempt to return to work failed because of anxiety and loss of self-confidence. With the loss of his job, he became increasingly depressed and felt guilty about the financial burden he was placing on his wife. He also complained of a complete absence of sex drive, which added to marital stress. At times he felt so helpless about his situation that he considered suicide.

Mr. K tried many different antidepressants, all of which failed to improve his panic attacks. Diazepam was somewhat helpful, but he encountered resistance from his psychiatrist when he asked for an ongoing supply. Group therapy provided some initial relief and support, but he was the only group member who did not experience significant improvement in his condition. He became more despondent and more withdrawn.

Mr. K returned to the group after a 1-month hiatus. He had experienced a complete remission of his panic attacks and depression and had returned to his job. A psychiatrist at another clinic thoroughly reviewed the patient's history and examination results, and ordered an EEG, which showed spiking in the temporal lobes. Having diagnosed the patient with TLE, the psychiatrist prescribed an anticonvulsant, which promptly led to remission of the patient's symptoms.

Diagnosis. Anxiety disorder due to a medical condition (temporal lobe epilepsy) with panic attacks (Axis I); temporal lobe epilepsy (Axis III).

Endocrine Disorders

Disturbances in the endocrine system affect the production of hormones, the human body's intercellular messenger system. Endocrine disturbances can profoundly affect the functioning of the CNS and produce psychiatric symptoms as a result.

Hyperthyroidism causes an increase in cellular metabolism in every organ system. In the CNS, this change can translate into a subjective sense of agitation, anxiety, and restlessness. Mania or psychosis may also result. **Hypothyroidism** can cause the opposite symptoms: depression with a sense of lack of energy (**anergia**), fatigue, a loss of interest and pleasure in normally enjoyable activities (**anhedonia**), and decreased sex drive. Hypothyroidism may also produce psychotic symptoms (called **myxedema madness**).

Brad F, a 24-year-old medical student, became depressed in the fall of his third year. He noticed that he had decreased energy, pervasive sadness, a growing sense of hopelessness and dread about the future, problems with concentration and short-term memory, and anhedonia. He and his friends advanced various psychological theories to explain his self-diagnosed depression: stress from the adjustment to clinical rotations, relationship problems, or seasonal affective disorder. A positive family history of affective disorders helped Mr. F to confirm his own diagnosis.

Mr. F's physician conducted a complete medical workup on him before prescribing antidepressants or psychotherapy and noted the following symptoms: mild weight gain, hair loss (alopecia) distributed throughout the scalp, and delayed return on testing of the patellar deep tendon reflexes (DTRs). Laboratory testing showed an elevated level of thyroid stimulating hormone (TSH). Treatment with a thyroid hormone replacement medication led to a rapid and complete remission of all physical and emotional symptoms without the prescription of antidepressant medication.

Diagnosis. Mood disorder due to a medical condition (hypothyroidism) with major depressive-like episode (Axis I); hypothyroidism (Axis III).

Diabetes can occur gradually and "silently," and as a result, may manifest with symptoms of depression or anxiety related to elevated serum (and thus CNS) glucose levels.

Florence G, a 53-year-old woman, was seen for severe depression 1 month after the death of her husband of 30 years. Worn down from supporting her husband through his protracted battle with metastatic lung cancer, Ms. G was extremely depressed and exhibited symptoms such as anxiety, insomnia, social withdrawal from family and friends, anhedonia, loss of sex drive, guilt, and poor self-esteem. She had gained 20 pounds over several months. She spent much of her days crying, and both her waking thoughts and dreams focused on her husband. She had become increasingly convinced that her life was no longer worth living and began considering ways that she might commit suicide.

Ms. G had no personal or family history of any psychiatric disorders. Her medical problems included hypertension and mild diabetes, for which she took a diuretic and an oral hypoglycemic. She refused referral to a support group but did not have the financial resources to pay for individual therapy more than once a month.

Under these circumstances, her psychiatrist prescribed antidepressants to treat her depression. To minimize side effects, she was started on the antidepressant fluoxetine, a selective serotonin re-uptake inhibitor (SSRI). Over the next few weeks, Ms. G's mood improved dramatically and most of the symptoms of her depression lifted. She did well for the next 3 months, but as the winter holidays approached, her depression returned with almost the same severity as before treatment. She asked if she could increase her fluoxetine.

Ms. G's psychiatrist discussed with her the relevance of her first Thanksgiving without her husband in 30 years, but that did not seem to help. The psychiatrist also inquired about Ms. G's general health. She reported that she was on a third course of antibiotics for a persistent bronchitis, and that she was increasingly thirsty, needed to urinate more frequently, and had occasional dizzy spells. The psychiatrist recognized that these symptoms strongly suggested an exacerbation of the patient's diabetes and recommended that she see her internist immediately.

A blood sample drawn at the internist's office indicated a fasting blood sugar level of 450 mg/dl, four times normal and potentially very dangerous. Ms. G's physician prescribed insulin injections, and within two weeks her blood sugar levels had normalized, and her bronchitis cleared. Ms. G's depression remitted completely despite the stress of the upcoming holidays.

Diagnosis. Major depression exacerbated by diabetes (Axis I); diabetes type II (Axis III).

Psychiatric disorders may also result from imbalances in endogenous corticosteroid levels. **Cushing's syndrome,** characterized by overproduction of corticosteroids, may result in symptoms of mania. **Addison's disease,** characterized by underproduction of corticosteroids, is likely to produce depression. Both diseases can result in personality changes or psychosis. Parathyroid disorders can also cause psychiatric symptoms.

Connective Tissue Disorders

Diseases such as **multiple sclerosis** or **systemic lupus erythematosus** can produce lesions in the central and peripheral nervous systems. Depending on their location, these lesions may cause a variety of psychiatric symptoms such as anxiety, psychosis, mania, or depression. These symptoms may appear months or years before physical symptoms of the diseases arise or become clinically apparent, and many patients are erroneously diagnosed with psychiatric conditions for several years. This problem may be exacerbated by the fact that connective tissue disorders tend to affect younger women, who may be more easily stereotyped as being "hysterical."

Cancer

Certain forms of cancer frequently cause neuropsychiatric syndromes. For example, patients who have pancreatic cancer often exhibit symptoms of depression. Other cancers of the gastrointestinal (GI) tract may also cause depression, perhaps by releasing neuropeptides that act as chemical messages to the CNS. **Pheochromocytomas** (rare benign tumors of the adrenal medulla) may cause anxiety or discrete episodes that can mimic panic disorder. Primary or metastatic cancer in the CNS can also produce psychiatric disturbances.

Infections

Infections can mimic psychiatric syndromes and also can cause dementia and delirium. HIV can cause mania, depression, or psychosis, as well as personality change and dementia either via cytotoxic effects to the CNS that result in neurotransmitter deficiencies, or by permitting opportunistic infections or tumors to affect the brain. **Neurosyphilis,** a CNS syndrome seen in advanced (tertiary) stages of syphilis, may produce similar symptoms.

Acute or chronic **meningitis,** a bacterial or viral infection of the structure that surrounds the brain, can produce depression and mild to severe problems with cognitive function, such as problems with memory and concentration. A lumbar puncture with analysis of cerebrospinal fluid for evidence of infection is considered diagnostic. Patients who have aseptic meningitis may present with subtle symptoms, and lumbar puncture samples may yield a negative or equivocal diagnostic result. Less common infections such as Lyme disease or rabies can also cause psychiatric symptoms.

Rosemary H, aged 25, was referred for a psychiatric evaluation for symptoms of depression that had worsened gradually over a 6-month period. Before the onset of her depression, Ms. H had been highly successful at work and was physically active on weekends. Now she complained of sadness, fatigue, diminished appetite, 20-pound weight loss, excessive sleep (hypersomnia), and difficulties with concentration and short-term memory so severe that she was in danger of losing her job.

Ms. H also complained of chronic pain in her

joints and occasional low fevers that started shortly after the onset of her depression. Her internist ran tests for connective tissue disorders such as lupus erythematosus and multiple sclerosis. All tests were negative except for sedimentation rate, a nonspecific indicator for possible inflammation. Ms. H's physician concluded that her depression was causing somatic complaints, and he prescribed the antidepressant fluoxetine. Ms. H noted minimal improvement, and her physician then referred her to a psychiatrist.

The psychiatrist learned that Ms. H had no family or personal history of mood or anxiety disorders. He performed a cognitive examination to test Ms. H's memory and concentration. Although he expected some impairment from depression, the psychiatrist noted that the deficits were unusually severe and also suspected an unrecognized medical problem. He recalled that the patient enjoyed camping in a part of the country where Lyme disease was prevalent and inquired about possible tick exposure. Ms. H remembered removing ticks from her dog 8 months earlier but did not recall being bitten herself.

The psychiatrist ordered a laboratory test for Lyme disease, which was positive. He relayed the information to Ms. H's internist, who recommended a course of antibiotic therapy. One month later Ms. H's depression, joint pain, and cognitive dysfunction had resolved. She stopped taking fluoxetine and remained free of all physical and emotional symptoms.

Diagnosis. Major depression due to a medical disorder (Lyme disease) (Axis I); Lyme disease (Axis III).

Medications

Medications are an important and common cause of psychiatric disturbances. The blood-brain barrier is permeable to many prescribed medications, and nonpsychiatric medications designed to treat one body system may have potent CNS side effects. For example, reserpine, an antihypertensive, produces severe depression in many patients; H_2-blockers such as cimetidine, a drug used to treat ulcers, can cause depression, agitation, dementia, or delirium; and oral contraceptives can cause depression in some patients.

Some patient populations are particularly at risk for psychiatric disorders due to medication: The elderly, individuals infected with HIV, and patients who have dementia are all more susceptible to CNS side effects. Women and some ethnic groups are poorly represented in all but the most recent drug studies, and side effects may occur more commonly in these patients. Also, new medications may not have known psychiatric side effects.

The same medication may cause a variety of symptoms in some patients and produce few or no psychiatric side effects in others. Steroids such as prednisone (frequently used in the treatment of asthma, severe contact dermatitis, or connective tissue disorders) can produce depression, mania, or psychosis in patients who have no prior psychiatric history.

Patrick J, aged 40, was hospitalized with leukemia. He was receiving aggressive chemotherapy, including prednisone, for the leukemia. His behavior became increasingly agitated and disruptive, and psychiatric consultation was requested when the nurses found him trying to adjust the controls on his IV infusion pump.

When he was interviewed, Mr. J was wearing very colorful clothing, and he had decorated the wall of his hospital room with dozens of crude drawings he had made in the past several days. Mr. J was talkative and at times spoke quickly and loudly, requiring the interviewer to redirect and focus him throughout the interview. As he talked he continued to draw. He seemed minimally disturbed about having been diagnosed as having cancer, and when asked whether he was shocked by the turn of recent events, he replied, "I have been shocked . . . and shocked . . . shocked by the insane actions of the President of the United States."

Mr. J went on to describe how the war between healthy and cancerous cells in his body was a "microcosm" of the current Persian Gulf War. At times he seemed to have loose associations but was not paranoid and gave no indication of hallucinations. His insight seemed poor; he recognized only fleetingly that prednisone might be responsible for his increased activity level and acknowledged his elevated mood was extremely unusual.

The dose of prednisone was lowered and Mr. J's mood, thought processes, and behavior returned to normal.

Diagnosis. Mania due to corticosteroids (Axis I); leukemia (Axis III).

Vitamin Deficiencies

Vitamin deficiencies can cause neuropsychiatric effects, including anxiety, mania, depression, psychosis, and personality change. A review of the patient's nutrition history is critically important. Those especially at risk include patients who are malnourished due to alcohol dependence, cancer, AIDS, anorexia nervosa, or other illnesses.

Alcohol & Drug Use

Substance use or dependence is one of the most common underlying causes of psychiatric illness and may be found in up to 50% of all psychiatric patients.

Not all of these patients will admit to using drugs or alcohol, prompting some inpatient and outpatient psychiatric services to automatically perform toxicology urine screens on patients.

Daniel R, aged 40, was referred by his internist for treatment of depression and panic attacks. He had long complained of a low-level depression (dysthymia), characterized by a lack of energy, self-esteem, sex drive, and interest in any activities. He dated the onset of his symptoms to his parents' death in a motor vehicle accident 7 years earlier, an event that left him with enough income that he could spend most of the year unemployed. He left several jobs after only a few months because he was "bored." His daily life consisted of watching television, playing his guitar, or idly passing the time. He had little contact with friends and complained of feeling isolated; but it was also clear that he frequently turned down invitations from friends to play tennis or have dinner. Mr. R wanted a romantic relationship but said he lacked the energy to pursue one.

Mr. R said he had tried psychotherapy once in the past for several months, without any improvement. He began to experience increased anxiety and the onset of panic attacks. These attacks followed textbook descriptions: episodes of mounting anxiety and dread with a crescendo quality over 20–30 minutes. They were accompanied by physical symptoms of heart palpitations, sweaty palms, upper extremity numbness, and hyperventilation. The panic attacks had worsened over time and occurred several times per week, mostly in the morning.

Mr. R had seen his doctor, who performed a physical examination to rule out any medical causes of depression and panic attacks. His physician also ordered a series of laboratory examinations, including thyroid function tests and routine blood chemistry and electrolytes. These tests were all normal. The physician prescribed a tricyclic antidepressant that he knew was effective in the treatment of panic attacks.

Mr. R's course was atypical for most people with panic disorder in treatment. Instead of experiencing rapid improvement, he continued to exhibit symptoms. Despite the gradual introduction of the antidepressant, he experienced problems with anticholinergic side effects (eg, blurred vision, dry mouth). Although these side effects usually fade after several weeks, Mr. R continued to experience them for months. The antidepressant could not even be increased to therapeutic levels, so the psychiatrist recommended changing to paroxetine, an SSRI antidepressant. This medication was better tolerated but led only to a partial resolution of Mr. R's panic attacks.

After 6 months in weekly psychotherapy, Mr. R continued to complain of depression and muted panic attacks. His life was no different than when he had started, and both he and the psychiatrist were frustrated with his lack of progress. Mr. R began each session by asking, "So, what are you going to do for me today?" Neither exploration about his parent's deaths, nor insightful interpretations linking the patient's current state to his childhood, nor attempts to engage the patient in the present seemed to have much impact.

Finally, the psychiatrist decided to devote 1 hour to completely re-taking the patient's history. When he reached the area of substance use, the patient again reported that he drank only "socially, a few drinks a week." Perhaps in order to be thorough, the psychiatrist inquired further, asking how much Mr. R had to drink the day before (Sunday).

Without any perceptible hesitation, Mr. R replied, "A six-pack of beer and a few shots of vodka."

"And Saturday?" the psychiatrist asked.

Mr. R replied that he drank about the same amount. In response to further questioning, Mr. R revealed that this was typical of his weekend alcohol intake, that he drank "somewhat less" during the week. When asked what the alcohol did for him, he replied that alcohol allowed him to "mellow out"—sometimes he had a drink in the morning to prevent a panic attack.

The psychiatrist ordered a new panel of laboratory tests and asked Mr. R to keep a log of his drinking, mood, and panic attacks over the next week. At the next appointment, Mr. R's record confirmed the suspicion that the panic attacks occurred on weekday mornings, probably due to mild withdrawal from alcohol. His liver function tests were mildly elevated in a pattern consistent with mild alcoholic hepatitis.

The psychiatrist explained that the patient's alcohol intake accounted for his continued depression, panic attacks, and lack of results in therapy. But he added that there was a good chance that these problems would resolve if Mr. R could join Alcoholics Anonymous, stop drinking alcohol, and continue in therapy.

Mr. R's reply was surprising: "That's what all of the other psychiatrists said, too." He then reported that he had seen "many" other psychiatrists over the past 5 years, all of whom ultimately recommended that he stop drinking alcohol. "I thought you could come up with something else to help me, so I guess I forgot to tell you about it." The psychiatrist reiterated the need for Mr. R to address his dependence on alcohol as part of the treatment plan and stressed the potential health risks of continued drinking.

Mr. R greeted this statement with skepticism. "I'm going on vacation for a couple of months," he said. "I'll call you when I come back and let you know what I think." The psychiatrist has not heard from Mr. R for over 5 years.

Diagnosis. Depression with panic disorder due to alcohol dependence (Axis I); alcohol dependence/abuse (Axis I); alcoholic hepatitis (Axis III).

Patients may not give an accurate substance use history for a variety of reasons. Some patients worry that if they are truthful they will not obtain treatment or that animosity on the part of health-care professionals will lead to a substandard level of care. Others do not consider their substance use to be problematic, or they may drastically underestimate their use of drugs or alcohol. Sometimes medical personnel may indirectly discourage adequate exploration of these issues.

Disruption of Sleep Cycles

Disruption of normal sleep may cause psychiatric symptoms. **Sleep apnea** is a disorder that drastically interferes with the normal sleep architecture—the pattern of different stages that correlate with brain wave activity. Relaxation of smooth muscles in the upper airway during REM-stage sleep causes **apneic episodes**—periods in which the patient does not breath, either because of obstruction or decreased output from respiratory centers in the CNS. The patient ceases breathing for up to 30–60 seconds; after that, the oxygen content of the patient's blood will decrease to 50% or less, the patient will turn blue, and finally will fully or partially waken to draw in a breath.

Patients may experience dozens, even hundreds of apneic episodes during a single night but may have no memory of interrupted sleep. As a result of nights with only minimal REM activity, they awaken exhausted and tired, and may struggle with lethargy and somnolence all day. This condition can easily produce depressive symptoms and personality changes. Common cognitive dysfunctions include short-term memory deficits and difficulty concentrating. Effective treatments include administration of forced air at night or surgery to remove excessive tissue from the palate and throat.

Gabriel J, a 60-year-old man who had morbid obesity and congestive heart failure, was admitted for a sleep study. The physicians involved in the case were becoming extremely worried about his medical condition, which placed Mr. J at high risk of cardiac arrest.

Mr. J was noted to nap during the day and seemed very tired and irritable. His concentration and short-term memory seemed grossly impaired. His family noted a gradual but drastic personality disorder over the past 10 years. A sleep study showed that Mr. J was experiencing over 100 apneic episodes (cessation of breathing) accompanied by significantly decreased levels of oxygen in his blood. Most alarming was the observation that the patient had cardiac arrhythmias during these periods of low oxygen.

Mr. J was given a treatment plan consisting of surgical removal of excess tissue in his mouth, a weight loss program, and a machine to provide CPAP (continuous airway pressure) to keep his soft tissues from collapsing at night. After treatment Mr. J reported dramatic improvement in his physical and emotional condition over the next 3 months and a return to his baseline personality.

Diagnosis. Personality change due to sleep apnea (Axis I); sleep apnea, morbid obesity, congestive heart failure (Axis III).

A significant proportion of people working night shifts or varying schedules (with work shifts rotating from days to evenings to nights) experience adverse psychological effects, including depression and personality changes. Cognitive dysfunction can occur and may be particularly dangerous in heavy machine operators, pilots, and physicians.

Rare Conditions

Psychiatric symptoms can also be the result of some uncommon medical conditions. Hereditary conditions such as **Wilson's disease** (abnormal copper metabolism), **intermittent porphyria** (abnormal hemoglobin metabolism), and **Huntington's chorea** (a progressive dementia) can produce symptoms of psychosis and dementia. Exposure to heavy metals in neurotoxins, at work or around the home, can also cause depression, anxiety, personality change, or dementia.

Diane M, a 23-year-old woman, was admitted to a psychiatric ward for treatment of schizophrenia, paranoid type. She had two previous inpatient admissions and on those occasions had responded well to aggressive treatment with an antipsychotic. On this admission, Ms. M was again floridly psychotic but refused treatment with the antipsychotic. She heard voices; occasionally admitted to visual hallucinations; and was extremely agitated, paranoid, and confused.

Neuropsychological testing showed that Ms. M had impaired concentration and visuospatial abilities. A review of her records showed that the diagnosis of schizophrenia had been assumed from the first admission, but laboratory testing had been incomplete. An MRI scan of her brain showed degeneration of the basal ganglia. A brownish "Kayser-Fleisher ring" from deposits of copper was noted around the periphery of Ms. M's cornea. Serum ceruloplasmin (a copper-carrying enzyme) levels were low, confirming a diagnosis of Wilson's disease. Treatment with penicillamine and a diet low in copper resulted in significant improvement of Ms. M's psychosis and cognitive functioning.

Diagnosis. Psychotic disorder due to a medical condition (Wilson's disease) with delusions (Axis I); Wilson's disease (Axis III).

TREATMENT

Definitive treatment for medically caused psychiatric syndromes always involves treatment of the underlying medical condition. For example, patients experiencing mania due to steroids should be taken off that medication; those who have depression due to hypothyroidism should be treated for that endocrine system disorder; and so on. Often psychiatric conditions will improve or completely resolve with correction of the medical problem. Some patients who use drugs or alcohol also experience clearing of their depression, anxiety, or other symptoms with abstinence from substances.

However, medically caused syndromes sometimes can take on a "life of their own." For example, a patient whose depression is caused by hypothyroidism may still have a major depression after his or her thyroid level has returned to normal, and as a result, would still require antidepressants or psychotherapy.

In other patients, psychiatric symptoms may lead to hardships or other hazards. For example, manic patients may spend so much money that they go into debt and need to declare bankruptcy, or their marriages may end because of infidelities that began during a manic episode. Even when patients intellectually know that their symptoms were caused by a medical condition, the psychological after-effects of psychiatric symptoms should be addressed.

EMOTIONAL REACTIONS TO PATIENTS

It is remarkable that despite their training, physicians often fail to undertake a thorough search for a medical etiology when patients exhibit psychiatric symptoms. Emotional reactions to symptoms such as anxiety, depression, mania, or psychosis may lead physicians to ignore possible underlying medical illness.

LEGAL & ETHICAL ISSUES

Most physicians and health-care analysts agree that the financial aspects of medical care will come under increasing scrutiny over the next decade. Until the 1980s physicians practiced with great autonomy and largely excluded economic concerns from clinical decision-making. Under the managed care systems so common today, certain procedures might not be reimbursed because of economic considerations. What happens when clinically based decisions collide with economic constraints, or when physicians no longer have the power to determine the extent of medical procedures performed? How should physicians weigh the cost of a test with the possible harm done if a medical illness remains undiagnosed? To what extent are physicians liable for missing a medical diagnosis if they are under constraints to perform fewer tests?

These issues may be even more complex in patients who have less accepted diagnoses, such as chronic fatigue syndrome, environmental illness, and Gulf War syndrome. Skeptics of these diagnoses protest that patients claiming to have these disorders are actually suffering from major depression or somatoform disorders, in which psychological stress leads to the production of symptoms that suggest a medical cause. Believers hold that these are actual physical illnesses that produce depressive states (eg, mood disorders due to a medical condition), and that patients are further depressed by the failure of the medical profession to acknowledge them. This issue is not an abstract chicken-and-egg controversy; many physicians are outraged by the notion that some providers are diagnosing and treating patients who have these disorders in a manner they feel is unscientific and unethical. Some patients feel "written off" by the medical system, labeled as "psychosomatic," and are forming groups to gain support and acceptance for their causes. The struggle for definition of these disorders has become as much political as it is scientific.

Ethical concerns may arise in attempting to determine whether patients are using drugs or alcohol. Given the high incidence of substance use in patients who have psychiatric disorders, some clinicians advocate frequent mandatory blood or urine tests to screen for substance use. What effect does this testing procedure have on trust between patients and physicians? In rare instances it may be necessary to violate patient confidentiality to protect public safety. For example, if a patient refuses a workup of symptoms of sleep apnea—including fatigue and drowsiness during the day, even while driving—the treating physician may be legally obligated to alert the state

Department of Motor Vehicles, even if the patient objects.

Some patients are unaware of the mental status changes certain medical conditions may cause. This unawareness or lack of insight may be the result of cognitive dysfunction, thought disorder, or denial. These patients may refuse further workup or treatment, and physicians will need to decide how to proceed. If a patient is unable to understand the implications of a particular illness and give informed consent for treatment, a family member may need to become a surrogate decision-maker. In the absence of family members, a medical conservator may be appointed by the local court to serve in the same capacity.

Finally, an unusual ethical issue may arise in the care of patients who have become manic from medication. These patients may request medication doses that let them feel somewhat euphoric. What final mood state should physicians accept as a goal of adjusting medication dosages? For example, should a patient with leukemia be allowed to take an extra 5–10 mg of prednisone per day so that he can feel less worried about his serious illness? This complex issue involves a consideration of how patients and physicians define optimal physical and emotional health and the extent to which physicians collaborate with their patients' wishes.

CONCLUSION

Many medical conditions can cause psychiatric symptoms, such as mania, depression, anxiety, personality change, or psychosis. Any patient presenting to a medical facility with such psychiatric symptoms should receive a thorough medical workup in order to rule out a medical cause for the symptoms. A full history should be obtained, and complete mental status, cognitive, and physical examinations should be performed, including any necessary laboratory tests. Treatment of the underlying medical disorder frequently results in full or partial resolution of psychiatric symptoms. Further treatment may be necessary, and the psychological, family, and cultural dimensions of psychiatric disorders due to medical conditions should always be considered.

REFERENCES

Buckley R: Differentiating medical and psychiatric illness. Psychiatr Ann 1994;24(11):584.

Cummings JL: Secondary and drug-induced mood, anxiety, psychotic, catatonic and personality disorders: a review of the literature. J Neuropsychiatr Clin Neurosci 1992;4:369.

Cummings JL, Trimble MR: *Concise Guide to Neuropsychiatry and Behavioral Neurology.* American Psychiatric Press, 1995.

Gadde KM, Krishnan K, Ranga R: Endocrine factors in depression. Psychiatr Ann 1994;24(10):519.

Lim L, Ron MA, Ormerod IEC, David J et al: Psychiatric and neurologic manifestations in systemic lupus erythematosus. Q J Med. 1988;n.s.66(249):27.

Pies RW: Medical 'mimics' of depression. Psychiatr Ann 1994;24(10):521.

Pine DS, Douglas CJ, Charles E et al: Patients with multiple sclerosis presenting to psychiatric hospitals. J Clin Psychiatr 1995;56:297.

Wyszynski AA, Wyszynski B: The patient on steroids. Chapter 5 in: *A Case Approach to Medical Psychiatric Practice.* American Psychiatric Press, 1996.

Delirium & Dementia

3

David Elkin, MD, & Kristine Yaffe, MD

Delirium is an acute, short-lived phenomenon that is characterized by global dysfunction of the brain. In contrast, dementia is a progressive chronic central nervous system (CNS) disease affecting higher cognitive functions. Both dementia and delirium have multiple potential causes and warrant full and rapid diagnosis and treatment.

DELIRIUM

Delirium is the accepted term for a variety of conditions, including encephalopathy and altered mental status.

INCIDENCE

The incidence of delirium is especially high in hospitalized patients, who tend to have serious underlying medical problems, or have had or are about to have surgery. In the general population of hospitalized patients, approximately 10% may be delirious; that percentage may rise to as high as 30% in surgical and medical intensive care units. Patients who have a higher-than-average risk of developing delirium include the elderly, those who have preexisting CNS disease (including dementia), and those infected with HIV. Patients who are taking multiple medications or who have sensory deficits (eg, hearing or visual impairments) are also at increased risk.

ETIOLOGY

Specific causes of delirium may vary depending on the hospital and patient population. For example, alcohol withdrawal is one of the most frequent causes of delirium in patients at inner city hospitals because of the high incidence of alcohol dependence in the population served by these medical centers. Medications also play a significant role in many cases; anticholinergic medications, opiates, and other pain medications can cause delirium.

Electrolyte abnormalities that disturb normal cellular functioning can easily produce delirium by affecting the cerebrospinal fluid (CSF) and, thus, the brain itself. Infections of the CNS, such as encephalitis or meningitis, can cause delirium, as can infections in other parts of the body (eg, urinary tract infections or pneumonia). Gross CNS disorders, such as stroke or post-seizure states, are another common cause. Head trauma may also result in delirium, as can hypoperfusion of the brain caused by cardiopulmonary disorders.

Thiamine deficiency is a potentially reversible cause of delirium (and dementia) that can occur with the re-feeding of malnourished patients in the hospital—since thiamine is a cofactor in metabolism, critically low levels can be depleted quickly when patients are finally given food. Patients who drink heavily (and therefore derive most of their calorie intake from alcohol) and patients who have chronic wasting illnesses such as cancer or AIDS are especially at risk for thiamine deficiency.

DIAGNOSTIC ASSESSMENT

Delirium usually develops quickly within hours or days in association with an underlying medical illness and often has a rapidly varying ("waxing and waning") quality. The mental status examination, in particular the cognitive examination, and the patient's history as supplied by family or nursing staff, are two important components in the diagnosis of delirium.

1. SIGNS & SYMPTOMS

The diagnostic criteria for **delirium** include reduced attention span, disorganized thinking, hallucinations, illusions, misperceptions, disturbance of sleep-wake cycles, disorientation, cognitive dysfunction, and a short history of onset with clear relation to an underlying medical factor. Delirium is often characterized by a variable quality in which the patient's mental state changes from normal to abnormal in hours, even minutes (and hence may confuse different members of the medical team).

2. MENTAL STATUS EXAMINATION

The mental status examination of the patient who has delirium is often markedly abnormal. These findings vary with the waxing and waning of the delirious state, so the examination may be different from hour to hour.

A. Appearance, Behavior, & Language. Patients who have **quiet** or **hypoactive delirium** may seem tired but overtly normal to hospital staff (but not to family members), whereas **agitated delirium** is grossly obvious to most examiners. The delirious patient often seems distracted because of problems with attention. Patients may have visible motor perseveration such as picking repeatedly at bedcovers.

B. Emotions. Affect may be restricted, inappropriate, or labile.

C. Thought Processes & Content. Thought processes are likely to show circumstantiality or tangentiality and may be marked by loose associations and disorganization in some cases. Hallucinations and illusions often occur. Tactile hallucinations increase the likelihood of alcohol or benzodiazepine withdrawal as causal factors. Paranoia is not uncommon.

D. Judgment, Insight, & Impulse Control. Judgment, insight, and impulse control may be markedly diminished.

E. Cognitive Examination. Cognitive dysfunction occurs in most cases of delirium. The patient's level of consciousness is often abnormal, with disorientation to location, date, and even time of day. Short-term memory, concentration, visuospatial skills, and abstract thinking are frequently compromised. Patients are often unable to follow or execute two- or three-step commands. A test for attention span can be particularly useful in assessing patients suspected of having delirium.

Tomb & Christiansen suggest a test that can be added to the cognitive examination to test a patient's attention span. The patient is asked to slap the table (or other surface) when he or she hears the letter "c" (any letter, word, or number can be used). The examiner then says, "c," and checks the patient's compliance. The examiner then proceeds to slowly give letters in, and later out of, sequence from the alphabet (eg, a . . . b . . . c . . . d . . . e . . . d . . . e . . . d . . . c . . . x . . . l . . . c). The delirious patient may have trouble learning the task because of deficits in short-term memory. However, once the patient learns the task, he or she may either fail to slap the table or slap indiscriminately after every letter. Attention may be so poor that the patient starts to attend to people walking by the door. In conjunction with other tests, this test provides some objective measure of the patient's cognitive status.

Psychiatric consultation was requested for Janice L, a 57-year-old woman hospitalized with pneumonia because, as the medical resident explained, "She's losing it—she seems pretty crazy. She seems like a real psychiatric case." Ms. L had been admitted several days earlier and had been placed on oxygen and antibiotics for her medical condition. She had no previous psychiatric history except for a brief consultation with a psychiatrist when she was hospitalized for surgical removal of her gallbladder 7 years earlier. She did not recall specific details about this consultation.

When seen, Ms. L was troubled by intermittent visual hallucinations. The day before, she had seen "tiny red devils" running through her room. Her response was to offer them a glass of ice water, "because they looked so hot." She also believed that a patient in an adjoining room had been murdered and that the staff was covering up the truth. She was convinced that she overheard the murder taking place and also heard hospital staff and "two other men—I think they were investigators" discussing the "cover up" in the hallway.

Despite assurances from the staff, Ms. L was alternately concerned, paranoid, or extremely anxious. The nursing staff noted that Ms. L's mental status appeared to fluctuate dramatically. Occasionally she seemed nearly lucid. At other times, especially when she was running a high (~103° F) fever, she was paranoid, agitated, and disoriented (eg, she thought she was in a church and when questioned gave the incorrect month and year). Ms. L's thoughts would become very disorganized with occasional loose associations, and her insight and judgment appeared very poor. Her sleep-wake cycle was highly disturbed: She took frequent naps during the day, sometimes in the middle of an interview, and was awake throughout much of the night.

Ms. L's medical condition improved dramatically over the next week as her pneumonia resolved. The periodic lapses in her mental status occurred less frequently and finally disappeared. Just prior to her discharge from the hospital, she realized that her hallucinations and delusions had been a result of her medical illness. "I don't remember it very well any more," she said, "Just a lot of weird ideas, and I guess I was seeing things, too."

Diagnosis. Delirium due to pneumonia (Axis I); pneumonia (Axis III).

DIFFERENTIAL DIAGNOSIS

Delirium is a condition involving CNS dysfunction that results from a medical cause. The medical cause(s) of delirium should always be sought so that treatment can be provided. Delirium often manifests with hallucinations, paranoia, and other symptoms commonly seen in other major psychiatric conditions, and these conditions also must be ruled out. Table 3–1 contrasts the key features of delirium and dementia with those of schizophrenia and depression.

1. DETERMINING THE CAUSE OF DELIRIUM

The patient suspected of having delirium should receive a full medical evaluation, including laboratory tests, in order to diagnose and treat underlying medical causes of delirium.

Delirium may present with agitation and excitability, which is readily recognized as an abnormal state by most observers. Patients who are agitated and confused may pose a danger to themselves or to others. Many delirious patients exhibit a "quiet," more subdued version of delirium, which may be mistaken for depression or may be missed entirely.

Isabel D, a 70-year-old woman who had colon cancer, was admitted to the medicine service for "failure to thrive." She had become extremely malnourished and dehydrated at home. The medicine team felt that Ms. D was very depressed. Family members confirmed that she had become withdrawn but felt that her mental status had changed drastically in the past several weeks. They denied that she had a history of alcohol use.

On examination, Ms. D was found to be confined to bed. She demonstrated marked psychomotor slowing; her affect was restricted, and she had few spontaneous thoughts. Her judgment and insight were poor. Cognitive testing showed her to be alert and oriented to place, month, and year. However, a nurse on the night shift noted that Ms. D seemed confused about where she was. Short-term memory deficits and concentration problems were noted.

Ms. D seemed to have poor constructional ability, as evidenced by her drawing of a clock that contained errors. She drew the number "3" on the clock several times before moving on to draw "4," and she repeated the phrase "If that is what must be done" in response to many different questions. Thus she demonstrated both motor and verbal **perseveration** (uncontrollable repetition of a response). She also exhibited marked **opthalmoplegia** (ie, she could not move her eyes left or right, but had to move her head instead to change her gaze).

Laboratory examination was remarkable for normal head CT scan and lumbar puncture, and negative rapid plasma reagin (RPR) to rule out syphilis. Ms. D had anemia, as well as electrolyte imbalances consistent with dehydration.

Table 3–1. Distinguishing between delirium, dementia, and major depression and schizophrenia.

	Delirum	Dementia	Major Depression and Schizophrenia
History			
Outset	Rapid (hours to days)	Insidious (months to years	Variable (days to years)
Course	Fluctuates over course of day	Gradual decline	Variable (may fluctuate or cause gradual decline)
Mental Status Exam			
Attention	Decreased	Normal	Normal
Level of arousal	Decreased	Normal	Normal
Orientation	Impaired	Normal exept in late stages	Normal
Sleep-wake cycle	Grossly disturbed	Variable	Variable
Hallucinations[1]	Often visual (especially illusions) or tactile	Often absent in late stages	Often auditory
Disturbance of affect, thought, personality	Present	Present	Affect abnormal in depression Thought process abnormal in psychosis
Cognitive function (memory, abstract thinking, judgment, concentration)	Disturbed	Disturbed	Often normal or near normal
Laboratory Exam			
—EEG	Diffuse slowing	Variable	Normal

[1]When disturbances of higher cognitive functions, visual hallucinations, or both are detected in the evaluation of any psychiatric condition (not just dementia), underlying medical cause(s) should be more actively pursued.

Total protein, a marker for nutritional status, was markedly low.

In spite of Ms. D's malnourished state on admission, the medicine team felt that she did not need thiamine on admission because there was no history of alcohol use. Now a week after admission, Ms. D was started on 100 mg of thiamine for 3 days. Her opthalmoplegia and her cognitive dysfunction cleared over the next few days. She became more alert, lively, and more aware of her situation.

Diagnosis. Delirium secondary to thiamine deficiency (Axis I); colon cancer, malnutrition, anemia, thiamine deficiency (Axis III).

Discussion. Although many clinicians associate thiamine deficiency with alcohol use, thiamine deficiencies can result from any cause of malnutrition. Ironically, hospitalization and medical care may precipitate a critical thiamine deficiency.

For example, a patient enters a hospital setting when malnourished, with very low levels of thiamine throughout his body. The patient receives intravenous fluids with glucose and is actively given food by health-care staff. It would seem that this treatment would help the patient's nutritional status. But thiamine is a necessary cofactor in the metabolism of food, so all of the remaining thiamine is used as the patient's body begins to utilize the nutrients and sugar. In the brain, as thiamine levels plummet to near-zero, CNS dysfunction occurs. The patient develops personality changes, then confusion, disorientation, fluctuating levels of alertness with lethargy or agitation, hallucinations, and other symptoms of delirium.

Opthalmoplegia, gait disturbances, and death may also occur as the condition progresses. This acute stage of thiamine deficiency is known as **Wernicke's encephalopathy.** While some patients make complete recoveries, others are left with permanent brain dysfunction. This form of dementia is called **Korsakoff's syndrome** and is characterized by impaired short-term memory and confabulation (unconscious acceptance of fabricated facts).

We know that Wernicke's encephalopathy and Korsakoff's syndrome can be prevented by administering supplemental thiamine either orally or intravenously. As in other cases of dementia and delirium, time is essential in preventing permanent cognitive dysfunction or death.

2. RULING OUT PSYCHIATRIC DISORDERS

Psychotic symptoms, such as hallucinations, paranoia, and disorganized thinking, can occur in delir-

ium and in psychotic states such as schizophrenia. The psychotic patient should have a normal level of consciousness and be alert and oriented, with normal vital signs and minimal cognitive dysfunction, in contrast to the delirious patient. Patients who have dementia or disorders such as schizophrenia or depression have normal attention spans, in contrast to patients who have delirium. When a psychiatric disorder is suspected, an electroencephalogram (EEG) may be helpful. Delirium usually produces characteristic diffuse slowing in all leads of the EEG tracing, while the EEG is normal or near normal in other conditions.

COURSE OF DELIRIUM

Delirium may first present with a **prodromal** (early) stage of several hours to days of irritability or personality change. Sometimes this stage precedes the clinical manifestations of the underlying medical problem. Any signs of personality change or mild signs of delirium should trigger a search for occult medical problems. For example, the patient who has AIDS who becomes abruptly more withdrawn, irritable, agitated, depressed, or confused should be examined carefully for an opportunistic infection such as Pneumocystis carinii pneumonia.

Figure 3–1 illustrates the various outcomes of delirium. Even in untreated cases, delirium may remit spontaneously when the underlying medical condition clears. Delirium may also linger, waxing and waning for weeks, or rarely may become chronic. Delirium is especially common in elderly patients or in patients who have AIDS or preexisting brain lesions or a history of head trauma. Delirium also carries a dramatically increased risk of morbidity and mortality. This risk is especially high for elderly pa-

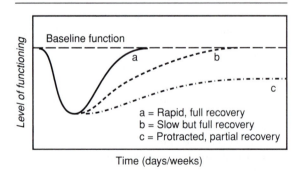

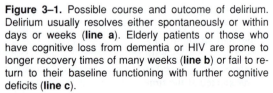

Figure 3–1. Possible course and outcome of delirium. Delirium usually resolves either spontaneously or within days or weeks (**line a**). Elderly patients or those who have cognitive loss from dementia or HIV are prone to longer recovery times of many weeks (**line b**) or fail to return to their baseline functioning with further cognitive deficits (**line c**).

tients and for patients who have chronic illnesses such as cancer or AIDS.

TREATMENT OF DELIRIUM

Basic principles for the treatment of delirium involve (a) the accurate diagnosis and treatment of underlying medical causes of delirium, (b) provision of a safe environment for the patient, and (c) treatment with antipsychotic medication (neuroleptics) or benzodiazepines for delirium due to alcohol withdrawal, when appropriate. Delirious patients often benefit from the presence of a family or medical staff member in the room throughout the day and night, or from materials to help them orient themselves, such as a board in their room showing the date and name of the hospital. Some delirious patients may need to be restrained to prevent them from wandering off, pulling out their IVs, becoming combative, or endangering themselves.

Antipsychotics should be prescribed when the patient's symptoms are particularly severe, for example, when the patient is paranoid or agitated. When antipsychotics are used, low doses are preferred. Because of the delirium, and underlying medical problems, the patient may not tolerate standard doses and may experience increased side effects. High potency neuroleptics have fewer built-in anticholinergic side effects that can make delirium worse. When delirium is due to alcohol withdrawal, benzodiazepines such as diazepam (Valium) or chlordiazepoxide (Librium) are the treatment of choice.

James R, aged 46, was brought to the emergency room by paramedics who rescued him after a car accident. He was admitted to the surgery service to have a broken femur repaired. Mr. R's wife denied that Mr. R had any history of alcohol use but acknowledged that he had been "pretty depressed and upset recently."

On his sixth day in the hospital, Mr. R became more alert but was agitated, screaming at nurses to "let me out on bail" and attempting to pull the IVs from his arm. He thought that the curtain was a wall of fire and complained of bugs running over his chest and legs. His pulse and blood pressure were markedly elevated, his temperature was above normal, and he was diaphoretic (sweating). He was placed in restraints and given intravenous neuroleptics. Although he became more sluggish his symptoms did not abate.

A medical team member interviewed several friends who came to visit Mr. R and learned that he had a significant history of alcohol use, which he and his wife tried to keep hidden from others. They added that Mr. R may have been intoxicated at the time of his accident. Based on this information, the surgical team discontinued neuroleptics and started benzodiazepines. Mr. R's mental state cleared within a day, and his hallucinations and paranoia vanished. He was alert and oriented, and amenable to alcohol rehabilitation after discharge.

Diagnosis. Delirium due to alcohol withdrawal, alcohol dependence (Axis I); fracture of femur (Axis III).

Alcohol dependence and withdrawal are commonly missed diagnoses, and physicians should be alert to their occurrence. Clues include visual or tactile hallucinations, disturbances of level of consciousness, and disorientation. Physical signs of autonomic nervous system hyperactivity, such as sweating and elevated pulse and blood pressure, are often prominent. An early sign of alcohol withdrawal is a subjective sense of needing to leave the hospital. Delirium due to alcohol withdrawal occurs within 2–10 days of stopping or reducing alcohol intake.

General anesthesia used in surgery may delay the onset of alcohol withdrawal. The additional administration of antipsychotics for alcohol withdrawal is not only unnecessary but dangerous, since antipsychotics lower the seizure threshold in all patients. [It is also difficult to screen for **neuroleptic malignant syndrome** (a complication of neuroleptics) in a patient who is already febrile.] For the patient who is in alcohol withdrawal, and therefore already at risk for seizures, these added risks are unacceptable. Moreover, adding antipsychotics offers limited benefit: When given in sufficient doses for alcohol withdrawal, benzodiazepines will completely alleviate symptoms of delirium, suppressing apparently psychotic symptoms, such as hallucinations or paranoia. If the patient's liver function tests are normal, diazepam or chlordiazepoxide can be used. If the patient has alcoholic hepatitis due to alcohol, lorazepam (Ativan) is better metabolized and has less risk of toxic accumulation.

PSYCHOLOGICAL ASPECTS OF DELIRIUM

Delirium may be extremely frightening both to patients and to their family members. Families and friends of patients who have delirium should be educated about the disorder before visiting. After recovering from delirium, patients often remember jumbled portions of their experience in the same way a person remembers a nightmare the next morning. Recovery from delirium may involve rebuilding self-esteem and confidence. The physician can facilitate healing by listening to the patient's and family members' fears and questions, by educating them about the nature of delirium, and by reassuring the patient that he or she does not have a long-term psychiatric illness.

Patricia J was a 29-year-old graphic artist whose mother and sister had schizophrenia. The sister had experienced her first psychotic episode while she and the patient were in their early 20s. Ms. J had been in therapy for 2 years, in part to address her fear that she too was destined to develop schizophrenia. She had read many books and articles and had reviewed research findings in medical libraries and on the Internet.

A bad cold had prompted Ms. J to take a combination of over-the-counter cold remedies that all contained strongly anticholinergic agents. Later that night she became mildly delirious, experiencing visual hallucinations of strange people observing her through her bedroom window. She began screaming and eventually woke the neighbors, who called the police.

Ms. J was extremely frightened, paranoid, and agitated when the police arrived, and they decided to initiate a 3-day psychiatric hold and bought her to the psychiatric emergency room. She was given a single dose of diazepam and slept for 10 hours. By the next morning her delirium had cleared, and she was no longer hallucinating or paranoid. However, she became convinced that the doctors were incorrect in their assessment that the cold medication had been responsible for her symptoms.

Ms. J believed the medications to be an unrelated factor, or that they had only "unmasked" her schizophrenia early, that her worst fear had been realized and she did indeed have schizophrenia. It took months of continued therapy to lessen Ms. J's anxiety and to reassure her that she had probably not experienced her first psychotic break.

DEMENTIA

Dementia may have many causes. It usually develops gradually over months to years but sometimes has a more acute onset. The following case is typical of **Alzheimer's dementia,** the most common dementing illness.

Philip B, a 67-year-old man, was brought to the family practice clinic by his wife, who said that she had noticed a change in her husband's behavior over the past 6 months. She said that her husband, an engineer, had become increasingly forgetful. As an example, she cited the day

before when she sent him to the store for milk, eggs, and other items. He returned 2 hours later but did not remember his wife telling him to pick up food. Instead, he had bought a rake and 8 boxes of plastic bags for leaves. When Mr. B's wife angrily asked him why he was thinking about raking leaves in April, Mr. B acted surprised, and replied that it was good to think of chores early.

After this episode, Mrs. B remembered other lapses in her husband's memory over the preceding months—needing to look up friends' phone numbers repeatedly, only to forget them minutes later; leaving important work assignments at home; keeping notes to himself all over the house, even in his clothes closet, with reminders about clearly outdated projects. At the same time he had forgotten important events at home, such as his anniversary, his son's birthday, and his new granddaughter's christening. Although she did not believe her husband was depressed, Mrs. B found him simultaneously more irritable as well as "distracted, not interested in me or much of anything."

Mrs. B then received a call from her husband's friend at work, asking if Mr. B was having difficulty at home. The friend informed her that Mr. B had been demoted the month before for failing to complete important assignments. This news had prompted Mrs. B to bring her husband to the clinic. Mr. B seemed more bemused than upset with his wife's summary of recent problems and insisted that he was "fine." His wife said that Mr. B rarely drank and did not take any over-the-counter medications. His neurologic and physical examinations were entirely normal, except that Mr. B was off by 2 days on the current date.

Cognitive testing showed that Mr. B had difficulties with concentration, short-term memory, and copying drawings. He had trouble naming common objects and had little insight into his difficulties. The medicine resident ordered a series of tests including an EKG; thyroid stimulating hormone level; RPR; vitamin B12 levels; and routine blood tests for electrolytes, toxicology, and red and white blood counts. All of the tests were normal.

Further neuropsychological testing demonstrated global deficits in immediate and delayed memory, visuospatial ability, with a normal level of verbal ability. These observations were consistent with a marked decline: verbal intelligence is so overlearned that it functions as a "watermark" of intelligence and a good indicator of baseline cognitive functioning. A lumbar puncture showed normal CSF fluid. An MRI of Mr. B's brain did not show focal defects such as strokes or tumors but was remarkable for general atrophy. Mr. B's clinical presentation, cognitive exam, head scan, and negative laboratory findings led his doctor to a diagnosis of probable Alzheimer's dementia.

Over the next 4 years, Mr. B's cognitive functions and behavior continued to decline. He was laid off from work after his job performance declined. His memory worsened, and his wife had to continually remind him that he had grandchildren, although by this time he had three. His wife and primary care physician demanded that Mr. B stop driving after he became lost driving home from across town and later went the wrong way on a one-way street. His wife needed to lay out his clothing the night before because he would otherwise dress in mismatched clothing, but he was still unable to dress without his wife's help. On one occasion he put his pants on backward, and another time his wife found him struggling to put on his pants over his shoes.

His behavior became more abnormal as well. At night he became more confused and sometimes belligerent when his wife tried to redirect his activities. He accused her of stealing his things when she rearranged furniture in the living room. He was arrested by police for urinating on a street corner and did not understand why bystanders had become upset. His wife awakened one night to find smoke filling the house; Mr. B had been trying to fry an egg, still in its shell, and had wandered off while the pan was still on the range. By this point, Mrs. B was exhausted. She was working two jobs to try to keep up with bills and could not find a home-care worker who would dependably care for her husband.

With much guilt but with the support of her family and the family practitioner, Mrs. B decided to place her husband in a nursing home. The move to the nursing home left Mr. B increasingly disoriented and paranoid. He was started on a low dose of high-potency antipsychotics, which helped to calm his behavior. In the last year of his life, he no longer recognized his children or his wife. His wife reluctantly agreed to "do not resuscitate" (DNR) status, and Mr. B succumbed to pneumonia 8 years after his illness began. Neuropathologic studies conducted at autopsy revealed changes consistent with Alzheimer's dementia.

Diagnosis. Alzheimer's dementia (Axis I).

Discussion. The onset of Alzheimer's dementia is very gradual and subtle, and family members may not notice the initial symptoms. The standard workup is often unrevealing, and there is no definitive test for the disease.

Alzheimer's dementia remains a diagnosis of exclusion to be confirmed at autopsy.

Dementia produces specific problems with memory. Several different types of memory are seen in the normally functioning brain. Immediate memory acts as a "notepad" in the brain, with a limited storage capacity of several minutes and rapid displacement by new material. For example, you may notice that you can retain a telephone number from a phone book for a short time before it fades, unless you practice the number repeatedly. Delayed (short-term) memory lasts longer, spanning information stored for hours or days at most. For example, you will probably recall what you ate for dinner yesterday, but it is unlikely that you could recall what you ate for dinner 1 month ago. Long-term memory is information that is highly over-learned, such as your birthday, your address in childhood, the school that you attended, the names and order of presidents during your lifetime. This information is thought to be stored in a more fixed, electrochemical pattern across the neuronal connections of the brain, coordinated by the hippocampus and temporal lobes.

Aging itself tends to result in mild neuronal loss and mild difficulties with concentration, attention, and memory retrieval. Other higher cortical functions such as verbal abilities, judgment, behavior, and long-term memory remain intact, however. Thus the stereotyped notion of the senile elderly patient owes more to youthful prejudice than scientific fact.

Dementing processes generally affect short-term memory. Long-term memory tends to be spared initially. Memory loss manifests itself with trouble learning new information (**anterograde,** or forward memory). **Retrograde amnesia** refers to the loss of recent memory as the patient gradually loses previously acquired memories. Memories closest to the present are most affected, but as dementia worsens, more remote memory is lost. For example, patients who have dementia will gradually forget the names or existence of new grandchildren or the results of recent elections. As the illness progresses, memory loss will extend further into the past, gradually erasing more information from recent years. Amnestic disorders that affect short-term memory but spare other cognitive abilities are also possible (see Chapter 10).

The most common forms of dementia affect the higher cognitive functioning of the brain. Some clinicians distinguish between cortical and subcortical dementias. **Cortical dementias** are characterized by difficulties with speech and visuospatial abilities. **Subcortical dementias** lead to slowing of speech, thought, and movement, with prominent apathy or mood changes. However, this distinction is controversial, since many exceptions, inconsistencies, and overlaps exist in this classification system.

Another important pattern to dementing illness is

the occurrence of **frontal lobe syndromes.** Dysfunction of the frontal lobes causes marked disinhibition and marked changes in personality, typified by apathy and lack of motivation, while sparing language centers that are located farther from the frontal lobes. **Pick's disease** causes a progressive dementia analogous to Alzheimer's in the frontal lobes.

Patterns of short-term memory also differ between forms of dementia. Patients who have cortical dementias have trouble learning (ie, storing) new information and have trouble recalling four items immediately. They are not often helped by category or list prompts at 5 minutes, and they tend to make up responses. In contrast, patients who have subcortical dementia perform well at immediate recall. At 5-minute recall, memory problems are evident, but the patient is often assisted by prompts. Thus the difficulty in memory dysfunction in subcortical dementia is mostly in memory retrieval of stored information.

Troy K, a 64-year-old man, was brought to the medical emergency room after being punched in the face. He had apparently asked a man ahead of him in line at the post office to drop his pants so that he could see what kind of underwear he had on. In the hospital, Mr. K was jocular and made frequent jokes with sexual references. He also attempted to fondle staff members on several occasions. Mr. K's family reported a significant change in his personality over the past year. Laboratory tests for various forms of dementia were negative, but an MRI scan revealed deterioration of the frontal lobes bilaterally, consistent with Pick's disease.

Diagnosis. Dementia, probably due to Pick's disease (Axis I).

Damage to the prefrontal areas (eg, from trauma, CNS bleeds, or tumors) causes an interesting clinical picture. Higher cognitive functions are generally spared, and the patient may perform well on tests of short-term memory and concentration. What is lost is considerably more subtle, yet critical to the patient's ability to function. The prefrontal areas correspond to executive functions that anticipate and plan for future events, and make possible the integration of emotions and cognition that allow individuals to make decisions based on what they think is best. Individuals whose brains have prefrontal damage often have normal intellectual abilities but function poorly in the world.

INCIDENCE

As many as 10 million people in the United States may have some degree of dementia. Four million people have severe dementia. Dementia is found in 60% of nursing home patients. The number of demented persons is expected to double in the next 25 years as the population of the United States becomes proportionately older because of increases in life expectancy and the "graying" of the large number of people born between 1945 and 1965.

ETIOLOGY

Dementia has many possible causes (Table 3–2). Alzheimer's dementia, the most common type, accounts for approximately 60% of all cases of dementia. The cause of Alzheimer's dementia is not known. Common features of the disease include decreased cholinergic neuronal activity, neurofibrillar tangles of abnormal protein, and "senile" plaques composed of amyloid (a protein).

Vascular diseases account for approximately 10% of all dementia cases. The most common example is **multi-infarct dementia** (MID), in which atherosclerotic disease causes many small areas of tissue death,

Table 3–2 Etiology of dementia.[1]

Psychiatric Disorder	Percentage of Dementia Cases Caused by This Disorder
Alzheimer's disease	55%
Vascular (multi-infarct) dementia (and mixed vascular/ Alzheimer's)	15%
Alcohol (usually due to thiamine deficiency)	5%
Brain tumors, Parkinson's disease, HIV, Huntington's chorea, trauma, and other rare causes	10%
Potentially reversible causes (with early detection and treatment)	
Depression (with mild cognitive dysfunction) (reversible)	<10%
Drug-induced, metabolic (electrolyte abnormalities, hypothyroid or other endocrinopathies states), infections/meningitis, subdural hematomas, or normal pressure hydrocephalus	<10%

[1]Note that etiologies vary in different medical settings.

or infarction, throughout the brain. Dementia may also present with mixed features of MID and Alzheimer's (as evidenced by history and brain scans), accounting for another 10% of dementia cases.

The remaining 20% of dementia cases result from a variety of conditions including alcohol use, AIDS, head trauma, and other disorders. Medications can cause cognitive slowing and is seen especially in the elderly.

Dementia associated with AIDS is probably the result of direct cytotoxic effects of HIV on the CNS. Dementia usually begins when CD4 counts (which correlate with progression of HIV disease) decrease to less than 100 and may be accompanied by symptoms of depression such as social withdrawal, lack of interest in usual activities, decreased energy, and psychomotor retardation. Antiretroviral agents may help to slow the progress of dementia by reducing viral load throughout the body.

In patients over age 65, the most common causes of dementia are Alzheimer's, MID, mixed MID-Alzheimer's dementias, and alcohol-related dementia. In younger patients, more common causes are HIV-associated dementia and head trauma.

DIAGNOSTIC ASSESSMENT

1. SIGNS & SYMPTOMS

The cardinal clinical features of dementia includes short-term memory loss combined with cognitive dysfunction, loss of abstract thought, behavioral or personality changes, and impairment of judgment.

2. MENTAL STATUS EXAMINATION

The mental status examination is critical in the diagnosis of dementia. The major findings follow:

A. Appearance, Behavior, & Language. Patients who have dementia may display signs of psychomotor slowing. There may be notable perseveration of speech or mannerisms.

B. Emotions. Affect may be restricted, labile, and inappropriate at times.

C. Thought Process & Content. Thought processes may be disorganized or notable for a paucity of spontaneous ideas.

D. Judgment, Insight, & Impulse Control. Judgment, insight, and impulse control are all likely to diminish with the progression of dementia. Judgment (the ability to anticipate difficulties and choose reasonable courses of action) is often diminished severely in demented patients. Insight is also compromised progressively. In the early stages of dementia, patients may be aware that their memory is failing, or that their behavior and personality have changed. As the illness progresses, however, the ability to observe and reflect on these differences—a feature of higher cortical function—is lost, and patients will deny any problems, even in the face of overt cognitive difficulties. The defense mechanism of denial may further prevent patients from being aware of their illness. Impulse control is also lost in advanced cases of dementia.

3. COGNITIVE EXAMINATION

The cognitive examination is of primary importance in diagnosing dementia. In the early stages of the illness, the patient is usually oriented to person, place, and date. While orientation to person rarely wavers (this information is too deeply ingrained in long-term memory to forget except in terminal cases), the patient may have increasing difficulty identifying the date as the illness progresses, often giving an earlier year when asked. Disorientation to place may result in the middle or later stages of dementia as higher cognitive functions are progressively lost. Level of consciousness is generally not affected, and disruption of sleep-wake cycles does not occur until the late stages of the illness. Long-term memory loss may be especially noticeable when the patient is asked to name the current president of the United States and then list previous presidents in reverse chronological order.

All cognitive examination questions should be interpreted in light of the patient's cultural and educational background. For example, a patient who has emigrated recently from a rural town in Southeast Asia may lack knowledge of the organization of the United States government, much less who currently holds the office of President.

Patients who have dementia will frequently have problems with cognitive tests, struggling for longer than expected, minimizing their difficulty. They may also confabulate (make up answers, believing them to be true). In contrast, depressed patients are likely to become upset because of their awareness of their performance, and anxiously ask, "Do you think I could have Alzheimer's?" Grading of responses also depends on educational background and intelligence. Assessment should be made in the context of known ability. For example, one AIDS patient had mild problems drawing a clock—but his background as an architect made this test result markedly abnormal.

Patients who have dementia will also tend to lose their ability to understand abstract concepts as their illness progresses. Asking a patient to compare items in a category will reveal "concrete" thinking. If the patient is asked, "A chair and a table are both pieces of furniture; how are an apple and an orange similar?" the patient may respond "I don't like oranges." Similarly, proverb interpretation, while notoriously prone to cultural bias, is likely to yield literal results:

When asked to explain the proverb "People in glass houses shouldn't throw stones," the demented patient may respond, "You can break the glass by accident." Or if asked the meaning of "Don't cry over spilled milk," the patient might say, "You should clean it up." Speech and language deficits should also be sought out, by having the patient repeat a sentence after the examiner, or by having the patient name common objects.

Testing for Memory Loss

Short-term memory disturbance is a hallmark of dementia, as mentioned above. In a standard test, the patient is given a list of four one-word items (eg, watch, pen, shoe, airplane) and is asked to repeat the list. The clinician should note whether the patient learns this list without difficulty. If the patient needs to hear the list one or more times before being able to recall it perfectly (which is common in dementias such as Alzheimer's), the test result is considered abnormal. The patient is told that he or she will be asked to recall the list at 5 minutes. When the time is up, the patient is given a minute or so to remember as many items as possible without prompting. The patient is told which were correct—many patients with dementia will confabulate, supplying items that are not correct, sometimes with a happy air of self-assurance that can make the examiner doubt himself or herself.

If the patient cannot recall the items spontaneously, he or she should be given **category prompts** (eg, "the first one is something that you would use to tell time"). If the patient does not recall the item, or supplies an incorrect response, a **list prompt** should be offered (eg, "Was it a watch, a clock, or a sundial?").

Testing Concentration Ability

Concentration can be assessed by giving the patient a set task, such as "serial sevens." In this test, the examiner directs the patient, "Take 7 from 100, and keep subtracting 7 from the result." If the patient has difficulty with math, serial threes (starting with 20) offer an alternative. Or a nonnumeric task can be given such as, "Name the months of the year, backward," or "Please spell 'world' backward for me."

Testing Visuospatial Ability & Memory

Other tests explore visuospatial memory ("Look at this drawing for 30 seconds; then copy it from memory.") or visuospatial ability ("Copy this figure," or "draw a clock, with all of the numbers, and set the hands for a quarter to two.").

Cognitive testing needs to be interpreted as a pattern rather than individual tests that are positive or negative. Also, testing establishes levels of neuropsychological functioning, but it often does not indicate specific neuroanatomic deficits. Sometimes a single dysfunction correlates with an anatomic location.

Alfred C, a right-handed 40-year-old man who had AIDS, exhibited psychomotor slowing and visuospatial difficulties, as evidenced by difficulty drawing a clock. Since visuospatial ability in right-handed individuals is usually located in the fronto-parietal area of the nondominant hemisphere, the psychiatry consultant was not surprised when an MRI of Mr. C's head showed a contrast-enhancing lesion several centimeters in diameter in that area on the right side of the brain. Subsequent lumbar puncture revealed toxoplasmosis, which responded gradually to treatment.

Abnormal findings in the cognitive examination, combined with the patient's history, provide a rationale for further workup.

DIFFERENTIAL DIAGNOSIS

1. DETERMINING THE TYPE OF DEMENTIA

Dementia may be caused by a variety of medical conditions, most commonly Alzheimer's dementia or multi-infarct dementia. The list of causes overlaps with the causes of delirium and other organic mental disorders. In urban hospitals, the four most common causes of dementia include Alzheimer's dementia, alcohol-related dementia (Wernicke-Korsakoff syndrome), multi-infarct dementia, and dementia associated with AIDS (either directly from the HIV virus or from complications such as toxoplasmosis, progressive multifocal leukoencephalopathy, or CNS lymphoma). Other causes of dementia include:

- infectious diseases: HIV, viral or bacterial meningitis, syphilis, Lyme disease
- CNS disorders: Normal pressure hydrocephalus (characterized by a classic triad of "magnetic" gait, urinary incontinence, and dementia); subdural hematoma
- systemic diseases: CNS lesions caused by systemic lupus erythematosus or multiple sclerosis
- other conditions: Trauma; brain tumors; Huntington's chorea; Pick's disease; Creutzfeldt-Jakob disease; vitamin deficiency syndromes; or toxins, especially prolonged exposure to lead, mercury, or other hazardous compounds

A psychiatrist spent one afternoon a week in an outpatient medical clinic and was assigned to observe and consult with one medicine resident each week. On one occasion, the observed resident told the psychiatrist, "I'm glad that you're here—this next patient is really strange." The resident went on to describe the patient, Jacqueline H as a "very sweet" 55-year-old woman whom she saw every 4 months for routine checkups and for follow-up of mild hypertension. What was odd, the resident noted, was that Ms. H had a mustache. The resident had never asked the patient in the year that they had worked together about the mustache. The psychiatrist felt that the mustache was potentially a clinical sign of psychiatric illness that warranted further investigation.

The psychiatrist proceeded with the resident's permission to ask Ms. H if she could examine her face. On closer examination, the psychiatrist noted that Ms. H did not have excessive hair on her upper lip after all. Rather, she had applied light-colored makeup to her entire face (which was dark-complected), except above her lip, producing the appearance of a mustache.

When asked about the "mustache," Ms. H exclaimed, "So that's it!" She had wondered why so many people stared at her when she went out. She denied symptoms of depression or mania, nor did she exhibit signs of psychosis such as auditory or visual hallucinations, paranoia, or ideas of reference. She had no significant medical illnesses except mild hypertension, took no medications, and had a negative family history for mental illness.

The psychiatrist proceeded to perform the cognitive examination. She found that Ms. H was alert and oriented, except that she was several days off on the date. Ms. H's remote memory was intact, but she had difficulty with immediate recall of one of four items. She could recall only two of those items 5 minutes later; she remembered one more with a category prompt.

Ms. H's concentration, as measured by her ability to perform serial sevens, was poor. She made frequent errors on the task, but she had not completed high school, a factor the psychiatrist took into account. Ms. H also had difficulty drawing a clock with numbers. The psychiatrist wondered if the patient's failure to apply makeup to her upper lip might constitute a form of visuospatial neglect, or **apraxia.**

Based on the cognitive examination, the psychiatrist strongly suspected a dementing process. The medical resident ordered a series of tests, including thyroid function tests, B12, electrolytes, a blood count, and a urine toxicology screen, all of which were normal. Serum was also sent for RPR and HIV testing, again for thoroughness since Ms. H denied having had any sexual contact in almost 30 years. Remarkably, the test for syphilis was positive, and a lumbar puncture was performed. A sample of lumbar fluid was sent for fluorescent treponemal antibody-absorbed (FTA-ABS) testing, which was also positive, indicating that Ms. H had neurosyphilis. Intravenous administration of penicillin for 6 weeks led to negative lumbar

punctures and an improvement in Ms. H's cognitive status over the next 6 months.

Diagnosis. Dementia secondary to neurosyphilis (Axis I); syphilis (Axis III).

2. RULING OUT MEDICATION-INDUCED COGNITIVE DYSFUNCTION

Medications such as cimetidine (Tagamet) may produce cognitive slowing. A thorough history of prescription and over-the-counter medications should be obtained from every patient.

3. RULING OUT PSYCHIATRIC DISORDERS

Delirium and dementia both manifest with cognitive dysfunction such as short-term memory loss and concentration difficulties. Both disorders can also produce behavioral changes and impairment of judgment and insight. The characteristics that help to differentiate dementia from delirium include level of consciousness, orientation, and attention (normal in dementia, except in severe late stages), and time course (months to years in dementia compared to hours to days for delirium). Delirium is especially common in hospitalized patients.

Depression typically causes mild cognitive dysfunction and behavioral change over a time frame of months to years, especially in elderly patients, but the concentration and short-term memory problems in major depression tend to improve with encouragement from the examiner. This state is sometimes referred to as "pseudo-dementia," but the term is inaccurate in that depression produces real (as opposed to "pseudo") but mild cognitive impairment. It may be difficult to distinguish between depression and mild dementia, which may occur with symptoms of depression. An EEG may help to make this diagnosis, as the EEG in depressed patients should be normal. If the clinician is unable to distinguish between depression and dementia, a trial of antidepressant therapy may be empirically helpful.

COURSE OF DEMENTIA

Dementia is often a progressive disorder with a variable course. In Alzheimer's dementia, the dementing process will tend to progress over 5–10 years, producing increasing loss of higher cognitive functioning. Behavioral and personality changes often occur; aggression and agitation may become problematic. Patients who have moderate to severe dementia may develop symptoms of psychosis such as auditory and visual hallucinations, paranoia, and delusions. Eventually these patients lose all insight and abstracting ability, short-term learning and concentration becomes minimal, and judgment and insight is lost. Patients require increasing amounts of help in activities of daily living (eg, dressing, preparing food, voiding). This may necessitate placement in a nursing home, or in a locked facility for patients at high risk of "wandering." Death is usually caused by another illness such as pneumonia or heart disease. In some demented patients, the decision is made not to take "heroic measures" to correct major medical problems, such as heart or kidney failure.

In contrast with Alzheimer's, vascular disease such as MID tends to proceed in a more rapid and step-wise fashion, with abrupt decreases in cognitive function alternating with periods of stabilization. The location of infarcts will determine the degree of physical incapacity experienced by the patient: Lesions in motor tracts will cause partial paralysis, whereas lesions in speech centers will cause **aphasias** (abnormal speech patterns marked by halting or nonsensical speech).

TREATMENT OF DEMENTIA

Treatment of dementia includes treating reversible medical problems, prescribing psychotropic medications to alleviate specific symptoms, assessing the patient's ability to live independently, and providing referral to long-term care facilities when appropriate.

In approximately 8–15% of cases, the underlying cause of the dementia is potentially reversible. Some reversible causes include normal pressure hydrocephalus, benign brain tumors, hypothyroidism, neurosyphilis, vitamin deficiency, depression, and medications. Early diagnosis and treatment is critical because dementia due to reversible causes may give way in time to an irreversible decline in higher cognitive functions.

It may be possible to slow the progression of dementia in some patients, and medications are being developed for this purpose. Tacrine (Cognex) and donepazil (Aricept) may boost acetylcholine levels in the CNS of patients with Alzheimer's, temporarily slowing the course of the disease. Estrogen replacement is being investigated for use in women who have Alzheimer's.

Patients who have alcohol-related dementia may benefit from referral to a rehabilitation program. Patients who have multi-infarct dementia may benefit from treatment designed to reduce stroke risk factors. Normal pressure hydrocephalus may be corrected by surgical implantation of a shunt to drain off excess CSF fluid; however, results are variable. Medications that lower the viral load may help slow the course of HIV-associated dementia.

Low-dose antipsychotics may be helpful with gross behavioral problems encountered in demented patients and for psychotic symptoms such as paranoia and hallucinations. Antidepressants may be warranted for treatment of depression, because depression can exacerbate cognitive problems and inhibit performance of activities of daily living in demented patients. If the diagnosis of dementia is uncertain and a diagnosis of major depression is a possibility, antidepressant medication is usually begun on a trial basis. The use of antidepressants in AIDS patients with dementia may lead to striking improvement, since the dementia associated with AIDS tends to produce many depressive symptoms.

Psychotropic medications should be used with care in patients who have dementia because these patients are more susceptible to side effects. Benzodiazepines may help to decrease anxiety and agitation but may disinhibit the demented patient and worsen cognition, leading to more behavior problems. Medications that have strong anticholinergic effects, such as the antipsychotic thioridazine (Mellaril) or the antidepressant amitryptiline (Elavil), can easily cause an anticholinergic delirium and other side effects.

Simplifying the patient's prescriptions may also help; many medications can cause indirect worsening of dementia. The elderly and patients who have AIDS are frequently the unintended recipients of **polypharmacy,** especially when multiple specialists are involved in their care. One clinician should always be identified as the central coordinator for patient care, to oversee all medications and treatment plans.

Patients who have dementia should be assessed for their ability to live independently. Patients can be tested for their ability to dress, take medications, and prepare meals (including important details such as turning off the stove or closing the refrigerator). Visiting nurse services may assist patients at home, or patients may need to be placed in a nursing home or board-and-care facility. The Department of Motor Vehicles should be notified of patients who are having difficulty driving.

EMOTIONAL REACTIONS TO PATIENTS

Demented and delirious patients often evoke powerful emotional reactions in medical personnel. Contact with agitated, disorganized, and disinhibited patients can easily cause house staff to feel angry and frightened. The cardinal symptom of dementia, short-term memory loss, may represent a special psychological threat to the tired intern or resident who is struggling to retain a multitude of names, facts, and lists. The student or house officer's angry or punitive feelings toward these patients may lead to overprescribing of powerful psychotropic medications, or the inappropriate use of physical restraints. Feelings of distancing or disinterest may cause medical staff to dismiss treatable medical problems. Others may feel compassion based on prior experience with dementia in family members. If unchecked, though, these feelings may lead to underrecognition and undertreatment of behavioral disturbances in these patients. Such feelings may also lead to behavioral problems leading to patients leaving the hospital against medical advice.

The emotional burden on families of patients who have dementia is similar but more protracted and difficult to bear, since family members are often left in roles of increasing responsibility for patients who may be only vaguely similar to the people they once were. These family members are at risk for guilt, depression, and burnout. The physician who detects, attends to, and openly addresses these issues—regardless of diagnosis—will alleviate suffering and help strengthen the patient's support network. Support groups can be very helpful for both the patient and his or her family members; it is often a relief for family members to share their rage, frustration, depression, or guilt with others in the same situation.

CROSS-CULTURAL ASPECTS OF DEMENTIA

Dementia is caused by biological factors with the exception of mild cognitive deficits resulting from depression. However, cultural variations in behavior may affect the prevalence of different types of dementia. The role of cultural factors, such as socially accepted behavior, partially accounts for variations in vulnerability to substance use. Notably, cultural or ethnic groups marked by social upheaval, political oppression, or economic depression may have an increased incidence of substance use. In other instances, behaviors influence the epidemiology of disease vectors and the spread of infectious agents that can cause dementia. This is true in the transmission of sexually transmitted diseases such as HIV and syphilis. The route of transmission of kuru, a disease caused by a slow-acting virus affecting the Fore tribe of New Guinea, was based solely on the practice of women and children feeding on the brains of deceased (and infected) tribe members. Attitudes toward acceptance of disruptive behavior and family and community care-taking of patients who have dementia also vary among cultural groups.

LEGAL & ETHICAL ISSUES

Legal and ethical issues frequently arise in the care of the demented or delirious patient. These issues in-

clude reduced capacity to give informed consent for medical procedures, involuntary hospitalization, end-of-life care and decisions, and research protocols for demented patients.

Diminished capacity for making medical decisions is often the result of the cognitive impairment that occurs in demented and delirious patients. The ability to give informed consent rests on the patient's understanding of his or her illness, and the risks and benefits of a medical procedure weighed against the possible outcomes of not having the procedure performed.

Lars F, aged 40, was brought into the hospital after being found unconscious in the street. On admission he was dehydrated and severely anemic. Later that day he was awake but was highly agitated, disoriented, thinking he was in a bus terminal and screaming, "Let me out of here!" His thinking was confused, disorganized, disjointed, and irrational. He was paranoid and refused to listen to the house staff's warning that he was in danger of dying from extreme blood loss.

Since Mr. F's stools were black, and he was vomiting blood, the residents were certain that he had an upper gastrointestinal bleed. Based on the rate of blood loss and Mr. F's declining blood pressure, the physicians estimated that he would go into shock and die within hours without treatment. It was clear that Mr. F's delirium, whether caused by alcohol withdrawal, blood loss, or hepatic encephalopathy, was interfering with his ability to make an informed decision.

No family members were known who could assist in specifying Mr. F's wishes in a non-delirious state. In a non-emergent situation, family permission would be sought. If no family were available, a petition would be filed with the courts to make the decision for the patient. In this case, the combination of lack of capacity to give informed consent and the presence of a medical emergency (defined as a danger of loss of life or limb within 24 hours) allowed the physicians to sedate Mr. F and proceed with their treatment plan.

Many hospitalized patients refuse some or all medical care, from medications and IVs to surgery. Some of these patients are delirious and need to be evaluated for their ability to give informed consent. Mildly delirius or demented patients are still capable of making informed decisions. Impaired cognition in more severe cases often precludes the patient's ability to understand their medical illness or weigh the risks and benefits of treatment options. In non–emergent cases involving reduced capacity, permission to proceed with medical treatment comes from family members or, in their absence, from the legal system. In some cases, delirium is either not diagnosed or its impact on medical decision-making is ignored because the patient agrees to treatment and signs consent forms to that effect. But obtaining consent in this manner is unethical and illegal, since reduced capacity to give informed consent precludes an individual's competency to make choices. Nor is it proper to wait until a patient becomes delirious so that a procedure can be performed without the consent that the patient refused to give in a nondelirious state. Clinicians who proceed with medical treatment on temporarily incapacitated patients in non–emergent situations may subject themselves to lawsuits filed by (or on behalf of) patients who are angry at having their rights violated.

The same issues arise in caring for a patient who has dementia. It is often necessary to confer with family members to make medical decisions for the patient who no longer has the cognitive ability to weigh alternatives. Whenever possible it is preferable to know the patient's wishes in advance by asking directly for instructions regarding DNR status and other treatment issues early in the course of dementia, while the patient retains his or her decision-making ability. So called "living wills" are becoming increasingly common. Delay in addressing these issues with demented patients and their families often results in confusion and emotional distress in patients, their families, and medical staff. Physicians should assist patients and their families in determining when treatment is likely to be futile.

Another ethical dilemma is posed by advances in medicine that make it possible to identify patients at risk for dementia, without offering the immediate promise of treatment. In recent years, several genes have been found to be associated with familial forms of Alzheimer's disease presenting in patients in their 40s and 50s. The apolipoprotein-E4 allele has been associated with an increased risk of Alzheimer's in the familial and nonfamilial forms. The E4 allele is not predictive of who will eventually develop Alzheimer's but only who is at risk. Future research is likely to determine more advanced but nonconclusive information about family members' risk for Alzheimer's and other types of dementia. Physicians will need to be mindful of the psychological impact of this information.

With the advent of new medications for cognitive decline comes the prediction that medications will soon be available to enhance thinking, memory, and concentration. The impact of such a discovery on society will no doubt make for a heated and interesting ethical debate on this subject.

CONCLUSION

Delirium is an acute form of brain dysfunction frequently encountered in inpatient medical settings that requires prompt evaluation and treatment. Dementia may be caused by a variety of diseases and is a chronic, often insidious and progressive brain disease that is sometimes reversible if detected early. The incidence of dementia is increasing rapidly with the aging of a large segment of the population. Both delirium and dementia present complex medical, ethical, and legal challenges for medical providers.

The disturbance of cognitive functions seen in dementia and delirium also informs us about the ways in which the brain processes and stores information. The biological basis of memory and its crucial role in preserving an individual's personal identity is one of the many mysteries that medical science has yet to fully comprehend.

REFERENCES

Alzheimers Disease: Literature citation and book reviews. http://moe.csa.com/alzcit.html

Cummings JL, Benson DR: *Dementia: A Clinical Approach*, 2nd ed. Buttersworths-Heinemann, 1992.

Doernberg M: *Stolen Mind: The Slow Disappearance of Ray Doernberg*. Algonquin Books of Chapel Hill,1989.

Hersh D, Kranzler HR, Meyer RE: Persistent delirium following cessation of heavy alcohol consumption: diagnostic and treatment considerations. Am J Psychiatr 1997;154(6):846.

Inouye SK, Charpentier PA: Precipitating factors for delirium in hospitalized elderly patients. J Am Med Assoc 199;275(11): 852.

Kaufman DM: Dementia. Pages 123–167 in: *Clinical Neurology for Psychiatrists*, 4th ed. Saunders, 1995.

Kim E, Rovner BW: Depression in dementia. Psychiatr Ann 1994;24(4):173.

Mace NL, Rabins PV: *The 36-hour Day,* revised ed. Johns Hopkins University Press, 1991.

Maldonado JL, Fernandez F, Sergio-Trevino E, Levy J: Depression and its treatment in neurological disease. Psychiatr Ann 199;27(5):341.

Meagher DJ, O'Hanlon D, O'Mahony E, Casey PR: The use of environmental strategies and psychotropic medication in the management of delirium. Br J Psychiatr 1996;168:512.

Murray GB: Limbic music. Pages 116–126 in: *Massachusetts General Hospital Handbook of General Hospital Psychiatry,* 2nd ed. Hackett TP, Cassem NH (editors). PSG, 1987.

Sacks O: The lost mariner. In: *The Man Who Mistook His Wife for a Hat.* Perrenial Library, 1987.

Shaughnessy R. Psychopharmacotherapy of neuropsychiatric disorders. Psychiatr Ann 1995;25(10):634.

US Federal Government agencies: Resources on Dementia (NIH searchable database). http://www.cais.com/adear/federal.html

Whitehouse PJ, Juengst E, Mehlman M, Murray TH: Enhancing cognition in the intellectually intact. Hastings Cent Rep 1997;27(3):14.

Schizophrenia

4

Cameron S. Carter, MD, David Elkin, MD, & Sophia Vinogradov, MD

Schizophrenia occurs in about 1% of the population and causes devastating symptoms that last for the lifetime of affected patients, often resulting in profoundly reduced levels of functioning. The causes of schizophrenia are not completely known, but recent studies suggest a combination of genetic and environmental factors, and a neurodevelopmental origin. The mental status examination of the patient who has schizophrenia is often marked by abnormalities in many categories, including affect, perceptions, and thinking. In diagnosing the disorder, clinicians first must rule out medical and psychiatric illnesses that can cause psychotic symptoms. Antipsychotic medication ameliorates symptoms and can improve the course of the illness but does not provide a cure. Psychotic patients are capable of inducing very strong emotional reactions in health-care providers, and their care may pose complex ethical and legal challenges.

CLINICAL FEATURES

Schizophrenia is characterized by a waxing and waning tendency to psychosis—a mental state notable for impaired reality testing, disordered behavior, and thought disturbances, such as loose associations or disorganized thoughts. Symptoms such as paranoia, delusions, auditory or visual hallucinations, and disturbances of emotion also may be present. Together these are known as **positive symptoms. Negative symptoms** include flattened affect, a loss of spontaneous thinking, social withdrawal, a lack of motivation, and other personality changes. Schizophrenia can be classified into five subtypes: paranoid, disorganized (hebephrenic), catatonic, undifferentiated, and residual. **Paranoid schizophrenia** is the most common type and is characterized by paranoia, delusions, and hallucinations in the absence of disorganization as prominent negative symptoms.

The five-type classification scheme dates back to early descriptions of the disorder as well as syndromes described by several other nineteenth-century psychiatrists. Historically, no distinction was made between various mental disorders, and people judged to suffer insanity were frequently housed and mistreated in asylums. The nineteenth-century psychiatrist Emil Kraeplin observed that some patients had episodes of impaired functioning but then returned to normal. These patients probably suffered from mood disorders. Kraeplin focused on patients who had episodes of psychosis but did not return to their premorbid level of functioning; these patients had dementia praecox, later termed schizophrenia, by Eugene Bleuler. According to Crow's more modern classification scheme, Type I schizophrenia is characterized primarily by good premorbid functioning, mostly positive symptoms, and response to antipsychotic medications; Type II is characterized by poor premorbid functioning, mostly negative symptoms, evidence of structural brain pathology (such as ventricular enlargement), and poor response to antipsychotics.

Other attempts to categorize schizophrenia into distinct types have focused on the predominance of negative symptoms in some patients who have schizophrenia. No single typology has been accepted broadly among clinicians or researchers; however, most clinicians in the field agree that schizophrenia is a clinically and possibly biologically heterogeneous syndrome.

INCIDENCE

Schizophrenia tends to have its onset in the second or third decade and is generally a lifelong condition. The incidence of schizophrenia in the United States is 0.3–0.6 per 1000 individuals. The lifetime prevalence is about 1.5%. Worldwide incidence figures are comparable when adjusted for differences in diagnostic criteria.

Because of direct health-care costs and the more indirect cost to society by lost productivity across the individual's lifetime, schizophrenia has been estimated to cost 2% of the Gross National Product of the United States annually. Beyond economic measures, the toll is devastating in terms of human suffering for patients, their families, and friends.

ETIOLOGY

Schizophrenia may be a single illness or a heterogeneous cluster of disease states, caused by a combination of biological, genetic, psychological, environmental, and developmental factors. The **stress-diathesis model** proposes that biological, psychological, or environmental stresses on an already vulnerable individual result in the clinical picture we know as schizophrenia.

Biological Factors

The **dopamine hypothesis** postulates overactivity of dopaminergic neurotransmitter pathways in the brain. Support for this theory lies in the therapeutic effects of **antipsychotics,** otherwise known as **neuroleptics** (or inaccurately as major tranquilizers), which block the neurotransmitter dopamine. These dopamine receptor antagonists have especially strong binding to D-2 receptors in the subcortical and mesolimbic tracts where the positive symptoms of schizophrenia are thought to arise. Consistent with this theory, dopamine agonists that increase dopamine in the brain, such as amphetamine or levodopa (L-dopa), can induce or exacerbate the positive symptoms of schizophrenia. Schizophrenia tends to occur in the late teenage years shortly after the dopamine system completes its development in the central nervous system (CNS).

Although they ameliorate the positive symptoms in 60% of patients, neuroleptics have little effect on the negative symptoms and cognitive deficits of schizophrenia. More recent formulations of the dopamine hypothesis propose that increased dopamine occurs in subcortical and limbic regions of the brain and underlies positive symptoms, while decreased dopamine function occurs in the cortex and may be related to negative symptoms and cognitive dysfunction.

The mesocortical and mesolimbic dopaminergic tracts in the CNS are the focus of intense research into the causes of schizophrenia. Some researchers are studying the nigrostriatal tract and basal ganglia, with their high concentration of D-2 receptors, while others have implicated norepinephrine, gamma-amino butyric acid (GABA), NMDA and glutamate function in the cortex in the development of schizophrenia. Computed tomography (CT) and magnetic resonance imaging (MRI) studies of patients who have schizophrenia show enlargement of the lateral and third ventricles in 10–50% of patients, and cortical atrophy in 10–35% of patients. MRI studies indicate that gray matter loss is particularly prevalent in the temporal lobes. Newer studies using positron emission tomography (PET) and functional MRI imaging have shown disturbances in frontal and temporal lobe function.

The anatomic changes in the brains of patients who have schizophrenia are present at or about the onset of the illness, suggesting that schizophrenia is a disorder of development rather than simply a degenerative disease of the cerebral cortex. Researchers do not yet know whether schizophrenia reflects a disruption of brain development in utero and/or whether it develops during the extensive brain reorganization that occurs in early adolescence. They also have yet to pinpoint the stresses to the fetus that might be responsible for problems in brain development 2 decades later. Studies show that in the northern hemisphere, most patients who have schizophrenia were born between January and April; a reverse pattern is found in the southern hemisphere, with the incidence of schizophrenia peaking in birth months of July through October. These researchers and others suggested a possible viral etiology for schizophrenia. Nonspecific perinatal trauma, malnutrition, and Rhesus factor incompatibility have also been linked to an increased risk for schizophrenia.

Genetics

Studies strongly support a hereditary basis for schizophrenia. The worldwide prevalence of schizophrenia is estimated at about 1%, but the risk increases to 10% in the presence of a first-order relative, and 50% for identical twins. The concordance rate of *only* 50% in identical twins suggests that environmental factors such as those described above must also contribute to the individual risk of schizophrenia. Some researchers have suggested that two kinds of schizophrenia exist—**familial** and **sporadic**.

Psychological Factors

Psychodynamic theory holds that the crucial defect in the patient who has schizophrenia is impairment of ego functions, which affects the interpretation of reality and the control of inner drives. A common feature of paranoid schizophrenia is the defense mechanism of **projection:** the unconscious displacement of unacceptable feelings and thoughts onto others. Thus, "I am angry" becomes "my roommates are angry at me and may hurt me." Many paranoid delusions also have grandiose features: For example, the patient who believes that the CIA is spying on her also believes that she is important enough to warrant government surveillance.

Social Science Perspectives

The incidence of schizophrenia shows a uniform prevalence worldwide. Schizophrenia generally results in "downward drift" through socioeconomic levels of society. The patient who has schizophrenia is much less likely to be able to hold a job or to engage in stable close interpersonal relationships. Social security disability benefits are available on the basis of mental illness, but a person who has schizophrenia is less likely to apply for these benefits, either through disorganization or paranoia. Depression or drug dependence may further impair functioning. Patients with schizophrenia also show better long-term outcomes in non-industrialized societies.

DIAGNOSTIC ASSESSMENT: MENTAL STATUS EXAMINATION

The important findings in the mental status examination of the patient who has schizophrenia are as follows:

A. Appearance & Behavior. Patients who have schizophrenia may appear disheveled, unkempt, agitated, or rigid. They may be uncooperative, seem suspicious or perplexed, or be distracted by unseen auditory or visual hallucinations. They may exhibit poor eye contact. Their overall behavior may be peculiar or bizarre, and they usually exhibit a decrease in facial expressions.

B. Language. Speech rate, rhythm, and pitch may be normal; however, patients who have schizophrenia may use unusual words that only they understand (so-called **neologisms**). Or they may produce nonsensical speech, in which word fragments remain intact; this is known as "word salad," from the analogy to taking words in sentences and tossing them about randomly. Clinicians may find it difficult to understand patients who are in a severe psychotic state.

C. Emotions. Affect is often disturbed in patients who have schizophrenia. The most common disturbance of affect is a general flattening or blunting of affective responses. Patients will therefore appear detached or distant during the interview. **Perplexity** is another common feature: a consistent emotional "tone" of puzzlement, in which patients appear confused about what they are saying or understanding. Incongruous affect is also common.

D. Thought Processes. The thought processes of patients who have schizophrenia can be illogical, circumstantial, or tangential, and are often characterized by loose associations. Such thought processes have been likened to the moves of the knight in a game of chess: jumping crookedly in a manner that is hard for an interviewer to follow. For example, in response to being asked where he was born, a psychotic patient might respond, "Born? I am under a lake, in the kid rash. . . live oaks toddling. . . my sister." A common experience is for the interviewer to realize that, after talking to the patient for several minutes, he or she cannot understand what the patient is saying.

E. Thought Content. Numerous abnormalities of thought content may be seen in patients who have schizophrenia. A **delusion** is a fixed, false belief that is not culturally endorsed. **Persecutory delusions** (eg, "the CIA is spying on me"); **ideas of reference** (eg, that special "messages" for the patient alone are contained in TV shows or books); and **thought broadcasting, insertion,** or **control** are common. There may also be **grandiose** or **religious delusions** (eg, "I am the next Messiah and will be elected president next year"). **Somatic delusions** may also occur, and some patients become obsessed with receiving medical validation of their physical complaints, often asking for repeated examinations and tests. Other delusions may be more bizarre, as in the case of a patient who repeatedly presented to the surgery clinic angrily demanding a head CT scan to locate a transmitter he thought had been implanted in his brain. A patient's delusions should be researched if there is a question of a partial basis in fact.

Max C, aged 25, was hospitalized for treatment of a broken leg. He claimed he was being pursued by a gang to which he previously belonged. Mr. C fearfully demanded police protection and a new identity to help him hide from the gang. Because Mr. C was agitated and had a history of psychotic episodes induced by amphetamine use, the medical team attributed his persecutory beliefs to his psychiatric illness and were surprised on the second hospital day by the appearance of police officers who were able to corroborate Mr. C's claims that he had testified as a witness to a gang-related murder. Mr. C had indeed been fleeing from gang members, some of whom later appeared on the medical ward asking for him by name. He was transferred to a different ward under an alias and under police protection.

F. Disorders of Perception. Hallucinations of all five senses have been reported, but auditory hallucinations are most common. The patient may hear a voice or voices, and these voices are frequently heard to be talking about the patient. The voices may be speaking in a derisive manner and sometimes will order the patient to attempt suicide or to harm others (so-called **command hallucinations**).

G. Judgment & Insight. Judgment and insight are frequently impaired in patients who have schizophrenia. Patients may act on bizarre ideas and have limited awareness that an emotional disturbance is responsible for their thoughts and feelings.

H. Cognitive Examination. Informal or bedside cognitive testing may be normal in many patients. However, specialized neuropsychological testing almost always reveals abnormalities in attention, executive-motor abilities, and/or memory. Since patients are frequently distracted or disorganized, their concentration and attention may be impaired. Their ability to think abstractly may be impaired. For example, when asked to interpret the proverb "People in glass houses shouldn't throw stones," a patient might respond, "Of course not, they'll break the glass." This is referred to as concreteness of thinking. Memory may also appear to be impaired when patients are actively psychotic.

Leona S, a 19-year-old single woman, presented to the emergency room of a large teaching hospital at the urging of her roommates. "It's like she's had too much drugs," said the friend who accompanied her. Ms. S's chief complaint was that she had been experiencing "voices and ESP." She related the gradual onset of auditory hallucinations (over the past 7 or 8 months), consisting primarily of lewd comments about people she encountered. These hallucinations caused her considerable distress, and she was afraid that she would actually repeat what the voices told her, or would say or do the (sexual) things that the voices instructed her to do.

Ms. S also reported that she had been communicating with her boyfriend and others telepathically. This telepathic communication began as a series of coincidences in which people would say things that she had been thinking. Now she felt that others were constantly behaving in such a way as to indicate that they knew what she was thinking. For example, when watching television two nights earlier, her boyfriend said to her, "How amazing," just after she had felt that the television was referring to her family. He also leaned forward and obscured the screen on several occasions, indicating to her that there were messages in the show that he was attempting to conceal from her or perhaps protect her from.

Ms. S's friends indicated that her behavior had become very erratic. For example, she talked constantly about her psychic experiences, did not pay her rent, left clothing all over the house, turned appliances on and off unnecessarily, and regularly burned newspapers on the stove.

Ms. S denied any previous psychiatric history. She reported that she was the oldest of two siblings. She indicated that she was a shy child and an average student in elementary and high school, although she reported some difficulty concentrating during her last year in school. Her parents had separated when she was 13 years old, and she had lived with her mother until she graduated from high school, when she moved in with her current group of roommates. She had a maternal aunt who had an unspecified severe mental illness.

Ms. S had smoked marijuana and drunk beer on the weekends since she was 14 years old, and during the past year she had used LSD, magic mushrooms, and intranasal cocaine on numerous occasions. She quit using these substances several months earlier when she began to hear voices and feel that she had ESP.

During her interview, Ms. S was surprisingly cheerful and engaging. She had limited eye contact, however, and her speech was spontaneous and not fully coherent. She described her mood as good, and her affect was quite inappropriately benign given the content of the experience she described. Her thought processes were somewhat tangential, exhibiting some loose associations. For example, she said "television can put thoughts into your head, producers, directors, actors, advertisers, they still have to work for a living." She admitted to hearing several male voices commenting on her behavior and instructing her to perform sexual acts with those around her. She was afraid that she would not be able to ignore the voices any longer and was embarrassed that others around her knew what the voices were saying. She had the ideas of reference described above, together with thought withdrawal. She was unable to provide a coherent explanation for why she was having these experiences.

Diagnosis. Schizophreniform psychosis (Axis I).

Discussion. The diagnosis of schizophreniform psychosis is used when schizophrenia is suspected but fewer than 6 months have elapsed since the onset of symptoms. Ms. S reported prominent hallucinations, delusions, and thought disorder. Because of her heavy substance use, a psychoactive substance–induced psychosis could have been considered, but this disorder was unlikely given that she had abstained from hallucinogens and stimulants for several months, while her symptoms persisted or worsened in the same period of time.

Prominent mood symptoms (depression or mania) had not been a feature of her illness. Her affect at presentation could best be described as inappropriate. Hence a mood disorder with psychotic features was unlikely. Ms. S's history and the findings at examination strongly suggested schizophrenia. Her illness began with a preliminary period of social and cognitive deterioration, followed by the development of hallucinations, delusions, and thought disorder, all of which are positive symptoms of psychosis. Laboratory tests ruled out a brain lesion, metabolic abnormalities such as Wilson's disease (a defect in copper metabolism), and infectious causes of psychosis and cognitive decline such as HIV disease. The presence of serious mental illness in Ms. S's maternal relatives was also consistent with the well-documented role of genetics in the etiology of schizophrenia.

DIFFERENTIAL DIAGNOSIS

1. RULING OUT MEDICAL CAUSES

Symptoms that suggest psychosis, such as visual and auditory hallucinations, delusions, and loose associations in thought processes, can be produced by a variety of psychological and medical states. The history and mental status examination help to distinguish between schizophrenia and other diagnoses. If the patient has symptoms of schizophrenia, the clinician should first rule out medical causes of psychosis and then consider other psychiatric disorders.

A variety of medical conditions can produce hallucinations, paranoia, and disorganized thought processes. Patients who have such symptoms will then present with a clinical picture identical to schizophrenia. Common diseases that can cause psychosis and thus mimic schizophrenia include the following:

- infectious diseases: HIV, neurosyphilis, herpes encephalitis, Creutzfeldt-Jakob disease.
- CNS disorders: cerebrovascular accidents (stroke), head injury, and brain tumors, especially in the temporal or frontal areas [particularly those that produce fluent (Wernicke's) aphasia and nonsensical speech].
- other medical conditions: epilepsy (especially temporal lobe epilepsy), acute intermittent porphyria, B12 deficiency, carbon monoxide poisoning, heavy metal poisoning, Huntington's chorea, Alzheimer's disease, systemic lupus erythematosus, multiple sclerosis, and other collagen-vascular disorders with CNS involvement, Wernicke's encephalopathy due to thiamine deficiency, myxedema (severe hypothyroidism), Wilson's disease, cerebral lipidosis, Fabry's disease, Fahr's disease, Hallervorden-Spatz syndrome, homocystinuria, and metachromatic leukodystrophy.
- medications, including steroids, H_2 blockers such as Cimetidine.

Even the most astute clinician cannot distinguish between schizophrenia and a psychotic disorder due to a medical condition without reviewing the patient's physical examination and laboratory test results. To rule out these medical conditions, clinicians should order a thorough medical workup for patients who exhibit a new onset of psychosis. This workup should include the following tests:

- routine laboratory work (including CBC, SMAC and sed rate)
- thyroid function tests (including T3RU, T4, TSH)

- rapid plasma reagin (RPR) test to rule out syphilis
- B_{12} and folate levels
- HIV test
- toxicology screen to rule out drugs
- heavy metal screen
- CT or MRI scan
- electroencephalogram (EEG)

Jesse P, aged 46, presented at a health clinic. He vaguely denied hallucinations, but mentioned sometimes smelling "burning rubber." Mr. P had a 2-year history of psychotic episodes. His wife reported that he frequently engaged in conversations with himself, at times apparently responding to internal voices. She also noted that her husband spent a great deal of time writing his ideas in notebooks and proselytizing about his religious beliefs to friends and strangers. He would become angry when his wife challenged him about his behavior. He had not worked in several years. Mr. P's wife also noted a complete absence of her husband's sexual drive over the same time period. There was no evidence of depression, mania, or substance use.

Mr. P agreed to admission to the psychiatry unit for evaluation. He spent most of his time on the unit writing in his notebooks and trying to get other patients to accept him as "the Son of God," and to vote for him in the next election." Laboratory testing was unremarkable. Mr. P was started on an antipsychotic, haloperidol (Haldol). Two days later, he became markedly more paranoid and agitated. The haloperidol dosage was increased. Several hours later, Mr. P began running down the hallway, screaming, convinced that he could see magnets in the wall pulling at him. He was placed in restraints.

A head CT scan revealed an old parencymal injury in the anterior pole of the right temporal lobe. A sleep-deprived EEG with naso-pharyngeal leads showed spiking seizure activity in the same area. A more careful review of Mr. P's medical records showed that shortly before he lost his last job, he had worked as a civilian on a construction crew refurbishing a naval aircraft carrier. Mr. P had lost control of an air-powered jackhammer, which rebounded into his face and fractured bones in his cheek and lip. Presumably the resulting contusion damaged his temporal lobe, setting up a seizure focus. Mr. P's symptoms diminished significantly after he was started on an anticonvulsant, carbamezepine (Tegretol).

Diagnosis. Psychotic disorder due to temporal lobe epilepsy (TLE).

Discussion. Mr. P exhibited the classic triad of TLE symptoms, including hyperreligiousity (also seen in schizophrenia), hypergraphia (extensive writing), and decreased sexual drive. TLE may produce strange emotional states or behavior during a seizure. Patients may report an aura or olfactory hallucinations at the onset of a seizure. Sometimes patients who have TLE will perform complex stereotyped behavior. Unlike generalized seizure disorders, seizure activity in the temporal lobes does not necessarily produce visible physical manifestations. TLE may also produce symptoms of psychosis, even between seizures. Such a chronic psychotic state will appear to an observer to match the presenting symptoms of schizophrenia. Anticonvulsants such as carbamezepine (Tegretol), valproic acid (Depakote), or phenytoin (Dilantin) are often used to treat TLE.

2. RULING OUT DRUG-INDUCED PSYCHOSIS

Common drugs that can cause psychosis and thus mimic the clinical presentation of schizophrenia include steroids, amphetamines, cocaine, hallucinogens (such as LSD), and PCP (phencyclidine). The phenomenon of **amphetamine psychosis,** first described in the 1940s not long after the synthesis of the drug, is one of the cornerstones of the dopamine hypothesis of schizophrenia. Amphetamine psychosis typically clears after days to weeks of abstinence, although it can occasionally take months for the syndrome to disappear completely. Antipsychotic medications will hasten the resolution of symptoms. Heavy (ie, daily) usage of methamphetamines over extended periods of time (ie, months to years) may produce chronic psychotic states that mimic schizophrenia even when the patient stops using the drug.

Bernard F, aged 28, was brought to the emergency room in shackles. He stated that he was being persecuted by the police. He was accompanied by two burly police officers, who reported that they found him cowering in a corner in a bus station, holding a loaded 38-mm handgun. Mr. F was hypervigilant, sweaty, and had a rapid pulse and elevated blood pressure. His speech was rushed and well organized. He was very frightened and stated that he had been followed for the past 2 weeks by government agents who were associated with the Mafia and were going to kill him. He reported that people had been watching him, talking about him, and mocking him. A single male voice had been calling his name, cursing at him and saying, "do it." According to Mr. F, this meant to shoot himself. He thought that the voice was that of Satan, and that he was supposed to kill himself before his enemies did. In the bus station, with his gun loaded, he was trying to resist this voice.

Mr. F admitted to one previous psychiatric hospitalization 2 years earlier. At that time he became "paranoid" after a heavy run of nasal methamphetamine use and stayed in the hospital for 3 days while he was treated with haloperidol. On questioning, he admitted that on most days he used half a gram of "crystal meth" and drank about a case of beer, and that over the past month had begun to use methamphetamine intravenously. He admitted to becoming suspicious, hearing a voice call his name, and wondering whether he was under surveillance.

Aside from the one previous admission, Mr. F had no previous psychiatric history. He had a long history in the judicial system, however, dating back to elementary school. He was frequently suspended from school for fighting, using drugs on campus, sexual assault, and carrying weapons. He spent 3 years altogether in Juvenile Hall and had been incarcerated 3 times as an adult for a total of 2 years in the county jail on petty theft, assault, and drug charges. His family had a history of depression and alcohol dependence.

Diagnosis. Psychotic disorder due to stimulant (methamphetamine) use (Axis I); consider antisocial personality disorder (Axis II).

Discussion. In all respects, Mr. F's symptoms—prominent auditory hallucinations and delusions—are typical of schizophrenia. However the presence of a known substance, methamphetamine, as a precipitating and maintaining factor for the psychosis militates against the diagnosis of schizophrenia in this case and suggests a psychotic disorder due to stimulant use.

A diagnosis of antisocial personality disorder should also be considered. A pattern of frequently violating the rights of others (eg, engaging in fights, theft, and sexual assault) established before the age of 12 strongly suggests this disorder.

3. RULING OUT PSYCHIATRIC DISORDERS

Psychotic states can occur in psychiatric disorders other than schizophrenia and the mental status examination alone is often not enough to distinguish the psychiatric illness. Psychosis seems to be a "final common pathway" that is the outcome of numerous illnesses. Psychotic states resulting from bipolar disorder, depression, personality disorders, drug use, or medical illness all tend to resemble each other, with hallmark symptoms of paranoia, disorganized thoughts, disturbed emotional responses, and hallucinations. The *DSM-IV* decision tree for psychosis is especially helpful in understanding the suggested process of clinical reasoning to distinguish between these diagnoses.

A. Mood Disorders. Patients who have either severe **mania** or **major depression** can develop psychosis. The presence of a depressed or euphoric mood in a patient may help the clinician to make these diagnoses. But a history of mania or depression, and a clear history of symptoms of mania or depression immediately prior to the current psychotic state, are most helpful in making either of these diagnoses. Family history of mood disorders is another helpful clue. Studies suggest that when the ethnicity of the patient and physician are different, patients experiencing mood disorders with psychotic symptoms are much more likely to be mistakenly diagnosed as having schizophrenia.

B. Schizoaffective Disorder. Patients who have schizoaffective disorder seem to have both schizophrenia and bipolar mood disorder. They frequently have episodes of psychosis, some of which occur after a period of depression or mania, and others not accompanied by mood changes (in keeping with schizophrenia). Treatment of schizoaffective disorder involves mood stabilizers and antipsychotic medication. If a patient is misdiagnosed as having schizophrenia, and a mood stabilizer is not taken, the patient will continue to have mood swings and frequent psychotic episodes. Given the confluence of two severe mental disorders, it is not surprising that patients who have schizoaffective disorder may have a very poor prognosis, compounded by poor psychosocial functioning, substance use, and suicide.

C. Schizophreniform Disorder. This disorder involves the symptoms of schizophrenia but lasts for fewer than 6 months. This diagnosis is often used after a patient has had a first psychotic episode. Many patients diagnosed with schizophreniform disorder have further psychotic episodes and are ultimately diagnosed as having schizophrenia.

D. Delusional Disorder. Delusional disorder is characterized by a fixed, false belief system but without the presence of other positive and negative symptoms found in schizophrenia, such as hallucinations, disorganized thoughts, or paucity of thought. Delusional disorder tends to occur around age 40 and has an incidence of only 0.02%, far less than schizophrenia. Patients present with one of three types of delusional systems. In the most common, the persecutory type, patients are hypervigilant for danger and believe that they are being persecuted by one or more people. In the somatic subtype, patients falsely believe that they have a physical dysfunction. In the erotomanic type, patients believe that someone—sometimes a celebrity—loves and desires them, in spite of a lack of proof or even evidence to the contrary. Antipsychotic medication may not be very effective for this disorder, especially for long-standing delusions, but supportive work that focuses on reality-based issues is often of benefit, as well as treatment for attendant depression and anxiety. Careful screening for suicidal (or homicidal) ideation are essential.

E. Induced Psychotic Disorder. Otherwise known as **folie à deux,** induced psychotic disorder occurs when a delusional or psychotic individual's mental state becomes shared with another person, usually a spouse or family member. That person will frequently take on the delusions of the first person. For example, the wife of a patient who has schizophrenia may suddenly claim that she believes, like her husband, that computers are organizing to take over the world and are speaking to them both through radio broadcasts. Treatment may involve couples counseling or a separation of the two affected individuals. Information from friends or family members helps clinicians to make this diagnosis.

F. Brief Psychotic Disorder. Short-lived psychotic episodes may occur in patients in reaction to severe stress, or uncommonly without apparent reason. Patients who have borderline personality disorder, who normally have grossly intact reality-testing, may develop brief psychotic states in response to emotional stress or drug use. Since patients who have borderline personality disorder have low thresholds for emotional stress, the stressor is often one too minor to have the same effect on the average person. For example, the patient who has borderline personality disorder, who is sensitive to issues of abandonment, might develop a week-long psychosis immediately after the breakup of an intense romantic relationship. Clues to this diagnosis include a history, often provided by friends and family, of labile mood, chaotic relationships with others, multiple suicide attempts, or self-destructive acts.

G. Late-onset Psychosis. Elderly patients, especially those who have lifelong personality disorders, may develop delusions and other psychotic symptoms in their 60s, 70s, or 80s. These symptoms may be associated with an early dementia and/or CNS abnormalities visible on CT or MRI brain scans, and low-dose antipsychotics help alleviate them.

COURSE

1. PRODROMAL SYNDROME

Prodromal syndrome refers to a period of minor symptoms that predate the onset of the full-blown disorder. Although schizophrenia can occur in personalities of all kinds, it is more likely to occur in the presence of some personality traits than others. The most classic findings are emotional and social detachment; these are people who seem shy, sensitive, and withdrawn. They avoid competition, tend to engage in solitary activities, have frequent and elaborate daydreams, and tend to retreat into fantasy. But many adolescents who do not develop schizophrenia match the preceding description; the association between these personality characteristics and schizophrenia is too weak to allow mental health professionals to predict whether specific individuals will develop schizophrenia.

2. ONSET

The acute illness is often so insidious that it cannot be said to have a definite beginning. In a typical case, family members will notice a decline in the patient's in-school performance and motivation. The patient may spend increasing amounts of time in his or her room, thinking about philosophic or religious ideas, and may socialize with friends less, becoming more solitary. Eventually, grossly psychotic symptoms emerge. For example, the patient might complain of hearing voices or might believe that government agents are monitoring his or her thoughts by radio. The development of these acute psychotic symptoms frequently follows a life stress such as the breakup of a relationship, or the move away from home for college or military service. The patient may be suicidal and is frequently hospitalized at this time for a "first psychotic break."

3. DISEASE COURSE

Approximately 10% of patients who experience a new onset of schizophrenia will recover and regain their premorbid level of functioning. Between 40 and 50% of patients have periods of remission but still experience occasional difficulties in social relationships and at work. Between 20 and 30% of all patients who have schizophrenia have a more severe form of the disorder and remain actively psychotic throughout their lifetimes, with very poor levels of functioning. Table 4–1 summarizes prognostic indicators for schizophrenia.

Although the prevalence of schizophrenia is about the same in both sexes, gender is an important predictor of course of the illness. On average, the age of onset is almost a decade later in women than in men. Women appear to function better with the disorder, as evidenced by the fact that they are more likely to be married and to be employed than are males. The mean dose of antipsychotic drugs required for maintenance treatment is also lower in females. Women make up the majority of patients who have "late onset" (age greater than 40 years) schizophrenia and are more likely than males to have mood symptoms (particularly depression) as a prominent residual symptom.

TREATMENT OF SCHIZOPHRENIA

Antipsychotic medications are an integral part of the treatment of schizophrenia. Supportive individual psychotherapy, group therapy, and vocational rehabilitation are also important treatment modalities. Patients who are so disorganized and paranoid that they pose a danger to themselves or others, or who are unable to care for themselves, may require inpatient psychiatric hospitalization. If a patient is not willing to be treated as an inpatient, he or she may need to be admitted on an involuntary basis, following legal guidelines that vary from state to state. Patients who repeatedly fail inpatient hospitalizations may warrant psychiatric conservatorship and hospitalization in a long-term facility for 6 months or more.

Clinicians should be alert to the development of either depression or obsessive-compulsive disorder in patients who have schizophrenia. Because patients often have blunted affect and strange thoughts clinicians often overlook major depression, which occurs in up to 60% of patients. Obsessive-compulsive

Table 4–1. Prognostic indicators for schizophrenia

	Good Prognosis	Poor Prognosis
Age of onset	Older	Younger
Onset of illness	Acute	Insidious
Precipitating factors	Obvious stressors	None
Premorbid social, sexual, and work functioning	Good	Poor
Affective disturbance	Depression	None or withdrawn
Marital status	Married	Single, divorced, or widowed
Family history	Mood disorder	Schizophrenia
Type of symptoms	Positive	Negative
Neurologic signs	None	Present
History of perinatal trauma	None	Positive
History of relapses	None or few	Many
History of assaultiveness	None	Present

symptoms are common in schizophrenia and may be worsened by the antipsychotic clozapine (Clozaril).

1. MEDICATION

Antipsychotics, also known as neuroleptics or major tranquilizers, control the symptoms of schizophrenia. Although they do not provide a cure, these medications can induce remission of psychotic symptoms within 7–21 days in acute schizophrenia and can also help to prevent recurrence of symptoms. These medications presumably work by blocking dopamine receptors, especially the D-2 type, in the mesolimbic system.

Side Effects

The older antipsychotic medications have many side effects based on their actions on receptors in the basal ganglia and hypothalamus. **Extrapyramidal symptoms (EPS),** such as painful contractions of muscles in the face, neck, and extremities, occur most frequently when antipsychotics are started or increased. These effects can be treated easily with anticholinergic drugs, such as benztropine mesylate (Cogentin) or diphenhydramine (Benadryl). **Parkinsonian side effects** that mimic Parkinson's disease may also occur during treatment with antipsychotic medication. Patients may exhibit gait abnormalities, masked faces, and difficulty initiating movement.

Akathisia is a subjective feeling of restlessness, sometimes manifested by behavior such as "restless legs." Often mistaken for the symptoms of anxiety, akathisia also occurs during initiation of antipsychotics and is treated similarly to EPS. In many patients beta-blockers such as propranolol (Inderal) may be more effective than anticholinergics for this symptom. **Gynecomastia** (breast enlargement) may result from longer-term use of neuroleptics. This is the result of dopamine blockade of the dopamine pathways in the tubular infundibulum leading to increased secretion of prolactin. Gynecomastia, **galactorrhea** (breast milk production), amenorrhea, and decreased sex drive are common side effects as are weight gain and photodermatitis.

Neuroleptic malignant syndrome (NMS) is a rare reaction to neuroleptics but constitutes a medical emergency since it carries a mortality rate of up to 30% if untreated. NMS usually occurs when starting or increasing the dose of an antipsychotic medication. Symptoms include fever with autonomic nervous system dysregulation, mutism, and muscle rigidity. Elevated serum creatine (phospho)kinase (CPK) levels can help confirm the diagnosis of NMS. Treatment consists of stopping antipsychotic medications, administering fluids, and providing supportive therapy.

In contrast to other side effects of neuroleptics, **tardive dyskinesia (TD)** occurs after cumulative exposure to medications, frequently after 10–20 years of treatment. Unlike other side effects, TD is irreversible, albeit with a waxing and waning course. It may paradoxically (and only temporarily) improve when neuroleptics are increased. The most common abnormal movement is oral facial dyskinesia. Women, (especially post-menopausal women), some ethnic groups, and the elderly appear at highest risk for developing TD, as early as 6 months after starting treatment. The best treatment for TD is prevention. Since cumulative exposure to neuroleptics determines the likelihood of developing TD, patients should be maintained on the lowest doses of neuroleptic possible without recurrence of psychosis.

Many patients receive antipsychotic medication, often in hospitals and nursing homes, sometimes inappropriately, and these patients (who are frequently medically ill or elderly) may be at high risk for side effects. Antipsychotic medications are not the only substances that can cause these side effects. Many medications for nausea have chemical structures related to antipsychotics. Patients taking these medications should be routinely asked about and examined for the symptoms of akathisia, NMS, and Parkinsonian syndromes.

Gwen T, a 36-year-old woman with kidney failure, was admitted to the hospital with dehydration and electrolyte imbalances. On the third hospital day she was extremely anxious. She received two doses of diazepam (Valium) in the afternoon but remained as anxious as before. Ms. T began pacing in the hallway and complained that even in bed she couldn't keep her legs still. When a consultation was requested the psychiatrist noted that the patient had complained of nausea when she was admitted and was given regular doses of two different antiemetic medications over the three days in the hospital. Her symptoms corresponded with akathisia. The patient was given diphenhydramine and reported dramatic relief from anxiety and restlessness in less than an hour.

Types of Neuroleptics

Neuroleptics are frequently classified by their potency (see Table 4–2).

Guidelines for Prescribing Neuroleptics

- Prescribe neuroleptics for individuals who have benefited from this type of drug in the past. If the patient's previous response is unknown, a family member's previous response to a neuroleptic may help predict efficacy.
- Select a neuroleptic that has desired effects and an acceptable side-effect profile. For example, a young agitated patient who has schizophrenia may benefit from the high level of sedation associated with lower potency medications such as thioridazine (Mellarel), or chlorpromazine (Thorazine), whereas the same drug may put an

Table 4–2. Neuroleptic potency classifications

	Potency		
	High	**Midrange**	**Low**
Example	Haloperidol (Haldol)	Perphenazine (Trilafon)	Thioridazine (Mellaril)
Incidence of EPS	High	Moderate	Low
Anticholinergic effects	Low	Moderate	High
Sedative effects	Low	Moderate	High

elderly patient at risk for falls as a result of over-sedation and low blood pressure, and for antipsychotic side effects.

- Educate the patient and family about typical side effects, how to identify them early, and what to do if they appear. This will greatly enhance compliance.
- A trial of 3–6 weeks of adequate doses is necessary before a dose change should be initiated.
- The simultaneous use of two or more neuroleptics from the same class is inadvisable.
- Always try to lower the dose after the acute phase of the illness is resolved. The risk of tardive dyskinesia is related to total cumulative doses of antipsychotics. Thus lower maintenance doses of neuroleptics are recommended after the acute phase of the illness has resolved. The use of high doses of antipsychotic medication is ill-advised, because studies have failed to show significant therapeutic benefits, while the risks of short- and long-term side effects are increased.
- Most patients who have schizophrenia will need pharmacotherapy indefinitely.

Atypical or Novel Antipsychotic Agents

Clozapine (Clozaril) is a new antipsychotic that acts by blocking D_2, D_3, D_4, and S_2 receptors. Because of the rare but potentially fatal side effect of agranulocytosis, weekly blood monitoring is necessary. Clozapine is not associated with TD, and sometimes produces remission in otherwise treatment-resistant psychotic patients. Risperidone (Risperdal), olanzapine (Zyprexa), and quietapine (Seroquel), are the latest antipsychotics to have received FDA approval. These three newer antipsychotics are as effective as the older agents, have fewer side effects, and represent an important advance in the medical treatment of the disorder.

2. PSYCHOTHERAPY

While antipsychotic medication is a mainstay of treatment for schizophrenia, it is only one aspect of treatment. The combination of psychotherapy and medication is more effective than either alone in reducing relapses in patients who have schizophrenia.

Patients who have schizophrenia benefit from a supportive approach that encourages them to share their concerns without necessarily trying to resolve or analyze them. A focus on real-life concerns (and a de-emphasis on complex fantasies) is recommended. Since these patients are emotionally "brittle," they must be prepared for changes and separations (eg, the therapist going on vacation) in advance. Many patients feel isolated and demoralized, and for these patients, group therapy may be helpful. Vocational rehabilitation programs may help to train patients for jobs that allow them to function with increased self-reliance and confidence.

Charles W, aged 39, had been diagnosed with schizophrenia almost 20 years earlier. He had been hospitalized infrequently for psychotic episodes, and his condition had stabilized on antipsychotic medications. In weekly psychotherapy sessions with a psychiatry resident, Mr. W discussed his frustration with his illness and his dislike for taking his medications. He had grandiose plans to build a laser to project a huge holographic image over the city in which he lived and had already begun purchasing parts for the project.

Mr. W was also convinced that a woman living in his apartment building was romantically interested in him, based on scant evidence (eg, "She said hello to me today; I think that she wants me to be her boyfriend"). Over several months of psychotherapy, Mr. W was better able to accept that he needed to take medication and had to develop more realistic ideas for pursuing friendships and romantic relationships. The psychiatry resident also encouraged Mr. W to build a scaled-down laser, which he built from parts and plans purchased at a local electronics store. Mr. W derived great satisfaction from the completed kit, which did indeed project a hologram over a tabletop.

Family members may be chronically stressed by their role in caring for the patient who has schizophrenia. Often family members have unrealistic ideas about the patient's prognosis, that is, they are certain the patient who has a poor prognosis will one day fully recover. Patients and their families can be helped to cope with chronic illness. Numerous studies have shown that including family members or significant others in the treatment of patients who have schizophrenia reduces patient and family stress and has a positive effect on the course of the disease.

Rachel C, aged 33, had her first psychotic break when she was 18 years old. Her parents, both attorneys, stressed education and achievement in their family; her three siblings were all professionals or were attending graduate programs. Ms. C was the youngest child and had been in her first year at a top university when she had to be hospitalized for the first symptoms of schizophrenia, including delusions, hallucinations, and suicidal thoughts.

Numerous trials on older antipsychotic agents failed to produce much improvement in her condition, and she spent much of the next 14 years living in residential programs for the mentally ill, averaging one psychiatric admission per year for exacerbations of her illness. Later she was started on clozapine. Within weeks her condition improved markedly. She was able to concentrate, and her thoughts became organized; she no longer experienced hallucinations or compelling delusions.

Ms. C's parents were thrilled when she was able to move into her own apartment 2 months later. They called and visited her frequently, punctuating their excitement and relief about getting their "old daughter" back by spontaneously and frequently hugging and kissing her. They also assumed that she would be thrilled to resume her college studies and enrolled her in summer classes at a nearby university. They focused on how she could "make up for lost time" by taking an accelerated college program for three years without breaks. Ms. C's protestations were drowned out by her parents' enthusiasm.

Two weeks after starting college courses, Ms. C became agitated and delusional, convinced that her family had planted eavesdropping devices in her brain and body to monitor her thoughts and movements. She was re-hospitalized, and her treating psychiatric team took a multipronged approach of adjusting her medication and offering individual psychotherapy to help her rebuild her self-confidence. They also convened several family sessions to allow her parents to express their sadness, guilt, and anger about their daughter's illness, and to educate them about how to engage with her in a supportive but less intrusive way. Ms. C made rapid progress and was able to live independently again after a month in a partial hospitalization program. One year later, she enrolled in college classes and began the process of completing her undergraduate degree, at a slower pace.

Education and support groups help to prevent "burnout" and have beneficial effects on the patient. Groups such as the National Alliance of the Mentally Ill (NAMI) act as both support groups and clearinghouses for information about services and treatments available to patients and their families. Case management, supportive psychotherapy, psychosocial and occupational rehabilitation, family treatments, and appropriate housing are all critical aspects of the long-term treatment of schizophrenia.

THE IMPACT OF SCHIZOPHRENIA ON SOCIETY

Patients who have schizophrenia are often dependent on nicotine and at risk for becoming dependent on alcohol or drugs, which complicates treatment. For example, clinicians must be aware of possible medication interactions with alcohol; substance-dependent patients are less likely to take prescribed medications and are more likely to miss follow-up appointments.

The morbidity and mortality rates in patients who have schizophrenia are much greater than in the general population. The incidence of depression, drug use, and untreated medical problems in patients who have schizophrenia is high. Over 30% of patients who have schizophrenia attempt suicide at some point during the illness, usually during a period of demoralization or depression associated with insight into the disability and loss associated with having the disease. The lifetime incidence of completed suicide in schizophrenia is 10–15%. Patients who have schizophrenia have frequently "fallen down" the socioeconomic ladder and often have limited access to medical or social resources, further imperiling their prognosis.

Patterns of health care for patients who have schizophrenia have changed significantly during the past 3 decades. Spurred by the discovery in the 1950s of the first neuroleptic, chlorpromazine, public policy changed to de-institutionalize patients who have schizophrenia by releasing them from locked mental institutions into the community. But because of reductions in funding for public health, and the high incidence of noncompliance with medication and follow-up care by patients, many patients have not received anticipated regular treatment at community mental health centers. At any point in time, 40% of patients with schizophrenia are not receiving treatment, and 15% of patients never receive any treatment during their lifetime.

Inpatient psychiatric admissions for patients who have schizophrenia have increased, and the likelihood of readmission within 2 years of a prior admission is approximately 50%. Patients who have schizophrenia occupy 25% of all hospital beds used in the United States annually and half of all mental health beds. Between 15 and 30% of all jail prisoners and over a third of the homeless population have schizophrenia. Clustering in urban areas and in the lower socioeconomic levels of society, individuals with schizophrenia have a high incidence of substance use, suicide, estrangement from families, and alienation from society as a whole.

EMOTIONAL REACTIONS TO PATIENTS

Patients who have schizophrenia frequently elicit strong emotional reactions from the people around them. Physicians may find themselves confused, emotionally distant, or angry as they interact with these patients, and may distance themselves from patients who have schizophrenia. The use of the term "schizophrenic" as a noun confuses the person with the illness itself, and diminishes the perception that an individual is suffering the illness. This derogatory labeling is commonly applied to patients who have psychotic or personality disorders (eg, "we admitted a wild schizophrenic last night"). Patients who have psychotic disorders often generate anxiety and discomfort among health-care providers because their symptoms—delusions, hallucinations, a break from reality—and subjective experience are very difficult for the provider to understand. This phenomenon is seen much less commonly in depression, mania, or anxiety states, where the patient appears to have more in common with the physician and is likely to generate a sense of empathy and understanding.

Spencer R, a 46-year-old patient who had a 25-year history of schizophrenia, was hospitalized with a severe lung infection. His paranoia hampered medical follow-up in the community, and he was only partially adherent to prescriptions of antipsychotics and antibiotics. The treating infectious disease specialists felt that Mr. R's only reasonable hope for survival was a lobectomy to remove the source of the infection. Mr. R agreed and appeared to understand the proposed operation; however, he remained very anxious and somewhat paranoid.

For example, he refused to use the bathroom in his hospital room, and took smoke breaks in isolated areas of the hospital. He turned the static on his TV up to a high volume to block out voices but refused additional antipsychotics to help with auditory hallucinations. He was told that he could not eat for 8 hours before surgery, and that he would not receive a breakfast tray. On the morning of surgery, however, Mr. R ate his roommate's breakfast. The surgery team was infuriated and decided to discharge him.

A psychiatric consultation generated another set of options. Mr. R welcomed a visit from his outpatient psychiatrist, who recommended diazepam to help with his anxiety. Mr. R agreed and was able to discuss his fear of surgery (particularly the fairly common fear that he would die during the operation). The surgeons were able to vent their frustration about Mr. R's ambivalence and his "general weirdness." Mr. R had his surgery 4 days later and made an uneventful recovery.

CROSS-CULTURAL ASPECTS OF SCHIZOPHRENIA

Cultural factors influence the expression of symptoms and community responses in all psychiatric disorders. Patients from Asian, Latin American, and African cultures have a greater incidence of visual hallucinations. Latinos may report more hallucinations and delusions involving religion, and hallucinations of God and saints are commonly encountered. The content of delusions is also influenced by cultural factors. Thus patients who have schizophrenia may believe that they are being pursued by the CIA in the United States, the KGB in the former Soviet Union, or witches or spirits in developing nations in Africa or Asia.

Misdiagnosis may also result from incorrect interpretations of symptoms or mental status examination findings. The patient's cultural background should always be ascertained and considered. African-American and Latino patients from lower socioeconomic groups whose depression or mania is complicated by psychotic features are often misdiagnosed as having schizophrenia. These patients often are then given too much antipsychotic medication and are not given needed antidepressants or mood stabilizers. African-American patients who have schizophrenia are often prescribed inappropriately high doses of antipsychotics, resulting in more side effects and a higher long-term risk of irreversible movement disorders. Patients from cultures that have a normative belief in witchcraft and supernatural explanations are also at risk for being misdiagnosed as having schizophrenia.

LEGAL & ETHICAL ISSUES

The care of patients who have schizophrenia involves many legal and ethical dilemmas. These include the need for involuntary hospitalization, and the impaired capacity these patients may have to give informed consent for medication, research protocols, and medical treatment.

Involuntary Hospitalization

A patient who is psychotic may be extremely disorganized, display disruptive behavior, or become suicidal or dangerous. In many states, patients may be held for psychiatric evaluation for up to several days at the discretion of a mental health worker (eg, social worker, psychologist, or psychiatrist). Such holds may be enacted for "danger to self" (suicide potential), "danger to others" (homicidal ideation), or "grave disability" (defined as the inability of the patient to provide for his or her own food, clothing, or shelter). The psychiatric hold often can be extended with judicial review.

Involuntary Treatment
With Medications

Some states make the distinction between grounds for involuntary hospitalization and competency to refuse treatment. Under these circumstances, patients who can explain the risks and benefits of receiving antipsychotic medications versus not receiving these medications cannot be legally compelled to take medications against their will, even if they are being held in the hospital. Exceptions are made for extremely agitated, suicidal, or aggressive patients. Some mental health professionals and advocacy groups suggest that this new law encourages better informed consent and communication between patients and physicians. Other psychiatrists argue that their hands are tied if they cannot treat patients with the medications that often provide dramatic relief from hallucinations, paranoia, and disorganized thinking.

Informed Consent
in Research Settings

The development and testing of new medications for schizophrenia raises difficult ethical issues. In a case involving trials of a new antipsychotic at a university research center, a family assisted their son in deciding to enter an experimental trial. Months later the patient's family protested that neither they nor their son, who had schizophrenia, were made aware of a phase of treatment that involved substituting a placebo for the patient's medication. During the first phase of the trial, the new medication greatly reduced the patient's delusions, but he experienced a rapid relapse when the antipsychotic medication was stopped. What safeguards need to be taken in research settings that involve patients who have schizophrenia? Are there potential problems when family members are asked to give their consent for treatment when a patient's judgment is impaired by psychosis? How can new medications be tested effectively if

drug trials are not conducted under "double blind" conditions?

Providing Medical Treatment

Patients who have schizophrenia may suffer a diminished connection to reality, through delusional thinking, ambivalence, or disorganized thoughts. This may result in a diminished capacity to weigh medical choices. The presence of delusions or hallucinations does not automatically mean that a patient is not capable of deciding rationally about medical treatment, although it certainly makes the situation more complex. Nor does involuntary psychiatric hospitalization suspend the patient's right to refuse treatment—a psychiatric hold does not make a patient incompetent to decide about medical treatment. Consider the following case, related by James Strain, MD:

A patient had a long history of schizophrenia. He had intermittent periods of psychosis but when functioning well was quite lucid and enjoyed painting as a hobby. His paintings were one day "discovered" and he became an overnight sensation in the city's art scene. The dramatic changes wrought by the patient's overnight success included public appearances at several highly touted showings of his artwork. The stress of his success led to an episode of psychosis in which voices commanded the patient to cut off his hand (the one that he used to paint). In his psychotic state, he had developed the belief that his hand was "evil." The patient arrived at a nearby hospital emergency room, agitated, bleeding, and in shock, and clutching a paper bag containing his severed hand. Before being restrained and sedated, and becoming unconscious, the patient shouted, "Don't put my hand back on!"

The surgeon and anesthesiologist thought that surgical reattachment of the patient's hand was contraindicated given his refusal to give informed consent and his expressed wishes to the contrary. They also worried about a lawsuit for disobeying the patient's wishes. But the consulting psychiatrist argued that in a psychotic state, the patient might be extremely ambivalent about his wishes. As evidence, he cited the fact that the patient had brought his severed hand in to the emergency room.

The patient's hand was reattached and was fully functional. After treatment with antipsychotic medication, the patient expressed his gratitude to the physicians for proceeding with the operation.

These issues bring up concerns about autonomy and physician beneficence. Is it possible to distinguish between the wishes of someone in a psychotic state compared to what that individual might want when thinking clearly? If you respect the patient's autonomy, how can you reconcile opposing wishes in a patient who is ambivalent about what he or she wants? At what point (if any) do the special needs of the psychiatric patient become "too much" for the system? And when—if ever—should a physician become a proponent for the health-care system, rather than for the patient?

Medical causes should always be ruled out when patients present with psychotic symptoms. Medication and psychotherapy help to relieve symptoms, but no cure is yet available. Physicians treating patients who have schizophrenia need to be aware of the powerful emotional reactions and legal and ethical issues that may complicate the care of these patients. The search for the definitive cause and treatment for schizophrenia remains one of the greatest challenges and sought-after goals of modern psychiatry.

CONCLUSION

Schizophrenia is a lifelong condition. Common symptoms include hallucinations, paranoia, delusions, social withdrawal, and personality changes.

REFERENCES

Andreasen NC: *The Broken Brain.* Harper & Row, 1984.

Carpenter WT: Maintenance therapy of persons with schizophrenia. J Clin Psychiatr 1996;57(Suppl No. 9):10.

Carpenter WT Jr, Schooler NR, Kane J: The rationale and ethics of medication-free research in schizophrenia. Arch Gen Psychiatr 1997;54:401.

Green MF: What are the functional consequences of cognitive impairment in schizophrenia? Am J Psychiatr 1996;153:321.

Johnstone EC, McMillan JF, Frith CD, Benn DK, Crow TJ: Further investigation of the predictors of outcome following first schizophrenic episodes. Br J Psychiatr 1990;157:182.

Jones PB, Guth C, Lewis SW, Murray RM: Low intelligence and poor educational achievement precede early onset schizophrenic psychosis. In: *The Neuropsychology of Schizophrenia.* David AS, Cutting JC (editors). Erlbaum Associates, 1994.

Keck PE, McElroy SL: The new antipsychotics and their therapeutic potential. Psychiatr Ann 1997;27(5):320.

National Alliance for the Mentally Ill. http://www.nami.org/

Practice guidelines for the treatment of patients with schizophrenia. Am J Psychiatr 1997;154(Suppl):4.

Rupp A, Keith SJ: The costs of schizophrenia: assessing the burden. Psychiatr Clin N Am 1993;16:413.

Schiller L, Bennett A. *The Quiet Room.* Warner Books, 1994.

Sheehan S. *Is There on Earth No Place for Me?* Houghton-Mifflin, 1982.

Shriqui CL, Nasrallah HA (editors): *Contemporary Issues in the Treatment of Schizophrenia.* American Psychiatric Press, 1995.

Torrey EF: *Surviving Schizophrenia: A Manual for Families, Consumers, and Providers,* 3rd ed. Harper Perennial, 1995.

Vaddadi K: Stress of caregiving for the chronically mentally ill. Psychiatr Ann 1996;26(12):766.

Mood Disorders: Depressive Disorders

5

David Elkin, MD, Louann Brizendine, MD, Adriana Feder, MD, & Sheldon Vile, MD

Most people experience a wide range of moods during any given period of time (hours to weeks). Individuals who have depressive disorders experience persistent sadness and other symptoms that result in impaired, pessimistic thinking, which in turn can lead to poor choices and worsening life circumstances.

Depressive disorders are the most common psychiatric disorders. They cause high economic burdens on society and emotional suffering for affected patients. Key symptoms include depressed mood; pessimistic thinking; and changes in sleep, weight, and appetite. The depressive disorders have their roots in biological, psychological, and social factors. They can manifest in a number of different clinical presentations, and medical illnesses that mimic depression must always be ruled out before a depressive disorder can be diagnosed conclusively. Variants of depressive disorders include minor, acute, or chronic forms. Psychotherapy and medication provide effective treatment for most patients. Despite the prevalence of depressive disorders—especially in medical settings—and the high response rate to treatment, underdiagnosis and undertreatment are common. Challenging legal and ethical issues also arise in the care of patients who have depressive disorders.

The two major categories of mood disorders are the **depressive disorders** and **bipolar disorder** (previously termed **bipolar affective disorder** or **manic-depressive disorder**). Mood disorders are also called **affective disorders.** Patients who suffer from one or more depressive episodes have **major depressive disorder** (or **unipolar depression**). Patients who have two or more episodes have **recurrent depression.** Depressive disorders may be complicated by anxiety or somatic complaints. Patients who have a severe depression may also exhibit psychotic symptoms. Patients who experience episodes of both elevated mood (mania) and depressive episodes have **bipolar disorder.**

Other depressive disorders include dysthymic disorder, adjustment disorder, and bereavement. **Dysthymic disorder** or **dysthymia** is a milder but chronic form of depression that persists throughout the patient's adult life. Patients who react to a stressful life event with mild symptoms of anxiety and depression that last for less than 6 months have an **adjustment disorder. Bereavement** refers specifically to the psychological response to the loss or death of a significant person in the patients life; like adjustment disorder it is a time-limited phenomenon for most people. Figure 5–1 shows a comparison of the duration and severity of adjustment disorder, dysthymic disorder, and major depression.

MAJOR DEPRESSION: CLINICAL FEATURES

INCIDENCE

Major depression has been well-studied in the general population, where depression is remarkably common. The annual prevalence of depression is 10%. The lifetime prevalence—the chance that any individual will have an episode of major depression—25% for women and 15% for men.

The incidence of depression is even higher in primary care settings. Many depressed patients exhibit increased morbidity and mortality from other illnesses, as well as physical complaints that result from emotional distress. Depression has been detected in 12–36% of patients seen in outpatient medical clinics, and in up to 40% of patients in similar clinics in urban public health settings. A majority of patients who have depression seek help from their primary care physicians and may not turn to mental health professionals or even family members for help because of feelings of shame, guilt, and embarrassment. Unfortunately, primary care providers detect depression (and other psychiatric disorders) in fewer

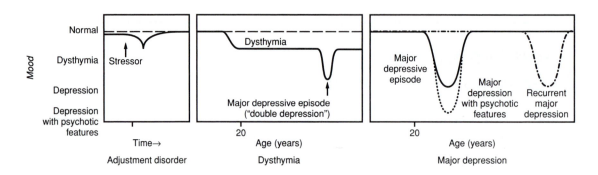

Figure 5–1. The duration and severity of depressive disorders. Adjustment disorder is a common time-limited syndrome of psychological distress that follows a major life stressor. Adjustment disorder presents with milder symptoms than major depression and lasts for fewer than 6 months. Dysthymia is a milder but more chronic depressive disorder that lasts most of the patient's adult life. Because of its chronicity dysthymic disorder often has profound effects on the patient's level of functioning and identity. Fewer than half of patients who have major depression have only one episode; more than half go on to have recurrent episodes. In most cases patients return to baseline functioning between episodes.

than half of all cases. Some patients receive inappropriate treatment, and others receive inadequate education about antidepressant medications, which can interfere with their adherence to the treatment plan. Only 5–10% of patients who have depression receive adequate care over their lifetime.

As one might expect, depression is more common among people who have no close personal relationships, and among divorced or separated people. There is no apparent correlation of socioeconomic status with depression.

The cost of depression for society is high. Depression causes more disability than do pulmonary disease or diabetes. Only cardiac disease results in more dysfunction. The direct treatment cost of depression is approximately $12 billion annually. An additional cost of $23 billion results from absenteeism, and premature death from suicide and worsening of other medical conditions costs an estimated $8 billion per year.

These financial costs should not overshadow the emotional cost of depression, for both patients and their families. Because the nature of psychological distress is different from physical manifestations of medical disease, the pain of the depressed patient is often unappreciated by families, friends, and physicians.

ETIOLOGY

Depression was previously classified as **reactive** to an external stressor or **endogenous** with a purely biological etiology. This division has been abandoned because of reporting biases in patients (who either downplay or exaggerate the importance of stressful events) and because the confluence of biological, psychological, and social factors that contribute to

the onset, maintenance, and recovery from depressed states is now more widely understood.

Biological Factors

A. Biogenic Amines. Mood disorders appear to be associated with heterogeneous dysregulation of the biogenic amines. Decreases in the levels of two of these neurotransmitters (norepinephrine and serotonin) are most often implicated in the pathophysiology of mood disorders.

B. Neuroendocrine Regulation. Abnormalities of the hypothalamic-pituitary-adrenal axis are commonly found in patients who have depression. Hypothyroidism sometimes appears as a depressive syndrome. Research has shown that hypercortisolism is common in depressed patients. Approximately half of depressed patients will therefore fail to exhibit a normal cortisol suppression response to a single dose of dexamethasone. This test is not diagnostically useful or routine because of high rates of false positives and negatives.

C. Neurophysiologic Abnormalities. The frontal and prefrontal lobes of most depressed patients appear to be hypoactive compared to normal controls. The degree of abnormal activity correlates roughly with the severity of the depressive episode. Subtle abnormalities of reduced volume of temporal and prefrontal lobes have also been noted, along with occasional small white matter abnormalities, especially in elderly patients.

D. Sleep Abnormalities. Sleep deprivation or disruption of circadian rhythms resulting from shift work or jet lag can lead to changes in mood and other symptoms of depression. Depression is associated with insomnia or hypersomnia (inadequate or excessive sleep, respectively) and with decreased REM sleep. Patients who have insomnia for more than 2 weeks without exhibiting other symptoms of depression are at increased risk of a major depressive episode. It is unclear whether sleep is a causal factor or a marker for depression.

E. Sunlight. Some patients who have depressive disorders and bipolar disorder notice that their depression worsens during winter months when total exposure to sunlight is decreased.

Genetic Factors

Twin, adoption, and family studies have shown that some patients may have a genetic predisposition toward major depressive disorder. The likelihood of having a mood disorder increases in first-degree relatives, compared to that of second-degree relatives. Patients who have early-onset illness (those who experience their first depressive episode before age 40) have greater familial risk factors than do those who experience late-onset illness.

Psychosocial Factors

A. Life Events & Environmental Stress. Stressful life events more often precede the first episodes of mood disorders than subsequent episodes. The loss of a parent before age 11 is the life event most often associated with the later development of depression. The loss of a spouse is the environmental stressor most often associated with the onset of an episode of depression. Other predisposing factors include lack of good social supports, experience of uncontrollable adverse events or trauma, and physical illness.

B. Psychoanalytic & Psychodynamic Factors. Various theories postulate the role of loss or threatened loss during childhood, an inability to express anger with consequent aggression turned against oneself, discrepancies between a patient's ideals and reality, and childhood deprivation or other factors that lead to lowered self-esteem and depression.

C. Learned Helplessness. The theory of learned helplessness views depression as the result of the subjects' perception of lack of control over their lives or environment. Experiments have shown that animals who are exposed repeatedly to inescapable electric shocks eventually give up and make no attempt to escape future shocks. Many depressed patients view themselves as having little control over their lives and see themselves as being at the mercy of other people or situations. According to this theory, depression can improve if the clinician helps the patient gain a sense of control and mastery of his or her environment.

D. Cognitive Theory. This theory views depression as a disorder of thinking. Depressed patients tend to be highly pessimistic and often think about themselves in a negative, self-defeating manner. Cognitive theory postulates that these negative thoughts lead to a depressed mood and the other symptoms of depression. Clinicians can help the patient to reconsider and control these negative thoughts.

Alice G, a 45-year-old legal assistant, came for her initial workup at a family practice outpatient clinic, stating that she was dissatisfied with her previous primary care physician. Records forwarded from the other clinic showed an increasing number of visits for various health problems over the year. Ms. G's complaints included fatigue and vague pains in her back, joints, and abdomen. Her appetite was decreased, and she had lost 20 pounds. Ms. G's previous physician could not find a physical basis for her symptoms and had written in one of his notes, "The patient is anxious and appears hysterical and hypochondriacal." However he did not request a psychiatry consultation or make a referral. He did prescribe diazepam (a benzodiazepine used to reduce anxiety) 1 month earlier, which Ms. G had found "helps me worry less, but I still have all of these problems."

Ms. G's new physician asked what she worried about. She asked the physician, "Do you think I could have cancer?" She became tearful and explained that her mother and husband had both died of cancer in the previous year. Thoughts of death and dying were becoming increasingly frequent and terrified her. She was upset about a recent demotion at work: "I always prided myself on my job performance, but I just can't think as clearly anymore." Her physician ran a brief screen for other symptoms of depression and learned that Ms. G had anhedonia, insomnia, and hopelessness, but did not have thoughts of suicide. Her sister and mother had histories of depression.

Recent tests for thyroid and other medical problems had been negative, and Ms. G's physical examination was not suggestive of any illness. Her new doctor explained that her symptoms were probably the result of depression. He prescribed an antidepressant, instructed Ms. G to taper off of the diazepam, and spent 15 minutes encouraging her to meet with a social worker about the clinic's depression and bereavement group. Ms G was skeptical but followed these recommendations. At her 6-week follow-up appointment, she had gained weight, appeared more energetic, and was pleased that her physical problems had resolved.

Discussion. Depressive disorders are common in medical settings but are often misdiagnosed. Ms. G's case had a good outcome, but earlier appropriate interventions could have spared her months of emotional distress and might have prevented her demotion at work. The savings in future inappropriate clinic visits and tests provide ample economic justification for the 15 extra minutes that her new physician spent addressing her depression.

COURSE OF DEPRESSION

The natural history of major depressive episodes is well-known from recorded histories of patients prior to the advent of effective treatment in the 1950s, and from the histories of patients who delay treatment for many years. Major depression is episodic in most cases, with resolution of symptoms and normal or near-normal mood and functioning between episodes. The average depressive episode lasts 7–14 months but may persist for longer than 2 years in up to 20% of depressed patients.

Broadly speaking, depressed patients follow one of three possible "trajectories." In almost half of all cases, a major depressive episode occurs only once in an individual patient's lifetime. At least half of patients who have a major depressive episode experience additional episodes of depression. Between 15 and 20% of all depressed patients have chronic rather than episodic depression; that is, the depression does not remit for more than brief periods without treatment.

Numerous studies have documented high levels of morbidity and mortality among depressed patients. Depression is closely linked to suicide attempts and completed suicides. Approximately 80% of suicide victims have histories consistent with depression. Of moderately to severely depressed patients, 15% commit suicide and many more make attempts. The severity of depressive episodes correlates with increases in suicide attempts and the rate of completed suicide, which was as high as 60% in one study of severely depressed patients.

DIAGNOSTIC ASSESSMENT

1. SIGNS & SYMPTOMS

The following symptoms often are observed in depressed patients:

- depressed mood (a pervasive sense of sadness) or signs of sadness evident to others (eg, tearfulness)
- **anhedonia** (loss of pleasure and interest in activities that the patient previously enjoyed)
- insomnia or hypersomnia
- appetite and weight disturbance (either increased or decreased)
- decreased energy (**anergia**) and a sense of fatigue or lethargy
- mild cognitive impairment of concentration, short-term memory, and decision-making ability
- social withdrawal
- decreased libido (diminished sexual drive)
- pervasive feelings and thoughts of guilt, shame, or pessimism
- frequent thoughts of death or suicide

The *DSM-IV* specifies that a diagnosis of depression requires that five or more of the above symptoms be present for at least 2 weeks. One of the five symptoms must be either depressed mood or anhedonia. Clinicians should also be alert to the following symptoms:

- anxiety symptoms such as feeling restless, worried, or fretful
- somatic complaints of diffuse and vague aches and pains
- psychotic symptoms, including auditory and visual hallucinations, delusions, or paranoia
- hypersensitivity to rejection
- excessive risk-taking behavior
- ruminations and obsessive thinking

Symptoms of anxiety such as worry and irritability occur in two-thirds of depressed patients. Major depression with psychotic features may manifest with psychotic symptoms ranging from subtle to overt. The presence of anxiety, rumination, and psychotic symptoms increases the likelihood that a depressed patient will attempt suicide.

2. MENTAL STATUS EXAMINATION

The important findings in the mental status examination of the depressed patient are categorized below. These findings tend to correlate with the severity of the depressive episode.

A. Appearance & Behavior. The depressed patient may be neat and well-groomed or may appear disheveled and exhibit poor hygiene. Posture and gait may be normal or slumped and slowed, respectively. Patients may look their stated age or older. They may appear thin, frail, or emaciated, or sometimes may be obese. Patients' facial expressions are usually sad, or their faces may seem motionless. Eye contact is often abnormal, with eyes turned downward or holding a fixed gaze and only intermittent contact with the examiner.

Slowed movements are common, but patients may seem restless in "agitated" depression. Specific mannerisms may be observed, such as hand-wringing, hair pulling or twirling, nail biting, pacing, and moaning or sighing in agitated depression. Patients usually cooperate with the interviewer, but they may indicate that they don't believe anyone can help them.

B. Language. Patients often talk slowly and may whisper, mumble, or speak in a monotone. Any difficulty with language comprehension should be noted, since this abnormality may indicate the presence of cerebral lesions.

C. Emotions. Patients usually report a sad mood, depressed mood or despair, hopelessness, guilt, self-loathing, or emptiness. Their emotional tone does not brighten even when talking about their favorite things (so-called **constricted effect**), or they may burst into tears seemingly for no reason (so-called **labile effect**).

D. Thought Processes. Patients' thought processes usually appear to be logical and goal-oriented. The rate and flow of ideas may be slower than normal, or a patient may say his or her mind is "empty of thoughts." Depressed patients often ruminate about an event, person, or specific concern, unable to shift their thoughts to another topic.

E. Thought Content. Depressed patients usually have an unrealistically low opinion of themselves. Their thoughts and ideas are often preoccupied with why they are bad or guilty. Other common preoccupations include death, dying, or bodily illness, even to a delusional extent. In cases of severe depression, patients may develop psychotic symptoms. The earliest sign is the experience of hearing one's name being called and turning to find no one there. Auditory hallucinations are more prominent in advanced cases of major depression with psychotic features; many patients hear people making derogatory comments about them. Paranoia may develop, with delusional thinking often centering around the patient's imagined guilt. Grandiosity and sensory/perceptual distortions are rare in depression. Suicidal thoughts occur frequently in depressed patients and should be explored fully (see Chapter 14).

F. Judgment & Insight. Depressed patients often exhibit impaired judgment as a result of distorted thinking. Insight varies from poor to good; some patients are aware that their thoughts are being influenced by depression, but with time and severity insight may be lost.

G. Cognitive Examination. Depressed patients are alert and oriented to person, place, and time. However, because they are often overwhelmed with emotions, they may have trouble concentrating. As a result, some cognitive tasks may be difficult, and immediate and recent memory are commonly impaired. In contrast to dementia, performance often improves with the interviewer's encouragement. Depressed patients of normal intelligence usually can give abstract responses to proverbs and similarities.

DIFFERENTIAL DIAGNOSIS

If a patient exhibits symptoms of depression, the clinician must first rule out medical causes, drug-induced depression, and other psychiatric disorders before diagnosing major depression.

1. RULING OUT MEDICAL CAUSES OF DEPRESSION

Symptoms that suggest depression, including weight loss, difficulty concentrating, and memory loss, can be produced by a variety of medical states. Medical mimics of depression may be suggested by the patient's history and the presence of either severe cognitive dysfunction or an abnormal physical exam (eg, alopecia, skin changes, slowed return on deep tendon reflexes in hypothyroidism). The following medical conditions can cause depression and must be ruled out before an accurate diagnosis of major depression can be made:

- infectious diseases: pneumonia, hepatitis, and mononucleosis are among the more common; meningitis, HIV, and Lyme disease are also potential causes
- cardiovascular diseases: myocardial infarction (heart attack), arrhythmias, and congestive heart failure
- cancers: tumors of the CNS, GI tract, or pancreas; leukemia; Hodgkin's disease
- CNS disorders: stroke, head injury, normal pressure hydrocephalus
- endocrine disorders: disorders of the hypothalamus, pituitary, thyroid, gonads, and adrenals
- systemic diseases: nutritional deficiencies, anemia, and autoimmune diseases such as lupus, multiple sclerosis, and acute intermittent porphyria
- other medical conditions: Huntington's chorea, Pick's disease, Alzheimer's dementia, and multiinfarct dementia

The clinician should perform or order a complete physical examination of the patient and a full laboratory workup, including the following tests:

- routine laboratory blood analysis for CBC, serum electrolytes, calcium, bilirubin, amylase, vitamin deficiencies, liver function tests, albumin, and total protein
- thyroid function tests (especially TSH)
- rapid plasma reagin (RPR) test to rule out syphilis
- HIV test
- toxicology screen to rule out drugs
- heavy metal screen
- electrocardiogram (EKG), if indicated
- head CT or MRI scan and electroencephalogram (EEG), if indicated

2. RULING OUT MEDICATION-INDUCED DEPRESSION

Common medications that can cause depression include steroids, methyldopa, oral contraceptives, and benzodiazepines. New data suggests that beta-blockers are not the CNS depressants they were once thought to be.

Alcohol, barbiturates, marijuana, amphetamine, cocaine, opiates, hallucinogens, and barbiturates can cause depression or may be used by depressed patients to self-medicate. Drug use is found in up to 50% of depressed outpatients, but many patients withhold this information from clinicians. If substance use is suspected, a serum or urine toxic analysis should be ordered.

3. RULING OUT PSYCHIATRIC DISORDERS

The following psychiatric disorders must be ruled out before depression can be diagnosed:

A. Adjustment Disorder. An adjustment disorder is a mild mood disturbance that occurs within 3 months of a stressful event and lasts no longer than 6 months. Adjustment disorder can be confused with major depression or a major depressive episode when it is associated with a depressed or anxious mood. Adjustment disorder is commonly seen in patients who are newly diagnosed with a medical illness or who have other life stressors such as divorce or job loss.

B. Bereavement. The symptoms of bereavement can be identical to a major depressive episode but follow the loss of a loved one for 2–3 months. Bereavement can result in sleep and appetite disturbance, as in major depression. The duration of normal bereavement can be culturally determined. In some cultures the phenomenon of seeing the deceased person is normal and is not evidence of psychosis.

C. Dysthymic Disorder. Dysthymic disorder is a form of chronic low-level depression that lasts for at least 2 years. Patients who have dysthymia are prone to superimposed episodes of major depression.

D. Bipolar Disorder. Over half of patients who have bipolar disorder are initially diagnosed as having another psychiatric disorder, usually major depression or schizophrenia. A depressed patient may later have an episode of mania and be diagnosed at that time as having bipolar disorder. Patients who have bipolar disorder type II have milder elevation of mood during hypomanic episodes, and as a result, the disorder may be misdiagnosed and incorrectly treated for many years. Antidepressants may "unmask" mania earlier in an individual's life than would have occurred naturally; however, antidepressants do not cause mania in patients who do not have bipolar disorder. If a manic episode results from antidepressant therapy, a diagnosis of bipolar disorder should be made.

E. Schizophrenia. It can be difficult to differentiate between depression with psychotic features and schizophrenia. Depressive symptoms in schizophrenia generally appear after the onset of psychosis, whereas in depression with psychotic features the mood disturbance comes before the onset of psychosis.

F. Schizoaffective Disorder. This diagnosis is given to patients whose symptoms and history demonstrate elements of both bipolar disorder and schizophrenia.

G. Personality Disorders. Individuals who have personality disorders do not tend to adjust well to life stresses and may have poor social networks. As a result, depression is seen more commonly in these individuals than in the general population. Patients who have obsessive-compulsive disorder (OCD) or borderline, histrionic, or dependent personality disorders are more likely to have a comorbid depressive disorder. The depression may also be chronic and fluctuating, often meeting the criteria for dysthymic disorder.

H. Anxiety Disorders. Many depressed patients also have severe anxiety; however, patients who have primary anxiety disorders such as panic disorder, OCD, and post-traumatic stress disorder have high rates of secondary depression. It may be difficult to distinguish between anxiety disorders and depressive disorders, although the patient's history, including the family history, may be helpful in determining the chronologic development of symptoms. Anxious patients also complain of somatic symptoms more often than do depressed patients.

I. Dementia. Depression can cause mild cognitive problems suggestive of dementia, and depression is common in the early stages of dementia. Sometimes it is impossible to distinguish between primary depression and dementia. Patients should then be started on empiric treatment for depression. A complete recovery eliminates the possibility of dementia.

TREATMENT OF MAJOR DEPRESSION

Most patients who have depression can be treated successfully as outpatients. Many depressed patients complain of suicidal ideation but can still be managed in outpatient settings if they have low risk factors for suicide. These factors include the ability to contract not to harm oneself, a negative past history of suicide attempts, lack of a suicide plan, and the absence of comorbid diagnoses associated with suicide risk such as substance use and borderline or antisocial personality disorders. Hospitalization may be indicated if the depressive episode is severe and the patient is highly suicidal, psychotic, catatonic, severely malnourished, or unable to care for himself or herself.

1. PSYCHOTHERAPY

For mild depressive episodes, certain forms of psychotherapy work well on their own. Therapy may be supportive in nature, for example, helping the patient to reidentify strengths and to increase self-confidence. Or therapy may be more insight-oriented, with the goal of having the patient learn more about his or her vulnerabilities to feelings of hopelessness and depression. Interpersonal psychotherapy and cognitive-behavioral psychotherapy are particularly effective.

Interpersonal psychotherapy uses the relationship between the therapist and patient as the curative agent. **Cognitive-behavioral therapy** (CBT) focuses on controlling pessimistic thinking so that the patient can break the cycle of negative thoughts, expectations, and actions. **Psychodynamic psychotherapy** focuses on past events and internal conflicts that may interfere with the patient's ability to achieve his or her full potential in the present. The therapist may be less interactive in this model. **Group psychotherapy** allows patients to receive support from others who can understand them, and to help patients achieve more effective relationships with friends, significant others, and at work. Group psychotherapy is cost-efficient and extremely effective, and may be increasingly utilized in an era of increased emphasis on cost control and managed care.

2. MEDICATION

In cases of moderate to severe depression, especially involving suicidal ideation, the presence of psychotic symptoms, or dysthymia, optimal treatment integrates psychotherapy and medication. Antidepressants are not addictive; however, patients treated with antidepressants alone tend to relapse when the medication is withdrawn. Psychotherapy appears to help patients address the root causes of depression and decreases the chance of relapse.

In choosing an antidepressant the clinician must consider the patient's previous history of response to an agent, family responses to medications, target symptoms, side-effect profile, cost, and the patient's suicide risk. Table 5–1 summarizes the different types of antidepressants, including their mechanisms of action and side effects.

The "art" of psychopharmacology involves forging a therapeutic alliance with the patient, understanding the symbolic value of medication, fielding questions and providing education, and helping the patient maintain hope for relief from depression while waiting for antidepressant medication and therapy to work. Adherence is related to the patient's education level and is inversely related to side effects. While physicians believe that 80-90% of their patients take their antidepressants as prescribed, only 40-50% of patients are actually adherent. Clinicians must decide when a patient's condition represents a partial or nonresponse to antidepressants and when to switch antidepressants or add or combine other agents such as lithium or thyroid hormone to achieve an optimal therapeutic response.

Once treatment has started, a response should be apparent to the patient and clinician within 2–4 weeks with most antidepressants. Many patients who believe that an antidepressant is not effective have not been on the medication for this minimum time period at maximally tolerated dosages necessary to justify this conclusion. Patients who have major de-

pression should take antidepressants for 9–12 months after achieving a complete remission of their depression. Although antidepressants are not addictive, stopping medications sooner often leads to a relapse.

Medications should be tapered slowly for several reasons. First, it may take several weeks or even months at a new dose level to achieve steady-state conditions, for brain receptors to adjust, and for depression to reappear. Second, stopping medications suddenly may result in a **discontinuation syndrome** with unpleasant flu-like symptoms. This is especially true for SSRIs with short half-lives such as paroxetine and fluvoxamine; the syndrome is rarely encountered with fluoxetine with its long half-life. Finally, the emotional impact of resurgent depressive symptoms may be disappointing and frustrating for the patient.

Clinicians should remember that depression is chronic in up to 20% of patients who may need to take antidepressants indefinitely after their first depressive episode and may need increased doses when stressed. No simple tests are available to determine when someone is ready to stop taking antidepressants, so dosages are gradually reduced to discover empirically if the patient is ready for a smaller dose or none at all. There have been no reports of adverse effects of long-term treatment with any antidepressant, although less data is available for the newer antidepressants.

There is currently no reliable way to predict which antidepressant will work in which dosages for any individual patient. A previous personal or family member's response to an antidepressant is predictive of a response. Otherwise the clinician must make the best choice based on the patient's symptoms and the mechanisms of action and side effects of each medication. Table 5–2 identifies some general guidelines for antidepressant use.

Types of Antidepressants

The oldest antidepressants are the **monoamine oxidase inhibitors (MAOIs).** They are effective in treating depressive episodes and yield superior responses compared to tricyclic antidepressants in the treatment of depression with atypical features and social phobia. Patients using MAOIs must strictly adhere to special diets free of foods containing tyramine and must avoid certain sympathomimetic medications and other antidepressants. Otherwise, a hypertensive crisis may result, possibly leading to a heart attack or stroke. These agents are rarely prescribed now that new agents are available.

Tricyclic antidepressants (TCAs) have the advantage of known safety, proven over decades of use. TCAs are more effective than are other antidepressants in the treatment of chronic pain syndromes, with or without associated depression. They are also inexpensive and probably just as effective as the newer antidepressants for depressive disorders, except atypical depression. However they have side ef-

Table 5-1. Types of antidepressants.[1]

Class	Generic Name	Trade Name	Mechanism of Action	Indications for Use	Usual Dosage Range	Side Effects	Comments	Potential Medication Interactions
SSRI	Fluoxetine	Prozac	Serotonin reuptake inhibition increases synaptic serotonin	Depressive disorders, anxiety disorders including OCD	10–80 mg/day	Nausea, headache, diarrhea, insomnia, sexual side effects	The first SSRI. Long half-life good for poor adherence and low chance of discontinuation symptoms. Very stimulating. Also approved for bulimia	Cytochrome P450 2D6, 2C, 3A4 (weak effect) All SSRIs may increase levels of TCAs, Bupropion, antipsychotics, type 1C antiarrhythmics, carbamazepine, and verapamil
	Sertraline	Zoloft			50–200 mg/day	As above. Slightly less stimulating. Discontinuation syndrome unlikely	Midrange in half-life and stimulation	Cytochrome P450 2D6 (weak effect), 2C (weak effect), 3A4 (weak effect)
	Paroxetine	Paxil			10–50 mg/day	As above. Least stimulating SSRI but can produce discontinuation syndrome	May be preferred to SSRIs for anxiety and insomnia	Cytochrome P450 2D6 (weak effect)
	Fluvoxamine	Luvox			100–300 mg/day in divided doses	As above. Discontinuation syndrome possible	Marketed only for treatment of OCD, but similar to other SSRIs	Cytochrome P450 1A2 (weak effect), 2C weal effect), 3A4 (weak effect)
TCA	Amitriptyline	Elavil	Block reuptake of norepinephrine and serotonin; also block histaminic, cholinergic, and α-1-adrenergic receptors	Depression, most anxiety disorders, adjunctive pain management	100–300 mg/day in divided doses	Dry mouth, blurred vision, constipation, urinary retention, delirium, worsening of narrow angle glaucoma, sedation, weight gain, postural hypotension, tremor, cardiac rate and conduction changes	Most anticholinergic TCA with most chance of sedation, orthostatic changes, and delirium	Caution advised with anticonvulsants, OCPs, cigarette smoking (lower TCA levels) Levels may be elevated by age, SSRIS, and antipsychotics
	Imipramine	Tofranil			100–300 mg/day in divided doses		First antidepressant discovered	
	Clomipramine	Anafranil			150–250 mg/day in divided doses		Only TCA approved for treatment of OCD. Almost as sedating as amitriptyline. Increased seizure risk.	
	Notriptyline	Pamelor			50–150 mg/day in divided doses		Can be titrated to therapeutic blood levels 50–150 µg/dl	
	Desipramine	Norpramin			150–300 mg/day in divided doses		Least sedating. Possibly stimulating in some patients	

Class	Generic	Brand	Mechanism	Indications	Dose	Side effects	Comments	Interactions
Other	Trazodone	Desyrel	Blocks serotonin reuptake, postsynaptic 5HT2A and histaminic receptors	Depression (see comment), sleep disorders	100–600 mg/day in divided doses	Extremely sedating, orthostatic hypotension. Priapism is rare, but is a medical emergency	Too sedating for use as a first-line antidepressant, but useful in low doses (25–100 mg) as a sleep aid. Somewhat effective as adjuvant treatment for pain, but less effective than TCAs.	Can increase levels of TCAs, triaz- and alprazolam, carbamazepine, astemizole
Novel agents	Nefazodone	Serzone	Blocks serotonin reuptake and postsynaptic 5HT2A	Depression, anxiety disorders	100–600 mg/day in divided doses	Lightheadedness, dizziness	Chemically related to trazodone but far less sedating. Few sexual side effects. May be especially useful for depression complicated by agitation and anxiety	Low potential for interactions
	Buproprion	Wellbutrin	Blocks serotonin and dopamine reuptake	Depression, possible use in adult ADHD	75–450 mg/day in divided doses	Headache, insomnia, nausea, irritability, seizure risk	Few sexual side effects. Stimulating; avoid in anxious patients. Higher risk of seizures avoidable using newer sustained release (SR) prepration.	
	Venlafaxine	Effexor	Blocks serotonin and norepinephrine reuptake	Depression, possibly anxiety disorders	75–375 mg/day in divided doses	Nausea, somnolence, dizziness, sweating, tremors, and hypertension (requiring weekly blood pressure monitoring)	Only antidepressant with shorter onset of action (1–2 weeks) and low protein binding	Neither an inducer or an inhibitor. However, metabolized by IDG pathway—quinidine, may increase venlafaxine levels
	Mirtazapine	Remeron	Increases serotonin and norepinephrine release. Blocks 5HT2 and 3. Histaminic antagonist	Depression, possibly anxiety disorders	15–45 mg/day in divided doses	Somnolence, increased appetite, weight gain, dizziness. Cholesterol and triglyceride levels, liver function levels may also increase	Sedating, anxiolytic in low doses, activating above 15 mg/day	Metabolized by most enzyme pathways Low potential for interactions
MAOI	Phenylzine	Nardil	Irreversible inhibition of monoamine oxidase	Depression (including atypical depression)	45–90 mg/day in divided doses	Postural hypotension, sexual side effects, weight gain, edema, myoclonus, paresthesias	Hypertensive crisis with stroke, heart attack possible if combined with tyramine-containing food or sympathomimetic medication. Strict adherence to tyramine-free diet necessary. Rarely used	Concurrent administration of sympathomimetics such as psychostimulants, amphetamines, decongestants, and TCAs can induce a hypertensive crisis
	Tranylcypromine	Parnate		anxiety disorders	30–40 mg/day in divided doses			

[1]Abbreviations: ADHD, attention deficit disorder with hyperactivity; MAOI, monoamine oxidase inhibitor; OCD, obsessive-compulsive disorder; SSRI, selective serotonin reuptake inhibitors; TCA, tricyclic antidepressants.

Table 5–2. Therapeutic guidelines for antidepressants.[1]

Depression with the Following Characteristics	Medication of Choice	Alternate Medication	Relative Contraindications
Uncomplicated depression	SSRI, TCA	Wellbutrin, Serzone, Effexor	
Prominent anxiety or insomnia	Low-dose[2] Paxil, Serzone ± benzodiazepine for anxiety ± trazodone 25–75 mg at night for insomnia	TCA, low-dose Prozac or Zoloft	High-dose SSRI, Wellbutrin
Elderly patients	Low-dose SSRI	Nortriptyline, desipramine, Wellbutrin, psychostimulants, Trazodone	TCAs with prominent orthotasis, anticholinergic effects
Chronic pain, fibromyalgia	TCA (effective for treating pain even in absence of depression)	(Wellbutrin, SSRI, Serzone not more effective for pain than placebo)	
Migraine	SSRI		
Cardiac disease	Low-dose SSRI	Wellbutrin	TCA (can cause arrhythmias, slowing)
Liver disease	Low-dose Paxil, Zoloft	Wellbutrin, Serzone, TCA	Prozac
Decreased libido	Wellbutrin, Serzone	TCA, SSRI (both classes may cause sexual side effects)	
Prominent fatigue	Prozac	Zoloft, Wellbutrin, Paxil, desipramine	Other TCAs
History of mania[3]	Wellbutrin	TCA, SSRI	
History of seizures[3]	Low-dose SSRI, Serzone	TCA (mild risk), Wellbutrin SR	Wellbutrin, clomipramine
Pregnancy[3]	Prozac	TCA after first trimester	MAOI
Concurrent substance use[4]	SSRIs		TCAs

[1]Abbreviations: MAOI, monoamine oxidase inhibitor; SR, sustained release; SSRI, selective serotonin reuptake inhibitors; TCA, tricyclic antidepressants.
[2]Low-dose SSRI = Prozac 10 mg every other day, Zoloft 12.5–25 mg/day, Paxil 5–10 mg/day.
[3]Psychiatric consultation strongly recommended.
[4]For an accurate assessment for mood disorder, the patient should abstain from substance use for >1 month before being evaluated. Some studies suggest SSRIs can be used with minimal risk in patients who have severe depression and suicidality and use alcohol if they are highly motivated to stop drinking.

fects that stem from their anticholinergic effects such as dry mouth, blurry vision, constipation, and urinary retention. These side effects may reduce adherence and necessitate more outpatient visits and more inpatient hospitalizations, thus driving up the overall cost of TCAs. They also have a low ratio of effective to toxic dose; the LD50 (average lethal dose) is as low as 750 mg, or a week's supply.

In the elderly and in patients with neuronal loss (eg, resulting from head trauma or HIV dementia), TCAs may cause anticholinergic delirium. In therapeutic doses TCAs have antiarrythmic actions similar to quinidine. A pretreatment EKG is recommended in older patients. At higher doses TCAs cause cardiac conduction delays with increased PR, QRS, and QT

intervals, bundle branch block, ventricular tachycardia or first, second, or third degree heart block. Most patients who attempt to commit suicide with a TCA overdose are therefore admitted to intensive care units to monitor their cardiac status.

Trazodone (Desyrel) is in a unique class of agents that possesses no anticholinergic action. It is extremely sedating and can also cause low blood pressure, which may result in falls (especially in elderly patients) and difficulty tolerating large doses. **Priapism** (a non-resolving penile erection) is a rare side effect, but it is considered a medical emergency. In a recent meta-analysis trazodone appears less likely to benefit patients than do other agents (effective in only 50% of patients). However trazodone is useful in low doses (25–100 mg) as a nonaddictive sleep aid for patients who have primary insomnia or insomnia as a side effect of other antidepressants.

The **selective serotonin reuptake inhibitors (SSRIs)** became well-known during the 1980s with the introduction of fluoxetine (Prozac) and are now the most commonly prescribed antidepressants in the United States. SSRIs block the reuptake of 5HT chemical transport system, thus increasing serotonin in the synaptic space. SSRIs are less toxic than TCAs and therefore much less likely to result in death during an overdose.

Initial side effects include nausea, headache, increased insomnia or agitation, and sexual dysfunction (decreased sexual drive or anorgasmia). SSRIs are expensive (approximately $2 per pill, with one to two pills per day as a standard dose), but they are associated with improved adherence and fewer outpatient visits and hospitalizations, which may place their overall cost-effectiveness on a par with TCAs. Up to one-third of patients on SSRIs will experience sexual dysfunction for the entire time that they are taking these antidepressants. Usual sexual side effects include decreased sexual drive, difficulty or inability to achieve erections in men or orgasms in women. These patients may need to change medications or else take another drug at the same time to counteract this side effect. Medications useful for this purpose include the antidepressant buproprion (Wellbutrin), the anxiolytic busprione (BuSpar), or the antihistamine cyproheptadine (Periactin).

In contrast to TCAs, SSRIs often produce robust responses at low doses but require upward titration to maintain the response, until the therapeutic dose is reached. Thus patients taking too low a dose of an SSRI will often complain that their medication has stopped working. Patients should be educated about this possibility and reassured that continuous dosage increases will not be necessary.

Fluoxetine has a long half-life and is advantageous for patients who frequently forget to take pills. Sertraline (Zoloft) and fluoxetine are termed "activating" because they increase patients' energy and are believed to be useful in patients who exhibit low energy and are sleeping more than usual (although no studies exist to support this). Because activating antidepressants may also produce insomnia and increased anxiety in susceptible patients, they should be used cautiously or avoided in patients who have anxiety, insomnia, or a history of panic disorder or sensitivity to caffeine.

Paroxetine (Paxil) is more sedating in some patients and is therefore useful in treating patients whose depression is associated with insomnia and anxiety. Fluvoxamine (Luvox) has been marketed and approved selectively for treatment of OCD but is most likely effective for antidepressant.

The SSRIs appear to have advantages in patients who experience ruminative thinking or aggression (which may be related to low serotonin levels) with their depressions. These medications are also useful for treating OCD (which is associated with low levels of serotonin in key areas of the brain) or dysthymia. Their low toxicity makes them safer in patients who are at high risk for side effects or suicide attempts.

Newer medications include buproprion (Wellbutrin), venlafaxine (Effexor), nefazodone (Serzone), and mirtazapine (Remeron). Buproprion produces no greater incidence of sexual side effects than does a placebo. It is activating and therefore contraindicated in depressed patients who have severe anxiety or panic attacks but is effective for depression. It is somewhat effective as a nonaddictive alternative to psychostimulants in the treatment of attention deficit disorder in adults. Care must be taken not to exceed 300 mg per day because the incidence of seizures rises to greater than 1 in 250, a problem avoided with the new SR (sustained-release) preparation. Venlafaxine has both noradrenergic and serotonergic activity and therefore a high side-effect profile, consistent with TCAs and SSRIs. However, it may be useful in patients who do not respond to initial trials of other first-line agents. Nefazodone is chemically related to trazodone but has fewer side effects and is helpful in treating patients who exhibit depression with prominent anxiety or insomnia. It also has a very low incidence of sexual side effects.

Approximately 60–70% of patients who have depression will respond well to the first or second antidepressant medication that they try. If a patient is not responding, the clinician should determine whether other factors are interfering with the patient's response, such as poor adherence, undiagnosed substance use, undiagnosed medical disorders such as hypothyroidism or sleep apnea, or comorbid psychiatric disorders (most commonly personality, anxiety, or bipolar disorders). If none of these factors is present, the patient is classified as "treatment resistant," or a "non-responder." These patients will need to try other strategies such as switching antidepressants, augmentation with other medications alone or in combination (see Table 5–3), or electroconvulsive therapy (ECT).

Table 5–3. Possible augmentation strategies for antidepressants for treatment-resistant depression.[1]

Change classes of medication (TCA → SSRI → Wellbutrin → Venlafaxine)
Combinations of medications
   SSRI + low-dose TCAs
   SSRI + Buspirone
   SSRI + low-dose Wellbutrin
Add to antidepressants
   LIthium carbonate
   Thyroid hormone
   Psychostimulants
   Phototherapy
ECT

[1]Abbreviations: SSRI, selective serotonin reuptake inhibitors; TCA, tricyclic antidepressants.

3. ELECTROCONVULSIVE THERAPY

Several antidepressant trials are typically completed before considering ECT; however, ECT is indicated for treatment-resistant depression and for patients who cannot tolerate medication side effects for various reasons, including medical illness or advanced age. ECT is also indicated for some cases of delusional or catatonic depression.

Alternatives have been sought to ECT because of side effects on short-term memory and its social stigma. **Transcortical magnetic stimulation** may be the next advance in the treatment of severely depressed patients. This procedure involves the generation of strong electromagnetic fields on the patient's scalp, which induces electrical stimulation of the cortex. Results in preliminary tests indicate high efficacy with fewer side effects than ECT.

4. ALTERNATIVE TREATMENTS FOR DEPRESSION

Physicians should be aware of alternative treatments for depression that their patients may be using. These treatments include herbs and over-the-counter remedies. Melatonin has achieved near-cult status and is widely used for sleep disturbances, jet lag, and depression. However, it has not been approved or studied by the FDA, and there are concerns that impurities in the preparation of melatonin could cause untoward side effects.

Some patients use herbal preparations to medicate their depression. Saint John's Wort and valerian root are the most common examples. Valerian can be taken in liquid, tea, or capsule form and is believed to have serotonergic properties and may have mild anxiolytic and antidepressant effects. Spirulina seaweed capsules contain L-tryptophan, the precursor of serotonin. These substances are naturally occurring and are considered safe to use. There is a theoretic risk of serotonin overload when serotonergic herbs are used with SSRIs. Scientific studies of the efficacy of alternative therapies have yet to be performed in the United States, although several German studies of St. John's Wort appear promising.

5. TREATMENT OF SLEEP DISORDERS ASSOCIATED WITH DEPRESSION

Sleep disorders occur frequently in depressive and anxiety disorders. Primary insomnia—insomnia not associated with another psychiatric disorder—is a common complaint among patients in medical clinics. Insomnia secondary to psychiatric disorders such as major depression or post-traumatic stress disorder (PTSD), or due to side effects from activating antidepressants may be very frustrating to patients and worsen complaints of sadness and decreases in concentration and energy.

Individuals who have persistent insomnia at any point in their lives—even when associated with a discernible stressor—are now known to be at high risk for later developing depression. Sleep disturbances may thus be an early marker for the ultimate manifestation of depressive disorders.

Low-dose trazodone is an effective sleep aid that does not interfere with sleep architecture (the proportion of Stage I–IV and REM sleep). Patients should also be encouraged to follow basic behavioral guidelines for sleep "hygiene":

- Wake at the same time every morning (preferably early).
- Do not take daytime naps even if tired.
- Spend a maximum of 20–30 minutes of unsuccessfully trying to sleep in bed. Get out of bed after that time and perform a relaxing activity (eg, reading, knitting) for half an hour and try to sleep again. This step loosens the association between the bed and anxiety about not sleeping.
- Get at least 20 minutes of light exercise (eg, walking), preferably in the morning.
- Consider bright-light or sun exposure in the morning to reset circadian rhythms.
- Minimize the use of alcohol.
- Avoid or minimize caffeine intake (including black tea, colas, and chocolate) after dinner.
- Take diuretics as late as possible in the day to minimize the need to urinate at night.

Patients may require encouragement with these behavioral prescriptions, which have been shown to be remarkably effective even in long-standing insomnia.

FACETS OF MAJOR DEPRESSION

Depression With Atypical Features

Depression with atypical features is marked by a reversal of the usual findings in major depression. For example, patients eat more, are likely to gain weight, sleep more, and easily feel rejected by others. Anxiety is also prominent, even more so than in patients who have major depression. SSRIs and MAOIs are more efficacious than TCAs in treating atypical depression.

Depression With Seasonal Component

Major depressive episodes and bipolar disorder may follow a seasonal and predictable pattern over the course of many years. Most commonly, symptoms of depression occur in the winter, and mania appears in the spring or summer months. A reverse pattern (ie, depression in summer) can occur but is not as typical. Increased sleep and appetite as well as psychomotor slowing are common. This seasonal pattern must be somewhat consistent and not due to environmental factors such as regular unemployment.

It also underscores the presumed biological mechanism believed to be responsible for the onset of this disorder. Seasonal depression is believed to be related to a decrease in melatonin production by the pineal gland during winter months.

Some clinicians have termed this disorder **seasonal affective disorder (SAD,** an appropriate acronym). Some degree of seasonal mood change is seen in the general population, and SAD is at the more pronounced end of the clinical spectrum. In a recent study based on meta-analysis of twins, seasonal depressions were seen to have a genetic association in almost one-third of the patients.

Antidepressants or light therapy (involving exposure to light of specific wavelengths and strength) are effective for treating SAD. Annual treatment or treatment that follows the illness' seasonal course is often necessary due to the recurrent nature of SAD. Patients may find it helpful to learn early signs of depression and to anticipate the need to resume or increase treatment.

Major Depression With Psychotic Features

If a major depressive episode goes untreated it may become so severe that psychotic symptoms develop. Hallucinations and delusions are usually of a mood-congruent nature. For example, patients may become convinced that they have done something wrong or are about to be punished, or a somatic delusion may develop involving the belief that the patient's body is breaking down or rotting from the inside out. The patient's history and family history should be used to rule out other psychiatric disorders such as schizophrenia or schizoaffective disorders.

Mina M, a 48-year-old woman, was referred to a psychiatrist by a friend after months of depression and somatic concerns. Ms. M had become increasingly upset over the previous 4 months and noticed problems with memory and concentration.

She had little energy, slept poorly, and was very anxious and ruminative. However, her complaints focused primarily on physical problems: aches in her back and extremities, headaches, sharp pains in her abdomen, and other gastrointestinal (GI) complaints. She saw numerous internists, general practitioners, and gastroenterologists and had multiple laboratory tests, GI series, and abdominal CT scans, which revealed nothing abnormal.

She remained convinced that she had a physical problem but agreed to meet with a psychiatrist, who noted that Ms. M was sad and tearful but did not describe herself as depressed. She mentioned feeling fearful at times, and related hearing her name being called, as well as furtive images of "seeing men out of the corner of my eye." On several occasions while alone she heard a low voice making derogatory comments about her.

Ms. M was started on low doses of perphenazine (Trilafon), an antipsychotic that has some sedating properties, for psychotic symptoms and an SSRI for depression. Within days her visual and auditory hallucinations ceased, and she was sleeping better. Perphenazine was stopped after 3 weeks. Her psychotic thinking did not return. After 4 weeks, she felt completely normal, with good energy and self-esteem and no somatic complaints. She accepted a referral to weekly group psychotherapy.

Diagnosis. Major depression with psychotic features (Axis I).

Discussion. Neuroleptics are useful for the treatment of major depression with psychotic features during the first few weeks, until the psychotic symptoms have cleared. Antidepressants are used concurrently. Treatment is otherwise similar to that used for uncomplicated major depression. ECT is also effective for depression with psychotic features. Failing to diagnose psychotic symptoms and treating patients with antidepressants alone (rather than adding antipsychotics) leads to treatment failure in 80% of the cases.

Depressive Disorder Not Otherwise Specified (NOS)

Other manifestations of depression include premenstrual dysphoria and depression that commonly occurs in other psychiatric disorders such as schizophrenia and delusional disorder.

Mild depressive disorders that meet fewer than five *DSM-IV* criteria for major depression would receive a diagnosis of depressive disorder not otherwise specified (NOS). Some clinicians have proposed a new diagnostic category called **subacute depressive disorder.** Patients who have this disorder exhibit higher rates of disruption of work and social relationships than do those without symptoms of depression. Other patients appear to have brief recurrent depressive episodes that last less than the 2-week minimum stipulated in the *DSM-IV.* Medication and psychotherapy appears to be effective in treating these disorders.

Depression in the Elderly

Symptoms of depression in the elderly, including decreased energy, insomnia, ruminations about death, anhedonia, social withdrawal, decreased sexual drive, and cognitive difficulties may all be underappreciated and dismissed as being somehow normal or age-appropriate. Depression may be more severe in elderly patients who exhibit psychotic or catatonic features. Dementia and medical mimics of depression are very common in elderly patients and should always be ruled out before treatment is started. Many depressed elderly patients are misdiagnosed as having dementia.

Previous clinical belief that the elderly would not benefit from psychotherapy has been disproved. Support groups may help relieve social isolation. As a result of misdiagnosis, many geriatric patients fail to benefit from readily available treatment.

Clinicians should remember to use lower dosages of medications in the elderly to compensate for lower metabolism and to avoid side effects. Tricyclic antidepressants should probably be avoided because of side effects.

Sarah D, aged 80, was referred to the psychiatry clinic after complaining to her internist about insomnia. A screen for symptoms of major depression revealed that Ms. D had additional symptoms of hopelessness, low energy, anhedonia, poor concentration, and a strong sense of guilt. She had become extremely withdrawn from her friends and had frequent thoughts of illness and death. She felt that the depression had developed relatively suddenly 3 months earlier. There was no previous psychiatric history and her history, physical examination, and laboratory testing ruled out medical illness. A cognitive screen was normal, eliminating dementia. Ms. D took few over-the-counter medications and denied substance abuse.

Ms. D was a retired schoolteacher whose husband had died 15 years earlier. She lived alone and prided herself on her fastidious nature, as well as an adventurous spirit that led her to travel extensively. She was extremely close to a single surviving sister who lived on the East Coast. Four months earlier, the sister had written to Ms. D, stating that she was breaking off contact with her because of a disagreement over their brother's will.

Ms. D was started in weekly psychotherapy, which was supportive in nature. She was asked to record her thoughts and learned to stop some of the negative thoughts that made her feel "like a bad person." She was also asked to take an inventory of her strengths and to reconnect with friends. After a negative EKG and cardiac exam, she was started on paroxetine (Paxil), and reported improved sleep within the first week and improved mood by the fourth week. Two months later, she was able to confront her sister in writing and to orchestrate a reconciliation. She ceased therapy 2 months after that to join a group of friends for a long cruise to the South Pacific and Asia.

Depression in Children

Depression in children may manifest in a very different fashion than in adults. Symptoms may include worsening school performance, truancy, behavior problems such as antisocial actions (eg, shoplifting or fire-setting) or outbursts of anger, sexual promiscuity, and regression. Children who have depression should be screened for medical illness, substance use, and other psychiatric disorders such as schizophrenia. Environmental stressors such as physical, emotional, or sexual abuse should also be investigated.

Alexithymia

One of the standard questions used to evaluate the diagnosis of depression asks about the patient's mood. But some patients do not seem to be aware of their mood at all. The term **alexithymia** comes from the Greek words for "no words for feelings." Alexithymia is not a diagnosis but describes a style by which patients fail to recognize their internal emotional states and therefore cannot answer questions about their mood. These patients are prone to express emotional distress with somatic symptoms and may be severely depressed, but an objective observer might only infer this from numerous physical complaints.

Patients who have alexithymia are likely to present at a health-care setting with somatic complaints that have no discernible physical cause. Since patients who have alexithymia are unable to give an account of their subjective mood states, evaluation and treatment should be centered on other symptoms of depression, such as sleep disturbance or fatigue. Psychotherapy may help these patients identify and talk about their emotions.

PREVENTION OF DEPRESSION

Psychotherapy, stress management, and cognitive restructuring may help prevent recurrent episodes of depression. Early recognition and treatment of trauma, child abuse, or loss in childhood may decrease the incidence of depression many years later. Genetic counseling may someday become appropriate.

DYSTHYMIC DISORDER: CLINICAL FEATURES

Dysthymic disorder or dysthymia is characterized by chronic, low-level symptoms of depression. Like depression, dysthymia is common but often underdiagnosed and undertreated. Unlike most cases of major depression, dysthymia is a lifelong rather than episodic disorder that starts in adolescence or early adulthood.

INCIDENCE

The annual incidence of dysthymia in the United States is 3% of the population. The lifetime prevalence of dysthymia for any individual is 6%. The 2:1

female-to-male ratio also seen in depression means that 13% of women will qualify for the diagnosis over a lifetime.

ETIOLOGY

The etiology of dysthymia is similar to depression, with a confluence of biological, psychological, and social causes.

COURSE OF DYSTHYMIA

Patients who have dysthymia often report that they never stop feeling depressed. Although they may be able to function, they are constantly sad, plagued by self-doubts and occasional bouts of despair. Patients often experience onset of the illness in their teens or early twenties. Their depression must include three of the depressive disorders criteria listed earlier and have lasted for at least 2 years in order for them to qualify for the diagnosis. Patients who have dysthymia tend to have appetite disturbance less frequently than do depressed patients (5% versus 53%). Anhedonia and difficulties concentrating are also much less common in dysthymia than in chronic major depressive.

Left untreated the natural history of dysthymia is unremitting and results in chronic feelings of low self-esteem and diminished self-confidence. The cost of dysthymia can be easily underappreciated by an outside observer. As one patient explained:

> Think back to the last time that you were experiencing a bad day, when everything seemed bleaker than usual, when your thoughts were more negative. You're pessimistic about everything, and the joy in life just isn't there. You have a hard time getting anything done, because everything is an effort. At the end of the day you doubt your resolve to have things be different, and worse yet you start to doubt yourself. The next day you feel better. But imagine that almost *every* day of your adult life is like that. You lose your perspective. You don't think, Oh, this is depression, it's a disease. You start to think, This is *me*, I'm lazy, stupid, and things are never going to be any better than this. You can see how hard life can be.

Patients who have dysthymia often feel that even if they accomplish as much as their peers they are exerting much more effort, as if they are moving through life with an anchor dragging behind them.

MENTAL STATUS EXAMINATION

The mental status examination of the dysthymic patient is similar to that seen in patients who have mild to moderate depression. Note that patients who have dysthymia do not exhibit psychotic symptoms unless they have a superimposed episode of major depression, drug use, or a personality disorder.

DIFFERENTIAL DIAGNOSIS

As in the case of other depressive disorders, dysthymia must be distinguished from medical causes, chronic and recurrent depressive episodes, bipolar disorders, and substance use. Patients who have dysthymia should also be screened for anxiety, personality, and eating disorders, all of which are common comorbid disorders.

TREATMENT OF DYSTHYMIA

Psychotherapy alone is only weakly effective for treating dysthymia; antidepressants combined with psychotherapy offer a much greater probability of success. The SSRIs have fewer side effects than do TCAs, but both are equally effective in treating dysthymia. Most clinicians agree that dysthymia requires a longer period of treatment with antidepressants than for major depressive episodes, probably longer than 1 year. Studies are in progress to determine the relapse rate of dysthymia following treatment and whether chronic treatment is necessary.

Sometimes dysthymia leaves the patient with an identity that is strongly tied to a depressive outlook on life. What may have been an eminently reversible disorder at age 25 may be much more difficult to change 20 years later.

> Bertram M, aged 46, felt that his life "wasn't going anywhere." Although he had done well in college and had graduated with a degree in engineering, he had held minimum wage jobs, had chronic low-level depression with poor self-esteem and motivation that ultimately led to his wife deciding to leave him. The separation precipitated an episode of major depression. He responded extremely well to fluoxetine and group therapy. Group members lauded him for his increased energy and enthusiasm. He began dating and participating in social events 4 times a week or more. He became more ambitious at work.
>
> After 2 months he appeared more depressed and told group members that he had stopped antidepressants, explaining, "it just wasn't me." In spite of objective improvement, he had spent his entire adult life with dysthymia and perceived his nondepressed state as alien. He left the group and infrequently called the psychiatrist, still complaining of feeling "stuck" but unwilling to restart antidepressants or therapy.
>
> **Diagnosis.** Dysthymic disorder (Axis I).

DEPRESSION DUE TO SUBSTANCE USE: CLINICAL FEATURES

Drugs and alcohol dependence and abuse are common in the United States, and depressed mood is often encountered in the setting of substance use. Depressive or dysthymic symptoms are associated with alcohol dependence and the use of other CNS depressants. Other drugs, such as heroin, produce euphoria in the intoxication phase but long-term use is associated with depression. The manic or psychotic states that often occur in intoxication from stimulants such as cocaine and methamphetamines are often followed by a "crash" with depressive symptoms, and the effects of long-term use of these substances often include depression.

The relationship between depressive disorders and substance use is complex. Researchers have postulated a number of possible relationships between drug use and depression. These relationships include the following:

- Depressed patients may "self-medicate" with drugs that ultimately worsen their mood disorder.
- Drug use can precipitate depression in patients who might not otherwise be vulnerable, and depressive symptoms may persist after drug use is stopped.
- Some patients may be genetically and psychologically vulnerable to both drug use and depression.
- Depression and drug use could occur independently of each other, and their association is coincidental.

Each of these theories may hold true in subsets of all patients who have depression. The clinician's challenge in treating depression in the face of substance use is to know when separate treatment for depression is warranted.

At one end of the spectrum are researchers and clinicians who advocate treating depressive symptoms aggressively immediately after patients stop using drugs or indicate their willingness to remain abstinent. This rationale is based on a desire to alleviate suffering and to eliminate depression as a risk factor for drug-use relapse.

Other physicians believe that patients should have abstained from taking drugs for at least 6 months before determining that depressive symptoms will not remit on their own. These physicians worry about the health risks posed by patients simultaneously using antidepressant medication and drugs, or of substituting one psychological "crutch" for another. Studies exist that support both views. The decision of whether and when to start antidepressants therefore remains a matter of clinical judgment. Most physicians wait for several weeks or months until sobriety is assured before prescribing medication.

Frank J, a 48-year-old salesman, was referred for a psychiatric evaluation after failing to respond to two trials of antidepressants. His medical history was notable for hypertension and occasional unexplained rises in his liver function tests.

Mr. J had become very depressed in the past 6 months, complaining of problems sleeping, weight loss, and prominent anxiety. He also expressed suicidal thoughts, which alarmed his referring family practitioner. The psychiatrist noted that Mr. J had numerous risk factors for substance abuse, including a positive family history of alcoholism and two motor vehicle accidents in the previous 20 months. When confronted with this possibility, Mr. J initially denied substance use but finally admitted, "I drink more than I like to think." He expressed his fears that he "can't handle my job without alcohol. It's stressful, and my customers consider it insulting to refuse to go out drinking after we meet." He also worried that he would not be able to sleep without "a couple of stiff drinks."

Treatment consisted of a referral to an alcohol treatment center, which the patient reluctantly accepted. Mr. J participated in group therapy and through individual counseling gained insight into the extent of his dependence on alcohol. Increased contact with his family led to a reappraisal of his life and a more detailed history of depressive symptoms in his early 20s shortly before he began drinking heavily.

Mr. J's first month of sobriety was marked by two slips as he experienced increased anxiety. At 6 weeks he remained depressed, and an SSRI antidepressant was prescribed. Mr. J was doing well at 1 year follow-up with good adherence to medication and therapy, improved mood, and only one other episode of drinking at a party to celebrate his promotion at work.

Diagnosis. Depression due to substance use (Axis I).

ADJUSTMENT DISORDER: CLINICAL FEATURES

Most people develop mild symptoms of psychological distress following any difficult transition or event. Common stressful events include divorce or the end of a close relationship, loss of a job, moving, starting college (or medical school), and medical illness. Attempts by researchers to quantify the impact of these stressful events has led to a widely used hundred point scale.

INCIDENCE

Everyone is believed to experience stressful life events at some time during their lives. The lifetime prevalence of adjustment disorder is therefore believed to be at or near 100%.

ETIOLOGY

The psychological impact of stressful life events depends on external variables such as the event itself and the circumstances in the patient's life. Important internal variables include the preexisting psychopathology and coping styles and strategies. A patient who has borderline personality disorder and a history of several episodes of depression and who tends to react with extreme emotional lability and catastrophic thinking (ie, "I will never make it through this!") is at much greater risk for developing an adjustment disorder following the break-up of a relationship than does someone with no previous psychiatric history.

COURSE OF ADJUSTMENT DISORDER

Adjustment disorder manifests with symptoms similar to those seen in major depressive episodes, such as insomnia, difficulty concentrating, feelings of sadness, and anhedonia. Suicidal ideation and feelings of worthlessness are less common. The symptoms seen in adjustment disorder are much less severe and pervasive than are symptoms of depression. By the *DSM-IV* definition, adjustment disorder begins within 3 months of the stressor and ends within 6 months after the stressor ends. Adjustment disorder has several clinical variants, manifesting with predominant symptoms of anxiety, depression, a mixture of anxiety and depression, or a disturbance of behavior.

Daniel M was a 20-year-old college freshman seen in student health services on his dormitory advisor's recommendation. Mr. M had transferred from a college across the country 3 months earlier. His girlfriend of 2 years had also agreed to transfer schools but announced at the last minute that she was breaking up with him and was not coming. Mr. M was now experiencing insomnia and difficulty concentrating on class assignments. He had no previous personal or family history of mental illness, denied substance use, and denied other symptoms of major depression such as anhedonia or suicidality.

Mr. M was given a prescription for Trazodone 50 mg at night for insomnia, and a copy of the clinic's sleep hygiene guidelines. Short-term psychotherapy focused on his adaptation to the move and the dissolution of his relationship.

Mr. M found the sessions helpful "as a place to talk about this stuff" and ended therapy after 8 weeks when his symptoms abated. He was doing well at 6-month follow-up, having received good grades and making a number of new friends.

Diagnosis. Depression due to adjustment disorder (Axis I).

TREATMENT OF ADJUSTMENT DISORDER

Adjustment disorder can progress to a major depressive episode, but most patients experience full relief within several months. During that time, however, patients may find that adjustment disorder symptoms such as insomnia and problems concentrating interfere with their relationships or job performance. Treatment often consists of brief, supportive psychotherapy focused on current emotional reactions and coping strategies.

Therapy has two goals: relieving symptoms and shortening the course of recovery. Most patients are relieved that they can expect complete recovery within a short time. Medication such as low-dose trazodone (Desyrel) is sometimes used as a sleep-aid. Benzodiazepines may be helpful for relief of acute anxiety, but their extended use is not recommended. In some cases, the severity of symptoms makes it impossible to differentiate between adjustment disorder and a major depressive episode. In these cases, a diagnosis of depression is often made and the use of antidepressants may be warranted.

BEREAVEMENT: CLINICAL FEATURES

Bereavement refers to the syndrome of emotional distress seen in most people after the death of a close friend, family member, or pet. Bereavement is similar in etiology, symptomatology, and course to adjustment disorder. Bereavement may intensify and become a major depressive epidsode, which may also follow the death of a friend or family member. However bereavement is rarely associated with decreased self-esteem or suicidality. Up to 50% of widows develop depressive symptoms in the first year after their spouse's death, and 15% are still depressed 2 years later. Bereavement may manifest with depressive symptoms with hallucinations of hearing or seeing the deceased person. Clinicians should consider major depression with psychotic features but should also realize that this phenomenon is both common and nonpathologic in some cultural groups. PTSD and somatization are also seen in bereavement.

TREATMENT OF BEREAVEMENT

Treatment of bereavement is similar to that for adjustment disorder. Bereavement support groups may help many patients. Bereavement groups are often coordinated by hospital personnel, especially in clinics and wards that have high death rates, such as oncology and AIDS clinics, or are sponsored by community organizations. Other family members may also benefit from support groups.

EMOTIONAL REACTIONS TO PATIENTS

Interactions with depressed patients often produce feelings of sadness, frustration, and hopelessness in those around them, including health-care providers. This effect may be especially helpful if a clinician can learn to recognize these feelings. These feelings may become useful as indicators of the presence of depression in patients or of comorbid anxiety and personality disorders or substance use. The physician may also use them to gain a window into the patient's experience of the illness.

Karl B, a 50-year-old engineer, came to the medical clinic very frequently, sometimes once or twice a week, with vague complaints of low energy, insomnia, and pain in his stomach, chest, joints, and extremities. He had been laid off from work recently. Questions about his mood went unanswered; Mr. B gave vague responses and failed to describe his emotions. Because his appointments were often "add-ons" to the drop-in clinic, he spent only 5–10 minutes with a physician.

One day Mr. B was seen by a medical student who again found no physical basis for his complaints. Although the student had been in a good mood earlier in the day, she found herself angry with Mr. B and depressed afterwards. Another medical student passed her in the hall and asked why she looked so glum. Suddenly she had a

flash of insight. It had all started when she interviewed Mr. B.

What if her thoughts and emotions had become attuned to him during their brief interaction? If this was even a portion of what he was experiencing, Mr. B might be very depressed. She had her supervising resident endorse her decision to refer Mr. B to the outpatient psychiatry clinic for a further evaluation.

Two months later, the student passed Mr. B in the hallway. He seemed like a different person, with a great deal more energy and enthusiasm than when she saw him in the clinic. He had started taking an antidepressant and was attending a support group. He thanked her for the referral to the psychiatry clinic. "I was in a bad space a few months ago, but I feel much better now. I'm trying to find work. And all of those aches and pains cleared up, too."

Diagnosis. Major depression (Axis I).

Providers may feel the desire or need to convince depressed patients that they should not be depressed. But because depression produces very negative, pessimistic thinking, patients may respond by trying to convince the physician that things really are as hopeless as they say. Physicians may become frustrated when patients do not follow through with their recommendations to exercise or participate in social activities. These efforts may produce an uneasy stalemate.

Part of the social stigma surrounding depression results from it sometimes being regarded as a character flaw, a sign of a moral failing, or simply laziness. Many physicians may pride themselves on having "willpower" to see their goals through. It may be difficult for them to be empathic with a patient who feels helpless and hopeless, and there may be a tendency to become angry with someone for "being weak" and "giving in" to the depression. In working with depressed patients, physicians may encounter their own personal and professional biases. These biases may also contribute to the low rates at which physicians detect depression. However interactions with challenging patients often provide an opportunity for physicians to examine their own values—conscious or otherwise—and to grow as a result.

CROSS-CULTURAL ASPECTS OF DEPRESSIVE DISORDERS

The clinical presentation and subjective experience of a major depressive episode may be influenced greatly by the patient's cultural background. In some groups of Native American and Southeastern Asian peoples there is no corresponding word for "depression." In many cultures depression is indicated by somatic complaints rather than self-reports of mood.

LEGAL & ETHICAL ISSUES

The treatment of depression may raise a number of legal and ethical issues. These include the involuntary hospitalization of patients who are at high risk for suicide or who are so severely depressed that they can no longer care for themselves. Legal protections exist to prevent patients' rights from being violated.

For example, a patient hospitalized against his or her will is entitled to a hearing within several days to petition for release. A court-appointed attorney testifies on the patient's behalf, and the burden of proof rests with the treating physician to demonstrate that the patient is truly incapable of caring for himself or herself. In some states patient rights are protected further by making the administration of medication a separate consideration. In these states a patient who refuses medication cannot be given antidepressants or ECT against his or her will without either family consent or a legal proceeding in which the patient must be shown to lack the ability to give informed consent.

Economic concerns and access to care present newer ethical challenges in caring for depressed patients. Most managed care and insurance companies have set limits on the number of psychotherapy sessions that a patient may have. Others attempt to limit coverage available to patients who have preexisting conditions, a particularly worrisome restriction given the recurrent nature of depression. Some clinicians may overuse the milder diagnosis of adjustment disorder to protect patients' future access to care.

Restrictions may also apply to the type of medication that physicians may select to treat depressed patients. Some health plans require trials of several TCAs before an SSRI may be prescribed. In some cases, patients who have been stable on one antidepressant have to switch to another medication when their health plan negotiates a contract for discounted prices, or are forced to pay out of pocket.

It may not be many years before medications are available that provide enhanced mood states for healthy individuals who do not have mood disorders. The ethical ramifications of such a discovery will no doubt be the subject of much debate.

CONCLUSION

Depressive disorders are both commonly encountered and frequently misdiagnosed by physicians. In spite of the advent of effective treatment and increasing responsibility for primary care providers to detect and treat depression, most patients fail to receive adequate treatment. Familiarity with the symptoms and classification of depressive disorders, and the basic principles of treatment, are essential skills for most physicians. The psychological and economic costs of depression and the adverse impact on physical health and the emotional well-being of families create an imperative for improved diagnosis and prompt treatment.

REFERENCES

Akiskal HS: Dysthymic and cyclothymic depressions: therapeutic considerations. J Clin Psychiatr 1994;55:(4): 46(Suppl).

Bliwise DL: Treating insomnia: pharmacological and nonpharmacological approaches. J Psychoact Drugs 1991;23 (4):335.

Docherty JP: Barriers to the diagnosis of depression in primary care. J Clin Psychiatr 1997;58(2):5.

Elfenbein D: *Living with Prozac (and Other SSRIs)*. Harper-Collins, 1995.

Jacobs S, Kim K: Psychiatric complications of bereavement. Psychiatr Ann 1990;20(4):314.

Judd LL, Mark HR, Paulaus MP, Brown JL: Subsyndromal symptomatic depression: a new mood disorder? J Clin Psychiatr 1994;55(4):18(Suppl).

Klein DN et al: Symptomatology in dysthymic and major depressive disorder. Psychiatr Clin N Am 1996;19(1):41.

Kocsis JH, Friedman RA, Markowitz JC et al: Maintenance therapy for chronic depression. Arch Gen Psychiatr 1996;53:769.

Kramer P. *Listening to Prozac*. Simon & Shuster, 1994.

Lejoyeux M, Ades J: Antidepressant discontinuation: a review of the literature. J Clin Psychiatr 1997;58(Suppl No. 7):11.

Manning M. *Undercurrents: A Therapist's Reckoning with Depression*. Harper-Collins, 1994.

Manson SM: Culture and major depression. Psychiatr Clin N Am 1995;18(3):487.

Quitkin FM, McGrath PJ, Stewart JW et al: Chronological milestones to guide drug change: When should clinicians switch antidepressants? Arch Gen Psychiatr 1996;53: 784.

Renner JA, Ciraulo DA: Substance abuse and depression. Psychiatr Ann 1994;24(10):532.

Robert MA, Hirschfeld MB, Keller SP, Arons BS et al: Consensus statement: the National Depressive and Manic Depressive Association Consensus Statement on the undertreatment of depression. CNS Spectrums 1997; 2(2):39.

Shelton RC, Davidson J, Yonkers KA et al: The undertreatment of dysthymia. J Clin Psychiatr 1997;58(2):59.

Styron W: *Darkness Visible*. Vintage Books, 1990.

Unipolar Depression (Duke University). http://www.duke. edu/~ntd/depression.html

Weiss M et al: The role of the alliance in the pharmacologic treatment of depression. J Clin Psychiatr 1997;58(5): 196.

Wells KB, Stewart A, Hays RD et al: The functioning and well-being of depressed patients: results from the Medical Outcomes Study. J Am Med Assoc 1989;262:914.

Web site for psychopharmacology tips: http://uhs.bsd. uchicago.edu/~bhsiung/tips/tips.html

Mood Disorders: Bipolar Disorder

6

David Elkin, MD

Bipolar disorder, formerly known as manic-depressive disorder, is a chronic disorder of mood regulation that results in episodes of depression and mania. Psychotic symptoms may appear at either "pole" of depression or mania. Like major (or unipolar) depression, bipolar disorder may be simulated by medical illness or substance abuse. Unlike major depression, almost all cases of bipolar disorder predispose the patient to episodes of depression and mania throughout the patient's life. Biological treatment consists of lifelong therapy with mood stabilizers such as lithium or anticonvulsants.

CLINICAL FEATURES

Bipolar disorder produces mood swings consisting of depressive episodes identical to those seen in unipolar depression and episodes of elevated mood known as **mania.** Manic symptoms exist on a spectrum from mild (hypomania) to severe (mania with psychotic symptoms). Episodes of mania and depression frequently have profound effects on a patient's self-concept, and on behavior as manifested at work and in social functioning. Between mood swings, patients frequently have a normal mood and often return to previous levels of psychosocial functioning. Without treatment, mood disturbances will usually recur throughout the patient's life after the first manic or depressive episode.

Variations of bipolar disorder include **bipolar disorder type I, bipolar disorder type II, rapid-cycling bipolar disorder,** and **cyclothymic disorder** (see Figure 6–1 for a comparison). In bipolar disorder type I, patients cycle between depression, normal mood, and full-blown mania, sometimes with psychotic features. In bipolar disorder type II patients' highs do not achieve the full extreme of mania but rather are hypomanic episodes. However patients do experience full-blown depressive episodes on their "downswing." Psychotic symptoms are possible at either extreme of major depression or mania; bipolar disorder type II patients thus do not experience manic symptoms as part of their elevated mood states. In rapid-cycling bipolar disorder, mood swings occur very swiftly, resulting in more than four episodes of depression or mania per year. Rapid cycling occurs in 15–20% of patients who have bipolar disorder. Cyclothymic disorder (also called cyclothymia) represents a milder form of bipolar disorder, just as dysthymia seems to be a more minor form of unipolar depression, in which patients cycle between periods of hypomania and mild depression. Thus the distinction between these variants can be seen as the differences in the severity and frequency of mood disturbance.

INCIDENCE

Bipolar disorder occurs in men and women with equal prevalence (unlike depression, which affects women twice as often as men). All mood disorders appear equally likely to occur in different ethnic groups, although misdiagnosis is likely across cultural lines. Bipolar disorder affects approximately 1% of the population and is found in slightly greater proportion in higher socioeconomic groups. This higher proportion may reflect more accurate diagnostic practices in wealthier patients, rather than an actual difference in incidence.

The economic impact of bipolar disorder is high even though the illness affects a smaller proportion of the population (1%) than do depressive disorders. Bipolar disorder results in over 150 million days of lost productivity in the workplace in any given year.

ETIOLOGY

The search continues for a specific genetic defect that might produce bipolar disorder. Meanwhile, a number of findings have been reported from neurochemical and neuroendocrine studies of mania. These

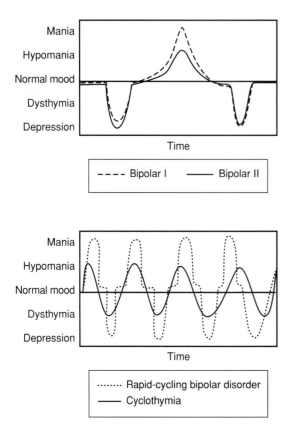

Mania
Hypomania
Normal mood
Dysthymia
Depression

Time

- - - - Bipolar I   ——— Bipolar II

Mania
Hypomania
Normal mood
Dysthymia
Depression

Time

········· Rapid-cycling bipolar disorder
——— Cyclothymia

Figure 6–1. A comparison of bipolar disorder type I (**dashed line, top**), bipolar disorder type II (**solid line, top**), rapid-cycling bipolar disorder (**dotted line, bottom**), and cyclothymia (**solid line, bottom**), with respect to intensity of mood disturbance (*y*-axis) and time (*x*-axis).

findings include a blunted response to TSH and TRH, increased dopaminergic activity, and the possible involvement of second-messenger systems such as cAMP in manic patients. Brain imaging studies are inconsistent, with the exception of a small subset of patients who have severe unipolar or bipolar disorders who have later onset, frequent hospitalizations, low IQ, and the presence of enlarged lateral ventricles on MRI scans. The anti-manic properties of anticonvulsants suggest the possibility of a "kindling" in the temporal lobes of patients who have mania. As in depression, dysregulation of the amine system (af-

fecting serotonin and norepinephrine) appears related to the presentations of mania and depression.

Bipolar disorders are seen in families, and genetic studies have demonstrated a much more robust relationship than in unipolar depression. One or both parents of about half of all bipolar patients have a mood disorder, most frequently unipolar depression. If one parent has bipolar disorder, the chances are one in four that any child will have a mood disorder (bipolar or unipolar). The chances rise to 50–70% if both parents have bipolar disorder. Adoption of children at risk does not reduce these chances, underscoring a biological etiology. Finally, monozygotic twins share a concordance rate for bipolar disorder of 70–100%; for fraternal twins concordance is only 20%.

DIAGNOSTIC ASSESSMENT

1. SIGNS & SYMPTOMS

Patients who have bipolar disorder cycle between episodes of depression, normal mood, and elevated mood. Some patients will demonstrate only slightly elevated mood (hypomania); in full-blown mania, patients may be purely euphoric or have a mixed presentation of elation and depression or irritability. In the most severe form of mania, patients may also develop psychotic symptoms. Table 6–1 shows the three stages of mania.

Hypomanic patients are often described as being upbeat, energized, extroverted, and assertive with others. At their best, they maintain insight and judgment and are able to channel their ideas constructively. In such a state, patients may generate and sort through many thoughts at a rapid rate and may be adept at problem solving. In bipolar disorder type II, patients alternate between depressive episodes, normal mood, and hypomania but do not enter the manic state (see below). Hypomania is frequently the idealized state for many patients who have bipolar disorder or cyclothymia.

In patients who have a fully manic presentation (seen in bipolar disorder I), mood may be elevated to the point of euphoria. Consequently these patients may exhibit grandiose thinking; occasionally they are paranoid or irritable as well. Mixed states of mania and depression are also possible. Paranoia and

Table 6–1. Stages of mania (summarized from Forster).

Hypomania (Stage I)	Mania (Stage II)	Mania with Psychotic Symptoms (Stage III)
Energetic	Euphoric/grandiose	Paranoid
Extroverted	Paranoid/irritable	Delusional
Assertive	Hyperactive	Confused/disorganized
		Hallucinations

grandiosity are often accompanied by delusions. These patients are often hyperactive and are much more likely to violate the personal space of people around them. In even moderate cases of mania, judgment and insight are compromised, and impulse control is reduced markedly. Patients who act upon plans or ideas that are influenced by their euphoric state can cause significant damage to relationships, jobs, or their financial status. Telephone and credit card charges are typically increased.

Some patients experience mood elevation to the point of reaching a manic state with psychotic features. In this condition, patients' thoughts are similar to those seen in other forms of psychosis: no longer just rapid, their thoughts are disorganized, characterized by loose associations or thought blocking. These patients may have hallucinations, grandiose or paranoid delusions, are frequently confused, and are unable to concentrate.

Eliza H, aged 35, though normally shy and reserved, was noted by friends and coworkers to have undergone a sudden personality change. Over a 2-week period Ms. H became more outgoing and extroverted. She spent thousands of dollars buying colorful clothing that seemed to match her new confidence and assertiveness. She gave pep talks to coworkers and began to bring them gifts. She joined a gym and began to work out almost every night, then spent the weekend at an all-day retreat to learn Spanish. She displayed increasing energy at work, staying until midnight to work on several innovative projects. She leaped over several administrative layers to promote these projects to the company vice president, which antagonized her supervisor. Formerly shy and uncomfortable around large groups of people, she gave several impressive talks at conferences. She commented, "I've never felt so good—I finally feel like my life is going somewhere."

By the end of the second week Ms. H's behavior had deteriorated. Her upbeat demeanor was now marred by irritability, sarcasm, and a growing sense of paranoia and grandiosity. "Everyone is after my ideas!" she complained. She had several angry discussions with her supervisor, who was now worried about her. She angrily quit her job, saying, "There are people who will pay millions for my ideas." She began to hear a male voice saying things like, "Go for it. You're the best. Don't let them stop you." Ms. H became increasingly hyperreligious and began looking through the bible for messages to her from God. She thought that she could understand what her cats were saying and could communicate with them. She became convinced that a national TV anchorperson was in love with her. When she tried to buy five tele-

visions at an electronics store, she was told she had exceeded her credit limit. She assaulted the manager when he attempted to confiscate her credit card. She was arrested and brought to the emergency room.

On examination, Ms. H was agitated, and her mood was labile (alternating between boastfulness and crying). Her thoughts were grandiose, paranoid, and disorganized. She tried to grab cigarettes from other patients and had to be pulled away from the telephone after repeatedly calling the mayor's office complaining that she was being kidnapped. Eventually she was placed in restraints and heavily sedated.

Diagnosis. Bipolar disorder, manic episode with psychotic symptoms (Axis I).

2. INTERVIEWING THE MANIC PATIENT

Several standard questions should be asked of the patient who is suspected of having bipolar disorder. In addition to routine questions about unipolar depression, questions similar to the following should be asked: Have you noticed any changes in your mood? Do you ever feel great, on top of the world, ready to take on anything? Does your energy level ever increase? Are there ever any times when you seem to require very little sleep and still wake up feeling good? Do you ever begin projects, or spend large sums of money, and realize only later that you have acted impulsively with a lapse of judgment? Have you ever been involved in legal problems or been arrested? Do people ever tell you that you seem "speeded up" or that they cannot follow your thoughts? Do your thoughts ever seem to "race," or do you sometimes find that people appear to be thinking much too slowly for you? Does anyone else in your family have a history of psychiatric illness, especially mood disorders? Do you have any medical problems? What medication do you take, both prescription and over-the-counter?

The patient's attitude during the interview will vary with the patient's mood. Hypomanic patients who are euphoric may be interested in explaining their ideas and plans to an interviewer. A patient who is in a full-blown manic state often speaks and thinks quite quickly and dominates the interview; the patient may be playful, joking (and determined to make the interviewer laugh), or extremely sexually provocative.

In cases where mania is mixed with elements of depression and anxiety (mixed mania), the patient may repeatedly beg for help and reassurance or become so irritable that he or she may try to provoke or embarrass the interviewer with sarcastic comments. The patient may give inaccurate information, lying to clinicians for amusement's sake or to exert power in the relationship. Since manic patients are potentially assaultive, clinicians need to avoid antagonizing the patient and should have ready access to help in the event of physical assault. Physical boundaries and other limits should be set as appropriate, and paranoid patients should be given extra physical and psychological "room" during the interview.

3. MENTAL STATUS EXAMINATION

The important findings in the mental status examination of the mood disordered patient follow:

A. Appearance & Behavior. The manic patient is often dressed in bright, colorful clothing, reflecting an elevated emotional state. If a patient enters a state of mania with psychotic symptoms, he or she may resemble a patient who has schizophrenia, appearing disheveled, disorganized, and confused. The manic patient frequently demonstrates psychomotor agitation, appearing excited, restless, or agitated. He or she may talk excitedly to other staff or patients, or may be engaged in numerous and frequent phone calls. The patient's interactions are frequently accompanied by dramatic speech and mannerisms, inappropriate sexual content, and frequent violations of personal space of the other party. The manic patient may be easily distracted by his or her own thoughts or the ideas of others.

B. Language. Speech and language in affected patients is often marked by loudness and "pressured speech" as the patient tries to keep up with his or her thoughts. The patient may also demonstrate creative uses of rhyme, association, or alliteration, applying a playful spirit to words and their usage (eg, "We are only prawns, and they're moving in for the krill."). Patients sometimes use new words (neologisms) to condense ideas. For example, a patient might describe him or herself as "flusterated"—a combination of frustrated and flustered.

C. Emotions. Patients who have mania may exhibit emotions on a spectrum from slightly elevated to frankly euphoric. Irritability, depression, and anxiety may appear in mixed states. Lability of affect is common, and inappropriate emotional responses may be seen.

D. Thought Process. The manic patient's thought processes will vary depending on the severity of the manic episode. In hypomania, patients note that their thoughts seem "faster," but they usually flow in a logical manner, with intermittent asides. In mania, patient's thoughts may seem to race as if the patient's speech cannot match the speed of their thoughts. The clinician may observe "flight of ideas," a condition in which the patient rapidly builds from one association to the next. An observer may understand the flow of a manic patient's thoughts if they can be sufficiently slowed or replayed. In mania with psychotic features, the patient's thought processes may resemble those seen in the patient with schizophrenia. For example, loose or bizarre associations,

neologisms, and clang associations (using rhyming words) may be noted.

E. Thought Content. The manic patient's thinking becomes progressively more grandiose, paranoid, and delusional as the patient nears a psychotic state. Mood-congruent hallucinations may also be present: Patients might hear "the voice of God" or a voice saying, "You're the greatest, you can do it." Ideas of reference also occur. Some patients who have bipolar disorder develop fixations about celebrities or world leaders. Note that people who threaten government officials are more likely to have bipolar disorder than any other psychiatric disorder.

F. Judgment, Insight, & Impulse Control. Judgment, insight, and impulse control can vary from good in mild cases of hypomania to extremely poor in a full-blown manic episode with psychotic features.

G. Cognitive Examination. The cognitive examination usually fails to reveal any problems in short-term memory or concentration, although extremely manic individuals may be so easily distracted that their concentration may be impaired.

DIFFERENTIAL DIAGNOSIS

Manic states can be seen in other medical and psychiatric illnesses. Medical, family, and past psychiatric histories may aid in differential diagnosis.

1. RULING OUT MEDICAL CAUSES

Several medical conditions can induce mania, including Cushing's disease (in which the body produces excess corticosteroids), hyperthyroidism, stroke, temporal lobe epilepsy, brain tumors (especially those involving the third ventricle), head trauma, HIV infection, and connective tissue disorders such as systemic lupus erythematosus or multiple sclerosis.

2. RULING OUT DRUG-INDUCED MANIA

Use of stimulants such as methamphetamine or cocaine can produce agitation, racing thoughts, flight of ideas, or psychotic symptoms that may easily be mistaken for a manic episode. When patients using these drugs "crash" and experience mood swings, they may appear to be following the course of mood swings seen in bipolar disorder. Patients who abuse psychostimulants may also use alcohol or tranquilizers to ease their descent from a drug high; these "downers" may accentuate the appearance of depression.

Medications can induce mania as well. Antidepressants can induce manic episodes in susceptible individuals who are destined to develop bipolar disorder.

Thus an episode of mania in response to antidepressants is considered diagnostic of primary bipolar disorder. In contrast, the development of mania in response to other medications does not place patients at higher risk of developing bipolar disorder. One of the most common examples of medication implicated in secondary mania (in part as a result of its widespread use) is prednisone, a corticosteroid that causes mania in some patients, depression or psychosis in others. Cimetidine (Tagamet), now available in over-the-counter form, can also cause mania, psychosis, or depression. Other medications implicated in the production of mania include levodopa (L-dopa) and bromocriptine (perhaps on the basis of their action of increasing dopaminergic activity in the brain); the muscle relaxant baclofen; and the anti-tuberculosis medication isoniazid.

3. RULING OUT PSYCHIATRIC DISORDERS

Mood swings are common symptoms in several psychiatric conditions.

A. Schizoaffective Disorder. Patients who have schizoaffective disorder often have histories of depressive and manic episodes. However, these patients have the chronic psychotic symptoms of schizophrenia, such as delusions and hallucinations, even during periods of normal mood and usually experience a progressive deterioration in functioning. Given the burden of having essentially two overlapping major psychiatric syndromes, it is not surprising that the prognosis for such patients is poor; a high incidence of substance use, homelessness, and suicide occurs among these patients.

B. Personality Disorders. Patients who have personality disorders may have mood instability. This is particularly true in "Cluster B" personality disorders, including histrionic, borderline, narcissistic, and antisocial personality subtypes. These mood changes may correspond to cyclothymia but often correspond to environmental factors. For example, a break-up of a relationship or a work setback may bring on a minor or major depressive episode, whereas hypomania may result from a positive event in the patient's life. Patients who have personality disorders may be misdiagnosed with bipolar disorder; however, mood stabilizers may still be effective in treating mood swings in these patients.

Leon J, a 50-year-old attorney, was hospitalized three times within an 8-month period for treatment of depression with suicidal ideation. Mr. J carried a diagnosis of bipolar disorder in his chart for several years. He rarely took lithium as it was prescribed or returned for follow-up appointments, although during each of the three admissions he insisted that lithium be prescribed.

Despite his reports of suicidal ideation, Mr. J never appeared more than mildly depressed or anxious, and immediately after each admission he was noted to "feel much better." He had difficult relationships with other patients and staff on the psychiatric unit. For example, he would monopolize the ward telephone, saying that he was conducting urgent business, and he was uniformly contemptuous of patients and staff unless he specifically wanted something from that person that day.

Mr. J's depression would melt away hours after he was admitted. At times he seemed hypomanic. On his last admission, Mr. J revealed (somewhat snidely) that he was claiming to be suicidal only to evade warrants issued by courts. It emerged that he would routinely abandon clients from whom he took large sums of money as a retainer. He would then fail to defend his clients and ignore subpoenas to appear in court, earning him a reputation among judges and other attorneys for being irresponsible. Mr. J appeared to have little remorse for his actions.

Mr. J. was eventually brought before the state bar where he chose to act as his own attorney and called on the treating psychiatrist as a witness. His defense consisted of the argument that bipolar disorder prevented him from appearing before the court on numerous occasions and that he was actively in psychiatric treatment. Mr. J waived his right to patient-physician confidentiality and brought his own psychiatric diagnosis into question. The psychiatrist was legally able to reveal to the bar that Mr. J had lied about his symptoms and probably did not have bipolar disorder. Mr. J was disbarred, but the psychiatrist saw him a year later on a TV talk show, where he presented himself as a world-famous author.

Diagnosis. Personality disorder, probably narcissistic with antisocial features; possible cyclothymic disorder (Axis I); malingering (V code).

C. Schizophrenia. Patients who have bipolar disorder are sometimes diagnosed as having schizophrenia, perhaps in part because of the presence of psychotic symptoms in mania, and the earlier age of onset that resembles schizophrenia. Such misdiagnosis is even more likely to occur when the patient and physician are of different ethnicity.

COURSE

Bipolar disorder manifests over time. The range of onset of bipolar disorder is childhood to 50 years of age; the mean age of onset is 30. The average patient (three-quarters of women and two-thirds of men) who has bipolar disorder has an episode of major depression preceding a manic episode. The first episode is likely to be depression in women and mania in men. Disease onset is also later in women. Bipolar disorder occasionally has an onset in childhood or adolescence, when it is likely to be misdiagnosed as attention deficit–hyperactivity disorder. At any age of onset, patients who have bipolar disorder are frequently misdiagnosed and wait years for appropriate assessment and treatment.

The average manic episode lasts 3 months if untreated; over time the interval between episodes decreases. This interval stabilizes after five episodes at approximately 6–9 months. Mood changes occur much more quickly in the rapid-cycling variant of bipolar disorder, with intervals averaging less than 3 months between mood swings. The average number of manic episodes over a lifetime is nine, although patients who have rapid-cycling bipolar disorder may have as many as 30 episodes. Fewer than 10% of patients have only one manic episode with no subsequent mood swings. Some patients have regular mood cycles throughout the year, just as a seasonal pattern can be seen in some depressed patients.

The prognosis for patients who have bipolar disorder varies greatly and depends on several conditions, including the natural course of the illness for the individual; degree of impairment of insight, judgment, and impulse control; and presence of psychosocial supports (eg, job, relationships). Patients who are unwilling to regard bipolar disorder as a lifelong illness, who are noncompliant with mood stabilizers, or who abuse drugs or alcohol are likely to have stormier courses with more episodes of depression and mania. Factors associated with poor response to mood-stabilizing medication include the presence of rapid-cycling bipolar disorder; dysphoric or mixed mania; episodic sequences of depression, mania, and normal mood; interepisode symptoms; and concomitant personality disorder. Some studies have indicated that the severity of manic episodes determines the likelihood of treatment response.

Bipolar disorder carries a poorer prognosis than does major depression. On follow-up with patients who have bipolar disorder, 15% of patients were completely well, 45% were doing well but had multiple relapses, 30% continued to have some symptoms (partial remission), and 10% were chronically ill with no decrease in their symptoms. Approximately one-third of patients who have bipolar disorder have chronic symptoms with evidence of social decline (eg, drop in socioeconomic status, loss of significant relationships).

Bipolar disorder is also associated with high rates of alcohol and drug use, in part because patients may attempt to use these substances to induce a hypomanic state. Studies estimate that up to 40% of patients with bipolar type II and up to 60% of patients with bipolar type I have a concomitant substance use disorder at some point in their illness. These rates are markedly higher than among the general population. Patients who have bipolar disorder and substance use are more likely to have mixed or rapid-cycling bipolar disorder with a poorer prognosis and decreased chance of responding to lithium.

As in unipolar depression, a significant risk of suicide is associated with bipolar disorder. Before the use of lithium, one person in five who had bipolar disorder committed suicide. The risk of suicide is reduced in patients on maintenance doses of mood stabilizers but remains much higher than that of the general population.

TREATMENT

Treatment of the manic patient presents special challenges. He or she may exhibit euphoria, irritability, grandiosity, or psychotic symptoms, such as auditory or visual hallucinations, and paranoia. Some patients are extremely agitated and potentially assaultive in their interactions with patients and staff. Patients in a depressed or mixed state may be suicidal. These patients are frequently placed on involuntary psychiatric holds as a danger to themselves or to others and admitted to a locked psychiatric unit. There they are treated with a combination of medications and behavioral therapy designed to curb their behavior. Severely agitated patients who are threatening or assaultive may require restraints and sedating medication.

The statistics on treatment for bipolar disorder remains sobering, however. Many patients do not realize that they have an illness; others are resistant to treatment. Ten years after their first manic episode, one-third of patients still have not sought treatment. Several studies found that at any given time only one-third of the estimated 2.5 million people in the United States who have bipolar disorder are actively receiving treatment for their illness. One-third of patients who have bipolar disorder cannot afford appropriate treatment.

1. MEDICATION

Lithium is effective for mood stabilization in bipolar disorder but takes weeks to months to work and is therefore not the treatment of choice for acute mania. Neuroleptics (antipsychotics) may be useful, especially for mania with psychotic symptoms. Their sedating side effects are often noted within hours, but it takes 3–7 days for their antipsychotic effect to begin to work. Benzodiazepines work within minutes to an hour depending on the means of delivery. Clonazepam (Klonopin), a long-acting benzodiazepine with additional anticonvulsant properties, may be especially effective in the acute management of agitated manic patients, perhaps more so than other benzodiazepines. Benzodiazepines and neuroleptics can then be stopped sequentially over days to weeks as mood stabilizers begin to work. Table 6–2 compares various medications used to treat mania.

Lithium was approved by the FDA in 1970 for the chronic treatment of bipolar disorder and won rapid acceptance by clinicians as the gold standard of treatment. Lithium is highly effective in preventing manic and depressive episodes. Unfortunately, lithium is also associated with a high incidence of side effects including tremors, mental sluggishness, hair loss, nausea and other gastrointestinal effects, weight gain, renal failure, and SIADH (syndrome of inappropriate antidiuretic hormone). It does not work for all patients who have bipolar disorder, so researchers have actively sought alternative agents for mood stabilization. The anticonvulsant carbamezepine (Tegretol) emerged as an effective second-line drug during the 1980s but was replaced by another anticonvulsant, valproic acid (Depakote), which had fewer side effects. Because of its efficacy and low incidence of side effects, valproic acid is considered by some psychiatrists to be a possible first choice in treating patients who have bipolar disorder. Valproic acid may offer better control of mood swings in patients who have rapid-cycling bipolar disorder, mixed manic states, and bipolar disorder complicated by alcohol dependence or drug use.

Maintenance therapy may reduce the severity (amplitude) of mood swings but still leave the patient vulnerable to attenuated episodes of mild depression or hypomania. Finding the correct dose of medication necessary to suppress mood swings with a minimum of symptoms is an ongoing dynamic process between physician and patient. Antidepressants can be used to treat breakthrough episodes of depression but always with a mood stabilizer in therapeutic doses to prevent overshoot into mania.

Samantha B, a 40-year-old dentist, was brought to the psychiatric emergency room by her husband. She was under the delusion that she had stumbled onto the "secret of life." She was extremely agitated and irritable, her thinking was grandiose, and she seemed very paranoid with her husband and the staff. She had previously been prescribed fluoxetine (Prozac) for depression. The antidepressant was stopped and she was started on clonazepam, a low-dose antipsychotic, and lithium. Her psychosis cleared rapidly over the next 4 days. Clonazepam was tapered off and stopped when she reported feeling sedated, and she was then discharged from the hospital. After 1 week the antipsychotic was stopped, and she was able to return to work.

Two weeks later, at her second outpatient appointment, Dr. B complained to her psychiatrist

of facial acne and a tremor in her hands that interfered with work. The lithium was stopped and replaced with valproic acid. She was doing well at 2-year follow-up.

One year later, Dr. B complained to her psychiatrist that her life was "boring," and she began to drink alcohol in increasing amounts. She then stopped the valproic acid and became hypomanic. Her psychiatrist found it difficult to convince her that she would need to be on the medication for the rest of her life. As she became increasingly manic she initiated an affair with a man she did not previously know and impulsively spent $10,000 treating both of them to a 2-week trip through the South Pacific. On her return, Dr. B was dismayed to find that her husband had filed for divorce and that she had been fired from her job. She was re-hospitalized with severe depression.

Discussion. Many people who have bipolar disorder will stop taking their medications to see if they still need them or because they are convinced that they no longer do. Alternatively they may be chasing a manic "high." When combined with euphoric mood and a lack of insight, this drive may lead to extremely poor compliance and continued difficulties. The results of behavior during manic episodes may also lead to consequences that are in themselves depressing, such as lost jobs, jeopardized relationships, financial burdens, or homelessness.

3. PSYCHOTHERAPY

Patients who have bipolar disorder may benefit greatly from psychotherapy to help them explore the impact and meaning of the illness in their lives. The use of support groups for patients who have bipolar disorder is extremely effective. Groups are led by mental health professionals or by individuals who have bipolar disorder who are insightful and more experienced with their illness. Group therapy, which provides newly diagnosed patients with education about their illness and a chance to air their concerns and watch others adjust to the diagnosis, should be a key part of every treatment plan. Families are often already affected by the patient's bipolar disorder and may benefit from family therapy or support and education from groups such as NAMI (National Alliance for the Mentally Ill).

One woman commented:

Nothing was the same after I turned 10 and my mother had her first episode of mania. My parents divorced, and I was raised by my mother. Sometimes things were great—she was like her old self. But then she would go off of her med-

Table 6–2. Comparison of medications used to treat mania.[1]

Medication (Trade Name)	Uses	Initial and Maintenance Doses	Side Effects	Serious Side Effects Warranting Possible Discontinuation	Possible Mechanisms of Action	Drug Interactions
Lithium (Eskalith, Lithobid)	Prevention and treatment of mania, hypomania, and schizoaffective disorder. Treatment and augmentation agent for unipolar depression. Treatment of impulsive and aggressive behavior	300 mg twice daily. Increase to reach serum concentrations of 0.5–1.4 gEq/L	Acne, hair loss, hand tremors, dry mouth, weight gain, increased thirst and urination, GI distress, weakness, mild cognitive problems (short-term memory, concentration)	Renal failure, hypo-thyroidism	Blocks inositol-1 phosphatase leading to decreased cellular response to multiple neurotransmitters	Lithium levels increased by dehydration, exercise, thiazide diuretics, neuroleptics and NSAIDs (eg ibuprofen)
Carbamazepine (Tegretol)	Prevention and treatment of mania, hypomania (not FDA approved). Treatment of impulsive and aggressive behavior	200 mg three times daily. Increase to serum concentrations 6–12 μg/dl	Blurred or double vision, fatigue, nausea, ataxic gait, mild cognitive impairment	Leukopenia (decreased white cell count), increased liver function tests, hyponatremia, agranulocytosis, aplastic anemia	Acts on neuron ion channels, reducing high-frequency firing. Affects many neurotransmitters including GABA, serotonin, dopamine and norepinephrine	Decreases serum levels of benzo-diazepines, TCAs, neuroleptics, and birth control pills
Valproic acid (Depakote, Depakene)	Prevention and treatment of mania, hypomania. May be more effective than lithium for mixed, rapid cycling BAD, mania due to medical conditions or comorbid substance use. Treatment of impulsive and aggressive behavior	250 mg twice daily. Increase to trough concentrations of 45–100 μg/ml	GI upset, tremor, transient hair loss, weight gain, asymptomatic decreases in platelets and white blood cells	Pancreatitis, agranulocytosis, severe hepatitis or liver failure	Increases concentrations of GABA, an inhibitory neuropeptide	Valproate levels increased by SSRIs. Valproic acid increases levels of TCAs, digoxin, and warfarin (all protein bound)

Gabapentin (Neurontin)	Possible treatment of hypomania and mania alone or with agents above (not FDA approved)	300 mg three times daily up to 3600 mg/day	Nausea, somnolence, fatigue, dizziness, GI distress, weight gain, double vision	Unknown. Binds to calcium channel with possible antagonist activity	Valproic acid may increase gabapentin levels
Lamotrigine (Lamictal)	Possible treatment of hypomania and mania (not FDA approved)	50 mg twice daily. Increase to 100 mg twice daily	Nausea, somnolence, dizziness, weight gain, rash	Stabilizes presynaptic membrane, inhibits release of excitatory neurotransmitters	Valproic acid may increase levels. Coadministration of carbamazepine may lead to reduced levels or neurotoxicity
			Toxic epidermal necrolysis (Stevens-Johnson syndrome)		
Verapamil (Celen, Isoptin)	Treatment of acute mania in patients who are responsive to lithium	90–360 mg twice or three times per day	Dizziness, flushing, increased heart rate, nausea	Blocks calcium channels, decreasing excitatory effect of neurotransmitters	Increased risk of neurotoxicity with lithium or carbamazepine. Increased risk of parkinsonism and slowed heart rate with lithium. Increased risk of parkinsonism with antipsychotics
			Parkinsonism		

[1]Abbreviations: BAD, bipolar affective disorder; FDA, Food and Drug Administration; GI, gastrointestinal; NSAIDs, nonsteroidal anti-inflammatory drugs.

ication, bring home scary men, act crazy, and leave me for a week while she spent all of the money we saved. Then she was too depressed to get out of bed for weeks, and I would have to stay home from school to take care of her. I never knew what to expect—it was like she was several different people, all in the same body, and I never knew which one would be my mother. When I was younger, I thought that the changes were somehow all my fault.

CREATIVITY & MOOD DISORDERS

A link between mood disorders and creativity has long been suspected. Many notable poets, artists, and musicians are suspected to have had mood disorders, including Edgar Allen Poe, William Blake, Vincent van Gogh, Georgia O'Keefe, Charles Mingus, Tennessee Williams, and Gustav Mahler. Some (eg, William Styron) have written about their experiences with mood disorders. Recent studies utilizing structured interviews, matched control groups, and strict diagnostic criteria demonstrate a strong association between mood disorders and creativity.

A 1970 study of 30 creative writers found that 80% had experienced at least one episode of major depression, while almost half reported hypomania or mania. A third of the accomplished British writers and visual artists included in another study had been treated for a mood disorder; half of the poets had needed extensive psychiatric care. In other studies, the rates of suicide, depression, and bipolar disorder in artists were up to 18 times as common as in the general population.

Many features of hypomania would appear conducive to creativity. Cognitive styles associated with hypomania, such as expansive thought and grandiose moods, can lead to increased production and speed of thoughts. Hypomanic individuals tend to use language more creatively than do normal controls. The ability to work with great energy and focus, to experience profound revelations and emotional depth, to transcend the mundane aspects of life and evoke a sense of meaning and higher purpose are all qualities that lend themselves to creative accomplishments. Patients who have bipolar disorder whose mood swings are well controlled may miss the creative insights afforded by manic episodes. Unfortunately, the association of mood disorders with substance abuse and suicide and the tendency to overestimate the productivity afforded by brief episodes of mania and discount the inevitability and impact of consequent depressive episodes represent some of the negative aspects of the link between mood disorders and creativity. This dilemma under-

scores the need for the therapist and patient to examine the effects of illness and treatment on creativity in an ongoing, dynamic manner.

EMOTIONAL REACTIONS TO PATIENTS

Manic patients are notorious for their ability to induce strong emotions in others. Among health-care professionals, trainees may have a particularly difficult time dealing with manic patients. These patients, especially those who are hypomanic, can be charming, interesting, and amusing, and frequently induce an initial feeling of good-humor and well-being among people who interact with them. However, even the most good-natured manic patient can overstep boundaries, causing annoyance and frustration. Patients who have more severe forms of mania, especially in mixed states where irritability is present, may be sarcastic, domineering, and manipulative. They may leave staff members feeling frustrated, angry, irritable, frightened, incompetent, or out of control. In the most severe case of mania with psychotic features, the treating staff's reactions may resemble those seen in working with patients who have schizophrenia. Staff may then feel disengaged, confused, or extremely frightened.

A third-year medical student interviewed a hypomanic patient in front of several of his peers. The patient, like the student, was in her early 20s. The interview began well as the student and patient spoke in a casual, open-ended way. But as the interview progressed the student tried to ask more structured questions. The patient became increasingly humorous and flirtatious, at one point leaning over as if to tickle the student and telling him he needed to "loosen up." The patient lost interest in the student and began to interact with the other students in the room. "Don't you think this guy's cute?" she asked the other students. "But he really needs to lighten up, right? Let's see if we can get him some help!" Meanwhile the student felt increasingly powerless, recognizing that he had lost control of the interview, and ashamed to have failed in front of his classmates. He made one more attempt to wrestle control back, saying, "I'm a doctor and I'm in charge here—I'm conducting an interview!" The patient laughed and replied, "Oh, did you learn to say things like that from that TV show 'ER?'" The rest of the students joined the patient in giddy laughter, and the student slumped in his chair with his ears and face burning.

CROSS-CULTURAL ASPECTS OF BIPOLAR DISORDER

Research has demonstrated that patients who have bipolar disorder with psychotic features may be misdiagnosed as having schizophrenia by clinicians who are from a different cultural background. This misdiagnosis often leads to mistreatment with antipsychotic medications at high doses for prolonged periods of time. Exposure to antipsychotics places patients who have bipolar disorder at enhanced and unnecessary risk of developing tardive dyskinesia, while at the same time missing the opportunity to start mood stabilizers. Thus patients are likely to experience continued symptoms and further psychosocial deterioration.

LEGAL & ETHICAL ISSUES

Ethical considerations in bipolar disorder are similar to those encountered in unipolar depression. Specifically, changes in mood are often accompanied by profound changes in judgment and insight. When patients are manic they may also be especially impulsive and therefore prone to act upon grandiose thoughts, spending large sums of money or engaging in high-risk sexual behavior. Moreover, mania may be ego-syntonic; that is the patient does not experience manic symptoms as being oppressive or even realize that anything is wrong. The treating physician may therefore be faced with the difficulty of wanting to involuntarily hospitalize a patient for the patient's protection.

In the case of manic patients who pose an assault risk, the patient may need to be hospitalized and possibly placed in restraints until medications take effect. If the patient is threatening a specific person the physician may also be legally obligated to contact the potential victim and the police. If the manic patient is engaging in high-risk sexual behaviors the physician may also feel compelled to warn the patient's spouse or significant other; if the patient does not agree the physician may be barred from breaking confidentiality. This situation may be especially problematic if the patient is manic and is infected with the HIV virus.

Tien V, a 50-year-old Asian male, was admitted to the inpatient psychiatric unit on a psychiatric hold. He had a history of a mania episode with psychotic features identical to this one that cleared promptly on antipsychotics, and was stable on lithium until he stopped taking the medication 1 week prior to this hospitalization. He expressed gratitude to the psychiatry staff during his previous episode for starting him on neuroleptics. At the time of his discharge he told the medical staff, "If I ever come in again, make sure that you give me the medication, even if I tell you not to." However, on this admission, he refused to take all medications, stating, "There's nothing wrong with me! I don't need medication, and I don't care what I said before!"

The unit psychiatrist argued that Mr. V should be restarted on his medications by hiding them in his food. His argument was based largely on the notion that he would be acting not only on behalf of Mr. V's best interests but also in accordance with Mr. V's wishes were he not psychotic.

The nursing staff thought that Mr. V should still have the benefit of a hearing to decide the best course of action. The hospital attorney recommended a legal hearing in the absence of a written "advanced directive" (also called a Ulysses contract) regarding medications.

Mr. V's previous wishes were upheld and he was given intramuscular injection of antipsychotics against his will. Hiding his medication was deemed inadvisable. After a week, his manic episode had cleared sufficiently for him to agree to take mood stabilizers. He thanked the psychiatry team for treating him involuntarily and adhering to his original wishes.

CONCLUSION

Bipolar disorder affects a small percentage of people worldwide yet remains a fascinating and important psychiatric disorder. The clinical features of hypomania, including increased energy and heightened self-confidence, motivation, and creativity, represent an idealized state for many people. The demonstrated links between mood disorders and creativity underscore the unique nature of the manic state. Yet the costs of untreated bipolar disorder and its uncontrolled mood swings are great. Effective treatment is now available for most patients who have bipolar disorder, but the chief obstacle in living with this psychiatric disorder is often the patient's reluctance to accept the disorder and the need for lifelong treatment. The clinician's challenge is to forge a working alliance with these patients, to manage their own countertransference, and to help patients accept both the benefits and implications of living with this disorder.

REFERENCES

American Psychiatric Association: Practice guidelines for the treatment of patients with bipolar disorder. Am J Psychiatr 1994;151(suppl.):12.

Bipolar Disorder (National Institutes of Mental Health gopher server). http://www.auburn.edu/~mcquedr/psych-info/bipolar.htm

Bowden C: Predictors of response to divalproex and lithium. J Clin Psychiatr 1995;56(Suppl. 3):25

Dubovsky S, Buzan RD: Novel alternatives and supplements to lithium and anticonvulsants for bipolar affective disorder. J Clin Psychiatr 1997;58(5):224.

El-Mallakh RS: New insights into the course and prognosis of bipolar disorder. Psychiatr Ann 1997;27:478.

Forster P: Bipolar disorder: assessment and definitive treatment in an acute care setting. *Bipolar Disorder Update* (Teleconference Program Synopsis), Annenberg Center Publication, 1996.

Gadde KM, Krishnan RR: Recent advances in the pharmacologic treatment of bipolar illness. Psychiatr Ann 1997; 27:496.

Goodwin FK, Jamison KR: *Manic Depressive Illness.* Oxford University Press, 1990.

Jamison KR: *An Unquiet Mind.* Knopf, 1995.

Jamison KR: *Touched By Fire: Manic-Depressive Illness and the Artistic Temperament.* Simon & Schuster, 1994.

Janicak PG, Levy NA: Rational copharmacy for acute mania. Psychiatr Ann 1998;28(4):204.

Swann AC: Manic-depressive illness and substance use. Psychiatr Ann 1997;27(7):507.

Anxiety Disorders

7

David Elkin, MD, & Cameron S. Carter, MD

Anxiety is an extremely common psychiatric symptom, as well as a normal emotion. Everyone experiences anxiety at some point during their lifetime. Anxiety is pathologic when it occurs in conjunction with other disorders such as depression, or when anxiety-related symptoms and behaviors are so severe and occur with such frequency that they interfere with work or relationships. The anxiety disorders include panic disorder, social phobia, generalized anxiety disorder, obsessive-compulsive disorder, and specific phobia. Post-traumatic stress disorder is also an anxiety disorder and is discussed in the next chapter. Key features of these disorders are reviewed in Table 7–1.

Experience in the diagnosis and treatment of anxiety disorders is an essential skill for all physicians. Patients who have these disorders, especially those who have panic disorder and generalized anxiety disorder, usually present in primary care medical settings seeking treatment for the physical symptoms associated with the anxiety disorder. Physical symptoms frequently include chest pain, headache, shortness of breath, dizziness, gastrointestinal distress such as stomach pains, or the sensation of having a lump in one's throat. Patients are usually more comfortable talking about the physical symptoms of panic disorder and other anxiety disorders. Over three-quarters of patients who have panic attacks present to medial settings, usually the emergency room or the office of their general or family practice physician.

Physical symptoms often lead to lengthy evaluations and diagnostic workups that are expensive and unrevealing. In some studies, up to five tests and procedures were performed per patient, who also received an average of two referrals to specialty services such as cardiology, gastroenterology, and neurology. Increasing economic pressures will increase the expectation that physicians who are in HMOs or who are contracting with managed care will both evaluate and treat anxiety disorders.

Considerable patient distress and physician frustration are inevitable if these diagnoses are missed. Patients who have anxiety disorders should be screened appropriately for medical illness that can mimic symptoms as well as major depression and substance use. Patients should be told to avoid caffeine or medications that might increase anxiety. Treatment for anxiety disorders usually consists of psychotherapy and medication, which are very effective in alleviating symptoms and preventing relapse.

PANIC DISORDER: CLINICAL FEATURES

Patients who have **panic disorder** suffer from repeated attacks of severe anxiety. The symptoms of these attacks increase with a crescendo-like quality for up to 20–30 minutes before resolving. The symptoms can be divided into three discreet categories.

First there is the **affective,** or emotional, experience of the attack. The patient feels extreme anxiety or fear, as if a threat were present. One patient described her emotions during an attack "as if there were a tiger roaring at me from just a few feet away—except there is no tiger, just the fear."

The typical patient describes multiple **somatic,** or physical, symptoms. These symptoms commonly include heart palpitations, rapid heart rate, shortness of breath, tingling of the extremities and face, sweating, dizziness or vertigo, a clenching or sinking sensation of the stomach, and the sensation of a lump in the throat. These physical sensations may predominate and lead patients to feel that they are physically ill.

Finally, many patients report a cognitive component, a terrifying thought that something terrible is about to happen. Often they feel that they are about to die, and the urgency of this thought coupled with their physical symptoms leads them to make multiple presentations to the emergency room or to the offices of internists, general practitioners, cardiologists, or neurologists.

Table 7–1. Clinical features of anxiety disorders.

Anxiety Disorder	Clinical Features
Panic disorders	Anxiety attacks are episodic and occur spontaneously with physical symptoms (eg, palpitations, shortness of breath, parasthesias)
Social phobia	Anxiety attacks occur in context of the patient feeling at the center of attention
Generalized anxiety disorder	Pervasive (not episodic) anxiety with physical and emotional symptoms
Obsessive-compulsive disorder	Obsessions and compulsions with accompanying anxiety (body dysmorphic syndrome may be a subtype)
Specific phobia	Extreme anxiety and fear associated with exposure to certain stimuli (eg, heights, insects, animals)
Post-traumatic stress disorder	Syndrome of anxiety following a life-threatening event (eg, disaster, car accident, crime) with numbing, panic, hypervigilance, and startle reflexes

INCIDENCE

Panic disorder affects 1–2% of the population. The modal age of onset is in the third decade, although it may occur at any age. The female-to-male preponderance ratio is approximately 1.5–2:1. Prevalence rates are as high as 10% of medical outpatients.

ETIOLOGY

Biological Factors

The anxiety attacks that characterize panic disorder are thought to reflect dysregulation of neural systems involved in normal anxiety, arousal, and nociception (perception of potential danger). Involvement of central catecholamines, as well as the inhibitory neurotransmitter GABA, is thought to underlie these abnormalities.

The high concordance rate of panic disorder in monozygotic twins (up to 90%) implies strong support for a biological etiology. Further evidence for the importance of biological factors comes from brain imaging studies, animal models, and the induction in affected individuals of panic attacks (with infusions of lactate or breathing carbon dioxide). The observed link between panic disorder and mitral valve prolapse, a common cardiac condition, has been known for many years, but the relationship between the two disorders is unclear.

Psychological Factors

Individuals who have anxiety disorders in childhood are more likely than the general population to have these disorders and depression in adulthood. Anxiety disorders in childhood predispose individuals to problems in adulthood by sensitizing the limbic system and by conditioning the individuals to react more strongly to internal emotional states. Alternatively, anxiety disorders may simply be lifelong conditions that make their earliest appearance in childhood.

DIAGNOSTIC ASSESSMENT

Panic disorder begins with the unexpected occurrence of a **panic attack,** a cluster of unexpected anxiety and physical symptoms that are frightening to the patient. The patient may seek urgent medical attention at this point. Most patients remember their first attack in great detail; many can give the exact date, location, and other minute details. Typically the symptoms recur and the patient begins to anticipate and dread their recurrence. This is known as **anticipatory anxiety.**

Sufferers also may begin to avoid situations in which they might experience an attack and not be able to easily get help or retreat without embarrassment. This is known as **agoraphobia,** and typical situations that are avoided include driving in traffic or on freeways, bridges, or tunnels; or being in crowded places or wide open spaces. The presence of anticipatory anxiety and agoraphobia can be important clues to the presence of panic disorder and should cue the examiner to inquire very carefully about panic phenomena.

Persistent and severe anxiety seriously undermines self-confidence and self-esteem. Many patients who have panic disorder and other anxiety disorders also complain of dissociative symptoms, which may consist of episodes of **derealization** (a feeling that the world is not real, but more like a dream) or **depersonalization** (the feeling of being outside of themselves, or as though parts of their body are not their own). Dissociative symptoms can be very frightening.

Dizziness is a common symptom in panic disorder and may be the focus of the patient's presentation. About one-third of patients being investigated for vestibular disorders who complain of dizziness have panic disorder. One clue to this diagnosis is that these patients do not describe vertigo. Rather they usually complain of an unsteady feeling, along with the feeling that they are going to fall over or collapse. They may actually sink to the ground in order to avoid a true collapse. The development of phobic behaviors, such as staying near a wall, furniture, or a companion who can offer physical support during an attack, is common. A careful history will reveal the complete panic phenomenology (four or more symptoms with a minimum frequency and duration of the disorder).

A common misperception about panic disorder is that attacks occur when patients are under stress. In fact patients are more often relaxing or engaged in some nonthreatening behavior or activity. By contrast, in social phobia and simple phobias, paroxysmal anxiety is triggered by specific stressors such as speaking in front of crowds. Although many patients report that exercise reduces their anxiety levels, a few patients will find that exercise can induce an attack.

Angela L, a 26-year-old single woman, was in her final year of medical school. She presented to her family physician, requesting a second opinion regarding persistent dizziness, a problem she had had intermittently for several weeks. She had seen a neurologist, who completed a physical and neurologic exam, a basic hematology and chemistry panel, and a computed tomography (CT) scan of the head, all of which were normal. She was then referred to an ENT surgeon who reported that tests of vestibular function were equivocal and reassured Ms. L that nothing serious was wrong.

When questioned, Ms. L described an initial episode of feeling unsteady on her feet, which occurred suddenly during morning rounds. She felt as though she would lose her balance and fall. This feeling alarmed her, so she promptly sat down. The sensation disappeared after 2–3 minutes, and she resumed rounds. About a week later, this experience recurred in the same setting, lasting several minutes, and prompted her to seek medical evaluation. She had subsequently experienced several similar episodes.

In addition to feeling unsteady and fearing that she would lose her balance and fall, Ms. L felt a sense of alarm, which she thought was appropriate to the circumstances. Her heart would beat rapidly, she would feel anxious and shaky, and a feeling of unreality would come over her. She usually sat down, if possible, during these episodes. She found herself very apprehensive about morning rounds and always took a position next to the wall, where she could lean if she felt unsteady. She called in sick for several days.

Ms. L's family physician then prescribed alprazolam, a short-acting benzodiazepine, which to Ms. L's surprise relieved the symptoms. By the time she was referred to a psychiatrist, Ms. L had begun taking one pill each morning before rounds and had not experienced an episode for several days, although she was beginning to constantly worry that one might occur.

Ms. L's continued anxiety led the psychiatrist to gradually shift her from benzodiazepines to the serotonin-selective re-uptake inhibitor

(SSRI) paroxetine (Paxil). Ms. L also joined a support group for patients who have anxiety disorders and was surprised and reassured that other people had the same condition. She was also relieved that she did not have a major medical problem and soon experienced resolution of all of her symptoms.

Diagnosis. Panic disorder (Axis I).

Panic disorder is often accompanied by a sense of shame and embarrassment. It may therefore manifest itself as a "family secret" that is not discussed until the patient raises the issue.

Richard W, aged 64, was coming to visit his daughter, a psychologist. He had had an "inner ear problem" for many years. The symptoms started when he was 31 and included extreme dizziness, palpitations, anxiety, and fear whenever he drove over a bridge. He would have to let someone else drive or would pull over and wait for the attack to subside, usually about 30 minutes. Over time the symptoms became more intense and frequent, occurring when he drove up or down steep hills. Mr. W would plot his route on a map, making sure to detour around bridges and hills, which would increase his trip times by up to 2 hours.

While in graduate school, Mr. W's daughter had taken a course on anxiety disorders and realized her father most likely suffered from panic disorder. Initially excited to explain the diagnosis to her father, she found that he was angry and hurt that she doubted the physical nature of his symptoms. "Listen to me," he said, "my heart pounds when I get these things, and sometimes it feels like it's going to give out; that's not a mental condition." He refused her suggestion to see a mental health professional.

Knowing that panic disorder can run in families, the psychologist asked family members and learned that four relatives on her father's side also suffered from "inner ear problems" with symptoms similar to her father's.

Diagnosis. Panic disorder (Axis I).

Anxiety disorders frequently manifest with significant somatic complaints. Patients may present to physicians with over a dozen physical symptoms and are often misdiagnosed as having somatization disorder (see Chapter 9). The average patient with panic disorder sees over ten physicians over more than a decade before being accurately diagnosed. Some patients are aware of an emotional component of their symptoms but are embarrassed or ashamed to report them.

Gino S, a 43-year-old executive, came to the emergency room asking to have his blood pressure checked. He had called the hospital on his car phone 20 minutes earlier because of persistent chest pain, which began as he was beginning his evening commute. As Mr. S pulled onto the freeway, he felt lightheaded, had difficulty getting enough air, and felt the onset of intense, sharp pain that started in his chest and radiated into his left arm. He also felt flushed, sweaty, and had a sense of unreality. He was afraid that he was having a heart attack and would lose consciousness at the wheel. He then pulled over and made the call to the emergency room.

Mr. S had a long history of labile hypertension and was taking captopril and a beta-blocker. On presentation he felt exhausted, but his pain was almost gone, and his other symptoms had resolved.

Mr. S described having these symptoms for almost a year. The chest-pain episodes occurred most often when he was working in his home office, driving, or flying, which he had to do more often during this period because his senior partner in business has been disabled following a heart attack. Mr. S had restricted his physical activity, particularly when he had frequent pain episodes, and as a result had gained 20 pounds over the past several months, with an associated worsening of hypertension. His internist had ordered an upper CT study, which was normal. An electrocardiogram (EKG) stress test (in which the patient exercises on a treadmill) failed to reveal problems with cardiac blood flow, despite the occurrence of an attack during the test.

Mr. S described himself as successful, optimistic, and highly productive. He was married, had five children, and was an active member of his community. He denied that he had significant stressors in his life, despite considerably increased demands at work. As part of a considerable commitment to his church, he had assumed foster care for a disturbed adolescent and just the night before had to take this young woman to the local community mental health center because she expressed suicidal thoughts. Mr. S noted that although he didn't worry, he was always "thinking" about events in his life, and as a result, he often had difficulty sleeping.

Mr. S's mother died after a protracted course with breast cancer almost 3 years earlier. His father, who was an alcoholic, died in an auto accident when Mr. S was 3 years old.

Diagnosis. Panic disorder with agoraphobia (Axis I).

Each year in the United States approximately 200,000 normal coronary angiograms are performed at a cost of over $600 million. Studies have shown that at least one-third of these patients have panic disorder. When patients are referred for noninvasive testing (usually because their symptoms are less typical of coronary artery disease), more than one-half of patients who have negative tests have panic disorder. The advantages for patients, as well as for the national economy, of recognizing and treating panic disorder after its onset are obvious.

An important question facing practitioners is to what extent coronary artery disease, a life-threatening illness, should be investigated before making the diagnosis of panic disorder. It is certainly possible to have both problems. The answer depends on the patient. In the previous case, Mr. S's age and persistent hypertension required that coronary disease be reasonably excluded. For a younger patient with atypical cardiac symptoms and no risk factors for coronary disease whose symptoms can be accounted for by a panic disorders diagnosis, proceeding with a trial of therapy for panic disorder would be the most rational approach to treatment. Instead, most patients who have anxiety disorders are told that "there is nothing physically wrong" with them but are not referred for education and treatment of an anxiety disorder. Left untreated, panic and other anxiety disorders can become associated with serious complications.

Rashad J, aged 27, had a history of "nervousness" and experienced the onset of panic attacks after he was laid off from work. He was walking through the deli of a local supermarket when he was overcome by palpitations, dizziness, shortness of breath, and a feeling that he was going to die. He sat down in the aisle, fearing that he was having a heart attack and might die if he moved. The attack lasted 15 minutes, by which time the store manager had contacted emergency services.

Mr. J was taken to a local medical emergency room, where a myocardial infarction was ruled out by a normal EKG and normal cardiac enzymes (serum creatinine kinase levels). Mr. J was told simply, "there is nothing medically wrong."

Mr. J was unsure what the episode had been but felt better upon discharge. However, when he went back to the supermarket the following week, he felt a growing sense of anxiety. What if the same problem returned? What if the doctors at the hospital were wrong and he did have a serious medical problem? What if it meant that he could not work again? How could he provide for his family? He found himself becoming increasingly anxious and on the verge of another attack. Sweating and with his heart pounding, he fled the grocery store.

Mr. J discovered that he was able to shop for his family at other grocery stores without experiencing a panic attack, at least for a few weeks. He avoided the original supermarket, even on walks through the neighborhood. He developed a growing sense of shame and embarrassment about his behavior, especially around his friends, and wondered if he might be "mentally sick."

Then the attacks began in the other stores. Mr. J was dismayed and took to shopping in smaller stores. His wife began to confront him about the large amounts of money he was spending on groceries in more-expensive convenience stores. He felt too embarrassed to tell her the reason, but eventually she learned the truth from one of his friends. Meanwhile, Mr. J was becoming increasingly anxious about leaving his house at all and was now having spontaneous panic attacks once a day or more.

Mr. J's wife and his friend convinced him to see an internist, who performed a thorough physical examination and ran tests to rule out hyperthyroidism and other medical disorders. His internist then referred Mr. J to a psychiatrist. After conducting a thorough evaluation, the psychiatrist prescribed an antidepressant. After 3 weeks on this medication, Mr. J experienced a marked reduction in the frequency of his panic attacks.

Mr. J also found significant relief from weekly psychotherapy sessions in which he could discuss his feeling of anxiety and shame about not being able to work. His own father had never held a job for very long and had abandoned his mother and him when he was 7 years old. These issues figured prominently in Mr. J's treatment.

Mr. J also benefited from group psychotherapy, where he was surprised to meet other people with similar symptoms. The group focused on education about panic disorder and a cognitive-behavioral approach to understanding his symptoms that included "homework" about writing down his thoughts when he was having a panic attack and learning how to stop them.

Mr. J gradually became encouraged to leave his house more and was even accompanied to the original supermarket by sympathetic members of the group. Mr. J was amazed that in spite of mild anxiety, the sight of the store no longer terrorized him. At a 3-month follow-up, he was doing well, was no longer having panic attacks or phobic behavior, and was working part-time while he looked actively for a new job.

Diagnosis. Panic disorder with agoraphobia (Axis I).

Panic disorder (and other anxiety disorders) can also be accompanied by dissociative symptoms such as depersonalization and derealization, which may lead to misdiagnosis as a primary dissociative disorder or even psychosis.

Patients who have panic disorder are more likely than other psychiatric patients to have family histories of anxiety, mood, and substance abuse disorders. Major depression is a comorbid diagnosis in about one-third of patients presenting for treatment. These patients are also at increased risk for substance abuse. For example, they might use alcohol to self-medicate when they are required to venture into a situation in which they feel likely to have a panic attack. An increased prevalence of labile hypertension occurs in patients who have panic disorder, and this group also exhibits increased cardiovascular mortality. Researchers were surprised to discover in the 1980s that as many as 10–20% of patients who have panic disorder attempt suicide.

Panic disorder has a negative impact on families. The sooner treatment is initiated, the better chance the patient has of avoiding significant comorbid depression, substance abuse, suicidality, or impaired functioning in work or social situations.

Susan C, aged 33, was admitted to a medical ward with acute pancreatitis brought on by heavy alcohol use. She received prophylactic treatment for alcohol withdrawal with diazepam (Valium) and was given multivitamins, thiamine, and folate. The medical student on the team requested that Ms. C receive a psychiatric evaluation after she revealed to the student that she had intermittent suicidal thoughts.

Ms. C told the consulting psychiatrist and medical student that she drank heavily to treat her "attacks." She described the attacks as lasting 20–30 minutes and characterized by palpitations in her chest, shortness of breath, dizziness, tingling in her hands and face, and the feeling that she was about to die.

Ms. C had suffered from these attacks since age 19. She could clearly remember her first one, which occurred when she returned to her parents' home to find no one there. Her father had been ill with cancer, and she had the immediate thought that her father had died. She suffered a paroxysmal attack, which ended spontaneously 30 minutes later. Her father's condition had indeed worsened, and he died the next day at the hospital.

Ms. C had her second panic attack after the funeral. The attacks did not recur for almost a year, leading her to think they had gone away. Then they began to recur, increasing in frequency and intensity over the years. Ms. C never sought treatment but gradually began to drink more alcohol to decrease her anxiety. She dropped out of college and worked for some time.

Eventually the panic attacks occurred when she drove her car, so she took public transportation. When she started to experience panic attacks on buses, she gave up her job. She became completely homebound (ie, agoraphobic) and dependent on her mother or sister to drive her to doctor appointments and had an increasing sense of depression and desperation. Although she had been seen by many different physicians over the years, few had asked about her symptoms, and no one had ever diagnosed panic disorder.

The consulting psychiatrist prescribed paroxetine, an antidepressant that has less initial stimulating effects (fluoxetine and sertraline may produce increased anxiety symptoms early in treatment). The panic attacks were much better at 2-week follow-up. One month later, Ms. C's depression was lifting. She had taken a bus to the beach and was thinking about returning to college. She had also started attending regular meetings of Alcoholics Anonymous, and except for one "slip" had stopped drinking alcohol. At 6-month follow-up Ms. C was doing extremely well, with a brighter mood and outlook.

Diagnosis. Panic disorder with agoraphobia; alcohol dependence (Axis I).

TREATMENT OF PANIC DISORDER

Approximately 80% of patients respond readily to treatment for panic disorder. Effective medications include tricyclic antidepressants, SSRIs, high-potency benzodiazepines such as alprazolam and clonazepam, and monoamine oxidase inhibitors (MAOIs). Specialized forms of cognitive-behavioral psychotherapy are also effective in treating these patients. These treatments help patients overcome their tendencies to catastrophically misinterpret the physical symptoms that occur and that may initiate panic. Behavioral therapy involving systematic exposure is the preferred treatment when agoraphobia complicates panic disorder. Many patients do best with a combination of pharmacologic treatment, cognitive therapy, and systematic exposure.

Sometimes anxiety disorders can be reinforced unintentionally through the efforts of well-intentioned health professionals, especially when the patient has dependent personality traits or a personality disorder. Physicians should be supportive but should refrain from behaviors that may encourage the patient's dependence on health professionals, for example, talking the patient through each panic attack.

SOCIAL PHOBIA: CLINICAL FEATURES

Social phobia is characterized by attacks of anxiety that are similar to those seen in panic disorder. The difference is that in panic disorder, anxiety attacks may occur spontaneously or are linked to social situations. In social phobia, attacks may occur when the patient is in a situation in which he or she may be scrutinized by others. This may be limited to a specific social situation, such as speaking, eating, or writing in front of others, or urinating in public rest rooms, or it may be generalized to include the majority of social encounters, or even speaking on the telephone.

INCIDENCE

Social phobia has been estimated to occur in 3% of the population. Its incidence is greater in women than in men.

ETIOLOGY

Biological Factors

The anxiety attacks associated with social phobia are thought to result from neurochemical imbalances in the CNS that cause the individual to experience anxiety and fear. Patients who have social phobia are more likely to have family histories marked by anxiety or mood disorders.

Psychological Factors

Social phobia is more likely to occur in adults who were fearful, shy, or anxiety-prone as children. Emotional, physical, or sexual abuse in childhood; adult trauma; and physical deformities that reduce self-esteem make social phobia more likely in adulthood.

DIAGNOSTIC ASSESSMENT

The diagnosis of social phobia was largely neglected until recent years and is still often dismissed as part of a personality disorder or misdiagnosed as panic disorder. In most respects, the emotional, physical, and cognitive symptoms that accompany the attacks are similar to those seen in panic disorder. A patient may have both panic disorder and social phobia (ie, panic attacks that occur both spontaneously and when the patient is the center of public attention). A subgroup of patients who have panic disorder appears to develop a social phobic pattern of avoidance behavior rather than an agoraphobic pattern. This pattern is referred to as **secondary social phobia.**

Social phobia may be complicated by other anxiety disorders, depression, substance use (usually alcohol or sedatives), and personality disorders (especially of the avoidant, dependent, borderline, and histrionic types). Patients who have these complications are more likely to exhibit significant impairment of social and work functioning, and they may be at increased risk for suicide attempts.

Anne P, aged 37, requested that her family physician refer her for treatment for panic attacks. After seeing a television talk show focused on panic disorder and agoraphobia, Ms. P believed she had the answer to a problem that had dominated her life since her teens: She was terrified of people. Whenever she had to speak with anyone outside of her immediate family, she became flushed and began to tremble. She felt ashamed that others would notice her blushing and stammering and would think she was making a fool of herself. When at home alone, she dreaded a knock at the door, because this meant she would have to face a stranger. Eye contact was the main cue for her intense anxiety. She avoided all social contact, and if she had to socialize with her husband's business contacts or attend meetings at her children's school, she would drink two or more glasses of wine "to get through it." She did not have anxiety attacks when she was alone.

Ms. P described herself as having been a shy child. Her father was eccentric and very frugal, insisting that she and her sister wear used clothes to school. She was unassertive and was teased frequently throughout elementary and high school. She worked briefly in an office until age 18, when she married her husband, who was 15 years older than she. She was a homemaker and kept the books for her husband's business.

Ms. P's family history revealed that her father had major depressive episodes, and her oldest son had both panic disorder and obsessive-compulsive disorder. Ms. P had never received any psychiatric treatment and until recently had not seen herself as more than "very shy." Her husband's business had experienced a downturn and she wished to find a part-time job to supplement the family finances but felt "paralyzed" whenever she thought about doing so.

Diagnosis. Social phobia (Axis I).

Discussion. Ms. P's symptoms and her anticipatory anxiety and extensive phobic avoidance seem to indicate panic disorder, but the critical distinction in this case is that Ms. P was anxious only in social situations where she feared the scrutiny of others.

TREATMENT OF SOCIAL PHOBIA

Social phobia responds best to a targeted combination of psychotherapy and pharmacologic treatment. The MAOI antidepressant phenelzine (Nardil) is particularly effective in treating social phobia. Patients must avoid medications such as pseudoephedrine (Sudafed) and meperidine (Demerol), which increase sympathetic nervous system activity, and they must follow a tyramine-free diet. These requirements may be daunting to the inexperienced clinician, but the benefits of this treatment are often dramatic and life-altering for patients.

Other effective and better tolerated pharmacologic treatments include SSRIs and high-potency benzodiazepines such as alprazolam and clonazepam. A few forms of social phobia, particularly fear of public speaking (if this occurs only occasionally in the patient's life), can be treated symptomatically with low doses of beta-blockers taken 30–60 minutes before a stressful event to block the autonomic symptoms of anxiety (ie, rapid heart rate, tremors, and sweating).

Psychotherapy for treatment of social phobia follows the same principles as the treatment of other anxiety disorders: cognitive restructuring and systematic exposure. Depression, poor self-esteem, and lack of assertiveness that have their roots in negative early childhood experiences often require a more dynamically oriented approach.

Ramona S, a 35-year-old businesswoman, presented for psychiatric treatment of panic attacks she would suffer before giving talks. Ms. S was called on to give business updates 3–5 times per week in company staff meetings. She reported that the attacks consisted of extreme anxiety, palpitations, dizziness, and shortness of breath. Ms. S would do fine at some talks and be paralyzed by fear and embarrassment at others. She was surprised that none of the meeting attendees knew when she was having an attack. She developed a system by which she could signal at the beginning of a meeting that her assistant would need to do the presentation instead. Ms. S was surprised that her assistant did not suspect that she was having difficulty; rather he believed that Ms. S was giving him last-minute assignments to keep him "on his toes" and to evaluate his performance.

This system worked for several years. Ms. S noted chronic feelings of mild depression, low self-esteem, and difficulty separating from friends and romantic interests who clearly took advantage of her generous nature.

In the year before she sought treatment, Ms. S experienced a number of stressors. She was promoted and was giving more talks to larger groups but could no longer switch off to an assistant. Her father, an alcoholic, suffered a stroke and Ms. S found herself unable to refuse his requests for her to visit him at his home 100 miles away at least twice a week.

She had also stopped drinking alcohol because she was worried that she was drinking too much to reduce her anxiety and was following in her father's footsteps. However, the alcohol had been an important means by which she had formerly modulated her anxiety levels. The attacks became more frequent, and Ms. S noted symptoms of worsening depression: She was losing interest in formerly pleasurable activities, her sleep was disturbed, and she had gained 30 pounds. She was initially hesitant to try antidepressants but was willing to try a beta-blocker that she could take before giving a talk. After using the medication about a dozen times, Ms. S felt an increased sense of control and reduced fear of having an attack.

In weekly therapy sessions Ms. S reviewed life-long feelings of low self-confidence, sadness, and fears of being alone. With the help of her therapist Ms. S was able to trace these feelings back to growing up with parents who abused alcohol, were erratically violent with each other and their children. They ultimately divorced when Ms. S was 11 years old. Ms. S's mother received custody of the children and forbade them from asking questions about their father. Ms. S found identifying and expressing her emotions in therapy to be helpful. She eventually agreed to try antidepressants in combination with psychotherapy, with good results.

Diagnosis. Social phobia; dysthymia, depressive disorder NOS (Axis I).

Because anxiety disorders are frequently complicated by other disorders, psychotherapy is often a useful means of "untangling" different disorders and probing the causes of anxiety disorders. Recent studies suggest that psychotherapy may also alter the longitudinal (lifetime) course of social phobia and panic disorder by reducing the likelihood and severity of future episodes.

GENERALIZED ANXIETY DISORDER: CLINICAL FEATURES

A discrete episode of persistent worry accompanied by insomnia, tension, or irritability lasting longer than 6 months suggests a diagnosis of **generalized anxiety disorder** (GAD). Patients who have GAD may also experience varied physical symptoms from overstimulation of the autonomic nervous system, including headaches, dizziness, heart palpitations, shortness of breath, diarrhea, diffuse aches and pains, restlessness, and fatigue.

INCIDENCE

GAD occurs with a female-to-male ratio of 2:1, although the ratio is 1:1 among those treated for the disorder, implying that women are either less likely to seek medical treatment or are more often misdiagnosed. The incidence of GAD has been estimated at 1–5% of the general population. A minority of patients who have GAD seek psychiatric treatment, but many individuals who have the disorder are commonly seen in outpatient medical settings. Most patients who have GAD patients are seen and treated by family or general practitioners; internists; or cardiac, pulmonary, or gastrointestinal specialists.

ETIOLOGY

Biological Factors

As in panic disorder and social phobia, abnormal neurochemistry is believed to play a major role in the production of anxiety-related symptoms in patients who have GAD. Genetic studies show higher rates of anxiety, alcohol use, and depressive disorders in relatives of individuals who have this disorder. The emotional and cognitive components of GAD imply dysfunction in both the limbic and frontal lobes. The efficacy of benzodiazepines and SSRI antidepressants in the treatment of GAD as well as other studies of neurotransmitter activity in humans and animals indicate underfunctioning of GABA and serotonergic neurotransmitter pathways in this disorder.

Psychological Factors

Patients who have GAD tend to be more vulnerable to stress and to have poor coping mechanisms. They are more likely to have had or to be at risk for episodes of major depression, alcohol dependence, and other anxiety disorders. Anxiety and insomnia can be associated with major depression and with dysthymia; therefore, these differential diagnoses must be considered. The presence of comorbid major depression or panic disorder will have implications for treatment. Medical causes should always be considered and ruled out.

DIAGNOSTIC ASSESSMENT

Symptoms of GAD last for at least 6 months and include autonomic nervous system hyperactivity such as sweating, palpitations, shortness of breath, and dizziness; motor symptoms including tension, restlessness, and muscle twitches; and subjective symptoms of irritability such as being "on edge," having insomnia, and having trouble concentrating.

For some patients, generalized anxiety is less an acute disorder than a facet of their personality. Patients who have GAD have a lifelong tendency to ruminate, meeting criteria for the disorder intermittently as life stressors supervene and overwhelm their ability to cope. As a result, some experts have proposed that GAD is a personality disorder; however, many patients have discrete, isolated episodes of generalized anxiety and then return to a nonpathologic baseline. These patients tend to worry excessively, and even if they are aware that their worrying is excessive, the level of anxiety becomes uncontrollable. In fact many GAD patients worry about worrying, which feeds into the vicious cycle of anxiety.

Owen G, a 41-year-old married physician, presented at a medical clinic asking for something to help him sleep. He reported that he had always been a poor sleeper. He admitted to feeling anxious every day and also said that he had always been an "uptight person," a "worry wart." This characteristic was associated with him being very organized, punctual, attentive to detail, and particular about his likes and dislikes. He indicated that he had a busy forensic practice and that he spent much of his time evaluating clients involved in litigation, preparing reports, and testifying in court. He had never been able to "leave work at work," but over the past year had spent more and more of his day worrying that he had forgotten important details, that he would miss deadlines or slip up in court, although none of these situations had occurred.

Dr. G was also increasingly worried about finances and had asked his wife to pay the monthly bills, because when he did it he would lay awake at night reviewing the family finances, which were quite solid. He was aware that his worrying was excessive, but he could not control it. Because of his fatigue on waking, Dr. G had switched from drinking tea to coffee during the past month and was drinking 4 cups per day. During the previous 12-month period he frequently felt tense and shaky, had palpitations, felt sweaty at night, and had frequent headaches. He also reported being irritable with his wife and 9-year-old daughter and increasingly demanding of his staff. Treatment included individual psychotherapy, low doses of a tricyclic antidepressant, and a gradual reduction in caffeine intake. Dr. D experienced a marked reduction in physical and emotional symptoms.

Diagnosis. Generalized anxiety disorder (Axis I).

TREATMENT OF GENERALIZED ANXIETY DISORDER

Many GAD patients respond well to psychotherapeutic treatments. Stress management, relaxation therapy, and cognitive therapy are often successful within weeks or months. For patients who have long-standing problems or whose tendency to expect the worst is rooted in developmental experiences, more dynamically oriented therapy is indicated.

Pharmacologic treatments include tricyclic and other antidepressants, which may be effective at doses considerably lower than those needed to treat depression, or the anxiolytic buspirone (BuSpar). Benzodiazepines may be helpful, but they should be used cautiously if the symptoms are long-standing because of the possibility that dependency might result.

OBSESSIVE-COMPULSIVE DISORDER: CLINICAL FEATURES

Obsessive-compulsive disorder (OCD) is marked by the presence of both obsessional thoughts and compulsive behavior. Patients who have OCD experience thoughts that have an extremely compelling and repetitive quality that goes far beyond rumination. These thoughts are experienced by patients as strange, alien, and originating from "outside" of themselves; the technical term for this quality is egodystonic. These thoughts are usually associated with increasing anxiety and generally fall into one of several categories, including fears of contamination, fears of being harmed or causing harm to others, sexual themes, or idiosyncratic ideas that lack obvious meaning.

INCIDENCE

Approximately 1–3% of the population of the United States are thought to have OCD. It occurs equally in men and women.

ETIOLOGY

Biological Factors

The advent of sophisticated techniques for investigating changes in brain chemistry and function has led to startling revelations about the pathophysiology of OCD. Positron emission tomography (PET) scans of patients who have OCD have shown marked decreases in metabolism in the head of the caudate nuclei, along with increased metabolism of the orbital frontal cortex. After several weeks of treatment with SSRIs, such as fluoxetine or fluvoxamine, or with cognitive behavioral therapy, these deficiencies disappear and correspond to improvements in symptoms. This observation suggests that serotonin may play an important role in brain circuits involved in limiting repetitive mental functions. Most patients who have OCD note the first onset of symptoms in early adolescence, when the serotonin system is becoming fully developed in the brain. Some studies suggest a connection with more neurologically based disorders such as Tourette's syndrome.

Psychological Factors

Psychological defense mechanisms may account for some of the manifestations of OCD. Isolation refers to the separation of thought from feeling and may account for the unshakable quality of obsessive thoughts without an awareness of their origin. Some patients are uncomfortable with their own aggressive thoughts at an unconscious level, either because of temperament or upbringing. Repression of feelings of anger at an individual may explain some repeated thoughts of harming that person. In some cases the object of aggressive thoughts is a different person entirely, further disguising the source of the feelings. Undoing refers to the need to reduce the anxiety that compulsive behaviors produce, at least temporarily by mentally "taking back" an unpleasant thought. The anxiety that accompanies obsessive thoughts is then banished for a brief period of hours or perhaps days. The use of a compulsive action to take back an obsessive thought also involves magical thinking, in which the patient knows logically that counting tiles in a room cannot reduce the chance of someone being harmed, but the irrational connection between the thought and the compulsion is reinforced by repetition.

The link between obsessions and compulsions, and their self-reinforcing quality, are explained by principles of learning theory. Obsessive thoughts initially have little emotional impact, because of isolation. With repeated experience the thoughts become increasingly associated with anxiety. Compulsive behavior produces temporary anxiety reduction. Patients soon find themselves locked into a positive feedback loop in which the compulsive behavior reinforces itself by rewarding the individual with temporary relief from anxiety.

DIAGNOSTIC ASSESSMENT

Compulsive behavior may involve repeated handwashing, checking of light switches or gas knobs, counting, tracing lines, or other stereotyped behaviors. Because the compulsive behavior makes the patient feel better almost immediately by temporarily relieving anxiety, the behavior will usually increase over time. Insight into the condition does not relieve the unshakable quality of obsessions and compulsions. In many cases, the patient will spend an increasing and significant amount of time engaged in these activities. Some patients find themselves locked into "loops" of obsessions and compulsions for hours, unable to leave the house, thus jeopardizing jobs and relationships. Embarrassment, shame, and concern that they are "crazy" or "insane" may prevent patients who have OCD from describing their problems to others, and the strange nature of the symptoms may cause others to distance themselves from patients.

Patients who have OCD typically do not seek medical attention until an average of 10 years after the onset of symptoms, and even then misdiagnosis is common. In one study, patients were not accurately diagnosed and treated for OCD until an average of 6–7 years after seeking medical treatment. The estimated annual cost of OCD in the United States is $8 billion, including $2 billion in direct care and almost $6 billion in lost productivity, sick days, and early retirement at work.

Conditions associated with OCD include depression; substance use; body dysmorphic syndrome (a conviction that a body part is deformed); depersonalization disorder; and more impulsive disorders such as gambling, sexual compulsions, an impulsive personality style or disorder (such as borderline personality disorder), and suicidal tendencies. Patients who have OCD may also have other anxiety disorders. OCD is sometimes found in patients who have schizophrenia and may be prominent in patients who have anorexia nervosa, an eating disorder in which patients restrict eating but frequently obsess about food and whose eating habits involve complex rituals.

Obsessions are distinguished from delusions by the presence of the patient's insight into the irrational nature of the obsessions. Most patients are aware of the strangeness of their symptoms and have an intact sense of reality. This distinction helps clinicians differentiate symptoms of OCD from schizophrenia. In an unusual subset of patients, OCD appears to have psychotic features. Patients who have schizophrenia may also have OCD, which may increase when patients are treated with clozapine (Clozaril). The distinction between obsessions and delusions is also important in the postpartum period, when puerperal psychosis may be present with delusions regarding the newborn infant. Unlike postpartum psychosis, in which mothers are in fact at risk for harming their infants, OCD patients virtually never act upon obsessions of harm, despite their fears that they will do so.

OCD is distinguished from generalized anxiety disorder by the association of anxiety with obsessions, rather than free-floating worry about life circumstances. Significant relief from anxiety is also provided by compulsive behavior, which is usually performed in response to an obsession (for example, compulsive washing in response to contamination obsessions, checking in response to obsessive doubt).

Jennifer E, aged 24, presented to her obstetrician with the complaint, "I think I'm losing my mind and am afraid I am going to kill my baby." Her baby was 7 months old, and Ms. E was troubled constantly by the intrusive thought that she would stab her infant with a kitchen knife. This thought first occurred to her several weeks after she delivered and was abhorrent and frightening to her. She had been struggling to stop the thought, but it entered her consciousness whenever she was not mentally involved with some kind of activity. She had always resisted the thought and had removed all sharp objects from the house. Moreover, she had been leaving the baby with her mother-in-law during the day when her husband was not home for fear that she would act on the thought. She was deeply ashamed of thinking such a thing and had told no one until she spoke with her obstetrician.

She was sleeping poorly, felt overwhelmed and hopeless, and had had fleeting thoughts of suicide during the previous week. When questioned, Ms. E admitted that she had had similar intrusive thoughts in the past. Starting at age 10, she had become preoccupied with symmetry, straightening objects in her room and her parents' home. She also had the impulse to count objects on a table or people in a room and had to check that the window in her room was locked at night 6 or 7 times before she could go to sleep. She recognized that these impulses and rituals were abnormal but kept them to herself and managed to contain her need for symmetry to her own room in order to avoid teasing from her family members. The need to count people and objects had gone away for the most part, returning only in stressful social situations. The checking behaviors had become part of life and had not interfered significantly with her functioning.

Diagnosis. Obsessive-compulsive disorder (Axis I).

TREATMENT OF OBSESSIVE-COMPULSIVE DISORDER

The psychotherapy of OCD relies upon the behavior principles of exposure and response-prevention. In a graded manner, patients are exposed to situations in which they are likely to experience their obsessions and then are required to resist the impulse to perform the compulsion. This method breaks the cycle by which patients rely on compulsions to reduce their anxiety. SSRIs provide effective pharmacotherapy for OCD. The SSRI fluvoxamine (Luvox) is approved for the treatment of OCD, and the other SSRIs (fluoxetine, sertraline, and paroxetine) are similarly effective. Clomipramine (Anafranil), a tricyclic antidepressant (TCA) that has serotonergic properties, is also effective for OCD but is associated with many anticholinergic side effects. Other antidepressants are not effective in treating patients who have this disorder. As with other anxiety disorders, the integration of pharmacologic and psychotherapeutic approaches results in the most effective and enduring treatment.

Another specific form of obsessive-compulsive disorder involves ritualistic behavior. For example, when the patient presents with compulsive hair-pulling, the condition is known as trichotillomania.

As in other obsessive-compulsive disorders, affected patients are often embarrassed or ashamed of their symptoms, which may delay or prevent their seeking treatment. Treatment often consists of a combination of psychotherapy, behavioral therapy, and medications that increase serotonin. The response rate is very favorable.

Karla H, aged 42, was referred for a psychiatric evaluation because her primary care physician was unable to determine the nature of localized alopecia (hair loss). Her physician had inquired about the multiple bald spots on a routine physical examination. Ms. H, a highly successful businesswoman, became extremely embarrassed and provided terse responses to her questions, usually "I don't know." As the physician expressed her concern and determination to characterize the history of Ms. H's problem, Ms. H began to tug on her hair, and the physician began to suspect a psychological etiology.

Ms. H was reluctant to see a psychiatrist but agreed to call for an appointment. She revealed to the psychiatrist that she had been tugging at her hair since she was 16 years old, shortly after her parents divorced. She had found that this habit at first decreased her level of anxiety. Later she realized the compelling nature of the hair-pulling but found herself unable to stop, particularly in stressful situations. She began to wear her hair up when she developed bald spots on her scalp. She was careful to minimize the behavior in business meetings but chose a career that allowed her to work from home in part to minimize the chances of being seen pulling her hair. She also reported other less-frequent ritualistic behavior such as repeated hand-washing, which had begun at age 11.

Ms. H was initially unwilling to try medication but eventually agreed to a trial of fluvoxamine (Luvox). Behavioral therapy focused on unlearning hair-pulling as a means of reducing anxiety. Her symptoms improved within several weeks. Three months later she had largely ceased to pull her hair and once again was wearing it loose. She also reported decreased anxiety overall and improved comfort in social situations.

Diagnosis. Obsessive-compulsive disorder with trichotillomania (Axis I).

Difficulties may emerge in the treatment of any psychiatric disorder. For example, the disorder may occur comorbidly with substance use or dependency that is likely to cause the patient to "cling" to his or her symptoms—and to health-care providers. Another scenario involves family members becoming enmeshed in the patient's disorder in a way that temporarily helps the family cope with stress or conflict, but often at the expense of the patient's improvement. A **systems approach** always includes assessment of social and family dynamics that may maintain the patient's symptoms.

Louis D, a 19-year-old college freshman, developed obsessive-compulsive disorder 2 years earlier, while in high school. His initial symptoms consisted of compulsive cleaning and counting activity but were mild enough not to interfere significantly with his life. In college, the anxiety, thoughts, and behaviors intensified, and he began to spend hours each day worrying or engaged in ritualistic behavior. Part of his anxiety around cleaning focused on germs and the possibility that he might die of a bacterial infection. He started to laboriously clean every eating utensil several times each day. He then had progressively less time during the day to study or socialize. By the end of his freshman year, his grades had declined and he was socially withdrawn. His parents convinced him to seek treatment through the student health center.

Mr. D had a modest initial response to psychotherapy and the SSRI antidepressant fluoxetine (Prozac). The fluoxetine dosage was increased gradually, and his obsessions remitted partially.

Mr. D's self-esteem had decreased markedly since starting college, and he had become much more withdrawn and socially isolated. He began to spend increasing amounts of time visiting his parents. His parents were meanwhile dealing with his mother's depression (exacerbated by her guilt that she had given her son "bad genes" that led to his OCD) and his father's alcohol dependence. They had experienced marital difficulties that were serious enough to make them consider separation and divorce. Now, with their son at home more, they were able to forget temporarily their own troubles as they focused on helping him.

The parents remained extremely troubled by Mr. D's symptoms and tried to convince him to "just stop doing those habits." They began to involve themselves in the rituals in an effort to help him. For example, if Mr. D removed a kitchen utensil from the drawer, he would regard all of the utensils in that compartment as "dirty" and would have to clean them in a time-consuming manner. Mr. D's mother began to clean all of the knives, forks, and spoons in the drawer after he touched any one of them so that he wouldn't "waste his time doing that silly stuff."

Mr. D developed new habits while at his parent's house, such as tracing all of the lines in the hardwood floor before going to bed. His father was unable to convince him to stop, so he joined the nightly ritual by tracing lines with Mr. D for an hour to "help get him to bed faster. We can do it in half the time if I help."

By the end of the semester, Mr. D was more depressed, dependent on his parents, and unwilling to return to school. The situation improved only when family therapy was recommended to help Mr. D regain independence. His parents resisted efforts to become less enmeshed with him, until they began couples therapy to help them with their own roles. They came to realize that by concentrating on their son's problems, they had unwittingly made his symptoms worse and that their over-involvement in his compulsions helped to mask their own emotional and relationship problems.

SPECIFIC PHOBIA: CLINICAL FEATURES

Specific phobia consists of the fear of a specific situation or stressor. Insects, small animals, heights, flying, and the sight of blood or needles are the most common stressors that invoke fear and terror to a degree that is far out of proportion to an expected reaction.

INCIDENCE

Between 3 and 5% of the United States population has been estimated to experience a simple phobia. The incidence of simple phobia is greater in women than in men.

ETIOLOGY

Overactivation of pathways in the brain that correspond to the emotional and cognitive components of anxiety are believed to lend a biological predisposition common to all of the anxiety disorders. Learning theory explains why patients avoid anxiety-provoking stimuli, and why their fear does not resolve with repeated exposure. What is less clear is why patients become frightened of a particular situation or object. Cultural factors may play a role, as in the fear of insects. For many patients, psychotherapy helps to reveal the symbolic nature of the anxiety, which may be linked to conscious or unconscious conflict about sexual or aggressive thoughts and feelings.

DIAGNOSTIC ASSESSMENT

Depending on the patient's work and home life, a specific phobia may produce varying degrees of dysfunction. For example, a fear of flying in a plane may not interfere with a patient's typical day. However, if that patient is given a promotion that involves frequent travel across the United States, the disorder may become a source of shame or dread and would quickly be identified as a strongly maladaptive trait. Accordingly, sufferers rarely seek treatment unless their life circumstances demand that they overcome their fears.

Pradeepa G, aged 24, presented to her family physician requesting referral to a psychologist because she was afraid of spiders. She had been afraid of them her entire life and had coped with this fear by careful avoidance. She and her husband recently moved to her husband's small family farm. The house, garden, and barn were filled with spiders, and to her chagrin Ms. G was unable to do much of anything around her new home because of her fear (already confirmed several times) of confronting a spider.

Diagnosis. Specific phobia (Axis I).

TREATMENT OF SPECIFIC PHOBIA

The treatment of specific phobia is behavioral, with systematic, graded exposure to the feared stimulus. For the fear of flying in the nonfrequent flyer, a benzodiazepine is a reasonable alternative or supplement to behavioral treatment.

Albert Y, aged 30, had a profound fear of heights (acrophobia) that began in childhood and had intensified since he took a job on the 23rd floor of an office building. Just thinking about being close to the windows made him feel dizzy and panicked. His coworkers and employers became aware of the problem and encouraged him to get help. Although Mr. Y approached psychiatric help with reluctance, he agreed to try a new form of treatment. At the start of each weekly session he placed a virtual-reality helmet on his head. A 3-D computer-generated image appeared around him, featuring a glass-sided elevator on the outside of a tall building. Mr. Y was able to "walk" into the elevator, press a virtual button, and ascend to the top of a virtual building. He was gradually able to tolerate heights with successively decreased anxiety.

Diagnosis. Specific phobia (Axis I).

Discussion. Psychiatrists have recently pioneered this treatment for **acrophobia** (fear of heights) and hope to expand its applications.

Support groups may help lessen patients' embarrassment about their fears. For example, some groups train for flying together by boarding parked airplanes.

DIFFERENTIAL DIAGNOSIS

Various medical and psychiatric disorders can produce symptoms similar to those seen in anxiety disorders.

1. RULING OUT MEDICAL CAUSES

Symptoms that suggest an anxiety disorder, including acute anxiety and physical symptoms, can be produced by a variety of medical states. These medical conditions must be ruled out before an accurate diagnosis of an anxiety disorder can be made. For example, patients who have hyperthyroidism and the much rarer pheochromocytoma and carcinoid syndromes often exhibit symptoms of panic disorder. Other medical causes, such as pulmonary emboli, cardiac arrhythmias, brain tumors in the third ventricle, and temporal lobe epilepsy, should be considered.

Routine screening measures used to rule out these disorders include a medical history with particular emphasis on the presence of symptoms indicating cardiovascular problems, as well as on the use of prescription or other drugs. The clinician should also order a complete physical examination of the patient and a full laboratory workup, including the following tests:

- serum electrolytes
- complete blood counts
- EKG
- thyroid function tests
- lumbar puncture, if indicated
- CT or MRI, if indicated
- EEG, if indicated

Appropriate tests are sufficient to rule out underlying medical causes, thus eliminating the need for inappropriate invasive and expensive evaluations such as coronary angiograms.

2. RULING OUT PSYCHIATRIC DISORDERS

Individuals suffering from major depression may present with anxiety that includes infrequent panic attacks. Patients who have social phobia and post-traumatic stress disorder (PTSD) may exhibit panic-like symptoms, triggered by social situations or trauma-related cues instead of occurring spontaneously. Generalized anxiety disorder is often associated with prominent autonomic symptoms that lack the acuity and intensity characteristic of panic attacks. Substance use—especially excessive caffeine intake, alcohol dependency, alcohol or benzodiazepine withdrawal, cocaine or methamphetamine intoxication, or marijuana use—commonly cause anxiety states.

EMOTIONAL REACTIONS TO PATIENTS

Because of the universality of the experience of anxiety, health-care providers, friends, and family members are usually able to understand and empathize with patients who have anxiety disorders. Paradoxically, empathy may leave medical interviewers feeling somewhat anxious themselves. The acuity and intensity of anxiety in panic attacks and simple and social phobia may strain the interviewer's ability to understand and believe the patient and may result in emotional distancing. The often bizarre symptoms seen in OCD may lead to feelings of disbelief, discomfort, and aloofness.

CROSS-CULTURAL ASPECTS OF ANXIETY DISORDERS

The primary impact of cultural factors is to increase the presentation of somatic symptoms in patients from backgrounds that stigmatize mental illness. Additionally, there is the danger of a health-care worker from a different cultural background diagnosing a patient who has an anxiety disorder as having psychosis or schizophrenia instead.

LEGAL & ETHICAL ISSUES

Ethical issues may arise in the treatment of patients who have dual substance use and anxiety disorders. Benzodiazepines such as alprazolam (Xanax), lorazepam (Ativan), and diazepam (Valium) may be extremely helpful in the treatment of anxiety disor-

ders, and the vast majority of patients do not abuse medications. However, in patients who have preexisting substance dependence or a family history of dependence, these drugs have a strong potential for tolerance, dependence, and abuse. The physician may be faced with the dilemma of managing a patient who has an anxiety disorder and active substance use. The physician may also be faced with the conflict between the tenet of doing the least harm and respecting the patient's desire to control his or her own treatment and for self-determination in weighing whether to start or continue medication when a patient is using substances intermittently.

CONCLUSION

The diagnosis and treatment of anxiety disorders is one of the most satisfying areas in medicine. Only a few decades ago, these disorders resulted in tremendous morbidity and disability, but the recent development of targeted pharmacotherapies and psychotherapies means a good prognosis for the majority of patients who have anxiety disorders. Because many such patients present to nonpsychiatric physicians, the primary care physician must have the diagnostic skills necessary to identify these disorders. Furthermore, it is increasingly within the scope of primary care practice to initiate the treatment of anxiety disorders such as panic disorder, social phobia, and generalized anxiety disorder and to then coordinate treatment with mental health professionals.

REFERENCES

Ballenger JC: Panic disorder in the medical setting. J Clin Psychiatr 1997;58(Suppl No. 2):13.

Bourne EJ: *The Anxiety and Phobia Workbook,* 2nd ed. New Harbingers Publications, 1995.

Carter CS, Servan-Schreiber D, Perlstein WM: Anxiety disorders and the syndrome of chest pain with normal coronary arteries: prevalence and pathophysiology. J Clin Psychiatr 1997;58(Suppl No. 2):70.

Eisen JL, Rasmussen SA: Obsessive compulsive disorder with psychotic features. J Clin Psychiatr. 1993;54(10): 373.

Goddard AW, Charney DS: Toward an integrated neurobiology of panic disorder. J Clin Psychiatr 1997;58(Suppl No. 2):4.

Hales RE, Hilty DA, Wise MG: A treatment algorithm for the management of anxiety in primary care practice. J Clin Psychiatr 1997;58(Suppl No. 3):76.

Katon WJ: *Panic Disorder in the Medical Setting.* American Psychiatric Press, 1991.

Kirmater LJ, Young A, Hayton BC: The cultural context of anxiety disorders. Psychiatr Clin N Am 1995;18(3):503.

National Institutes for Mental Health, Anxiety Disorder for Professionals. http://208.231.11.108/nimh/resource/index.htm

Yonkers KA, Warshaw MG, Massion AO et al: Phenomenology and course of generalized anxiety disorder. Br J Psychiatr 1996;168:308.

Zajecka J: Importance of establishing the diagnosis of persistent anxiety. J Clin Psychiatr 1997;58(Suppl No. 3):9.

Post-traumatic Stress Disorder

8

David Elkin, MD, Emily Newman, MD, Cameron S. Carter, MD, & Mark Zaslav, PhD

Post-traumatic stress disorder (PTSD), one of the five anxiety disorders described in the *DSM-IV,* refers to the psychiatric syndrome that develops in some individuals after exposure to a major stressor or trauma. Psychological results of trauma have been well-documented. In the United States, special attention has been paid to this phenomenon during wartime. The *DSM-I,* which was developed after World War II, described a **gross stress reaction** in soldiers, but later theories minimized the impact of trauma. This assessment changed drastically in the aftermath of the Vietnam War, when PTSD was more closely observed and described in military veterans.

Since the 1980s the concept of PTSD has been broadened to include the results of traumatic events encountered by the general populace, with a growing appreciation for the frequency of trauma encountered in modern society. The women's movement has contributed significantly to an appreciation of the frequency of sexual abuse. Medical conditions and invasive treatment for illness are now known to produce PTSD. Research has also led to a better appreciation of long-term results of trauma, including the high incidence of other psychiatric disorders such as depression and anxiety disorders, and the long-lasting impact of trauma on some patients. Researchers have also demonstrated the significant difference between children and adults in their response to trauma.

Psychologically traumatic events such as rape, military combat, earthquakes, airplane crashes, and torture evoke some symptoms of distress in almost anyone who experiences these events. Usually these reactions are mild, nonspecific, and short-lived and would not be considered psychopathological. However, depending on the individual affected and the traumatic event, a characteristic psychopathological syndrome may develop—the post-traumatic stress disorder. Post-traumatic stress disorder reflects an ongoing maladaptive response to trauma that may become chronic.

Individuals responding to any stressful event and the anxiety with which the event is associated will demonstrate emotional responses and adaptation over time. The anxiety generated by an exposure to trauma is moderated by psychological defense mechanisms. During the initial minutes and hours after trauma, individuals may report feeling overwhelmed, confused, dazed, or dissociated. In most cases, denial and repression reduce awareness of the trauma, thereby providing an emotional buffer in the days following the event. A high degree of emotional numbing immediately following the trauma actually predicts the development of more severe PTSD.

Over time, some patients become aware of the significance of the trauma and experience break-through anxiety and intrusive thoughts and images about the trauma. Symptoms that occur during the first month after trauma are defined in the *DSM-IV* as **acute stress disorder** that includes the same symptoms as PTSD but is marked more by emotional shock, anger, depression, and emotional dissociation or numbing. Acute Stress Disorder usually resolves within the first month after exposure to trauma. Acute stress disorder in many ways reflects a healthy, adaptive response to trauma, where the individual is able to work through and eventually integrate the psychological effect of the trauma.

In PTSD this process is more prolonged and resolution does not always occur. Psychotherapy can often help to accelerate this process of recovery from trauma. By definition, PTSD occurs one month or more after the traumatic event and is characterized by symptoms such as flashbacks, nightmares, insomnia, anxiety, and emotional numbing.

Repeated exposure to trauma produces a different and more complicated psychological response as the patient's psychological defenses are frequently overwhelmed. The psychiatric syndrome that develops after repeated trauma may be much longer lasting and more difficult to treat, often producing lifelong symptoms. This syndrome has been termed **complex PTSD** or **disorders of extreme stress.** Figure 8–1 illustrates the relationships among the variants of PTSD.

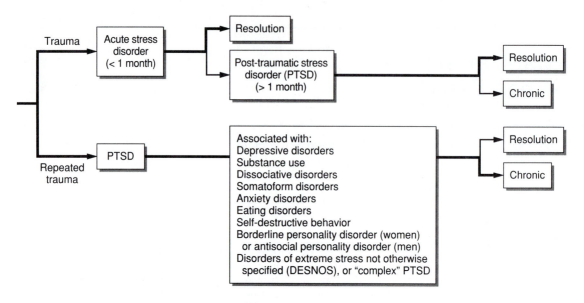

Figure 8–1. Relationship between trauma, acute stress disorder, PTSD, and complex PTSD. Most patients exposed to a traumatic event develop a time-limited psychiatric syndrome known as acute stress disorder. Patients who still have symptoms beyond 1 month after the event are diagnosed with post-traumatic stress disorder (PTSD). Some patients have symptoms for many months or years (chronic PTSD). Repeated trauma, especially in childhood, often leads to a more chronic, complex clinical syndrome associated with other serious psychiatric diagnoses. This has been termed disorders of extreme stress not otherwise specified (DESNOS), sometimes called complex PTSD. **Darker arrows** indicate usual course or outcome.

Stress disorders are widespread in society and are often present in patients seen in medical settings. PTSD may manifest with different clinical presentations, sometimes masked by somatization, substance use, and other psychiatric symptoms. Effective treatment exists for PTSD, but physicians must be familiar with the basic clinical definitions and assessment tools used to identify this important syndrome.

INCIDENCE

As many as 5–10% of Americans will at some time in their lives satisfy the full criteria for PTSD. Women are more likely to be affected than men. The incidence of PTSD resulting from any episode of trauma is estimated at 25% but is not well studied. For example, the risk of PTSD resulting from a motor vehicle accident is unknown, even though hundreds of thousands of such accidents occur annually. Risk factors for PTSD include certain occupations (police, military, paramedics, and body handlers), certain situations (residence in high-crime areas, lower socioeconomic status, immigration from war-torn countries), age (children and the elderly), previous history as a victim of crime, and a past history of trauma. PTSD occurs in 57–80% of all rape victims and may be even more likely in displaced populations exposed to war and political oppression. Homeless individuals

have a high incidence of PTSD (one-fifth of men and one-third of women in one study). The reason for this incidence may be that PTSD (especially when associated with depression and substance use) may lead to work impairment and precipitate homelessness or homeless populations are exposed to more traumatic events.

The level of severity and duration of the traumatic event correlates with a greater chance of developing PTSD, as does the patient's proximity to the event. Physical injury with lasting medical problems, such as scarring, fractures, or chronic pain or paralysis, also increases the likelihood that an individual will develop PTSD. PTSD is likely to be encountered in surgery wards and clinics, where a large proportion of patients are seen for treatment of physical injuries. Physicians have only recently realized that PTSD is common among medical patients who have had multiple intrusive procedures performed to treat a medical illness.

ETIOLOGY

Biological Factors

In clinical studies, diminished serotonergic effects, reduction in cortisol release, and hypersuppression of cortisol to dexamethasone inhibition distinguish patients with PTSD from control subjects. As is true in other anxiety disorders, PTSD is thought to involve impaired α_2-adrenergic receptor feedback inhibition. This mediates the stress-induced release of norepinephrine from the locus coeruleus. Progressive behavioral sensitization and generalization develops to stimulus cues associated with the original trauma, resulting in patients "learning" anxiety-based behaviors, thoughts, and feelings. Studies of the psychobiology of PTSD have also begun to examine the links between emotions and memory. Increased noradrenergic activity at locus coeruleus projection sites in the hippocampus and amygdala facilitates learning of fear-based memories that persist and resist extinction. Studies demonstrating higher concordance of PTSD in monozygotic and dizygotic twins exposed to trauma suggests a genetic vulnerability to trauma.

Psychological Factors

Studies have identified individuals who are more vulnerable to stress and therefore more likely to develop PTSD following a traumatic event. Psychological risk factors for the development of PTSD include a past psychiatric history of depression or previous trauma. Personality characteristics of high neuroticism and extroversion or a history of behavioral problems in childhood also increase the likelihood of PTSD developing after exposure to trauma. However, the disorder may also develop even when there are no predisposing factors, especially when the stressor is extreme.

Social & Environmental Factors

Environmental factors play a significant role in any psychiatric disorder but are especially important in PTSD. Enhanced social support will tend to ameliorate or even protect against the development of PTSD. In contrast, isolation and invalidation of the patient's experience will increase the likelihood of psychopathology, as in the case of the patient whose family refuses to believe his or her account of spousal abuse or in the patient whose parents deny sexual abuse. The lack of validation has also been implicated in the higher incidence of PTSD in Vietnam veterans compared to veterans of World War II. Living in an environment with repeated exposure to traumatic cues—such as a victim of assault returning to his or her apartment in a high-crime area where gunshots can be heard—is likely to exacerbate PTSD.

The Nature of the Trauma

Traumatic events traditionally were defined in the context of combat trauma in wartime and later as an event occurring outside the realm of normal human experience. Because traumatic events are in fact common, trauma now refers to any potentially life-threatening situation, even if an individual is not physically harmed. Threats of physical violence, as occur in stalking, or situations in which natural disasters threaten cities but fail to do any immediate danger are nonetheless capable of engendering acute and post-traumatic stress disorders. Physical injury from trauma such as fractured limbs, burns, or paralysis may serve as a potent reminder of the trauma and increases the risk of PTSD.

Recent studies have focused on the likelihood that television broadcasts of disasters and crime can serve as traumatic stimuli, especially in children. Trauma or threats of violence by human beings is more likely to produce emotional distress than will natural disasters. It may be less threatening to one's world view to experience an earthquake or hurricane than to accept the possibility of human aggressiveness and cruelty.

ACUTE STRESS DISORDER & POST-TRAUMATIC STRESS DISORDER: CLINICAL FEATURES

Patients may develop significant anxiety after exposure to extreme trauma. The reaction may occur shortly after the traumatic exposure (acute stress disorder), or it may be delayed in time and subject to recurrence (PTSD). In both syndromes, individuals experience a number of key symptoms, which often impair work performance or social functioning. These symptoms include four main categories: avoidance, anxiety, re-experiencing, and hyperarousal:

- **Avoidance** of emotions and thoughts can manifest as derealization, depersonalization, numbing or detachment, loss of emotional responsiveness, or memory loss (eg, being unable to recall specific aspects of the trauma). Other avoidance behaviors attempt to reduce exposure to stimuli that precipitate recollections of the trauma, such as avoiding the location of the trauma or people connected to the traumatic event. Patients may actively avoid discussing the trauma to avoid emotionally painful thoughts or feelings.
- **Anxiety** symptoms include episodes of panic or chronic anxiety, insomnia, poor concentration, irritability, or restlessness.
- **Re-experiencing** of the trauma involves dreams, nightmares, or vivid "flashbacks" in which patients feel as if they are momentarily reliving the event, with thoughts or images of the trauma.
- **Hyperarousal** symptoms include motor restlessness, hypervigilance (constantly scanning one's environment for potential danger when no threat is discernible), and a startle response such as jumping in response to hearing a car backfire.

Other symptoms include feelings or behaviors associated with depression, poor self-esteem, crying spells, changes in appetite, feelings of powerlessness or hopelessness, reduced energy and motivation, and a foreshortened sense of the future. Mood swings may be present, usually ranging from normal to very depressed. Dissociative phenomena may also occur, including partial amnesia about the traumatic event. Patients may also vacillate between feeling emotionally numbed and having episodes of extreme rage and sometimes violence. Phobias and avoidance may lead some patients to become completely isolated or homebound. Sometimes patients who have PTSD engage in high-risk behavior. Symptoms may be converted into physical complaints or lead to an exaggeration of physical symptoms. PTSD is also associated with suicide attempts in some cases, especially in rape victims.

Horowitz has postulated a spectrum of possible responses to trauma, in which a "normal" reaction includes many of the symptoms listed above. Intensification of these symptoms are also possible. Uncommonly, temporary psychotic states immediately follow the trauma and may be associated with disorganized thoughts, paranoia, and delusions. Severely anxious patients may develop panic disorder or ritualistic behavior suggestive of obsessive-compulsive disorder. Some patients may seek to enhance emotional numbing by using alcohol or other substances. This behavior is very likely if substance use was a problem before the trauma, leading to tolerance, dependence, or relapse in former substance users. Benzodiazepine dependence may result when physicians overprescribe these antianxiety medications.

Edward H, aged 29, was in a convenience store with his 2-year-old son. He went to the restroom and was surprised by two young men brandishing guns. They demanded his wallet, watch, and wedding ring. As he fumbled to give them his valuables, his assailants began to scream at him to hurry. One of the men held his gun inches from Mr. H's face and told him that he would shoot him if he did not comply. The robbery was interrupted by several other patrons entering the store, and the gunmen fled.

Afterwards Mr. H filled out a police report. He felt strange, almost numb. The incident was so sudden and surprising that he did not feel that he had time to react, and did not remember feeling in danger. He ruminated about the present for his wife that he had forgotten to buy. He went home and continued to feel "unreal, like I was in a trance. Everything felt so strange."

Mr. H had difficulty sleeping and eating for the next 2 weeks. He had nightmares about the robbery in which he was shot or his son was injured. During the day he found himself distracted and prone to thinking back on the assault with increasing anxiety and dread. His anxiety

increased when he passed by any convenience store. It was difficult for him to concentrate at work. During the third week, however, he noted that the incident seemed more distant and that he was mentally replaying the crime less and less frequently. By a month's time he had no residual symptoms.

Diagnosis. Acute stress disorder (Axis I).

SURVIVAL GUILT

Guilt is a common symptom in the survivors of catastrophes in which others were injured or killed. Patients may believe that they should have acted to protect others, that their own death would have saved other lives, or that they were for some reason less deserving to live.

EXISTENTIAL ISSUES SURROUNDING TRAUMA

Exposure to life-threatening event often gives rise to pressing questions about existential issues. These issues include the most difficult concerns of human existence: the nature of death, the meaning of life, the conflict between responsibility and freedom, and the limits to closeness between an individual and other people. The urgency and poignancy of these issues may confront patients exposed to trauma and leave them feeling even more isolated from friends and family members who are not as engrossed in these matters.

PTSD IN CHILDREN

PTSD in children has become increasingly regarded by psychiatrists, public health officials, and child advocacy groups as a public mental health emergency. It has been estimated that 3 million children are exposed each year to traumatic events, including emotional, physical, and sexual abuse; accidents; burns; crimes; medical procedures; and disasters. Adolescents are more likely to experience traumatic events particular to this age group, such as motor vehicle accidents, rape, violence in schools or in the streets, suicide, or serious illness in their peer group. There is considerable controversy over the impact of violence portrayed on television on the mental health and well-being of children.

PTSD in children differs significantly from adult PTSD in both clinical symptoms and the effect of trauma on psychological development. Immediately after trauma, children may appear withdrawn, unresponsive, or "robot-like" in their behavior. Children may exhibit many of the same symptoms of PTSD seen in adults but may also demonstrate oppositional behavior and problems at school, including falling academic performance. Regression to earlier developmental stages may occur. For example, previously mastered fears may return. Some of these symptoms may overlap with depression and attention-deficit disorder. Some studies suggest that boys tend to become more aggressive as a behavioral consequence of PTSD, while girls tend toward passivity. Others have observed trauma reflected in children's play many months or years after the original trauma.

As in adults, treatment consists of psychotherapy, including behavioral desensitization. Antidepressant medications are sometimes used, although carefully controlled studies of the efficacy and safety of these medications in children is lacking. Play therapy and drawing may also allow children to express their feelings about traumatic events. Some families may be resistant to therapy. This is especially problematic in the case of children who have been abused by family members. Family therapy may help restore normal support, structure, and communication. As is true for traumatized adults, therapeutic interventions at an early stage are critically important.

Tami S, a 3-year-old girl, was seen by the pediatric consultation service 3 weeks after a motor vehicle accident in which she received minor lacerations. Her mother had been driving and Tami was in the back seat when an intoxicated driver broadsided their car. While she gave police a report of the accident, Tami's mother said they had seen the driver of the other car being moved to an ambulance "screaming in pain and covered with blood."

Tami's behavior changed markedly after the accident. At night she would awaken moaning or screaming from "bad dreams" and would insist on sleeping with her mother. Although she had been toilet-trained for almost a year she began to have "accidents" and asked to wear diapers again. Her mother described her as being defiant, "like she was in her 'terrible twos' all over again," sometimes screaming at her mother in arguments. Tami had punched a classmate at preschool when he refused to share a toy. She had refused to get into a car since the accident, and her mother was "at wit's end" over daily battles to get Tami to preschool.

Therapy consisted of the medical student and child psychiatry fellow being assigned to the case and began by meeting with Tami twice weekly. Tami gradually came to trust the student enough to start play therapy. Offered a choice of toys, Tami chose two cars and began to violently crash them together, screaming, "Bad man! Bad man!" She also drew crude pictures of cars and mangled bodies. Over several weeks the pictures became less violent. Meetings with Tami's mother, who felt guilty for

"not doing something to prevent the accident" led to a referral for individual therapy and advice to resume normal habits and structure in caring for her daughter.

Tami's behavior gradually returned to her pre-accident baseline, and her symptoms became less pronounced. She was symptom-free at a one year follow-up visit.

Diagnosis. PTSD (Axis I); minor injuries from a motor vehicle accident (Axis III).

Some researchers and clinicians have speculated that the prompt treatment of acute and post-traumatic stress disorders in childhood may reduce the risk of patients developing anxiety disorders in adulthood.

PTSD IN RESPONSE TO RAPE

Most people who are raped experience some or all of the symptoms of PTSD. Rape is not a sexual crime but rather a crime of violence and aggression, and the perpetrator may be an acquaintance, friend, or colleague. As might be expected, the most frequent and marked symptoms are recurrent thoughts and nightmares of the assault and insomnia. Victims of rape often feel responsible for having failed to prevent the assault. Again, PTSD symptoms usually immediately follow the event, diminish over time, and in most victims, return on the anniversary of the assault. PTSD may also be exacerbated by secondary trauma entailed in physical examinations in hospital emergency rooms, or in dealing with the legal system in which patients may see the suspect, or find themselves verbally assaulted by defense attorneys. Rape is associated with a very high incidence of PTSD; up to 80% of victims meet criteria for PTSD in the months after the rape.

THE PSYCHOLOGICAL AFTERMATH OF GENOCIDE

The persecution and murder of Armenians at the turn of the century presaged the rise of genocide, the attempted mass murder of entire religious, political, or cultural groups that has haunted the 20th century. The Holocaust of World War II claimed an estimated 11 million lives, including 6 million Jewish Europeans, as well as millions of Poles, gays, physically and mentally disabled persons, and members of other groups. The past 30 years have witnessed the decimation of millions in Timor and Cambodia, "ethnic cleansing" of Bosnian Muslims, and murderous strife between ethnic groups in Rwanda. The combined stresses of witnessing large-scale brutality and the impact of forced immigration make severe, chronic forms of PTSD highly likely. Profound impacts on interpersonal behavior have been observed, including on parenting. Numerous studies have documented the impact of genocide across generations, many years and thousands of miles from the original events. The psychological effects on children of survivors include an increased incidence of anxiety and other psychiatric disorders.

GROUP ASPECTS OF TRAUMA

The psychological effects of trauma on a group of people differ from PTSD in individual patients. Often trauma survivors are able to validate and support each other's experiences, especially following a natural disaster.

> The 1991 wildfire in the wooded hills of Oakland, California, was the worst urban blaze in United States history and claimed over two dozen lives and hundreds of homes. Survivors of the fire rapidly established organizations for support and to share information. Support groups provided psychological assistance and shared problem-solving.
>
> The combined political activity of survivors accelerated reimbursement from insurance companies for the rebuilding of homes and helped solicit funding and community support for several monuments to those who perished in the fire. One such memorial consisted of hundreds of tiles, many designed and hand-painted by children, each depicting a survivor's tale, including escaping the flames, being reunited with family pets, and tributes to those who perished in the fire. These activities helped greatly to ameliorate the severity of psychological aftereffects.

While survivors of disasters often form strong interpersonal bonds, a psychological barrier can often form quickly between survivors of trauma and those trying to help them. Clinicians must provide interventions before this so-called **trauma membrane** forms.

> Immediately after the 1989 Loma Prieta earthquake near San Francisco, the University of California at San Francisco Medical Center's Psychiatry Department organized a phone bank, staffed by psychiatry trainees, who answered telephone calls from traumatized individuals throughout the area. Many people benefited from reassurance that their symptoms of shock and dissociation were normal and should pass within days. They were also educated about the possibility of developing PTSD and were given phone numbers of nearby mental health clinics in the event that they began to exhibit symptoms of PTSD.

COURSE

The onset and duration of an individual's response to trauma varies considerably. Some patients may not experience any symptoms of PTSD despite exposure to considerable stress. Some patients may emerge from significant trauma with little clinical symptomatology or may pass through the stages of acute stress disorder, denial, and intrusive PTSD symptoms in hours or perhaps days.

The symptoms of acute stress disorder usually begin shortly after the event. Sometimes several months to several years may pass before any manifestation of the illness appears. During this period, an individual may appear to be remarkably unaffected by the traumatic experience. PTSD can also become a chronic condition, especially when complicated by depression or substance abuse and may last for many months or years. Alternatively, PTSD symptoms may resolve, but the traumatic response can reemerge on an anniversary of the event or after another trauma.

> Mary L, aged 47, was injured by a hit-and-run driver as she was driving to work. She was hospitalized on the surgery service for repair of her broken pelvis and needed to have her leg in traction for several weeks. During the first week, she was noted by the nursing staff and surgery team to be sleeping poorly and crying during the day. An evaluation by psychiatry confirmed other PTSD symptoms of anxiety, restlessness, feelings of vulnerability, flashbacks, and nightmares.
>
> The flashbacks and nightmares were not about the accident, however. Instead Ms. L was experiencing a resurgence of PTSD symptoms related to being raped by a high school classmate 30 years earlier. These symptoms had persisted for months after the rape and had finally been relieved by individual psychotherapy almost a year later.
>
> Ms. L was given a series of relaxation exercises, trazodone for sleep, and daily supportive psychotherapy sessions in the hospital. Her symptoms did not fully resolve until several weeks after her discharge from the hospital.
>
> **Diagnosis.** PTSD (Axis I); multiple fractures due to a motor vehicle accident (Axis III).

The onset of PTSD may also be delayed by many months or years. Delayed cases of PTSD are often precipitated by a major life stressor such as another traumatic event, divorce, the death of a family member or friend, or life-threatening illness.

> Arthur M served in World War II at age 16 by lying about his age. His unit was sent to Europe where they engaged in fierce combat with

German soldiers as they crossed through France. On one occasion Mr. M had fired at a figure that he believed was a sniper. The "sniper" was later found to be a young woman clutching her son, both of whom died from their wounds.

Although Mr. M denied significant symptoms of PTSD, he described himself as "anxious" as an adult. His wife noted that he kept to himself and was not forthcoming with his emotions. At age 75, Mr. M was diagnosed as having leukemia. He then decided to go to Europe with his wife. On his trip he noted the onset of symptoms of PTSD, including severe insomnia, feelings of guilt for having survived his tour when so many of his friends had died, and nightmares and flashbacks so vivid that "I swear I feel like I'm back there, I'm 16, and I'm ready to fight for my life all over again."

Mr. M. was treated with an antidepressant, which helped with his insomnia and flashbacks. He was referred to a support group for military veterans who have PTSD and reported significant improvement 3 months later.

Chemotherapy produced a remission of his leukemia, and he noted that his relationship with his wife was marked by better communication. Mr. M commented that he had not realized how much he "held back from people."

Diagnosis. PTSD (Axis I): leukemia (Axis III).

ASSOCIATED CONDITIONS & DIFFERENTIAL DIAGNOSIS

PTSD increases the risk of depressive disorders and of alcohol use. Clinicians should screen for these disorders by inquiring about depressive symptoms, which may overlap significantly with symptoms of PTSD, and substance use. Standard treatment for depression should be attempted if it is not possible to distinguish between the two conditions.

When substance use occurs, recovery may be significantly delayed or precluded. Alcohol and CNS depressants such as benzodiazepines are the most commonly abused drugs.

Anxiety, somatoform, and dissociative disorders may also occur in the aftermath of trauma, although these disorders are more likely in cases of repeated trauma. Somatoform disorders are often evidenced by health concerns and repeated visits to physicians for medical complaints that yield no physical etiology. Clinicians can identify dissociative disorders by asking questions about the patient's feelings of emotional numbness, derealization, and depersonalization; and about complaints of "blackouts" or lost time. Patients sometimes feign exposure to trauma

and symptoms of PTSD in factitious disorder or malingering. These patients tend to overemphasize intrusive phenomena and are less skilled (or knowledgeable) about avoidance symptoms. Collaboration from family members, a review of previous medical records, and neuropsychological testing often help to reveal the deceptive nature of these clinical presentations.

TREATMENT

Acute Stress Disorder

Acute stress reactions are usually self-limited, and treatment typically involves only short-term supportive/expressive psychotherapy. Many patients will question whether their symptoms of insomnia, poor concentration, and feeling confused or "numbness" are normal. Education and assurance about the normal and usually time-limited nature of most symptoms of acute stress disorder are most helpful at this point. Patients often benefit from psychotherapy that emphasizes support, understanding, and validation as the patients recount the trauma along with their changing emotional responses. Therapists can also help patients to review and use coping strategies, such as encouraging patients to call friends or family members or to resume stress-relieving activities such as exercise or hobbies.

Patients bothered by sleep disturbances may benefit from behavioral techniques to minimize insomnia known as sleep hygiene. This includes avoiding caffeine or alcohol at night, trying to keep to a routine sleep and waking schedule, and getting out of bed after 30 minutes if sleep is not achieved. If patients request medication for sleep, short-acting benzodiazepines such as lorazepam or temazepam can be prescribed. Patients should be warned of the addictive potential of benzodiazepines when used daily, especially if the patient or family members have histories suggestive of substance use or personality disorders.

There is anecdotal concern that benzodiazepine use in the first few days after a trauma may actually correlate with more severe PTSD symptoms at a later time, perhaps because of the medication's effect on changing normal sleep cycles and the reduction of REM stages of sleep. Trazodone, a sedating antidepressant, may be a superior choice to treat symptoms of insomnia as it is nonaddictive and does not adversely affect REM sleep. Antidepressants are usually prescribed only when symptoms of acute stress disorder are intense and interfere with daily functioning.

Finally, preventive efforts should be directed to educate patients about possible maladaptive coping strategies such as the use of alcohol or social isolation. Clinicians should encourage patients to avoid substances and to seek treatment if they experience more delayed symptoms of PTSD weeks or months after the original trauma.

PTSD

The nature of PTSD, and chronic PTSD in particular, requires a more complex approach using medication and behavioral treatments. Because substance abuse (especially of alcohol) frequently is associated with PTSD, patients should be questioned closely about their drug and alcohol use. Drug treatment programs may be an essential first step for patients experiencing PTSD complicated by substance use.

Tricyclic antidepressants, such as imipramine and amitryptiline (Elavil), and the SSRIs (fluoxetine, sertraline, paroxetine) can all reduce anxiety, symptoms of intrusion, and avoidance behaviors. There are no controlled studies comparing the efficacy of these agents, but SSRIs are generally better tolerated because of their lower side-effect profile. As is true for the treatment of other anxiety disorders, less activating agents such as paroxetine and trazodone frequently are used at night to help with symptoms of insomnia. Carbamezepine and valproate have also independently produced symptomatic improvement in some patients in uncontrolled trials and may help with mood swings and visual flashbacks. Recent studies have identified buspirone as a useful adjuvant to antidepressants, especially for anxiety symptoms. Beta-blockers or clonidine are sometimes used to help modulate autonomic arousal and anger. Benzodiazepines are not believed to be as effective for PTSD and are contraindicated in patients at risk for developing tolerance. Neuroleptics are generally not used except in unusual cases of PTSD complicated by psychosis.

Individual psychotherapeutic strategies are used in treatment of PTSD to help patients overcome avoidance behaviors and demoralization and to help them master their fears related to the trauma. Therapies that encourage patients to "dismantle" avoidance behaviors through stepwise focusing on the experience of the traumatic event are often very effective. Many victims of assault report that during the course of successful therapy the contents of their dreams change. Early dreams of passively submitting are often replaced by dreams in which they fight back or even annihilate the assailant.

Psychotherapy for PTSD focuses on coping strategies but also emphasizes an understanding of the patient's life, including previous conflicts, ability to trust others, and any previous traumatic experiences. Therapy generally follows several stages including the establishment of a safe environment and emotional stabilization, emotionally processing the trauma through the gradual retelling and re-experiencing of the traumatic event and its aftermath, and finally the re-integration of normal psychological processes and relationships This last stage frequently involves a reappraisal of the patient's world view and

a resolution of existential issues, including the patient's sense of meaning and trust in other people.

PSYCHOLOGICAL CONSEQUENCES OF MULTIPLE TRAUMATIC EVENTS

Most people who develop acute stress disorder or PTSD after a single traumatic event will return gradually to pre-event functioning and will experience a diminishing or disappearance of symptoms over time. Repeated exposure to trauma, however, often produces a more complicated and long-lasting psychological response. People who experience multiple traumas, such as childhood physical or sexual abuse, domestic violence, community violence, or war-related trauma, often suffer numerous psychiatric and physical symptoms, and may meet criteria for several Axis I and Axis II diagnoses in addition to PTSD. Judith Herman initially proposed a new diagnostic category, **complex PTSD,** to describe the most common clusters of symptoms encountered in these patients.

The committee that worked to define PTSD for *DSM-IV* also suggested adding a separate diagnostic category, **disorders of extreme stress not otherwise specified** (DESNOS) to more completely describe patients who had experienced multiple traumas. The decision was made to include a description of this syndrome under the "associated features" section of PTSD, rather than as a separate diagnostic category.

INCIDENCE

Because the response to chronic trauma is complex and varies according to the nature of the individual's traumatic experience and other factors, no single incidence figure is known. Childhood sexual and physical abuse, as well as domestic violence, are widespread, but underreporting is suspected. Researchers in the trauma field are attempting to quantify the most common results of these traumatic experiences. Individuals at special risk include families and relationships in which one or more individuals are engaging in substance abuse or have antisocial personality disorders. Refugees from war-torn countries or from nations where human rights violations are frequent also have a high incidence of exposure to traumatic events.

ETIOLOGY

Repeated trauma overwhelms psychological defenses. If repeated trauma occurs in childhood, healthy defenses may never develop. Instead, children may learn to manage overwhelming emotions by relying on primitive coping strategies, such as dissociation or self-harming behavior. These patterns of maladaptive coping may persist into adulthood, and other strategies, including substance abuse, somatization, or bulimia may develop. The normal pattern of psychological development is often skewed. Patients often develop difficulties trusting others, and feelings of extreme shame, guilt, and self-blame are common. Patients may also come to identify with the aggressor. Some patients become attracted to abusive relationships or place themselves in danger. Most of these patients are thought to be driven by unconscious compulsions to re-experience earlier traumatic events, perhaps in an attempt to master the trauma, but instead become trapped in cycles of abuse.

COMPLEX PTSD: CLINICAL FEATURES

Patients who have experienced multiple traumas suffer difficulties with emotions, behaviors, and interpersonal relationships. Emotional symptoms generally include poorly regulated extremes of anxiety, anger, depression, or numbing. Behavioral disturbances include avoidance and social isolation, and mood-regulation strategies such as bingeing and purging, self-harming by cutting or burning, or substance use.

Interpersonal relationships are often significantly disrupted. Chronically traumatized patients have repeatedly experienced the malignant misuse of power by others. When this abuse occurs at the hands of a parent or other adult in a care-taking role, subsequent interactions with others, particularly authority figures, can be extremely difficult. Adult survivors of childhood abuse use their experience as a template for forming expectations about how other people are likely to behave. Therefore they will have difficulty with trust, expecting others to be untrustworthy and inattentive to their needs, and they will expect to be victimized by having their physical and emotional boundaries violated.

At the same time, traumatized patients often also have a set of compensatory wishes: that others will be totally, perfectly trustworthy and that all their needs will be anticipated and taken care of. In addition, patients who have experienced chronic trauma may also have an unconscious identification with their perpetrator, and may fear their own violent impulses. These complex perceptions and expectations are often directed at physicians, particularly when patients are also dealing with the stress of medical illness and may be more emotionally regressed.

Maria G was a 38-year-old single Latina woman. She was born in Mexico and grew up in a family in which she was frequently severely physically punished and neglected. At age 6, Ms. G was sexually molested by a man in her neighborhood. The sexual molestation continued throughout her childhood, and the man would take money from other men to have sex with her. At age 16, Ms. G escaped to the United States, where she worked in prostitution and began using crack cocaine. She decided to leave prostitution and stay clean and sober after she spent 6 months in jail.

Ms. G began to experience multiple symptoms, including flashbacks, nightmares, panic attacks, dissociative episodes, and suicidal ideation. She also engaged in cutting herself when she felt overwhelmed, and would be subject to attacks of rage and physical violence when she perceived a threat. She decided she wanted to have a child, viewing this as a way of creating something positive in her life. However, because of chronic pelvic infections from her abuse, Ms. G. was infertile. She became enraged at the doctor who gave her this news and began using crack again.

Diagnosis. PTSD, panic disorder, major depressive episode, dissociative disorder NOS, cocaine abuse (Axis I).

ASSOCIATED CONDITIONS & DIFFERENTIAL DIAGNOSIS

In addition to PTSD, patients who have experienced chronic trauma often meet criteria for multiple psychiatric disorders. Major depression is the most frequent comorbid diagnosis. These patients report sleep disturbances, hopelessness, poor self-esteem, and suicidality. Dysthymia is seen frequently, as are panic disorder, social phobia, obsessive-compulsive disorder, and generalized anxiety disorder. Eating disorders (anorexia and bulimia) are common in this population. Patients also often describe somatic symptoms, for example, pelvic pain or nonspecific gynecologic or gastrointestinal complaints, some of which may represent "body memories" of traumatic experiences. Somatoform disorders are also reported. Substance abuse is a particularly common comorbid condition in patients who have experienced chronic trauma. Patients who experience chronic hyperarousal and intrusion may turn to alcohol, benzodiazepines, or opiates; patients most troubled by numbing or dissociative symptoms may use stimulants.

Dissociative phenomena, including memory lapses and depersonalization, frequently occur; dissociative identity disorder (formerly defined as multiple personality disorder) is a less common diagnosis associated with particularly severe childhood physical and sexual abuse. Patients may experience psychotic symptoms, the most common being auditory hallucinations, usually of the perpetrator's voice. Physical trauma often involves head injury and brain damage, and some patients may experience symptoms of temporal lobe epilepsy. Self-harming behaviors such as cutting and burning can represent acting out of angry impulses, traumatic reenactments, self-punishing, or can be a way for patients to calm themselves down.

Behavioral and interpersonal difficulties (lability of mood, behavior, and thoughts; unstable self-identity; suicide attempts; and volatile relationships) overlap with the diagnostic criteria for borderline personality disorder. Some patients—especially males—with abusive and traumatic experiences who identify with the perpetrator will also have antisocial personality disorder and may recount a history of abusing others.

Minh H, a 50-year-old Vietnamese man, was admitted to the hospital for the treatment of pneumonia. He was extremely fastidious and kept to himself during the hospitalization. The nursing staff grew concerned when they witnessed him pulling on his hair with great force on several occasions.

A psychiatric consult, performed with a Vietnamese interpreter, revealed that Mr. H was extremely depressed and anxious. He had been an engineer in South Vietnam, and because of his professional background he was judged to be a political "enemy when the country was unified." He was sent to a "retraining" camp for seven years. There he was tortured, and he witnessed the murder of his wife and daughter. He came to the United States in 1988 and had frequent flashbacks and nightmares about these events, which he did not discuss with anyone in his family.

His compulsive hair-pulling (trichotillomania), which served to decrease his feelings of anxiety, was the only overt sign of severe post-traumatic stress disorder. Other symptoms of depression, such as hopelessness, anhedonia, and weight loss, were present.

Diagnosis. Post-traumatic stress disorder; obsessive-compulsive disorder (Axis I); also consider major depression.

TREATMENT OF COMPLEX PTSD

Chronically traumatized patients may never have experienced a positive interpersonal relationship, particularly with an authority figure. This makes establishing a therapeutic alliance a difficult, but not impossible task. The structure of the patient-physician relationship should be described explicitly and demonstrated as well as explained to the patient as a "working partnership." Whenever possible, patients should be empowered by being offered choices and opportunities to exercise reasonable control. For example, a patient can be offered a choice of where to sit, what time to meet, and whether her or she needs to pause during an interview if feeling emotionally overwhelmed.

It is also helpful for the provider to reduce anxiety and fear of the unknown by explaining the purpose and planned structure of an interview. For example, "This interview will take about 30 minutes. I am going to be asking you some questions about your symptoms and how you are doing in general. The reason I am asking these questions is so that I can work to help you feel better. If you begin to feel like this interview is too difficult, or you are not comfortable answering certain questions, just let me know and we can take a break."

For particularly sensitive questions, the context for asking should be provided: "I am going to ask you about any unwanted sexual experiences you may have had. I am asking about this because these experiences may relate to symptoms you are having now."

Students and residents in busy clinic or hospital settings may have trouble keeping expected appointments, so attempts should be made to inform patients of delays. If it isn't possible to meet with a patient as planned, a brief phone call or message delivered by the ward clerk will help to decrease the patient's anxiety and demonstrate the clinician's trustworthiness. Flexibility must be balanced with realistic limit-setting. When inevitable disappointments do occur, patients may react with extreme anger and express feelings of loss of trust. It is important to listen to these reactions and validate the feelings of disappointment.

Psychiatric medication can be helpful in treating patients who have experienced chronic trauma. Psychopharmacological intervention should always be directed at target symptoms. Antidepressants, particularly the SSRIs, are useful in treating symptoms of depression and anxiety. Low-dose, mid-potency neuroleptics can be used to treat psychotic symptoms. Mood stabilizers, particularly valproate and carbamezepine, are useful in helping modulate extreme affective states and may be helpful in reducing impulsive behavior and dissociation.

Although benzodiazepines may produce immediate reduction of anxiety, they should be avoided because of the risks of disinhibition (which may increase impulsive or suicidal behavior) and physical and psychological dependency. Particular care should be taken to warn patients about side effects of all medications prescribed, since chronically traumatized patients are likely to be vigilant, fearful, or paranoid about adverse effects of any intervention. Medications should be started at very low doses and increased slowly. The risk of suicide should always be weighed when prescribing medication that have significant toxicity, such as TCAs or lithium.

EMOTIONAL REACTIONS TO PATIENTS

Clinicians who work with patients who have acute stress disorder or PTSD may experience a variety of emotions, ranging from over-identification to emotional distancing. Clinicians may sometimes experience feelings similar to those of the traumatized patient, such as denial, disbelief, fear, rage, or numbing.

Several common reactions may occur unconsciously in clinicians who work with chronically traumatized patients. The clinician may take on the role of victim, where he or she feels "held hostage" by the patient; the perpetrator role results in the clinician feeling like he or she is punishing or hurting the patient; and in the most common role of rescuer, the clinician feels and acts overly responsible for the patient. Herman also describes the common phenomenon of blaming victims, understanding this as a way for providers to distance themselves from the painful realization that the world is often unpredictable, uncontrollable, and dangerous. Clinicians who work with traumatized patients are susceptible to emotional burnout and should seek support from their colleagues and plan time to discuss the difficulty of their work. Therapeutic neutrality in the clinical setting is different from ethical and legal impartiality. The clinician is still free to affirm that the transgressor has committed a crime and express his or her own outrage to the patient.

CROSS-CULTURAL ASPECTS OF PTSD

Many features of PTSD are dependent on the patient's cultural background and experience. Traumatic experiences themselves are seen in extremely high rates among immigrants to the United States from Central America, Eastern Europe, the former Soviet Union, and Asia, where political turmoil and violence have resulted in the detainment, torture, and deaths of millions. Pre-immigration conditions and trauma experienced during the flight from other countries further increase the likelihood of PTSD. The stresses inherent in the experience of the newly arrived immigrant (ie, exposure to different customs, language, and values) also contribute to all anxiety disorders. The expression of anxiety as somatic symptoms is frequently seen in patients from rural backgrounds who have lower socioeconomic and educational status. Support groups for patients

with similar backgrounds may help to ease the sense of alienation and loss associated with PTSD.

LEGAL & ETHICAL ISSUES

Legal and ethical issues encountered in treating patients who have PTSD often involve conflicting responsibilities for the physician between medical and legal obligations, the confidentiality of information and the assessment of the impact of trauma on the patient's abilities to function at work.

State laws may require that physicians report many crimes to the police, including domestic violence, which can violate the patient's confidentiality if he or she does not agree. Physicians are legally required to inform child protective services of cases of possible child endangerment. This does not mean that clinicians need to investigate and be certain of abuse, only that they suspect abuse. It is always preferable to advise patients in advance that their right to confidentiality may be compromised, even if this warning results in delays in forming a therapeutic alliance. Otherwise, patients may feel betrayed on learning that they have disclosed information that is no longer confidential.

Roberta F, a 19-year-old college sophomore, was seen at student health services for multiple physical complaints. The astute medical student performing the interview and physical exam noted that the somatic symptoms were vague and primarily involved the patient's abdominal and pelvic areas, and that Ms. F seemed depressed and anxious. Based on these findings, the medical student asked if Ms. F had ever been sexually abused. Ms. F asked if her response would be confidential. The medical student assured her that the information she gave would be known only to the student and her supervisor, an internist at the clinic.

Ms. F then revealed that she had been sexually molested by her stepfather for the past 6 years. She had never reported the abuse to anyone except her mother, who did not believe her. Ms. F worried that her stepfather might now be molesting her two younger sisters, ages 12 and 15.

The supervising internist joined the patient and medical student for the rest of the visit. After the medical student finished presenting the case, the supervisor told the patient that the clinic was legally required to inform child protective services about possible abuse of her sisters. Ms. F was furious and shouted at the student, "You promised this would be confidential!" The student and the supervisor apologized to the patient and explained that there were limits to confidentiality that they should have explained. The attending physician offered Ms. F the option of making the call to police while still at the clinic in an effort to empower her. Ms. F did so and also accepted a referral to a psychotherapist.

Competing duties to patients and agencies can also arise in military situations and employee assistance programs, where physicians may need to report on the mental health condition of a patient to the patient's superior officers, decide whether the patient is mentally fit to return to work, or establish the extent to which a patient has been traumatized to determine work-related benefits. Cases involving legal issues such as worker's compensation and other disability proceedings may also involve conflicts between the physician's allegiances to patients and insurance companies, or to the judicial system.

Clinicians should also be mindful of the need to maintain confidentiality, especially in the case of media coverage of catastrophes and other forms of trauma.

An emergency room was flooded with dozens of children who were rescued from a school bus accident. The local news sent a camera crew to the hospital. The crew was banned from the emergency room but waited outside in hopes of interviewing medical staff or families.

The news anchor approached a third-year student as he left the building and asked how the children were doing. The student began to describe the physical and emotional state of the children and their families but was interrupted by a nurse who was leaving the unit. She reminded the student that the families had not given their consent to release information and that the student was breaking confidentiality in discussing their condition.

CONCLUSION

PTSD has emerged in past decade as a disorder that had been poorly understood and underdiagnosed. PTSD is associated with significant impairment in some cases, complicated by depression, substance use, declines in occupational or social functioning, and even suicide. Fortunately, PTSD can be effectively managed and treated: The key is in prompt diagnosis and referral to mental health professionals. Research continues into the psychological and biological basis of PTSD, as well as the most effective forms of therapy for the disorder.

Because medicine and psychiatry tend to focus on psychopathology, relatively little attention has been paid to the concept of resiliency, and to the characteristics of those individuals and groups who emerge from single or repeated trauma psychologically unscathed. The study of these individuals may permit clinicians to move into the practice of preventing PTSD by "immunizing" vulnerable population groups exposed to trauma. The most effective prevention strategies, however, may be public health efforts to decrease the incidence of trauma itself.

REFERENCES

Blanchard EB, Hickling EJ: *After the Crash: Assessment and Treatment of Motor Vehicle Accident Survivors.* American Psychiatric Association Press, 1997.

Cardena E, Speigel D: Dissociative reactions to the San Francisco Bay Area Earthquake of 1989. Am J Psychiatr 1993;150(3)474.

Goleman D: Trauma and emotional relearning. In: *Emotional Intelligence.* Bantam, Doubleday, Dell, 1995.

Herman JL: *Trauma and Recovery.* Basic Books, 1992.

Horowitz MJ: Disasters and psychological responses to stress. Psychiatr Ann 1985;15(3):161.

Janoff-Bulman R: *Shattered Assumptions: Toward a New Psychology of Trauma.* Free Press, 1992.

Marmar CR et al: Characteristics of emergency services personnel related to peritraumatic dissociation during critical incident exposure. Am J Psychiatr. 1996;153(7): 94 (Suppl).

Marshall RD, et al: A pharmacotherapy algorithm in the treatment of posttraumatic stress disorder. Psychiatr Ann 1996;26(4):217.

National Center for PTSD: Research and Education on PTSD (includes link to searchable PILOTS database). http://www.dartmouth.edu/dms/ptsd

Schwartz ED, Perry BD: The post-traumatic response in children and adolescents. Psychiatr Clin N Am 1994;17(2):311

Terr L: Childhood traumas: an outline and overview. Am J Psychiatr 1991;148:10

Terr L: *Too Scared to Cry.* Harper & Row, 1990.

Tomb D: The phenomenon of post-traumatic stress disorder. Psychiatr Clin N Am 1994;17(2):237.

van der Kolk B, McFarlane AC, Weisaeth L (editors): *Traumatic Stress: The Effects of Overwhelming Experience on Mind, Body, and Society.* Guilford, 1996.

Wilkinson A: A changed vision of God (Cambodia's Holocaust). New Yorker 1994; Jan 24.

Somatoform Disorders & Abnormal Illness Behavior

9

David Elkin, MD

Physical (**somatic**) complaints that are psychologically based or that are exaggeration of existing physical illness are commonly encountered in hospitals and outpatient clinics. The classification of disorders involving somatization involves several different categories. First, there is somatization that occurs commonly even in healthy individuals and is not considered a sign of psychopathology. Most people have had transient episodes of milder forms of somatization, such as feeling sick to one's stomach when interviewing for a job, or getting out of a social obligation by calling in sick.

In medical clinics patients who have mild, chronic medical concerns are known as the **worried well.** However some patients have somatic complaints that are so severe that they interfere with the patient's ability to work and affect their relationships with friends and families. These disorders may develop with or without the patient's awareness and are often associated with other psychiatric illnesses. They are sometimes so chronic and debilitating that patients become partially or completely disabled.

Figure 9-1 shows the relationship of the three major categories of abnormal illness behavior. When patients are unaware both that they are producing symptoms and the goals of this behavior, the patient has a **somatoform disorder.** In **factitious disorder,** patients consciously produce symptoms but are unaware of the objectives of doing so and appear to be motivated only by a desire to be patients in a medical setting. **Malingering** describes the behavior of patients who consciously feign physical symptoms for the goals of obtaining pain medication or financial compensation.

Patients who have these disorders comprise a small percentage of outpatients who somatize but may make extraordinarily frequent and expensive use of the health-care system. A disproportionately large share of health-care dollars and physician efforts are expended on these patients. Their frequent office and emergency room visits often result in frustration on both the patient's and physician's parts, as well as

raising the clinical dilemma of how aggressively to investigate symptoms. Recognition, evaluation, and treatment are critical steps in the management of these disorders.

Somatic complaints that are psychologically based or that are exaggerations of existing physical illness are commonly encountered in hospitals and outpatient clinics. Recognition, diagnosis, and treatment are critical steps in the evaluation of possible symptoms of somatization. Patients with somatoform disorders make up a small percentage of outpatients farther out on the spectrum of patients that comprises the "worried well" but may make extraordinarily frequent and expensive use of the health care system. Their frequent office visits may result in frustration on both the patient's and the physician's part, as well as raising the issue of how aggressively to investigate patient complaints. A disproportionately large share of health-care dollars and physicians' efforts are expended on these patients.

SOMATOFORM DISORDERS

There are six types of somatoform disorders: conversion disorder, somatoform pain disorder, hypochondriasis, somatization disorder, body dysmorphic syndrome, and undifferentiated somatoform disorder. In these disorders, both the production of symptoms and the goals of the illness behavior are not consciously known by the patient.

INCIDENCE

Hypochondriasis is the most common somatoform disorder; it affects an equal number of men and women. The most broad definition of the disorder

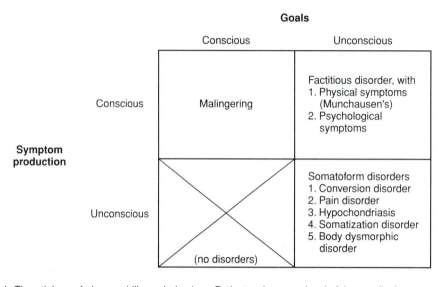

Figure 9–1. The etiology of abnormal illness behaviors. Patients who consciously feign medical symptoms for financial gain or to obtain drugs are said to malinger. Patients who have factitious disorder often present to many hospitals, clinics, and emergency rooms (factitious conversion). These patients also simulate symptoms consciously but are unaware of their goal, which is only to become a patient in a medical setting. Patients who have somatoform disorders (conversion disorder, pain disorder, hypochondriasis, somatization disorder, or body dysmorphic syndrome) have physical complaints. However, these patients are unaware (unconscious) of their goals or that their perceived physical problems are psychologically based.

would apply to half of all patients in outpatient medical clinics. The lifetime risk of somatization disorder is less than 3% in women and is even less common in men. The incidence of the other somatoform disorders is low. Conversion disorder and somatoform pain disorder are more common in women than in men but are experienced by less than 1% of the population. However the incidence of all of these disorders is much higher in medical settings, due to the concentrating effect of frequent medical appointments for patients who have multiple physical complaints. Body dysmorphic syndrome is also rare and is most often encountered in plastic surgery clinics.

The high costs of somatization are primarily due to the expense of evaluating physical complaints. Approximately 10% of all medical and surgical patients have no physical evidence of illness or disease. Most of these patients have anxiety or somatoform disorders. According to a 1991 study the cost of evaluating and treating these patients was $30 billion per year; this figure does not include the added costs of disability. Economic constraints in health-care delivery will increasingly emphasize the role of the primary care provider in screening and treating patients who have physical complaints that are psychologically based.

ETIOLOGY

Somatization (the process of producing symptoms suggesting a physical illness) is the defense mecha-

nism common to all of the somatoform disorders. According to the psychodynamic model, somatization wards off anxiety arising from conflicting and unacceptable drives in the unconscious, and preserves a cohesive sense of self. The process of somatization can occur in a variety of patients and settings but may also arise in the context of extreme psychosocial stressors that are intolerable at a conscious or unconscious level.

For example, on the eve of a major battle a soldier might struggle unconsciously with the drive to kill (to stay alive) and the belief that the taking of life is morally wrong under any circumstance. This soldier might find that his or her hand is paralyzed, suggesting a neurologic disorder. But on physical examination, the paralysis would not correlate with any known pattern of neurologic deficits, and all physical tests (eg, EMG, MRI) would be unremarkable. The soldier would have unconsciously produced a physical symptom (paralysis) enabling him or her to avoid both physical and emotional conflict. The symptom serves two purposes. First, the patient's anxiety is decreased—this is called primary gain. Secondary gain is derived from taking on the sick role; in this case, the soldier's paralysis excuses him or her from battle and other responsibilities.

Somatization is a remarkably common phenomenon that exists on a spectrum ranging from what most clinicians would regard as normal to the more psychopathologic states considered here. An example of somatization that may be familiar to many readers is "medical student disease," in which medical students (typically in their second or third year) come to believe that they have an illness they have been studying. Physical problems, such as an ache or a sprain, may be drastically over-interpreted—for example, a student who has lower back pain from exercise believes she has ankylosing spondylitis (a progressive disorder that fuses the spine), or lymph node swelling following a head cold becomes Hodgkin's disease (a form of lymphatic cancer). The intractability and resistance to rational assurance resembles a somatic delusion (a false, fixed belief that something is wrong with a body part, organ, or function), which are sometimes found in the somatoform disorders and are often embellished by the student's knowledge of the disease. The timing of the appearance of this syndrome in medical school has led to theories that some students use somatization as a defense against the anxiety created by the exposure to the body's vulnerabilities and other stresses associated with medical training.

Somatization is often a culturally sanctioned expression of depression and anxiety and may also be seen to rise during times of social stress, for example, in an economic downturn. There appears to be an inverse relationship between cultural tolerance for the acceptance and discussion of mental illness and somatization.

CONVERSION DISORDER

In conversion disorder, patients exhibit symptoms that suggest a neurologic disorder, but laboratory tests are negative, and physical examination may reveal symptoms that are inconsistent with the body's anatomy. Symptoms may include paralysis, seizures (with normal EEG), incontinence (with normal sphincter tone on testing), blindness, and so on. Onset may follow an acute stressor. The prognosis is good if symptoms have not lasted very long (eg, days to weeks) but is worse for chronic cases.

Gloria R, a 22-year-old senior nursing student, was admitted to the neurology unit for evaluation of a seizure disorder that began 3 months earlier. Laboratory tests performed on an outpatient basis were all negative, including blood serology and chemistry, head CT scan, and EEG. Because seizure disorders may not show up on an EEG (false negative results are common) Ms. R was admitted to the neurology unit for 24-hour **telemetry.** This procedure uses a camera to videotape the patient's behavior while EEG leads simultaneously record the patient's physiologic responses.

Ms. R described multiple psychosocial stressors to the neurology team. The youngest of several children and the self-acknowledged "baby" of the family, she had taken an extra year to grad-

uate from nursing school. She had been finding the training stressful and was frightened and ambivalent about the prospects of assuming the responsibilities of a full-fledged registered nurse. She had been very disturbed by her psychiatry rotation at a state hospital 6 months earlier. She felt extremely anxious working with psychotic patients and was frightened by their uncontrolled, bizarre behavior. Ms. R had married an old boyfriend in the past 6 months, despite her misgivings that she was not ready to "settle down and assume all of those responsibilities." She and her husband had difficulty adjusting to married life, and when the seizures began, she took an extended medical leave from school and they moved back in with her parents. She and her husband were now having difficulty dealing with her family in such "close quarters."

Ms. R had never seen a mental health professional. However, in the past she had episodes of anxiety, depression, and poor self-esteem. Her medical history was remarkable for chronic abdominal pain at age 15. An exploratory abdominal laparotomy was normal at that time and the abdominal pain remitted after 6 months.

During the 24-hour observation period, Ms. R had two seizures. She had minimal post-seizure symptoms, and her movements were atypical of those found in most seizure disorders. Most significant, the EEG tracings remained completely normal during the seizures, except for artifacts from the patient's movements; no spiking activity was observed, confirming the diagnosis of conversion disorder. Ms. R was shown the telemetry results, and the findings were explained as a symptom of stress. Ms. R reacted with shock, anger, and disbelief that her seizures were not physiologically based, insisting "I'm not faking it." She later accepted a referral to a psychotherapist.

Diagnosis. Conversion disorder (pseudoseizures) (Axis I).

In 10–50% of patients diagnosed with a conversion disorder, a physical disease process will ultimately be diagnosed. For example, because symptoms of connective tissue disorders such as multiple sclerosis or system lupus erythematosus often occur at different times and in different locations in the body, such disorders are often initially misdiagnosed as psychological problems. Biases within the medical system, and on the part of some individual practitioners, against women, economically disadvantaged, or ethnically diverse patients may contribute to inadequate workups and the premature diagnosis of conversion disorder in the presence of actual disease.

Louise H, a 25-year-old woman in her final month of pregnancy, presented in the emergency room with a complaint of unilateral blindness. She appeared frightened and anxious, and one physician described her in the chart as "hysterical." Her vital signs showed an elevated blood pressure and pulse rate, judged to be normal for an anxious patient. The patient's anxiety made examination of her eye and retina with an ophthalmoscope difficult, but the medical student conducting the examination thought she "saw something funny" in the affected eye. The resident on call listed the eye examination results as "unremarkable."

An inventory of the psychosocial aspects of Ms. H's life made the resident increasingly suspicious of a conversion disorder. Ms. H was 36 weeks pregnant and ambivalent about the pregnancy. The biological father was a boyfriend who had abandoned Ms. H after learning of the pregnancy. She had considered an abortion but felt it was against her religious beliefs and was now upset about the prospects of caring for a child and considered putting up the baby for immediate adoption.

Ms. H was discharged from the emergency room after several hours with a presumptive diagnosis of conversion disorder without treatment. She had a prenatal clinic visit scheduled for the next week. She refused a psychiatric outpatient appointment and was visibly angry and upset as she left the emergency room, still complaining of poor eyesight.

Ms. H returned 2 days later with continued reduction of vision in her right eye and onset of a severe, throbbing right-sided headache. Ophthalmoscopic examination now clearly showed thrombosis (clotting) of the right retinal vein, which presumably was present on her previous visit. The baby was delivered several days later, but the patient's vision remained impaired.

Diagnosis. Right retinal venous thrombosis (Axis III). No psychiatric diagnosis.

Childhood sexual abuse can commonly manifest with conversion disorder. Conversion disorder can also occur in the "identified patient" within a chaotic, dysfunctional family. (The identified patient is labeled as having the "problem," distracting the family—and often the physician—from more disturbing, shameful family problems such as alcoholism, domestic violence, or sexual abuse.) Another potential pitfall occurs when a conversion disorder overlaps with an existing medical illness.

Maribel G, a 12-year-old Latina girl, was admitted to the neurology unit for evaluation of seizures. The seizures occurred even when Maribel was taking therapeutic levels of anticonvulsants, as confirmed by her parents' supervision of medication and blood levels. The neu-

rology resident noted that Maribel had been noncompliant with anticonvulsants in the past, when her seizure disorder was first diagnosed and had several seizures documented on EEG. The seizures now were different, with more violent muscle contractions that seemed purposeful at times—for example, she sometimes struck out at some family members preferentially. The resident and nursing staff shared a growing suspicion that Maribel was conscious during the seizures they saw during this hospital admission.

A psychiatric consultation with Maribel was remarkable for the absence of psychiatric symptoms, except that Maribel was noted to be emotionally immature for her age, giggling and laughing during the interview. There were no signs of depression or psychosis, and no evidence of sexual abuse.

Maribel's family was then interviewed. The family was experiencing numerous psychosocial stressors. Both parents were working on farms for low wages, far from their own families. They were barely able to support their four children, and their work hours left them with little time for parenting. Family members were arguing with each other, and the parents had become physically violent with one another several times in the previous month. Maribel's seizures had returned during these arguments, after 2 years of good seizure control.

An EEG recorded during one of Maribel's seizures showed normal traces in all leads, without the spiking characteristic of true seizures. Her parents were advised to continue antiseizure medication and were given a referral to a family therapist.

Diagnosis. Conversion disorder with seizures and convulsions (pseudo-seizures) (Axis I); seizure disorder (Axis III).

PAIN DISORDER ASSOCIATED WITH PSYCHOLOGICAL FACTORS

Pain disorder associated with psychological factors is analogous to a conversion disorder in which pain is the symptom for which the patient seeks treatment. A psychogenic basis may account for some or all of the pain. This disorder can also occur in patients who have sustained significant physical injury but in whom the pain seems out of proportion or unexpected given the known extent of physical damage. Again, the prognosis is inversely related to the chronicity of the syndrome; pain syndromes that persist for months or years may be especially intractable to treatment and pain reduction. Unresolved legal action, workers' compensation hearings, or disability status are also associated with a chronic course. It may be difficult to evaluate any form of conversion disorder, but this is especially true in the case of pain, where few objective tests are available and health care workers have a marked tendency to underestimate the patient's subjective experience. The patient's response to pain medications does not help to discriminate physically based pain from psychogenic pain because narcotics often produce relief from psychogenic pain.

A third-year medical student was assigned to evaluate a cardiology patient for a psychiatric consultation. The patient, a 32-year-old man, was experiencing chest pain that responded well to nitroglycerin. A treadmill test with a simultaneous EKG did not demonstrate changes consistent with cardiac ischemia, despite the patient's complaint of chest pain responding to nitroglycerin. The cardiologists believed that on the basis of an unconvincing patient history and negative laboratory tests the patient probably had pain of psychological origin and requested a psychiatric consult.

When the medical student arrived to see the patient, he learned that the cardiologists had already decided to proceed with coronary angiography, to visualize any blockage of the coronary arteries. The student tracked down the patient in the waiting area of the cardiac catheter laboratory. The patient was scheduled for the next available room and was lying on the gurney with his eyes closed. He had been given intravenous opiate pain medication and a benzodiazepine minutes before and was sleepy. He understood that the student was with the psychiatry service and said, "I think this pain is psychosomatic—my father died from a heart attack in his 30s, and now I'm worried I might have one." Before the student could ask further questions, the patient was taken into the laboratory for the catheterization.

The following day the student went to the patient's room to complete the interview and psychiatric assessment. The catheterization test results had shown no coronary artery blockage, definitely eliminating a physical cause of the patient's chest pain. The patient seemed puzzled to see the student and did not recognize him or his name. When the student reminded the patient of his statement from the previous day, suggesting that he knew the pain was psychogenic and related to his father's death, he became agitated and angrily demanded that the medical student leave the room.

Diagnosis. Pain disorder associated with psychological features (Axis I).

Discussion. Short-acting benzodiazepines such as diazepam have an effect similar to alcohol and are used in many procedures specifi-

cally for their amnestic effects. The patient in this case probably was able to give such an unusually informed and insightful answer just before catheterization because of the disinhibiting effect of preoperative medication. Once the medications wore off the patient once again lacked insight into the psychological cause of his pain. When the student inadvertently broached these psychological defenses, the patient reacted with fear and anger.

HYPOCHONDRIASIS

A certain amount of concern about one's health is considered normal and adaptive. Patients with **hypochondriasis** are overly concerned with being sick, far beyond the usual spectrum of concerns and in a manner that is maladaptive for themselves and those around them, especially their physicians. They tend to misinterpret normal physical signs. For example, to a patient who has hypochondriasis, a gurgling stomach becomes stomach cancer. Obsession with illness may result in significant interference with work and social relations. These patients make frequent trips to physicians, tending to present their complaints in a ruminative manner. They sometimes suggest that negative test results are incorrect, that they are certain something is wrong, and that they need more tests and examinations. These patients may have strong family history of hypochondriasis. Patients who have hypochondriasis usually present with a detailed manner of processing information that is closer to that of a patient who has an obsessive-compulsive personality as opposed to the more histrionic style typically seen in somatization disorder (see next section). As in other somatoform disorders, physicians need to be reassuring and not feed into patients' fears by working up every complaint, but they must also deliver appropriate care.

SOMATIZATION DISORDER

Somatization disorder is characterized by a variety of complaints in multiple organ systems: one or more conversion disorders, diffuse aches and pains, gastrointestinal (GI) disturbances such as nausea and vomiting, and genitourinary complaints (see Table 9–1). Somatization disorder frequently begins in the patient's 30s and tends to be chronic, interferes with work and social relations, and is resistant to psychological interventions. Patients who have this disorder may be on disability and tend to have impaired, intense, and unstable relationships with resulting poor social support systems. Their behavior may be highly chaotic and unstable, and they may elicit from their physicians strong countertransference reactions, including anger or rage. There is a correlation between

Table 9–1. Core features of somatoform disorders.

Somatoform Disorder	Key Clinical Features	Associated Disorders	Comments
Conversion disorder	Symptoms suggesting a neurological disorder	PTSD	Physiology etiology missed in 10–50% of patients (eg, those with lupus, multiple sclerosis)
Pain disorder	Pain completely or partially psychologically based	PTSD, depression	Physiological etiology missed in some cases; requires a multidisciplinary approach
Hypochondriasis	Persistent, vague complaints and concerns about physical illness	Major depression, dysthymia, obsessive-compulsive disorder, personality disorder, or traits	Mild form seen in up to half of medical outpatients; only somatoform disorder with equal gender incidence
Somatization disorder	Multiple complaints in many organ systems; begins in patient's 20s; chronic	Borderline personality disorder, PTSD from childhood physical and sexual abuse, substance abuse, and suicide attempts; male siblings often have antisocial personality disorder	Often frustrating disorder for patients and clinicians; mild neuropsychologic deficits suspected
Body dysmorphic disorder	Pervasive, often chronic belief that a body part is malformed	Depression, dysthymia; suicide attempts possible	Closely related to obsessive-compulsive disorder; effective treatment with SSRI antidepressant, cognitive behavioral therapy
Undifferentiated somatoform disorder	Multiple physical complaints that do not meet criteria for disorders above	Depression, borderline personality disorder	Newly defined but may apply to many patients who have persistent health complaints

somatization disorder, depression, borderline or histrionic personality disorder, and eating disorders such as anorexia or bulimia.

Some studies have documented language abnormalities and other cognitive dysfunctions in patients who have somatization disorder. Patients suspected of somatization disorder should be evaluated for a history of childhood sexual abuse since somatization may represent a form of chronic, complex posttraumatic stress disorder (PTSD) in which genitourinary and other pain serve as intrusive somatic (ie, physical) memories of abuse. Patients with somatization disorder are also a greater risk for substance use and self-directed destructive acts such as suicide.

Joan C, a 31-year-old white female being evaluated for a number of GI symptoms in an outpatient GI clinic, repeatedly refused consultation with a psychiatrist. She had been seen every 2–3 weeks for the past 2 years and wanted to be seen weekly. She was placed on disability by another physician and so did not work. She was estranged from her family and had no friends, explaining angrily, "I can't trust any of them."

Ms. C had numerous complaints, which she described in detail at each appointment, eliciting anger and frustration from the GI fellow assigned to her case. She insisted that she had been diagnosed in Europe with pancreatic insufficiency. The GI fellow could not convince Ms. C that she did *not* have pancreatic insufficiency in spite of tests performed in the clinic that repeatedly failed to show any GI problems. He decided to start Ms. C on pancreatic enzymes, which are relatively harmless (but of no value to the patient who doesn't have insufficiency), "just to get her off my back."

Instead of being calmed by this action, Ms. C became furious and threatened to sue the clinic: If the fellow felt that she needed enzymes for pancreatic insufficiency, why had he withheld this treatment for 2 years, and why did he lie to her during that time? Ms. C proceeded to write a long, scathing letter accusing the GI fellow and the clinic of mistreating her by lying about her diagnosis and failing to find the cause of her numerous other physical complaints. Figure 9–2 shows Ms. C's illustration of her health complaints.

Ms. C refused a referral to a psychiatrist, shouting, "Now you're telling me it's all in my head!" She then demanded Valium, "because you doctors are stressing me out." Shortly afterward, Ms. C changed her care to another clinic,

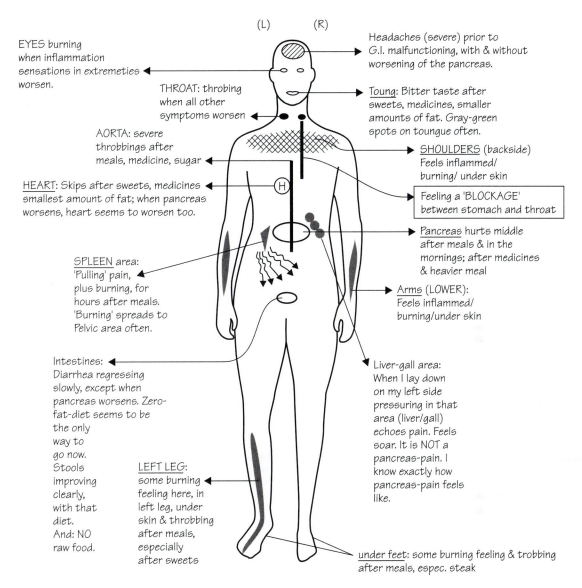

(L)   (R)

EYES burning when inflammation sensations in extremeties worsen.

THROAT: throbing when all other symptoms worsen

AORTA: severe throbbings after meals, medicine, sugar

HEART: Skips after sweets, medicines smallest amount of fat; when pancreas worsens, heart seems to worsen too.

SPLEEN area: 'Pulling' pain, plus burning, for hours after meals. 'Burning' spreads to Pelvic area often.

Intestines: Diarrhea regressing slowly, except when pancreas worsens. Zero-fat-diet seems to be the only way to go now. Stools improving clearly, with that diet. And: NO raw food.

LEFT LEG: some burning feeling here, in left leg, under skin & throbbing after meals, especially after sweets

Headaches (severe) prior to G.I. malfunctioning, with & without worsening of the pancreas.

Toung: Bitter taste after sweets, medicines, smaller amounts of fat. Gray-green spots on toungue often.

SHOULDERS (backside) Feels inflammed/ burning/ under skin

Feeling a 'BLOCKAGE' between stomach and throat

Pancreas hurts middle after meals & in the mornings; after medicines & heavier meal

Arms (LOWER): Feels inflammed/ burning/under skin

Liver-gall area: When I lay down on my left side pressuring in that area (liver/gall) echoes pain. Feels soar. It is NOT a pancreas-pain. I know exactly how pancreas-pain feels like.

under feet: some burning feeling & trobbing after meals, espec. steak

Figure 9–2. Self-portrait by a patient who had somatization disorder. The patient was a 32-year-old woman who made many visits to the gastrointestinal specialty clinic. She demanded treatment for multiple health problems shown in her drawing, despite a lack of evidence for a physical cause. Note the spelling and grammatical mistakes and the reversed orientation of the drawing (**right** and **left**). Some patients who have somatization disorder show evidence of problems with information processing. Patients who have this disorder also have a high comorbidity with borderline personality disorder and post-traumatic stress disorder from physical and sexual abuse in childhood.

eliciting marked relief from the fellow and staff at the clinic.

Diagnosis. Somatization disorder (Axis I); consider borderline personality disorder (Axis II).

BODY DYSMORPHIC SYNDROME

Patients with **body dysmorphic syndrome** are convinced that some part of their anatomy is malformed. This condition may seem ridiculous or comical to observers but may result in incapacitating stress for patients, some of whom will go to great lengths to avoid mirrors or social contact, or to obtain surgery. Cultural factors may play a significant role, especially in United States, where a youthful appearance is considered desirable. Patients with this disorder often seek consultation with plastic surgeons, but they are unlikely to be satisfied with the results of surgery (and may request and sometime receive repeated procedures).

Body dysmorphic syndrome seems to share many

features with obsessive-compulsive disorder. Many patients respond well to antidepressants that have specific anti-obsessional activity [eg, serotonin-selective re-uptake inhibitors (SSRIs) or clomipramine (Anafranil)]. Cognitive therapy, which helps patients to change thoughts and behaviors provides another useful treatment modality.

Glenn B, a 43-year-old white male, was seen by the psychiatric consultation service because he was convinced that his nose was disfigured. Plastic surgeons saw no abnormality but could not convince Mr. B that his nose was not malformed. Mr. B was persistent and received plastic surgery, then campaigned successfully for a second surgery because he was certain that his nose was still deformed. Unfortunately, he was no more pleased with the results of the second surgery and mounted an effort to have a third surgery on his nose. At this point, the surgeons, who had been ambivalent about performing the second surgery, realized that Mr. B was unlikely to benefit from any further operations for his nose and referred him to psychiatry.

Mr. B was a slight, balding man who cooperated with the psychiatric evaluation, believing the psychiatrist might be a useful advocate in convincing the surgeons to perform a third operation. He was pleasant, soft-spoken, and self-effacing but became strident when describing the need for more surgery. Mr. B was angry with the surgeons, and the psychiatrist noted some symptoms of dysthymia and anxiety, but there was no evidence of psychosis or personality disorder, and if the patient's concerns about his nose were delusional, no other delusions were detected.

The psychiatrist felt that Mr. B might benefit from psychotherapy and introduced him to a resident who would be his therapist. Mr. B agreed somewhat reluctantly to return in 2 weeks for an appointment. Meanwhile, he learned that the surgeons had emphatically rejected his request for a third operation. When Mr. B's case was presented and discussed in the outpatient clinic several days later, the staff of the clinic—and later the surgeons—joined the psychiatrist in laughing about the patient's concerns about his nose.

Mr. B reluctantly entered into psychotherapy. Over the next several months he came to trust the psychiatry resident. With shame and embarrassment he disclosed the extent to which his symptoms consumed his waking hours. He said that he had been so distressed and hopeless about his physical appearance when he was in his 20s that he made several unsuccessful suicide attempts by overdosing on pills, but he had not received medical attention after these attempts.

Given the severity and duration of Mr. B's symptoms the psychiatry resident advocated a trial of antidepressant medication. Mr. B agreed with trepidation but experienced marked relief from his depressive symptoms within a month of starting fluoxetine (Prozac), an SSRI. He was also amazed to find that his concern about his appearance decreased as well; he spent less time looking at himself in the mirror and was much less upset by his appearance. Mr. B was referred to group psychotherapy, where he explored his relationships with others. At 1-year follow-up he reported only mild concerns about his face and was starting to date.

Diagnosis. Body dysmorphic syndrome, dysthymia (Axis I).

Discussion. Mr. B's case illustrates the significant degree of impairment associated with somatoform disorders. Emotional reactions may lead physicians to underappreciate the patient's emotional distress. This is unfortunate since treatment for these disorders is often helpful— perhaps especially so in body dysmorphic syndrome. As in the case of panic disorder, studies have only recently led to a recognition of increased suicidality in patients who have body dysmorphic disorder and other somatoform disorders.

Body dysmorphic syndrome appears to be closely related to obsessive-compulsive disorder and is believed to have biological and psychological roots. But society's attitudes toward the aesthetics of appearance greatly influence an individual's standards, and body dysmorphic syndrome may represent an extreme form of culturally sanctioned narcissism. Computer-enhanced images of attractive models fill the media, inundating women and men with repeated messages about the desirability of youth and beauty. Plastic surgery (now available on monthly installment plans) puts changing one's physical appearance within financial reach of many more people. There is a great difference between changing one's appearance out of choice or repeatedly seeking surgical modification of a body part because of obsessions and compulsions, and a spectrum exists between these two behaviors.

UNDIFFERENTIATED SOMATOFORM DISORDER

Undifferentiated somatoform disorder is the latest category to be added to the somatoform disorders. The diagnosis applies to patients who have multiple somatic complaints but do not meet the full criteria for somatization disorder; it may be very common. This new diagnostic category may apply to patients who have a milder form of somatization disorder, and implications for etiology and treatment appear to be similar.

DIFFERENTIAL DIAGNOSIS

Patients who complain of somatic symptoms should always be evaluated first for the presence of physical illness. Even after physical illness is ruled out, the possibility of an underlying medical disorder should be regularly reassessed.

These patients should next be screened for major psychiatric disorders. Major depression may be associated with multiple, vague somatic complaints, or with somatic delusions in major depression with psychotic features. Patients who exhibit alcohol or drug dependence or abuse may also make frequent visits to physicians for vague physical complaints. All patients should routinely be asked about substance use. Anxiety states such as panic disorder, social phobia, and PTSD may also be associated with somatic symptoms. Patients with schizophrenia may be convinced that there is something physically wrong with their body. Patients with a history of sexual abuse in childhood, or personality disorders, may present with multiple physical complaints.

TREATMENT OF SOMATOFORM DISORDERS

The treatment of somatoform disorders remains a challenge for physicians. Treatment for body dysmorphic syndrome is perhaps the most easily implemented, since patients who have this disorder are more apt to accept referral to psychiatric services and are more likely to respond to anti-obsessional agents such as SSRIs and cognitive-behavioral therapy. Hypochondriasis may be treatable in a similar manner.

Patients who have other somatoform disorders are likely to refuse psychiatric services since they experience such referrals as invalidation of their diseases. Antidepressant or antianxiety medication and therapy may be very useful if dysthymia, depression, or anxiety disorders are diagnosed concurrently.

What seems the most helpful to patients who have somatoform disorders is an ongoing relationship with a caring physician who can empathize with them. Regular appointments should be scheduled to avoid the behavioral rewards of increased physician contacts for more physical complaints. At the same time, the physician must set realistic boundaries for medical care and avoid either extreme of overzealously pursuing tests and examinations of every symptom or uniformly ignoring every physical complaint without any workup.

Patients with somatoform disorders sometimes have an undiagnosed physical ailment or become ill with other diseases. Physicians must be able to contain patients' frustration and anger, which are often vented at the health-care system or at the physician. Patients who have somatization disorder are likely

also to have borderline personality disorder or traits and may be especially difficult to treat without giving in to reciprocal feelings of anger and hostility.

Patients who have somatoform disorders are frequently in search of a meaningful connection with other people. They often feel rejected, misunderstood, and alienated from others. Group psychotherapy may offer relief from some of these feelings, especially when patients are allowed to help each other express and validate their frustrations. Group therapists can also guide patients with a cognitive-behavioral approach, helping patients to see the connections between their emotions, thoughts, and physical symptoms, and their interactions with health-care providers.

OTHER ABNORMAL ILLNESS BEHAVIOR

In the somatoform disorders, patients are unaware that they are producing symptoms and are not conscious of their goals in doing so. Other presentations of physical complaints not based on actual medical illness are also possible. Malingering occurs when patients feign illness for conscious (and often criminal) objectives such as obtaining money or addictive medications. Factitious disorders are uncommon psychiatric disturbances in which patients are aware that they are falsely reporting physical symptoms but seem intent on no other goal than to be a patient in a medical setting. Both syndromes are clinically important. Malingering is common in many medical settings and is included in the differential diagnosis for many other disorders. Factitious disorders are believed to be relatively rare but carry a high burden of morbidity and mortality either due to the disorders themselves or to coexisting depression or personality disorders.

MALINGERING

In **malingering,** the patient consciously produces symptoms for obvious goals, such as financial gain or to obtain narcotics. Malingering is often associated with antisocial personality disorder and may be difficult to diagnose. Collaborative sources of information, such as police reports and medical records from other hospitals, may be very helpful.

Doug N, a 35-year-old white male, presented to the emergency room with the complaint that he had AIDS and needed AZT and "plenty of codeine" for pain. He said he had been treated in New York City at a clinic where his condition was diagnosed and where he routinely received this medication. He said he had moved to town the week before, and when asked whether he brought hospital records with him, he became angry and told the resident who was examining him, "Don't bother calling—the clinic burned down, so you have to believe me!"

Mr. N insisted he did not remember the names of any of his doctors or nurses in New York. He repeatedly refused a physical examination and became angry and upset when he was told that his demands for codeine would not be met until he agreed to a physical examination and laboratory tests. "At the clinic in New York they let me get my medications in the emergency room and said I had enough blood tests already." After several more insistent demands for codeine, he stormed out, refusing follow-up at the AIDS outpatient clinic. He said he was going to the "nearest newspaper office to complain about how you treat AIDS patients in this city."

Another resident had gone to medical school in New York City and was familiar with the public health-care system there. He was able to reach an ex-classmate in an emergency room in New York City and learned that the patient was on their "look-out list" for making similar demands for medication and free housing in many emergency rooms throughout the city. His HIV test was negative on at least one occasion. He was also well-known to the police for a long history of burglary and assaults related to opiate abuse since age 14. He had a history of stealing medication from hospital pharmacies and lying to medical personnel and threatening them with violence if his demands for pain medications were not met. He carried a presumptive diagnosis of antisocial personality disorder.

Diagnosis. Opiate dependence and abuse (Axis I); probable antisocial personality disorder (Axis II); malingering (V code).

TREATMENT OF MALINGERING

The treatment of malingering is a matter of continued controversy. Patients who are found to be malingering should be informed that they will not receive treatment for their condition and why. Because malingering is often associated with antisocial personality disorder, two or more staff members should probably confront such patients, in case they become hostile and threatening. Some clinicians regard malingering as criminal behavior and believe that these patients should be excluded from treatment, and that the doctor-patient relationship is violated by the patients' behavior. They argue further that criminal behavior should be reported to insurance companies, police, or other authorities. A decision to maintain or to break patient-physician confidentiality—such as circulating a warning about the patient to other hospitals and clinics—rests on the physician's judgment on a case-by-case basis.

FACTITIOUS DISORDERS

Patients who have **factitious disorders** consciously produce either physical or psychiatric symptoms, but they are not aware why they are doing so. These patients tend to present at many different hospitals and clinics, frequently giving false histories in attempts to obtain treatment. Here the objective of the behavior is unclear; the only goal seems to be a patient in a medical setting. Some clinicians have found that these patients have had previous contact with the health-care system in childhood and some have worked as health-care professionals.

Munchausen syndrome is a factitious disorder in which the patient presents with physical symptoms. (Baron von Munchausen was a reputed pathologic liar who traveled from tavern to tavern, spinning tales of his glories in battle. He had a reputation for moving on to a new inn when confronted by the falsity of his tales.) Since many patients do become very ill or even die from their actions (or complications of repeated surgeries), this disorder is considered dangerous. Other patients present with feigned psychiatric symptoms, endorsing symptoms of depression or anxiety. Patients with factitious disorder tend to flee to new geographical areas when confronted with the nature of their problem, and so are poorly studied. The disorder may be complicated by substance abuse, borderline personality disorder, and self-destructive behavior.

Jorge S, a 47-year-old man, presented at the emergency room and said he had been diagnosed with colon cancer and had been given only 6 months to live. He appeared thin and depressed, and there were several healed scars on his abdomen, partially consistent with the gastrointestinal surgery he described. He had been seen in many of the medical emergency rooms in the city in which he lived, asking for laboratory tests and chemotherapy for his cancer. However, many of the details of his history were inconsistent and led the emergency room staff to call to some of the medical centers where he said he had been treated in the past.

Mr. S's "hospital trail" was traced to Arizona, where records showed he was treated for a self-inflicted abdominal stab wound several years earlier. Since then he had been to dozens and perhaps hundreds of emergency rooms across the country. All of the visits were similar, and the patient had never been known to seek disability payments or pain medications, so there was no obvious secondary gain to his behavior. His chief complaint was always colon cancer, and he frequently asked for surgery "to find out what else can be done."

Diagnosis. Factitious disorder with physical symptoms (Munchausen syndrome)(Axis I); history of laparotomy for self-inflicted abdominal stab wound (Axis III).

Munchausen by proxy is a form of factitious disorder found in children. In this syndrome, one or both parents produce symptoms in their children rather than themselves; inducing seizures, fevers, or hypoglycemia is not uncommon. A recent study revealed parents on hidden videocameras smothering their hospitalized children to simulate apneic episodes. As in the adult version of the disease, the parent(s) are aware that they are producing symptoms in their children but not why they are doing so. And, as in adults, there is a significant danger of morbidity or death.

Chloe D, a 40-year-old divorced nurse, brought her 3-year-old daughter to the medical emergency room for treatment of repeated episodes of hypoglycemia. In two episodes the hypoglycemia led to seizures that had to be treated as well. Ms. D's behavior was always initially angry and rude to the medical team, but she would then become overly friendly and solicitous, showering them with presents and praising their diagnostic abilities—even though they were unable to establish an etiology for the hypoglycemic episodes. She begged with the doctors to "save my baby—she's all I have" and also alluded to the death of an older child several years before.

One day a nurse saw Ms. D injecting something into her daughter's IV line. Tests of the later-confiscated syringe confirmed that Ms. D had been injecting her daughter with insulin. Laboratory testing on stored blood samples from her first child revealed the presence of synthetic insulin. Ms. D was arrested on suspicion of child abuse, endangerment, and the murder of her first child. Her daughter was placed by child protective services in foster care.

At trial Ms. D admitted injecting both children with insulin that she stole from the hospital where she worked. But she defended her actions by claiming that both children had illnesses that doctors could not diagnose, and that she had induced hypoglycemia only in an effort to have doctors take their medical problems seriously.

Her defense attorney attempted to portray her as being "not guilty by reason of insanity" but failed. Ms. D was convicted on all charges and sent to prison.

Diagnosis. Child: none. Mother: probable borderline personality disorder (Axis II); factitious disorder with physical symptoms (Munchausen by proxy) (Axis I).

TREATMENT OF FACTITIOUS DISORDERS

Treatment of factitious disorders often involves confronting the patient with the physician's suspicions. A face-saving meeting can be convened between the patient and the health-care team. This meeting also discourages the patient from attempting to pit health-care team members against each other by letting the patient see that the team is unified in their communication and treatment plan.

Roberto F, a 46-year-old divorced man with a long history of intermittent pancreatitis, was admitted to the medicine service. The latest flare-up appeared related to his ongoing alcohol dependence. Mr. F's pancreatitis had a complicated course, including fevers of unknown origin and an infection around his intravenous catheter site. He quickly became the bane of the medical staff's daily existence. He was rude, hostile, demeaning, and demanding. The nursing staff had to bring in ancillary staff to work with Mr. F because he had "burned out" most of the staff with his abusive behavior. At the same time, several nurses defended him as "sweet" and "misunderstood."

The cause of Mr. F's fevers was finally revealed: He was caught changing the temperature on the nursing chart. In spite of being observed changing the mark with a pencil and eraser, he denied ever doing so. Meanwhile, infections sprang up at every site where blood had been drawn for cultures. Examination of pus at each site revealed enterococcal bacteria, most commonly found in human feces. Apparently Mr. F had repeatedly inoculated himself with fecal material.

A psychiatric consultation was obtained. Mr. F was initially guarded and hostile but later became increasingly friendly and hopeful that the psychiatrist could help him get "better care around here" because he felt the hospital staff treated him like "a criminal."

A detailed history revealed that Mr. F was ignored by his mother and physically and emotionally abused by his father, a surgeon. When he was 11 years old, Mr. F had begun to complain of pain on urination. His father refused to take him to a pediatrician, insisting he was imagining his symptoms. His parents left to vacation in Florida for several weeks, leaving him and his sister with a house sitter. One morning while his parents were gone he noticed blood in his urine. He was hospitalized for several weeks on a pediatric unit for a severe urinary tract infection. His father spoke with his treating pediatrician but did not return from his vacation. Mr. F came to regard his hospital stay as "the happiest time" in his childhood, remembering the doctors' and nurses' "loving care" with fondness and longing.

The psychiatrist convened a meeting of the entire treating team: nurses, doctors, specialists. He allowed them to express their anger (and fear) about the patient's medical and psychiatric condition. He then brought them all into Mr. F's room, having first prepared Mr. F for the meeting. The psychiatrist explained again that the medical team was there to improve their communication with the patient. He conveyed the team's concern about Mr. F's downward course in the hospital and also mentioned the finding of inoculation of his wounds with fecal contaminants.

Mr. F was indignant, saying, "How could that happen? It must be one of your defective toilets in this place." The psychiatrist explained that the cause of the infection did not matter. What was significant was that there was a definitive diagnosis (pancreatitis and skin infection) and a definite plan (hydration and antibiotics). The medical team had every confidence in the treatment plan and expected the patient to be ready for discharge in 5 days. If the patient continued to experience unexpected complications, the staff would have to assume that an emotional problem was preventing recovery and a psychiatric hospitalization would be pursued. Mr. F grew stone-faced and rejected this plan. He also refused further contact with the psychiatrist and was sullen and contrite with the medical team. However, his infections promptly resolved. He left the hospital against medical advice 1 day prior to his scheduled discharge date.

SOMATIZATION IN GROUPS

Medicine tends to focus on individuals, but the same psychological mechanisms can manifest in group situations. In fact, it is possible for a group of people to "share" a conversion disorder. Berton Re-

ouche reported the following case of group somatization at a college campus:

The infectious disease consultation service at a university medical center was asked to collaborate with the US Centers for Disease Control (CDC) in evaluating an epidemic at a nearby college campus. Hundreds of people were in the dining hall eating lunch when a student fainted. He was quickly revived and taken to the student health clinic. There was considerable excitement among the rest of the students, and rumors began to circulate that "poison gas" was leaking from the chemistry center into the dining hall. Many students noticed a strange odor in the air, and another student collapsed. Within 20 minutes dozens of students were complaining of shortness of breath, nausea, palpitations, and tingling sensations in their hands. An hour after the first student collapsed, almost 200 students were lying prostrate on the floor of the dining hall or on benches in the plaza outside. The campus was in a state of near-pandemonium, with students and faculty members demanding action and local news crews arriving to interview students about a presumed toxic spill.

However, evaluation by the student health service and infectious disease specialists from the medical center and CDC was puzzling. The students who were examined showed few physical symptoms other than anxiety, and the cases did not seem to follow any pattern related to where the students had been sitting in the dining hall or which foods they had eaten. The odor turned out to be the usual smell of Sterno cans used to keep food warm. Tests and history from the first student to collapse were consistent with a mild case of the flu compounded by dehydration from a basketball game that morning. Apparently his fainting had triggered a mass somatoform disorder. When the consulting physician announced the investigation's findings at a campus meeting she was shouted down with cries of "Cover-up!" and "We want answers now!" Eventually the students began to recover, the crowds and media disbanded, and by the next day the campus was again calm.

Diagnosis. Somatoform disorder NOS (Axis I).

Research and publicity on indoor air pollution has led to consideration of **sick building syndrome,** a condition in which workers in a single building develop the same symptoms. Whenever there is an outbreak of illness, a group conversion disorder is always a possibility, but as in any disorder, physical causes should be eliminated first. These can include a number of infectious and toxic agents, which tend to achieve higher concentrations in newer buildings that are outfitted with the latest insulation materials that keep both air and heat inside.

AREAS OF CONTROVERSY

The differentiation between physical illness and symptoms resulting from psychogenic causes depends on available scientific knowledge and laboratory tests. But this knowledge is far from complete, and medical history is littered with theories erroneously ascribing various conditions to psychological causes. Chronic fatigue syndrome, environmental illness, sick building syndrome, and Gulf War syndrome are currently the subject of intense controversy and scrutiny.

Patients who claim that they have **chronic fatigue syndrome (CFS)** insist that their illness has a physical cause, such as a virus, and that if they are depressed it is the result of a medical cause, compounded by the medical community's dismissal of their plight. Critics note that the symptoms of CFS include depression, fatigue, anhedonia (lack of interest in regular activities), and decreased sex drive, overlapped with symptoms of depression. These critics cite studies failing to demonstrate a physical etiology and showing high rates of psychiatric disorders in patients who have CFS both pre- and post-morbidly. The fact that chronic Epstein-Barr and other viruses can and do cause such syndromes further complicates a firm diagnosis in many cases.

Angelo S, aged 55, was admitted to the hospital for a 2-week research protocol to determine the effects of high- and low-calorie diet on various physical parameters. Mr. S revealed that he had enrolled in the study because he had read that a low-calorie diet might benefit someone with chronic fatigue syndrome. He had been treated for syphilis 5 years earlier. A lumbar puncture showed the presence of *Treponema pallidum* in his cerebrospinal fluid, confirming a diagnosis of neurosyphilis.

Mr. S responded well to intravenous antibiotic therapy, but neuropsychological testing showed apparently fixed but mild cognitive deficits in memory, concentration, and visuospatial skill. Mr. S's overall IQ score remained high in the 150 range. He had also developed a depression that did not clear with treatment for neurosyphilis. He became convinced that the doctors were either wrong or were misleading him in their diagnosis. He developed the un-

shakable conviction that he suffered from chronic fatigue syndrome and felt that CFS was the cause of his cognitive problems and multiple vague physical complaints in almost every organ system.

Mr. S refused to take antidepressants even though a brief trial several years earlier had relieved some of his symptoms, stating, "It's just another way of doctors to invalidate this disease. Sure I might be less depressed, but it would just be covering up the damage that the CFS is causing." Mr. S was so convinced of his worsening health status that he contacted Dr. Jack Kevorkian to explore assisted suicide, though apparently he was rebuffed. Any rational discussion with Mr. S quickly devolved in a struggle over his diagnosis. He completed the study and refused all psychiatric follow-up, vowing, "I'll give it another year, but if I can't find a cure I'll have to think about ending my life."

A similar controversy surrounds **environmental illness (EI),** a disorder afflicted patients claim is a type of allergic reaction to twentieth-century chemicals. These patients exhibit a variety of symptoms, including fatigue, headaches, and intermittent paralysis. Patients insist that their symptoms are closely tied to exposure to toxins in the environment, in the home, and in the workplace. Many move to rural locations, wear natural fibers exclusively, and live in homes that are free from as many modern chemicals as possible. Critics suspect that these patients actually suffer from major depression or somatization disorder and cite arguments similar to those used to criticize CFS.

The latest addition to the list of disorders that lack a proven clinical etiology and have conflicting evidence for either a psychological or physical basis is the so-called **"Gulf War syndrome."** The term has been applied to veterans of the 1991 Gulf War who exhibit a vague syndrome with multiple physical manifestations as well as neuropsychiatric symptoms of depression and cognitive dysfunction. Earlier studies found no evidence for a physically based problem, and the United States Department of Defense denied reports that soldiers were exposed to chemical or biological weapons, as some soldiers claimed. Recent reports have contradicted this conclusion. It is now believed that at least 100,000 United States soldiers and their allies were exposed to low levels of nerve gas that were incinerated. Researchers are also considering whether the immunizations that soldiers received could be responsible for their health complaints, especially given the experimental nature of some of the vaccines. Uncertainty continues about the soldiers' health problems, despite years of investigation into this clinical entity.

How should a physician approach a patient without the certainty of knowing if the patient's symptoms are physical or psychological in nature? First, a broad-minded approach is recommended; physicians often fall back in defensive postures of unfounded dogmatism in the face of the unknown, insisting exclusively on either a medical or a psychiatric etiology. It is also valuable for the patient to see open-mindedness modeled by a treating physician. If depression or anxiety disorders can be diagnosed, the patient should be encouraged to seek treatment, but as in the somatoform disorders, psychiatric diagnoses and treatment should be uncoupled from the notion that "it's all in the patient's head." Rather, one can truthfully tell a patient, "We do not know the nature of this illness, but we do know that every illness has a psychological aspect, including the stress of coping with an unknown. We also know that stress, anxiety, and depression leave patients less able to cope successfully with challenges and may impair the body's immune function as well. Let's try to work on both sides of the problem, without getting caught up in a struggle about putting you or your illness in a fixed category."

EMOTIONAL REACTIONS TO PATIENTS

Patients who have somatic complaints that lack a physically discernible cause frequently engender very strong reactions from physicians. These reactions frequently include disbelief, emotional distancing, and often anger based on the notion that these patients are attempting to somehow take advantage of physicians and the health-care system. J. Burack has suggested that a physician's anger at a patient who has a somatoform disorder may stem from the physician's own frustration at his or her difficulty in distinguishing between psychological and physical disease processes. Physicians may also be led by these emotions to provide too much care and attempt to perform medical and emotional "rescue." More commonly, however, physicians may find their treatment of patients who have somatoform disorders affected by their own emotional reactions.

A 25-year-old patient was admitted to the neurology service with urinary incontinence and a possible seizure disorder. A seizure disorder was ruled out with a series of three negative EEGs. The patient continued to experience urinary incontinence without a detectable physical cause, much to the consternation of the treating team.

The psychiatric consultant was surprised to find that the patient was given the equivalent of adult diapers to wear in the hospital and not offered a urinary catheter. The neurology team responded that they did not want to "encourage" the patient's symptoms. The psychiatrist then pointed out that the neurology team had included a diuretic medication in the patient's daily medical orders, without a notation (or logical reason) in the chart. The neurology resident sheepishly responded, "I guess that was a mistake," and crossed out the order.

Discussion. Although mistakes do occur in medical care, placing a patient who has urinary incontinence on a diuretic seems too psychologically over-determined to be an accident. This case illustrates that physicians—especially overtired and overburdened residents and medical students—may be prone to unconscious reactions toward frustrating patients. In this case, the treating team's unrecognized frustration, anger, and hostility led to their punitively "acting out" against a patient.

The challenge of appreciating patients' subjective experiences with somatoform and factitious disorders in a sense represents the Rosetta Stone between mind and body. It is often tempting to dismiss patients' somatic complaints as unreal and overwhelming. But level-headed and empathic physicians can utilize these physical symptoms, along with their own emotional responses, to build a "vocabulary" to help patients translate their physical complaints into a more accessible language to describe and treat emotional distress.

LEGAL & ETHICAL ISSUES

A number of legal issues commonly encountered in the care of patients who have somatoform disorders appear in the cases above. Access to information about a patient's previous medical history is extremely helpful, but in some instances, physicians at different hospitals and clinics exchange confidential information about problematic patients even in the absence of signed release forms from these patients. However, physicians who suspect factitious disorder involving a child—Munchausen by proxy—are obligated by law to break confidentiality and alert Child Protective Services.

The treatment of somatoform disorders also raises ethical issues. Many patients who have somatoform disorders are highly suggestible. In some cases, patients who have conversion disorders are given placebo injections or pills as treatment, along with suggestions that they will feel better very soon. This treatment method violates the principle of informed consent, because the physician would undermine the efficacy of the treatment if this information was disclosed to the patient.

Theresa W, a 46-year-old woman with a low-normal intelligence level, presented to the medical emergency room after losing her vision. She had come home from work early to find her husband in bed with a neighbor. She ran to a friend's home in a very agitated state, saying that she had "gone blind." Ms. W's friend drove her to the emergency room where medical staff noted that she was able to anticipate obstacles such as chairs and benches by walking around them and at one point picked up a brush to comb her hair without hesitation. Her physical examination was completely normal, including pupils that were reactive to light and changes in distance. The friend told the emergency room resident that Ms. W was prone to becoming extremely upset and tended to develop physical complaints when she was emotionally distressed. Ms. W's father died when she was a child, and when she was 13, her mother died from complications of diabetes, which included renal failure and blindness.

Ms. W was given a saline injection in the emergency room, along with the suggestion that the "special shot" would cure her. Thirty minutes later she exclaimed, "I can see again! The shot worked!" The medical staff made no attempt to explain to her that she had an episode of hysterical blindness without a physiologic cause, or that the cure that she received was a placebo.

Diagnosis. Conversion disorder (Axis I).

The preceding case illustrates the difficulty raised in treating a patient who is not completely aware of the nature of his or her medical illness. It may be difficult for a health-care professional to decide how honest to be when he or she knows that a patient's physical problems are psychogenically based? Somehow the professional must ensure that the patient receives the best care, with the least harm from unnecessary procedures and prescriptions. It may be difficult to satisfy the requirements for informed consent and to respect the patient's autonomy. Should a patient be informed of his or her psychiatric diagnosis after the symptoms have passed? There is no agreed-upon standard of whether deceit (or telling a patient a "partial truth") is justifiable when the physician holds the patient's best interest in mind, and whether the "ends" ever justify the "means" in providing relief from physical symptoms, real or imagined. A patient may also suffer emotional distress, humiliation, and a sense of betrayal if he or she learns the true diagnosis later from some other source such as a new doctor or a consultant who is reviewing the case.

Physicians' powerful emotional reactions to patients who have somatoform disorders, especially when complicated by personality disorders, can lead them to behave in unusual ways that violate the ethical and legal standards of physician conduct.

Mary F, a 23-year old woman, had been repeatedly sexually abused as a child, had multiple physical complaints corresponding to the abuse and was in search of a "protector" in her life. Her physician was an orthopedic surgeon who had recently separated from his wife and who quickly rushed in to "rescue" the patient, including ordering unnecessary tests, loaning her money, and promising to keep her hospitalized until she could straighten out her chaotic housing situation.

The surgeon's promise led to a hospitalization of over 6 weeks. The surgeon's colleagues became aware of the dilemma and forcefully pointed out his inappropriate behavior. The chagrined physician was angry at himself and the patient and swiftly moved to discharge her from the hospital, thus breaking his previous promises to her. She angrily left the hospital, blaming the doctor for betraying her trust in him, only to be admitted the next week with a broken leg that she sustained falling off the wheelchair-loading platform on a transit bus. The surgeon's colleagues intervened to take over the case. The surgeon agreed with a mixture of relief and resentment.

CONCLUSION

Somatoform disorders, factitious disorders, and malingering are a fascinating set of related conditions linked by the boundaries of medical illness, psychological defense mechanisms, and cultural norms for illness behavior. Physicians entering any area of medicine are likely to encounter patients who have these disorders, and in treating these patients, are likely to encounter diagnostic and ethical dilemmas. Accurate assessment and management of these conditions is essential. Delays in treatment for the somatoform disorders in particular is likely to result in a more prolonged course, with further complications of depression, suicidality, and unnecessary clinic and emergency room visits and surgeries. Future challenges remain in elucidating the causes of chronic fatigue syndrome, environmental illness, and Gulf War syndrome, which may represent a combination of medical and psychiatric factors.

At the same time, the disorders described in this chapter represent only a fraction of the larger field of psychosomatic illness. The first half of the twentieth century was marked by investigation into so-called psychosomatic illnesses, medical diseases that were believed to have a partial psychological cause (eg, ul-cers, asthma, ulcerative colitis). Links were made between levels of stress and physiologic functioning. Currently this line of investigation is being pursued in studies of immune function and stress, and other "mind-body" relationships. Much more can be learned about the relationship between mind and body, an area of clinical research that is likely to be challenging but richly rewarding for many years to come.

REFERENCES

Burack J: Provoking new epileptic seizures: The ethics of deceptive diagnostic testing. Hastings Center Report. 1997;27(4):24–33.

Dr Marc Feldman's Munchausen Syndrome and Factitious Disorders Page. http://ourworld.compuserve.com/home-pages/Marc_Feldman_2/

Escobar JI: Transcultural aspects of dissociative and so-matoform disorders. Culture and major depression. Psy-chiatr Clin N Am 1995;18(3):555.

Ford CV: Illness as a lifestyle: the role of somatization in medial practice. Spine 1992;17(10):173(Suppl).

Hahn SR, Thompson KS, Wills TA, Stern V, Budner NS: The difficult doctor-patient relationship: somatization, personality and psychopathology. J Clin Epidemiol 1994;47:647.

Jorge CM, Goodnick PJ: Chronic fatigue syndrome and de-pression: biological differentiation and treatment. Psy-chiatr Ann 1997;27(5):365.

Kaufman DM: Psychogenic neurologic deficits. Pages 25–33 in: *Clinical Neurology for Psychiatrists,* 4th ed. Saunders, 1995.

Kirmayer LJ, Robbins JM (editors): *Current Concepts of Somatization: Research and Clinical Perspectives.* American Psychiatric Association Press, 1991

Kroenke K, Spitzer RL, deGruy FV III, Hahn SR et al: Multisomatoform disorder: an alternative to undifferenti-ated somatoform disorder for the somatizing patient in primary care. Arch Gen Psychiatr 1997;54:352.

McElroy SL, Philips KA, Keck PE, Hudson JI, Pope HG: Body dysmorphic disorder: Does it have a psychotic subtype? J Clin Psychiatr 1993;54(10):389.

Min SK, Lee BO: Laterality in somatization. Psychosomat Med 1997;59(3):236.

Sadler JZ. Ethical and management considerations in facti-tious illness: one and the same. Gen Hosp Psychiatr 1987;9:31.

Dissociative Disorders

10

David Elkin, MD, & Claudia E. Toomey, PhD

The **dissociative disorders** develop as a result of a failure in the normal integration of perception, consciousness, memory, and identity. They include depersonalization disorder and the amnestic disorders: dissociative amnestic disorder, dissociative fugue disorder, and dissociative identity disorder.

Figure 10–1 illustrates the spectrum of dissociative disorders. **Depersonalization disorder** is characterized by persistent and distressing feelings of detachment and numbing and changes in perception of oneself and the environment. **Dissociative amnesia** is marked by an inability to remember important personal information following trauma. Patients who have **dissociative fugue** disorder suddenly travel from home with a gap in memory and may be confused about their personal identity or assume a new identity. Individuals who have **dissociative identity disorder** (previously known as multiple personality disorder) possess two or more distinct identities or personalities that can control their behavior. They are also unable to recall important personal information.

There is a strong relationship between dissociative disorders and trauma. Most people can recall mild episodes of dissociation in their lives. These states may even be adaptive under some circumstances. However the dissociative disorders almost always represent responses to traumatic experiences. Often dissociation is used as a defense in an effort to ward off overwhelming feelings of anxiety and powerlessness. Histories of physical and sexual abuse are noted frequently among those who develop dissociative syndromes. Individuals who have been involved in life-threatening events such as war, natural disasters, and crime are more likely to experience dissociative symptoms. Patients should be screened for medical illnesses as well as for possible cultural determinants of their behavior.

EVIDENCE FOR STATES OF AWARENESS OUTSIDE OF CONSCIOUSNESS

Dissociative disorders are fascinating in and of themselves and also for what they reveal about the functioning of the human mind. Dissociative states are extensions of psychological phenomena that occur in everyday life. The concept of dissociation rests on the premise that the human brain can operate, sometimes simultaneously, at different levels of consciousness. Dissociation of mental functioning reveals some of the elements of consciousness that are normally integrated and of which most people are not aware. Although this chapter is concerned with psychopathologic states in which perceptions or memory are severely compromised, milder dissociative phenomena can be observed regularly in healthy individuals. Such phenomena include the experiences of daydreaming or being lost in one's thoughts to the point that it requires an effort to "come back to real life" afterward.

Beyond being adaptive, altered states of consciousness may be beneficial. For example, most people have experienced the pleasure of losing oneself in a book, a movie, a long drive, or some other activity. Relaxation or meditation exercises often enable people to feel rested and recharged. Csikszentimihalyi studied so-called **peak experiences,** in which individuals had brief, intense episodes in which they felt and functioned at their best. The individuals would become totally immersed in an activity to the point that their concentration was highly focused and all distractions dropped away. This experience occurs across many disciplines and activities, usually to people who have spent years practicing a skill (eg, a surgeon in the operating room, a musician performing a difficult piece, or an experienced rock climber who climbs without safety ropes). These individuals describe a loss of the normal passage of

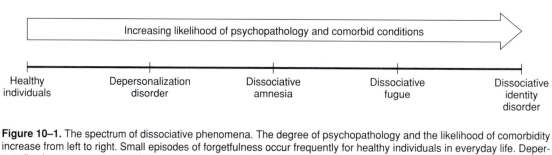

Figure 10–1. The spectrum of dissociative phenomena. The degree of psychopathology and the likelihood of comorbidity increase from left to right. Small episodes of forgetfulness occur frequently for healthy individuals in everyday life. Depersonalization symptoms occur frequently in patients who have acute stress disorder and borderline personality disorder. Dissociative amnestic disorder can occur in response to overwhelming trauma and results in a larger period of lost time. In dissociative fugue disorder both memory and identity are partially compromised. Patients who have dissociative identity disorder (formerly known as multiple personality disorder) frequently have a history of extreme physical and sexual abuse in childhood, leading to the formation of multiple personalities.

time and intense feelings of concentration, confidence, and energy, with a loss of self-consciousness and self; a feeling of being completely "in the moment." This experience may be closely related to Eastern concepts in Zen called **satori.** This is a state of mind that makes it possible for someone to perform at or above their highest expectations and may briefly illustrate the boundaries of human potential.

A growing body of research indicates that the human mind is capable of processing information at many different levels of awareness. Consider this example: Find the error in the following phrase:

> Paris in the
> the spring.

If this phrase is shown in a classroom, many individuals will fail to realize that the word "the" is repeated. Even if told that the phrase contains an error, many people will be unable to detect the problem until it is pointed out. This example demonstrates that the human brain is configured to selectively *not* notice or attend to observations or facts that do not fit with expected patterns.

The use of scientific research provides more evidence that human beings are capable of processing information outside of consciousness. In one study, words were displayed on a computer screen for intervals of approximately 40 ms. Subjects observing the screen immediately knew that they had seen something and that it was probably a single word, but they did not consciously recognize the word. This is a strange sensation, akin to having a word stuck on the tip of one's tongue. If subjects were told to select the target word from a list of three similar words immediately afterward, they insisted they could not, because they did not see the target word. Yet they consistently selected the word that was presented subliminally earlier. Thus another system of information processing is capable of recognizing information and feeding it into consciousness for future recognition and analysis.

Further evidence of a parallel system of processing information comes from a study of Vietnam War veterans who have post-traumatic stress disorder (PTSD). The subjects were also shown words on a computer screen for intervals short enough to preclude conscious recognition. They were shown two kinds of words. The first type had no emotional significance, but the second type included emotionally charged words that evoked feelings about the war (eg, "incoming," "wounded," or "choppers"). Even though the veterans denied recognizing any words, they were unable to perform simple tasks immediately after seeing the words related to the war.

In a study that took this research one step further, veterans from the Vietnam War were shown similar words while being monitored for autonomic nervous system activity changes in heart rate, blood pressure, and galvanic skin response. When they were exposed to subliminal words that were related to the war, the subjects' hearts would race, they would break out in a sweat, and were clearly responding with a fight-or-flight response, even though the trigger was outside of their awareness. Again, these studies suggest that individuals can attend and respond to information in the environment without being consciously aware of the input, with emotional and physiologic consequences.

In an intriguing experiment, researchers questioned whether patients undergoing gastrointestinal surgery could respond to suggestions given to them while they were anesthetized. The researchers told the unconscious patients that they would recover quickly from their surgery, with a rapid return of normal bowel function. Compared to the control group (who did not receive such suggestion while undergoing surgery), these patients made more rapid recoveries from surgery and were even discharged home several days earlier.

Hypnosis is also based on the phenomenon of dissociation. Hypnotic and related states can best be described as altered states of consciousness in which normally integrated functions of consciousness are dissociated, resulting in a highly focused and suggestible state of attention. Essentially, the clinician performing hypnosis helps the patient achieve a dissociated state in which he or she is more receptive to suggestions. Patients can learn to assume partial control over autonomic body functions to reduce blood pressure or pain. Many clinics specializing in the care of patients who have cancer, burns, or chronic pain utilize hypnosis to help patients achieve better control of pain and anxiety with less medication.

Ethan Z, aged 25, was admitted to the hospital with second-degree burns on his lower body as a result of a car accident. During his 3-month hospitalization, Mr. Z required increasing doses of opiates to achieve partial pain relief. This situation caused tension between Mr. Z and the staff, who felt that Mr. Z was too demanding and dependent. Mr. Z worried that the staff would not respond quickly enough when he was in pain.

A consulting psychiatrist met with Mr. Z daily for 2 weeks to lead him through a series of relaxation exercises. Mr. Z was instructed that his hands were like "magic wands" that could reduce pain by waving them over any part of his body. He became more relaxed and experienced diminished levels of pain that let him become less dependent on opiates for pain control. His partial mastery over his anxiety and pain led to increased self-esteem and improvement in his relationship with the staff.

Thus the process of dissociation is helpful in understanding facets of information processing and alternate states of consciousness that occur in healthy and traumatized individuals.

DEPERSONALIZATION DISORDER: CLINICAL FEATURES

We usually regard human consciousness as a unified state. Our subjective experiences confirm this, for we each perceive ourselves as a sole agent in charge of our lives, with no discrepancy between our minds and bodies. For example, when you move your hand, the action is not experienced as thousands of separate nerve or muscle impulses firing. You do not feel that the frontal lobe of your brain is ordering your hand to move.

In depersonalization disorder the normally integrated perception of experience is disturbed. Patients may note changes in any of their five senses; such as muted sounds, tunnel vision, or diminished pain perception. They often feel "numb" and have diminished awareness of their immediate surroundings. Patients feel that parts of their body are not their own or that they are "outside" of their body. Some describe the sensation that their body is a "puppet" that they are controlling from a separate vantage point.

Derealization involves the loss of the normal perception that the world itself is "real." Patients often describe this feeling as "dreamlike," or they report that they suddenly perceive that the world "is like a movie, that it just isn't 'real.'" Feelings of unreality and detachment frequently cocoon with other symptoms such as anxiety and panic. Although patients frequently complain that they are "going crazy," reality testing is intact and patients are not psychotic. However depersonalization disorder results in marked distress and impairment in relationships and work.

INCIDENCE

Episodes of depersonalization and derealization occur in healthy individuals and are frequently seen as symptoms in anxiety disorders such as acute stress disorder, PTSD, panic disorder, social phobia, and in borderline personality disorder and substance use. The isolated disorder of depersonalization is uncommon.

ETIOLOGY

Experiences of depersonalization or derealization are thought to be based on **dissociation,** a defense mechanism used to ward off anxiety. Among healthy individuals, dissociation may be associated with exhaustion, boredom, or sensory deprivation. Depersonalization often occurs as a response to psychological stress or physical trauma, or in individuals who have a history of past trauma. For example, prisoners of war and hostages have sometimes constructed elaborate fantasies to escape the stress and boredom of their situations.

Isolated dissociative phenomena are considered to be a normal part of psychological functioning. If these episodes become more discrete, frequent, and pronounced, they then meet the criteria for depersonalization disorder. Most commonly, depersonalization and derealization are encountered as a result of medical factors or as a feature of another psychiatric disorder.

DIFFERENTIAL DIAGNOSIS

A variety of medical and psychiatric conditions can simulate the symptoms of depersonalization disorder. Medical problems can simulate the sensations of depersonalization and derealization. Medical causes should be excluded before the clinician considers primary and associated diagnoses.

1. RULING OUT MEDICAL CAUSES OF DEPERSONALIZATION DISORDER

Medical conditions that can mimic the experiences of derealization and depersonalization include

- neurologic disorders: epilepsy, migraine, brain tumors, cerebrovascular accidents, cerebral trauma, encephalitis, connective tissue disorders (such as SLE or multiple sclerosis), Alzheimer's dementia, Huntington's chorea, spinocerebellar degeneration
- metabolic causes: hypoglycemia, hypoparathyroidism, and hyperventilation
- reactions to toxins: carbon monoxide, botulism, mescaline intoxication
- medications: anticholinergic medications or antihistamines

2. RULING OUT SUBSTANCE USE DISODERS

Most substances can cause episodes of derealization and depersonalization. These substances include marijuana, hallucinogens (eg, LSD, mescaline), PCP, glue, opiates, and alcohol. The patient's use of these substances must be determined before a conclusive diagnosis can be made.

3. RULING OUT PSYCHIATRIC CAUSES

Depersonalization disorders can occur on their own but most often are a minor feature of one of the following psychiatric disorders:

- schizophrenia
- affective disorders: mania and depression
- anxiety disorders: acute stress disorder, PTSD, obsessive-compulsive disorder, social phobia, and panic disorders (less common in generalized anxiety disorder)
- personality disorders (especially borderline and other cluster B personality disorders such as histrionic, narcissistic, and antisocial)
- delirium

Episodes of depersonalization often occur with the intense anxiety that is a hallmark of panic disorder, social phobia, or simple phobia.

Bernard H, aged 19, experienced the onset of panic attacks 1 month after leaving home for college. These attacks occurred daily, often while Mr. H was relaxing, and were accompa-nied by such classic signs as palpitations, sweating, hyperventilation, tingling sensations, mounting anxiety, and a sense of impending doom. Mr. H stated that while the anxiety itself was difficult to bear, he was more disturbed by other strange feelings: "It's like I'm numb, strange, like I'm not myself, really." He also described the sensation that his hands "didn't feel like they belonged to me—they felt like they weren't connected to me. I keep staring at them, but it's as if my hands aren't mine. I can make them 'move,' but they seem to belong to someone else."

Although he knew other members of his family who had panic attacks, the accompanying episodes of depersonalization made him question whether "something more serious is going on—could I be having a nervous breakdown or something?" Psychotherapy and treatment with antidepressants produced rapid improvement, and Mr. H's panic attacks and the episodes of depersonalization ceased.

Diagnosis. Panic disorder (Axis I).

Dissociative phenomena, including depersonalization, are also common during and after an overwhelming traumatic event and are important features of acute stress disorder. Dissociative symptoms are common in anyone experiencing life-threatening events including disasters, crime, or even medical procedures. Patients who experience dissociative symptoms during the initial stages of trauma are more likely to develop PTSD.

Yvonne L, aged 56, was traveling with friends on a tour bus when the bus went out of control on a steep curve and crashed into a stand of trees. Ms. L never lost consciousness and remembered the details of the crash vividly. When the bus started to slide, she thought, "This can't be happening." Everything seemed to happen in slow motion, and the screeching of the bus's brakes and screams of the passengers seemed muted and distant.

Ms. L had a moment of panic when she thought that she was going to die. Then she experienced the anxiety abruptly lifting and felt as if she were observing the crash "like someone would watch a movie." She reported thinking, "It's just a dream and I'll wake up soon."

Ms. L was treated for minor bruises in the emergency room, where she reported still feeling "dazed and numb." She entered psychotherapy 2 months later after continuing to experience persistent flashbacks to the crash and feelings of depersonalization.

Diagnosis. Acute stress disorder, post-traumatic stress disorder (Axis I).

Patients who have borderline personality disorder often experience instability of emotions, thinking, and interpersonal relationships as well as episodes of depersonalization. These patients often have a history of childhood trauma and are prone to anxiety disorders and substance use. They often engage in self-destructive behavior or repeated suicide attempts.

Marjorie S, aged 31, came for an initial medical clinic appointment but was reluctant to have a physical examination. She relented eventually, and the medical student giving the examination noted many linear parallel scars on Ms. S's left wrist, as well as a series of healed circular scars on her left arm and her thighs. When questioned about the scars, Ms. S. was initially angry, almost shouting, "It's private, I don't want to talk about it." The student explained that although Ms. S did not have to answer the questions, the information would help her obtain the best care possible.

Ms. S replied, "I hate when students try that doctor stuff with me. I'll tell you anyway." She explained that she became upset with her current boyfriend of 1 month when they had a fight. When Ms. S had the slightest reason to believe that her relationships were threatened, she would become "really angry—screaming, throwing stuff, feeling suicidal. It really frightens me."

She managed these feelings by cutting her wrist with a razor and burning herself with cigarettes. She found that she felt minimal pain: "It's like I'm floating outside of myself, not really in my body. My room looks kind of funny too—the angles are strange, and everything seems far away and quiet."

Ms. S revealed that she had experienced several similar episodes dating back to adolescence. She found that cutting or burning herself made her anxiety decrease dramatically for up to several hours. She described this feeling as "an incredible release. I'm peaceful and serene—it's the only time I feel in control." Ms. S expressed interest in a referral to the psychiatry clinic but did not show for her appointment.

Diagnosis. Borderline personality disorder (Axis II).

TREATMENT OF DEPERSONALIZATION DISORDER

The treatment of all dissociative disorders, including depersonalization disorder, involves correcting underlying medical disorders, first and foremost. In the absence of organic factors, treatment should be provided for major psychiatric disorders, if present. Treatment for these primary conditions frequently

will result in a resolution of the sense of depersonalization and derealization.

Treatment usually consists of psychotherapy and possibly antidepressant medication. Group therapy is often very helpful because the shame, fear, alienation, and embarrassment associated with dissociative disorders frequently abates when the patient hears others discussing their own experiences. Other nonpharmacologic interventions include "prescriptions" for rest, exercise, avoidance of alcohol and drugs, and relaxation exercises such as meditation, deep breathing, or biofeedback. The net effect of these interventions is to lower stress and give patients a greater sense of control over their emotions and thoughts.

AMNESTIC DISORDERS: CLINICAL FEATURES

Dissociation can also affect the normal process of integration of memory from consciousness, resulting in dissociative amnesia. Again these disorders are expansions of dissociative phenomena that occur in healthy individuals. Most people have had the experience of feeling frustrated by misplacing an object, forgetting that they have already picked up the wallet for which they are searching, or being unable to remember the name of an acquaintance. Patients often report that they "forgot" to take their medication or cannot remember the directions or explanations provided by their physician. Larger gaps in memory can be more disconcerting.

Arlene K, a 24-year-old medical student, was driving home from a 30-hour shift at the hospital on her surgery rotation. On the 20-minute trip she found her thoughts drifting to the day's events and then to her parents' upcoming visit. Suddenly she realized that she was only a block from her apartment and had no memory of the last 15 minutes of the trip. As she pulled into the parking lot, she wondered what had happened. Had she been asleep?

This was unlikely, because she had to have passed through several traffic lights, crossed a narrow bridge, and negotiated a sudden curve. How could she have executed these complicated procedures without crashing? But if she had been aware of what she was doing, where was the missing memory?

Diagnosis. None (minor dissociative episodes are not pathologic and occur in most healthy individuals).

Discussion. This situation will be familiar to many readers. Most people can relate similar experiences, finding a vagueness or "hole" in their memory for a brief period of time. In amnestic disorders, however, there is not a vagueness about loss of time but a complete inability to recall what happened for a more significant period of time. Typically the memory loss is related to traumatic or stressful life events such as rape or marital discord. For example, someone might wake up to find a new car in the driveway and then find the receipt for the car but have no recollection of purchasing the vehicle. Someone who has dissociative fugue disorder might find himself or herself living in a different part of the country with no memory of the previous 6 months.

INCIDENCE

The incidence of these disorders is very low. Dissociative amnestic disorder and fugue disorder are rare phenomena. Dissociative identity disorder has been given wide ranges of occurrence from rare to up to 3% of all mentally ill patients. These disorders may increase during times of war, natural disasters, or severe social upheaval. The increase in the incidence of these disorders in the past 25 years is believed to be due to reporting errors, suggestibility of patients, overdiagnosis, or possibly greater recognition of the existence of dissociative phenomenon.

ETIOLOGY

The psychodynamic model of the mind conceptualizes mental functioning with both conscious and unconscious processes that function in parallel. In this model, unconscious conflicts or any other threat to a cohesive sense of self generate anxiety. Speigel distinguishes between dissociation and repression. Dissociation is a defense mechanism that is used to block the conscious realization of anxiety and conflict related to a specific trauma for a discrete period of time. In contrast, **repression** is more enduring, stems from nontraumatic conflict, and involves less easily discernible content. However, there is some "cost" of using these defenses, that is, the odd sensation of being cut off from part of one's affect, memory, or identity.

This is the explanation invoked for dissociative amnesia, in which psychological defense mechanisms produce gaps in memory. Such gaps are seen in cases of dissociative amnesia as well as after trauma (eg, in acute stress disorder and PTSD) and in somatization disorder. In dissociative fugue or dissociative identity disorders (see below), memory gaps are so severe that the patient's identity is also compromised.

DIFFERENTIAL DIAGNOSIS

1. RULING OUT MEDICAL CAUSES OF AMNESTIC DISORDERS

The presence of any psychiatric symptom warrants a full workup, beginning with the elimination of possible medical causes for the symptoms. A physical examination that includes a thorough neurologic examination is critical for ruling out medical causes of memory problems. Some of the more common medical causes of dissociative amnesia, fugue, and identity disorders are listed below. Many of these medical conditions are extremely serious and warrant accurate and rapid diagnosis and treatment.

- CNS disorders: cerebral infections (encephalitis, meningitis, herpes simplex affecting temporal lobes), cerebral neoplasms, cerebrovascular accidents (especially in the limbic and frontal portions of the brain)
- metabolic disorders: uremia, hypoglycemia, hypertensive encephalopathy, intermittent porphyria
- other disorders: transient global amnesia (TGA), trauma, anoxic damage, electroconvulsive therapy, temporal lobe epilepsy

Of these disorders, transient global amnesia (TGA), can have interesting consequences. TGA is an unusual and fortunately brief condition that produces profound amnesia and impaired learning (short-term memory). It clears within hours, tends not to recur, and is believed to be the result of an interruption of blood flow to the hippocampus and other CNS structures critical to memory. Harold Klawans, a neurologist, wrote a fascinating account of a surgeon who developed TGA—in the middle of performing surgery. His surgical skills were still intact, but he could not remember one moment to the next. The operating room nurse had to guide the surgeon through the rest of the procedure.

The following standard battery of medical tests should be used to screen for these medical conditions:

- standard blood tests for serology (electrolytes) and CBC (to check blood volume, white cell count, and platelets)
- toxicology screen
- head CT or MRI scan, and lumbar puncture, when clinically indicated
- EEG, to rule out seizure disorder, when clinically indicated

2. RULING OUT DRUG-INDUCED AMNESIA

Memory loss can be induced by various drugs, including alcohol, barbiturates, benzodiazepines, PCP,

LSD, and steroids. A toxicology screen should be ordered to identify any drugs or medications that the patient might have taken.

DISSOCIATIVE AMNESIA DISORDER

Dissociative amnesia disorder is characterized by a sudden inability to recall personal information that is usually related to trauma. This inability is too pervasive and extensive to be explained by normal forgetfulness and may be associated with depression, personality disorders, suicidality, and conversion disorder. Dissociative amnesia can occur in children, adolescents, or adults and may predispose an individual to future episodes of amnesia under stressful conditions. Chronic or continuous memory loss is an infrequent outcome, and most individuals gradually regain their memory. Let us consider a severe example of memory loss and dissociative amnesia:

Caroline R, aged 32, was involved in a traffic accident in which she was badly injured and her 5-year-old son died. In the hospital she was perfectly lucid and alert, with all senses intact. But her knowledge of all events, personal and general, ended sharply 6 years before the present. She gave her old address and her age from 6 years before. She could name presidents up to the current administration. She was unable to provide any details about the accident and insisted that she had never had any children. Her last memory was planning a trip to Hawaii with her husband.

At first Ms. R's physicians wondered if she might have sustained a head injury that would account for her memory problems. But she had no physical findings to suggest a head injury and was not noted to be unconscious at the scene of the accident. Her neurologic examination was unremarkable, and an MRI of her head was normal. There was no history of drug or alcohol use (which should always be considered in motor vehicle accidents); a toxicology screen was negative.

A consulting psychiatrist was called in. She performed a cognitive examination, including tests of concentration (serial sevens), attention, and short-term memory. Ms. R performed well on all portions of the examination, including recall of four items at 5 minutes without prompting. Thus, Ms. R's ability to remember forward in time seemed unaffected. The consultant found no evidence for delirium; the patient was alert, and showed no signs of cognitive impairment or of waxing or waning of consciousness.

Preexisting dementia was considered extremely unlikely given the normal examination and Ms. R's relative youth. The psychiatrist was impressed by the abrupt cessation of Ms. R's long-term memory at a date 6 years before the accident, and by the normal cognitive examination. She later learned from Ms. R's husband that the trip she had referred to was the one on which her son was conceived.

Diagnosis. Dissociative amnesia (Axis I).

Discussion. A thorough history, mental status examination, and laboratory testing failed to provide evidence for a medical cause for memory loss such as delirium or postconcussive syndrome. It appeared that the patient had used dissociation to cope with the profound emotional impact of her son's death.

The patient gradually recovered memories in individual psychotherapy. Experiencing and integrating staved-off memories and associated feelings of guilt, depression, anger, and loss are important elements of the therapeutic process.

Memory provides the continuity to our lives that is essential for maintaining a stable personal identity. When memory is severely compromised, as in dissociative fugue and dissociative identity disorders, disturbances of personal identity also occur.

TREATMENT OF DISSOCIATIVE AMNESIA DISORDER

Memory loss due to dissociative amnesia can sometimes be accessed using sodium amytal or lorazepam (Ativan) or through hypnosis. These techniques presumably bypass defense mechanisms by lowering internal levels of anxiety. The same effect may be accomplished with psychotherapy but at a slower rate. There are some advantages to therapy, though, and some distinct dangers of using hypnosis and other more direct routes of access to the patient's unconscious. Hypnosis may provide a means to recover memories, but because of the plastic nature of memory and the suggestible nature of hypnotized subjects, information recovered in this manner is usually inadmissible in courts of law.

Goeffrey V, a 48-year-old African-American Vietnam veteran, was seen at the Veteran's Administration hospital for treatment of depression and symptoms of PTSD. He had been involved in many combat situations during the war, and 15 years later continued to experience intrusive flashbacks, feelings of anger and guilt, and episodes of anxiety that bordered on panic. He rarely slept through the night and he had frequent nightmares about the Vietnam War.

Mr. V was admitted for 2 weeks on the inpatient unit. He was started on antidepressants but seemed to benefit most from his relationship with the unit psychologist, who led him through relaxation exercises that helped him feel less anxious and more confident. The psychologist noted that Mr. V seemed to be able to enter a light trance very easily and rapidly achieved a relaxed state. Group psychotherapy offered Mr. V the chance to listen to and be accepted by a group of his peers who also fought in Vietnam.

At the end of his 2-week stay, Mr. V had experienced significant improvement in his mood, PTSD symptoms, and interpersonal functioning. He was invited to enter a long-term (up to 6 months) inpatient program that specialized in the treatment of Vietnam veterans. He accepted the offer and left for the program immediately.

After Mr. V was admitted to the new program, the staff read the psychologist's reports and decided that Mr. V was an excellent candidate for hypnotherapy. He was asked about his most difficult moment in Vietnam, so that he could therapeutically "relive" the experience under hypnosis. This technique is sometimes used to help patients realize that they truly performed to the best of their ability under difficult circumstances and may help relieve feelings of guilt.

Earlier, Mr. V had tearfully described an incident in which his friend was mortally wounded but still alive as Viet Cong soldiers advanced on their exposed position. Mr. V had refused a direct order so that he could stay behind with his friend until he died, at risk to his own life as the North Vietnamese soldiers advanced. He felt proud that he had been there for his friend.

Under hypnosis, Mr. V revealed a profoundly different account. His friend was indeed badly wounded, and the North Vietnamese soldiers were approaching. At this point, the men in Mr. V's company realized that they could not let the injured soldier be captured to be tortured, nor could they afford the time to carry a dying man. So Mr. V stayed behind briefly . . . to ensure his friend's quick death by shooting him.

Mr. V was not instructed under hypnosis to return to his presumably false memory of events and retained the memory he recovered in hypnosis. He was furious at the staff for exposing these events and angrily left the program that day.

Diagnosis. Post-traumatic stress disorder (Axis I).

DISSOCIATIVE FUGUE DISORDER

Dissociative fugue is encountered in individuals who are under extreme stress. The fugue state is often marked by a physical as well as mental "flight."

These patients will sometimes take on a new identity and start a new job and relationships far from their original home, appearing to have no awareness or memory of their previous life. During a fugue state, patients function normally and do not appear to suffer any distress. However they are often brought to treatment when their memory loss is noted by someone else. Some patients take on a new identity in a fugue state that is more outgoing and confident than their usual personality. Most patients do not have an entirely new identity but instead lack key personal information. These patients may be distressed by their lack of self-knowledge. The episode may last days or months and tends to resolve rapidly. Differential diagnosis, including ruling out a medical disorder, is the same as for dissociative amnestic disorder.

A man who appeared to be in his early to mid 20s was brought to the emergency room by police after he was found wandering in a confused state. He claimed that he did not know his name or any other personal information and that he had no past, except for the previous day, when he found himself wandering the city.

In the emergency room, the patient received a full physical examination and laboratory testing, which were normal. He was in perfect health. A toxicology screen showed that he had no drugs or alcohol in his blood. He voluntarily agreed to an inpatient admission to psychiatry, where he received the name "Mike" and a battery of neuropsychologic testing.

Testing revealed no patterns of dementia or other organic brain syndromes. Mike's short-term memory and concentration were intact, and he possessed above-average intelligence. His long-term memory was intact for most information, such as past presidents, current events, and geographical knowledge, but he had no personal history. Questions about his place and date of birth, family members, schools attended, and names of childhood friends all drew blanks. An amytal interview failed to reveal personal details as well. It was as if the patient literally had been "born yesterday." Psychological testing revealed that Mike was naive and inclined to hysterical reactions, but there was no indication of malingering or other conscious fabrication of symptoms.

Mike was in the hospital for several months, during which time he received antidepressants and supportive psychotherapy for mild depression. The working diagnosis was that he had experienced a loss of memory due to a traumatic event, and that in time his identity would be regained. To that end he was set up in local housing.

Mike was featured several months later on a national TV talk show. He told his story and shortly thereafter received a phone call from his parents in the Midwest. He had evidently been raised in a small, conservative community, where he had fallen in love with the town sheriff's daughter. When she became pregnant, the sheriff quickly organized a shotgun wedding. Mike, caught between his desire to flee and his sense of honor and responsibility, left town in a dissociated fugue state. He returned to the Midwest without a dramatic return of memory and was lost to follow-up.

Diagnosis. Dissociative fugue disorder (Axis I).

TREATMENT OF DISSOCIATIVE FUGUE DISORDER

Hypnosis may provide access to important memories of triggering events and conditions. Benzodiazepines may be somewhat less effective. Generally fugue states resolve with the conclusion of stressful conditions. Psychotherapy focuses on gaining more familiarity with internal mood states and uncomfortable thoughts. Prognosis for the resolution of the fugue state is excellent, although patients may be at risk for future psychiatric disorders when under stress.

DISSOCIATIVE IDENTITY DISORDER

A history of severe emotional, physical, or sexual abuse in childhood, particularly repetitive trauma, predisposes some patients to develop multiple personalities. These patients often have a passive core personality with severe difficulties in dealing with normal stresses in addition to other partially formed personalities (so-called **alters**) who often have complementary emotional make-ups. Thus a mild-mannered patient usually has an angry, violent, or capable alter.

Of interest is the profound differences in physiologic functioning between patients when expressing different personalities. Researchers have shown alterations in handedness, resting pulse rate, and blood pressure when different alters are present.

There is typically no awareness of other personalities when any given personality is interviewed—only an awareness of blackouts or periods of amnesia into which the patient has little insight. In partially treated individuals, personalities can become aware of each other.

Mary E, aged 24, was referred to psychotherapy for depression and anxiety. Her childhood was marked by frequent beatings and sexual abuse by her father. She was employed by a university in a mid-level position but felt stressed at work and at home, where her husband was pressuring her to become pregnant. During therapy, she disclosed that she had plans to go on a long trip and that she had just purchased a gun. The therapist was disturbed by Ms. E's blithe assurance that everything was under control. At one point, the therapist mentioned that Ms. E might require inpatient hospitalization if she were a danger to herself or others. Ms. E's eyes abruptly rolled back into her head and she fell back in her seat.

A minute later, Ms. E looked slowly around the room and said in a Southern accent, "Where am I? I need to get out of here." Her mannerisms and appearance were remarkably different. She got to her feet unsteadily and, appearing very confused, attempted to leave through the closet door. The therapist gently suggested that given her unsteadiness, Ms. E should sit down and relax. He added that she would feel better shortly after a brief rest.

Ms. E was resistant but eventually returned to her seat. She closed her eyes and appeared "dazed" for several minutes before "awakening" minutes later. She appeared frightened and was aware only that she had become anxious and "then I was sitting here with you staring at me." Subsequent inquiries with the patient's family and friends (with the patient's permission) revealed accounts of amnesia and the identity of several different personalities.

Diagnosis. Dissociative identity disorder (Axis I).

Any report of memory loss should also raise the possibility that a patient is consciously simulating amnesia. This may occur in malingering or in factitious disorder with psychological symptoms (see Chapter 9). The ability to know of or communicate with other personalities or the potential for obvious secondary gain should raise the possibility that the patient is malingering.

Kenneth Bianci, the "Hillside Strangler," was arrested and charged with serial murders in Los Angeles in the early 1980s. He was examined in prison by forensic psychiatrists and psychologists on the suspicion that he had an alter-ego who had committed the crimes. Bianci himself denied knowledge of the crimes but dropped subtle clues about another person who did. When hypnotized, he revealed another personality, who recounted the murders in chilling detail.

Bianci's deception was detected by Dr. Martin Orne of the University of Pennsylvania, who watched videotape interviews of Bianci with other psychiatrists. He suspected Bianci was not truly in a hypnotized state and was feigning dissociation between "good" and "evil" personalities. Orne decided to test Bianci to see if he would change his behavior based on a suggestion in an unhypnotized state.

When introduced to Bianci for an interview, Orne feigned surprise that Bianci "only had one other personality." He dropped a hint that most people with dissociative identity disorder have at least two other personalities. When Orne proceeded to hypnotize him, Bianci promptly produced a third "personality." Orne also had Bianci "see" his attorney in the room. Bianci went one step further and spontaneously shook hands with the nonexistent visitor. Orne pointed out that tactile hallucinations are very rare and noted that Bianci repeatedly drew indirect attention to physical clues to his alternate personality after hypnosis (eg, saying "Look at these cigarettes! Who smoked this—I don't smoke cigarettes this way!"). Orne concluded that Bianci was only pretending to be hypnotized and did not actually have dissociative identity disorder.

It was later discovered that Bianci feared arrest and the death penalty and planned his defense of "not guilty by reason of insanity" by researching the topic in college psychology courses. A search of his basement revealed numerous books about abnormal and forensic psychology, dissociation, and multiple personality disorder.

Diagnosis. Probable antisocial personality disorder (Axis II); malingering (V Code).

TREATMENT OF DISSOCIATIVE IDENTITY DISORDER

Treatment goals in dissociative identity disorder focus on the integration of all personalities, which may take years of intensive therapy. Because individuals who have dissociative identity disorder frequently have a history of repeated physical, sexual, or emotional trauma in childhood, many of the same treatment issues seen in PTSD and borderline personality disorder arise.

Establishing trust and safety in the therapeutic alliance is critical. Antidepressant medication may help with depression, anxiety, or intrusive symptoms of PTSD. However, a tendency may remain for the patient to dissociate under periods of extreme stress.

THE CONTROVERSY OVER REPRESSED & RECOVERED MEMORY

Barbara A, aged 29, was asked to participate in relaxation exercises at her workplace. The exercises were led by a consultant who was famed for running encounter groups in the 1970s. Participants laid on mats on the floor for extended periods of time, hyperventilating. As Ms. A did the exercises and hyperventilated, she became increasingly anxious and frightened. Suddenly she was confronted by memories of being sexually abused by a close family relative, memories she was completely unaware of until then. She became extremely agitated and paranoid, and was taken to the psychiatric emergency room for evaluation.

Ms. A's psychosis cleared within several days, and she gave an unremarkable history, which was negative for all signs of major psychiatric disorders, including psychotic or affective disorders, or substance dependence. She was discharged from the hospital and began weekly psychotherapy, gradually integrating memories of trauma that she had forgotten for almost 2 decades.

Diagnosis. Dissociative amnesia, brief reactive psychosis (Axis I).

The area of repressed memory has become controversial in the past several years. Dissent over the issue within the mental health community has been picked up in the popular press. Many therapists argue that even allowing for the malleability of memory, it is still possible for traumatic memories of childhood to be walled off, repressed from consciousness until they are recovered in adulthood.

Critics argue that it is impossible to repress significant memories for such a long time and that patients claiming to have recovered memories are either fabricating their stories knowingly or perhaps believe what they are saying but are merely confabulating. Others fault mental health professionals for either manipulatively or naively "implanting" in highly suggestible patients false memories of sexual abuse by family members. This concept has been termed **false memory syndrome,** and a False Memory Syndrome Foundation has been started by family members who claim to have been unjustly accused of sexual abuse.

This controversy has an historical heritage in the beginnings of psychoanalysis. At the turn of the century Sigmund Freud saw large numbers of young women from upper-middle-class families who were coming to him with somatic complaints and dissociative disorders. Many reported being sexually abused by their fathers, stepfathers, or family friends. While Freud initially accepted their stories as fact he was given pause by the sheer number of such patients in his practice. If they were truly representative of his community, incest and sexual abuse was rampant in upper-middle-class Vienna and, by extrapolation, perhaps epidemic throughout all societies. Freud decided that this was simply impossible, so he changed his theories to speculate that these women must have *fantasized* about the sexual experiences. Since these experiences neatly fit Freud's theories about unacceptable unconscious drives (ie, the women wanted to have sex with prohibited male figures), he was able to account for their neuroses. Freud offered hope for cure if these women could consciously become aware of and accept their forbidden impulses.

To our dismayed late-twentieth-century mentality, Freud's so-called "abandonment of the seduction" theory is a terrible misstep by a man who could have drawn society's awareness to the widespread sexual abuse of children almost 100 years earlier. This view should be tempered by Freud's limitation in perspective. He was the product of his times, a repressive society that was used to turning a blind eye to many forms of social inequity and was already a pariah for his theories about the unconscious. Whatever the extent of Freud's historical culpability in delaying society's recognition of sexual abuse, ample forces in our current society would like to sweep under a collective rug what we have come to see. Some of the proponents of repressed memory see the pendulum shifting back from awareness of childhood abuse to renewed societal denial. If true, the controversy over repressed memory is more than an academic argument; it is a political power struggle over the extent to which our society will tolerate self-awareness and has implications far beyond therapy.

DISSOCIATIVE PHENOMENA IN GROUPS

Modern medicine tends to focus almost exclusively on the individual, but it is interesting to consider the phenomenon of dissociation in groups. There are examples of how dissociation is perhaps purposefully induced in malls and supermarkets to encourage shopping. There are also extreme examples of how human beings can function in groups as if they are in a trance—the phenomenon of mob psychology, for instance. Robert Jay Lifton studied "psychic numbing" in the survivors of Hiroshima, and the form of "group think" that allowed physicians to serve under the Nazis in World War II. Restrictive groups (eg, cults) frequently use techniques such as hyperventilation and sleep deprivation to induce dissociative states in new recruits.

Some theorists such as Noam Chomsky see society as a whole as being extremely susceptible to the influences of special interest groups via the media. James Loewen, a sociologist who carefully studied a dozen leading high school history textbooks, concluded that our view of history is severely biased to avoid cultural dissonance. Thus we read and learn a great deal more about the early history of the United States than about controversial events such as the socially turbulent 1960s and the Vietnam War. Even our knowledge of historic figures appears to be filtered carefully to avoid dissonance. In Loewen's view our cultural values are a narrative that not only is determined by the past but also influences what facts we do and do not accept. Just as an individual person will "forget" and edit his or her own life history, so our cultural narrative defends us from unpleasant ideas from our collective past.

EMOTIONAL REACTIONS TO PATIENTS

Patients who have dissociative disorders can evoke feelings of dissociation in their health-care providers. This can include feeling lost or "spaced-out," not thinking clearly, or having difficulty focusing one's attention. Sometimes these disorders engender feelings of disbelief or anger from medical professionals.

CROSS-CULTURAL ASPECTS OF DISSOCIATIVE DISORDERS

In many societies, cultural factors help individuals to enter a trance state. Aids to dissociation in other cultures may include fires, music, singing, chanting, and dancing. Some observers would argue that in the United States, television and shopping malls are the culturally sanctioned means of achieving a dissociated state. Trance states may be viewed as a tribal or communal phenomenon that may take on religious or spiritual dimensions, much as "speaking in tongues" at Pentecostal gatherings. Culture-bound phenomena include individuals who develop "amok" in Indonesia or "Latah" in Malaysia. These phenomena would be classified by the *DSM-IV* as dissociative disorder NOS (not otherwise specified), and do not necessarily indicate psychopathology.

Another unusual form of dissociative disorder is **Ganser's syndrome,** which occurs in prisoners and others in high-stress situations. In this syndrome, patients appear dazed and give approximate answers to questions. For example, the patient asked to perform serial sevens from 100 might start answering "92." Medical conditions and malingering are important considerations in the differential diagnosis of these conditions.

LEGAL & ETHICAL ISSUES

Several ethical dilemmas are encountered in the treatment of patients who have dissociative disorders, particularly those affecting the patient's memory and identity. It may be difficult for the treating physician to preserve patient autonomy when working with a patient whose identity is partially or wholly split into conflicted parts. What are the ethical ramifications of trying to do what is best for a patient? Do you ally yourself with that aspect of the patient that is conscious, to help protect the patient from what you know must be painful, even dangerous to his or her consciousness? Or do you opt to share the truth, respecting the possibility that at some level the patient might be capable of tolerating painful knowledge? Should the physician be the one to decide what is right for the patient, or is there a way to work with the patient that allows this power to be shared? These are the same dilemmas that the physician encounters with many patients, but the dissociative disorders throw these challenges into sharp relief.

Max D, aged 24, was in therapy for several months for the treatment of severe depression. He improved with psychotherapy and antidepressants but displayed traits consistent with borderline personality disorder such as impulsivity, difficulties regulating his mood, and turbulent relationships. These behaviors were consistent with either a personality disorder or the effects of repeated trauma in childhood.

Mr. D had few memories of his childhood. He said that he had a vague memory of his stepfather taking him for a drive, and "then I felt like something bad was going to happen, and then I don't remember anymore." Mr. D wanted to know if the therapist thought that he might have been sexually abused. The therapist had considered this possibility herself and was worried that Mr. D was emotionally vulnerable and suggestible and was unsure of how to proceed.

She decided to tell Mr. D that he should wait to see what would develop in therapy. But 2 weeks later Mr. D announced that he wanted the therapist to hypnotize him to see if he could remember actual memories of abuse. The therapist suggested to Mr. D that if he had something to remember, he would do so in good time, but Mr. D was insistent, stating, "you are here to help me proceed in therapy any way I choose—I can ignore your advice if I want to. Besides, if you won't hypnotize me, I'll find someone who will, but I'd rather it be you since I trust you."

The therapist refused to hypnotize Mr. D, and

he dropped out of treatment. The therapist wondered if she had made the correct decision.

DISSOCIATION & THE MEDICAL PROFESSIONAL

Dissociative phenomena lie on a continuum that ranges from part of normal mental functioning to a form of psychopathology. Dissociation may also be a desirable state in certain settings. Individuals who are going to be exposed to extreme stress may be taught to function in an "automatic" fashion with suppressed emotions in order to better cope with the stressful situation. However, functioning in a depersonalized state has longer-term emotional costs.

The sleep deprivation, emotional and physical stress, and emphasis on objectivity that are common to medical training can lead to dissociative phenomena. One critical goal of medical training is to produce physicians who can function smoothly under extreme stress. Examples include ignoring cultural taboos by inserting needles and tubes into skin and bodily orifices, looking at and examining people when they are naked, and thinking and responding logically and objectively to life-threatening emergencies without becoming overly empathetic or emotional.

It is perhaps not surprising that there are many similarities between military and medical training, including the use of military metaphors such as the "war on cancer," "blasting" bacteria with antibiotics, "magic bullets," and "zapping" tumors with X-rays. "Teams" of medical students and residents "take hits" (admissions) and work "in the trenches" together. The same psychological processes used to mold men and women into soldiers are utilized in medical training. Furthermore, medical training involves a strongly hierarchical chain of command, long hours, uniforms, and repeated exercises.

Socialization is the term used to describe the process by which premedical students gradually accumulate not only medical knowledge but the professional identity of a physician. Students are exposed to progressively more stressful situations and given increasing levels of responsibility in medical school, and the process continues in residency and fellowship training. Stein has suggested that medical training utilizes the stress of medical training and rituals such as CPR training, morning report, and case conferences to help forge professional identities. This process includes having medical students become indoctrinated in the values of medicine. In this manner, boundaries are created; physicians-in-training learn to separate cognitive tasks (analyzing the patient's symptoms and history, constructing a differential diagnosis) from empathy for the patient's plight.

A third-year medical student on his rotation in surgery was on call. His team had a very busy call, and he had not been able to sleep for 36 hours. Toward the end of the shift, the team was called to resuscitate two patients almost simultaneously. Both attempts at CPR were unsuccessful and the patients died. Intrathoracic massage of the heart was attempted for the second patient, a 25-year-old car accident victim. The medical student had enjoyed working with the patient; now he found himself inserting his hand into the opening in her chest and performing cardiac compressions. Although he was initially anxious and nauseated by his role in the procedure, he suddenly felt "numb," "like I was a robot," he later reported. The feeling persisted throughout the day. The medical team never discussed the deaths of the two patients, saying only, "It's been a rough day. Let's go home and get some rest, because tomorrow morning we do this all over again."

The student returned to his apartment and continued to feel "strange, on autopilot" as he fixed his dinner and prepared for sleep. He tried to watch television but continued to feel emotionally "flat." He woke up feeling "almost normal" the next morning. He was too disturbed and embarrassed to tell anyone on his medical team about the strange feelings from the day before.

Medical students are taught that the physician's goal is to become objective, and they are frequently warned about the risks of becoming too emotionally involved with patients. In contrast, students are not alerted to the dangers of becoming too distanced from patients and their own feelings. The overuse of psychological mechanisms to dampen emotional responses and the lack of forums to discuss stressful events may contribute to the high incidence of depression, substance use, divorce, and suicide among physicians. While most students concentrate on memorizing and accumulating facts, an equally important challenge may be to complete medical training with one's values and identity intact and to learn to balance objectivity with compassion and empathy for patients, families, colleagues, and oneself.

CONCLUSION

The capacity for self-awareness, for conscious thought, and the intricacy of parallel systems of conscious and unconscious thought and their interplay is an integral part of human psychology. Neuroscientists, philosophers, and mental health professionals are attempting to understand how the brain integrates thoughts and emotions. Their work is being studied by computer scientists and artificial intelligence experts who are designing neural networks that eventually may simulate human intelligence. The complexity of mental functioning illustrated by dissociative phenomena provides fertile ground both for the appreciation of the development of psychopathology as well as for the richness of human thought and experience.

REFERENCES

Cohen L, Belzoff J, Elin M: *Dissociative Identity Disorder.* 1996

Csikszentmihalyi M: Flow: the psychology of optimal experience. Harper & Row, 1990.

Damasio AR. Descartes' Error: Emotions, Reason and the Human Brain. Grosset/Putnam, 1994.

Escobar JI: Transcultural aspects of dissociative and somatoform disorders. Psychiatr Clin N Am 1995;18(3): 555.

Flanagan O: *Consciousness Reconsidered.* MIT Press, 1992.

Goleman D: *Simple Lies, Vital Truths.* Touchstone, 1985.

Hilfiker D: Clinical detachment. Pages 120–131 in: *Healing the Wounds.* Pantheon Press, 1985.

Hofstaeder D, Dennett W: *The Mind's I: Fantasies and Reflections on Self and Soul.* Basic Books, 1981.

International Society for the Study of Dissociative Disorders. http://www.issd.org

Loewen J: *Lies My Teacher Told Me.* Touchstone, 1995.

Rosenfield I: The Strange, Familiar and Forgotten: An Anatomy of Consciousness. Knopf, 1992.

Schacter DL (editor): *Memory Distortion: How Minds, Brains, and Societies Reconstruct the Past.* Harvard University Press, 1995.

Speigel D: *Dissociation, Mind and Body.* American Psychiatric Press, 1994.

Stein H: Socialization and the process of becoming a physician. In: *American Medicine as Culture.* Westview Press, 1988.

van der Kolk BA: The body keeps the score: memory and the evolving psychobiology of posttraumatic stress. Harvard Rev Psychiatr 1994;Jan/Feb:253.

11

Substance Use

Kalpana I. Nathan, MD, Robert P. Cabaj, MD, & David Elkin, MD

Most people at one time or another have used at least one psychoactive substance such as caffeine, nicotine, or alcohol. Users of such substances usually have experienced some temporary adverse consequence that resulted directly or indirectly from the substance. These temporary problems do not necessarily constitute disorders, and usually fairly stringent criteria are applied to make diagnoses of abuse, dependence, withdrawal, and intoxication.

Substance dependence is one of the world's major health and social problems and is one of the most challenging—and rewarding—treatable illnesses in the practice of medicine and psychiatry. Personal attitudes of medical providers are often barriers to the accurate diagnosis of substance abuse and to the humane and adequate treatment of the identified substance abuser. All health-care providers have their own attitudes about the use of abusable substances—whether shaped by family influences, religious beliefs, political beliefs, personal experience with friends or family members, the providers' own use of alcohol or drugs, or direct clinical experience working with substance abusers. Medical providers must overcome these personal attitudes if they are to provide the highest quality ethical care for substance users.

Providers must understand two key concepts in order to offer such care. First, substance abuse is indeed an illness, just as is diabetes or other medical conditions. Second, some treatment interventions are successful with substance users, whereas others may fail.

The *DSM-IV* defines **substance-related disorders** as being related to the taking of drugs of abuse, to the side effects of medication, and to toxic exposure. Table 11–1 summarizes the classification of substance-related disorders. Tables 11–2 and 11–3 outline the *DSM-IV* diagnostic criteria for **substance abuse** and **substance dependence.**

Substances likely to be abused are classified into the following 11 categories:

- alcohol
- amphetamines and other sympathomimetics (stimulants)
- caffeine
- cannabis
- cocaine
- hallucinogens
- inhalants
- nicotine
- opioids
- phencyclidine and similarly acting arylcyclohexylamines
- sedatives, hypnotics, or anxiolytics

INCIDENCE

A 1991 survey by the National Institute of Drug Abuse, the most extensive review of the use of substances to date, reported the following statistics for the "age 18 and over" population in the United States:

- lifetime prevalence of a diagnosis of abuse or dependence: 16.7%
- lifetime prevalence of alcohol abuse or dependence: 13.8%
- lifetime prevalence of non-alcohol abuse or dependence: 6.2%
- use of one or more illicit substances in lifetime: 37%
- use of illicit substances in the last year: 13%
- use of illicit substances in the last month: 6%
- use of alcohol over lifetime: 85%
- use of alcohol over last month: 51%
- use of marijuana over lifetime (ages 12 and up): 33%
- use of marijuana currently: 5%
- use of sedatives, hypnotics, or anxiolytic agents over lifetime: 12.5%
- use of sedatives, hypnotics, or anxiolytic agents over last month: 1.6%
- use of cocaine over lifetime: 11.5%
- use of cocaine over last month: 0.9%

Table 11–1. Substance-related disorders.

Substance use disorders
  Substance abuse
  Substance dependence
Substance-induced disorders
  Substance intoxication
  Substance withdrawal
  Substance-induced delirium
  Substance-induced persisting dementia
  Substance-induced persisting amnestic disorder
  Substance-induced psychotic disorder
  Substance-induced mood disorder
  Substance-induced anxiety disorder
  Substance-induced sexual dysfunction
  Substance-induced sleep disorder

- use of hallucinogens, inhalants, and heroin over lifetime: < 9%
- use of hallucinogens, inhalants, and heroin over last month: < 1%

The 1995 National Household Survey on Drug Abuse reported that an estimated 12.8 million Americans were illicit drug users (ie, they used an illicit drug in the month prior to the interview). This statistic represents 6.1% of the population 12 years and older. Marijuana is the most commonly used illicit drug, used by 77% of current illicit drug users. Of Americans age 12 and older, 111 million had used alcohol in the past month (52% of the population). About 32 million engaged in binge drinking (defined as 5 or more drinks consumed on at least one occasion in the past month), and about 11 million were heavy drinkers (defined as drinking five or more drinks per occasion on 5 or more days in the past 30 days). An estimated 61 million Americans were current smokers in 1995 (29% of the population). Among smokers in 1995, 12.6% were heavy drinkers and 13.6% were illicit drug users, while among nonsmokers 2.7% were heavy drinkers and 3% were illicit drug users.

The costs to society of alcohol and drug use, including tobacco, have been conservatively estimated at $166 billion annually in 1991. The economic impact of substance use is based upon consideration of 1) emergency room and other direct medical costs, 2) lost productivity, 3) criminal behavior, and 4) the increased incidence of HIV infection and AIDS. Alco-

Table 11–2. *DSM-IV* criteria for substance abuse.

A. Maladaptive pattern of substance use leading to clinically significant impairment or distress, with one or more of the following occurring within a 12-month period:
  Recurrent substance use resulting in a failure to fulfill major role obligations at work, home, or school
  Recurrent substance use in situations in which it is physically hazardous
  Recurrent substance-related legal problems
  Continued substance use despite having persistent or recurrent social or interpersonal problems caused by effects of the substance

B. Symptoms do not meet criteria for dependence

Table 11–3. *DSM-IV* criteria for substance dependence.

A. Maladaptive pattern of substance use leading to clinically significant impairment or distress, with three or more of the following occurring within a 12-month period:
  Tolerance
  Withdrawal
  Substance is taken in larger amounts or over a longer period of time than was intended
  Persistent desire or unsuccessful efforts to cut down
  A great deal of time is spent in activities necessary to obtain the substance
  Important social, occupational, or recreational activities are given up to obtain/use the substance

B. Substance use is continued despite knowledge of having a persistent physical or psychological problem that is exacerbated by the substance

hol has also been estimated to contribute to half of the 50,000 fatal motor vehicle accidents in the US annually, and to hundreds of thousands of non-fatal accidents. The costs of substance use among patients with Medicaid (federal medical insurance for impoverished patients) constitute almost 20% of the inpatient medical budget of the Medicaid program.

ETIOLOGY

Biological Factors

Substances that are addictive stimulate the **neural reward pathway,** which activates the limbocortical region of the brain, which in turn regulates the most basic emotions and behaviors. The activation of the reward pathway through behaviors as diverse as feeding and copulation conferred a survival advantage through evolution. The same structures persist today and provide a physiological basis for our subjective perception of pleasure. Substances of abuse stimulate these reward pathways and thus instigate humans and animals to sacrifice other pleasures or endure pain to ensure that the substance is administered as much as possible. Substance abuse and dependence are rooted in the normal neurobiology of reinforcement. The magnitude of reinforcement varies among different addictive drugs and is correlated directly with the amount of drug that reaches the brain and with the speed with which the drug's concentration rises.

Evidence indicates that genetics plays a role in alcoholism. Family studies of alcoholism have consistently shown higher rates of the disorder among first-degree relatives of individuals who are dependent on alcohol. Twenty-five percent of fathers and brothers of alcoholics become dependent on alcohol. Compared with control subjects, relatives of alcoholics are more likely to exhibit depression, criminal behavior, and antisocial personality disorder. Monozygotic twins have a higher concordance rate for alcoholism than do dizygotic twins. Adoption studies have shown that biological relatives of alcoholic probands are significantly more likely to become dependent on alcohol than are the relatives of control adoptees.

Environmental & Social Factors

Individuals are also influenced by multiple social and environmental factors that play important roles in the development of dependence. The personality traits of the individual appear to be important as well. Although no definite personality patterns predict substance abuse, certain personality disorders such as antisocial personality disorder are more likely to be associated with substance dependence.

At the earliest stages of use, experimenters or casual users who go on to develop dependence on substances are generally indistinguishable from their peers with respect to the type and frequency of substance use. The cheaper and more readily available drugs, such as alcohol, nicotine, and marijuana, are viewed as **gateway drugs,** and the use of such drugs often leads to experimentation with other illicit drugs. Early onset or regular use of gateway drugs, and early evidence of aggressive behavior, intrafamilial disturbances, and association with substance-using peers, contribute to and predict continued substance use and the subsequent development of abuse and dependence.

TREATMENT
OF SUBSTANCE USE DISORDERS

Treatment of substance dependence includes an assessment phase, the treatment of intoxication and withdrawal when necessary, and the development and implementation of an overall treatment strategy. The assessment includes the following elements:

- a detailed history of the patient's past and present substance use and its effect on cognitive, psychological, behavioral, and physiologic functioning
- a general medical and psychiatric history and examination
- history of prior psychiatric treatments and outcomes
- family and social history
- screening of blood, breath, or urine for abused substances
- other laboratory tests to help confirm the presence or absence of comorbid conditions frequently associated with substance use disorders (such as HIV disease, hepatitis, and tuberculosis)

Substance use disorders affect many domains of an individual's functioning and frequently require treatment that incorporates biological, psychological, and social interventions. Goals of treatment include reduction in the use and effects of substances or

achievement of abstinence, reduction in the severity and frequency of relapse, decrease in morbidity and sequelae of substance use disorders, and improvement in psychological and social functioning.

Detoxification plays a key role in early stabilization, but by itself is not effective in sustaining abstinence. The key internal factor for recovery is motivation and the most significant external factor is structure. The term **recovery** specifies that in addition to abstinence from drugs and alcohol, there is substantial change of behavior, thoughts, and feelings. While early recovery focuses on abstinence, relapse prevention forms the crux of treatment intervention for substance dependence.

Relapse prevention techniques help the individual to develop new ways of coping with stress and to cultivate new activities that do not involve substance use. Traditional **12-step models** of treatment are structured programs that urge the patient to seek abstinence. After the AIDS epidemic began, the **harm-reduction model** became widely used. The goal of this approach is to initiate treatment at the level at which the patient is currently using substances, and to strive for future reduction of harm to self and society. Although abstinence is the long-term goal and remains the foundation for continued therapeutic work, the harm-reduction model acknowledges that patients need different kinds of help, depending on where they are in the change cycle, described below.

The **stages-of-change model** was popularized by Prochaska and DiClemete. In this model, there are five stages of change:

1. precontemplation
2. contemplation
3. determination
4. action
5. maintenance

In the stage of **precontemplation,** a person is not aware that there is a problem related to substance use and is not considering a change; in **contemplation,** the person begins to recognize the existence of a problem but is ambivalent about change; in the phase of **determination,** something has occured, usually a crisis of some sort, that tips the balance in favor of change; this leads into the stage of **action,** when there is active treatment; the stage of **maintenance** compounds relapse prevention. As recovery is a process, so is relapse. It is helpful to view relapse as being one step closer to recovery and not as a negative process. Table 11–4 lists several interventions that clinicians might use. The first group of interventions are helpful; the second group should be avoided.

Many patients who use, abuse, or are dependent on substances may have concurrent psychiatric diagnoses, so called **dual-diagnosis patients.** Though a patient who has a substance use disorder and a personality disorder could be considered a dual-diagno-

Table 11–4. Intervention guidelines for treating patients who have substance-related disorders.

The provider should

Encourage constructive expression of feelings and listen

Express caring and concern for the individual

Ensure that there are consistent consequences for negative behaviors

Realize personal limitations as a professional, not trying to be "all things to all people"

Hold the individual responsible for his or her own actions

Talk to the individual about specific actions that are disruptive or disturbing

Monitor personal reactions to client's behavior for possible interference with the treatment relationship

Communicate plan of action to other staff

The provider should not

Minimize or avoid talking about abuse or the results of it

Avoid confrontation

Compromise personal values or expectations

Make excuses for continuing drug or alcohol use

Save the client from feeling the results of his or her addiction

Try to "protect" the patient from alcohol or drugs

View alcoholism or addiction as a weakness rather than an illness

Try to find the cause, hoping that the disease will go away when the cause is found

Encourage the use of "willpower" or other over-simplified "cures"

Express anger, frustration, blame, or disappointment toward a patient who continues to use drugs or alcohol

Gossip about the patient to others

sis patient, the term usually applies to someone who has a substance use disorder and an Axis I major psychiatric illness, such as schizophrenia or major depression. Accurate diagnosis is difficult but crucial for the best treatment planning. Though debate still rages over the best approaches to treating dual-diagnosis patients, it seems evident that the substance use and the mental illness need to be treated simultaneously, focusing on one first if it interferes with the treatment of the other. For example, a patient who has schizophrenia and uses cocaine may be suffering from intense auditory hallucinations and be very paranoid and suspicious; without attempting to intervene on the cocaine use, it is unlikely that the patient will be able to trust the provider enough to use antipsychotic medications, and the efficacy of the medications will be undermined by the cocaine.

DIFFERENTIAL DIAGNOSIS

The differential diagnosis between anxiety, depression, and psychosis and the effects of intoxication and withdrawal from a substance is quite difficult. In general, without a clear and supported history of a major mood disorder, a condition with psychotic features, or a major anxiety disorder, a definitive diagnosis is impossible when there is current or recent

heavy drug or alcohol use or abuse. Ideally, a patient would be free of all drugs or alcohol for a minimum of 2 weeks before symptoms could be attributed to a mental illness versus the effects of the substance. A past history of psychiatric conditions and treatments and family histories of mental illness may help the clinician make an accurate diagnosis, but, again, with recent or active substance use, a conclusive diagnosis of a mental illness is not warranted. A working diagnosis may help shape treatment, but the provider should wait until the patient is clean and sober or has dramatically reduced the drug or alcohol use before a valid diagnosis is determined.

Though difficult to diagnose, if a concomitant major mental illness that responds to psychopharmacology is discovered, medication treatment is warranted. Medications that are likely either to be abused or to induce a return to drinking, such as the benzodiazepines or many psychostimulants, should be avoided entirely or used only with caution and close monitoring; most other psychotropic medications are safe and essential in successful treatment of both the substance abuse and the mental illness.

ISSUES RELATED TO SPECIFIC SUBSTANCES

These sections review different forms of substance use, including alcohol; sedatives, hypnotics, and anxiolytics; stimulants such as cocaine and methamphetamines; opioids; hallucinogens; phencyclidines; inhalants; caffeine; marijuana; and nicotine.

ALCOHOL

Alcohol consumption is common throughout the world. In the United States, 90% of all adults drink alcohol, more than 40% of men and women have temporary alcohol-induced problems, and 10% of men and 3–5% of women develop pervasive and persistent alcohol-related problems (dependence). The typical individual who has an alcohol use problem has a family and a job, and only 5% of individuals who are dependent on alcohol fit the skid-row stereotype.

Biology

The development of tolerance to alcohol illustrates the biological and genetic components of the disease of **alcoholism.** Figure 11–1 shows the development of tolerance to alcohol in the person who is destined to become alcoholic. The social drinker, that is, one who does not develop alcohol dependency or abuse,

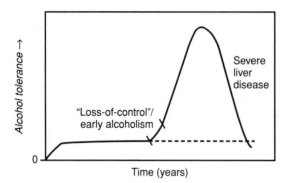

Figure 11–1. The development of tolerance to alcohol over time. The solid line is the course for the alcoholic; the dotted line is the course for the social drinker. The curve indicates the number of drinks needed to feel the same effect of the alcohol over time and is different for each individual.

learns to tolerate alcohol and then levels off at an idiosyncratic tolerance level throughout life—a certain number of drinks will cause a certain, desirable effect; drinking more than that will cause intoxication or unpleasant effects.

The potential alcoholic begins in the same way, learning to tolerate the effects of alcohol and leveling off until roughly 10 years of regular exposure to alcohol (not necessarily daily). At that point, the person begins to need more and more alcohol to achieve the desired effect, and his or her tolerance rises. The alcoholic can tolerate large quantities of alcohol accordingly, and alcohol blood levels may exceed levels that would be fatal for the nonalcoholic. Normally, one drink is cleared by the liver in one hour. As the liver deteriorates with exposure to alcohol, the alcohol is not processed by the liver as quickly. Thus tolerance decreases as liver disease progresses; more alcohol stays in the bloodstream longer, and the person does not need to drink as much. Once the tolerance begins to increase, it stays at high levels until the patient develops liver failure. If someone who has stopped drinking resumes alcohol use even years later, the tolerance will be at the same level it was at when the person stopped drinking.

Screening & Assesment

Most patients respond to the question "Do you drink alcohol?" with the answer, "Yes. Socially." Two follow-up questions are useful: "Have you ever had a drinking problem?" and "When was your last drink?" A drink within the last 24 hours is a "red flag" that should lead to further evaluation. A series of questions known as the CAGE questions are also helpful in identifying individuals who abuse or are dependent on alcohol:

- Have you ever tried to **C**ut down on your drinking?
- Have you ever been **A**nnoyed by others' comments about your drinking?
- Have you ever felt **G**uilty or worried about your drinking?
- Have you ever had an **E**ye-opener drink in the morning?

Two positive answers indicate possible alcoholism and should alert the physician to follow up with further inquiry and possible intervention. The AUDIT (Alcohol Use Disorder Identification Test) developed by MJ Bohn and colleagues is an alcohol screening tool that also highlights some of the physical symptoms or traits of alcohol use or abuse to look for in the physical examination and review of systems. Such physical symptoms include head injuries after age 18, broken bones since age 18, conjunctival injection (eg, redness from enlarged blood vessels), hand tremor, tongue tremor, hepatomegaly, or high GGT value (a blood test for liver enzyme function; this value is elevated in patients who have hepatitis from any cause including alcohol).

Clinical Effects

The effects of alcohol depend in part on the amount of ethyl alcohol or ethanol consumed per unit of body weight. In general, 340 ml (12 oz) of beer, 115 ml (4 oz) of nonfortified wine, and 43 ml (1.5 oz or a shot) of an 80-proof (40% alcohol by volume) beverage each contain about 10 g of ethanol; 1 pint of an 80-proof beverage contains approximately 160 ml, and 1 liter of wine contains 80 g of ethanol. In the United States, legal intoxication requires a blood alcohol concentration of at least 80 to 100 mg/dL (0.1 g/dL), although behavioral, psychomotor, and cognitive changes may be seen at levels as low as 20–30 mg/dL (after one or two drinks).

The essential feature of alcohol intoxication is the presence of clinically significant maladaptive behavioral or psychological changes that develop during or shortly after ingestion of alcohol. In addition, one or more of the following signs and symptoms may be present:

- slurred speech
- incoordination
- unsteady gait
- nystagmus (rhythmic oscillation of eye movement)
- impairment in attention or memory
- stupor or coma

Pathologic intoxication is characterized by an excited, combative, psychotic state in a susceptible individual after minimal alcohol consumption. The belligerent intoxicated patient must be assessed for potential violence. Administration of benzodiazepines along with low-dose antipsychotics may be required for management of increased agitation.

Alcohol withdrawal syndrome consists of two or more of the following signs and symptoms:

- autonomic hyperactivity
- hand tremor
- insomnia
- nausea or vomiting
- transient visual, tactile, or auditory hallucinations
- psychomotor agitation
- anxiety
- grand mal seizures

The first stage of withdrawal occurs 6–8 hours after discontinuation of drinking. The signs include mild tremulousness, nervousness, and occasional nausea. The second stage begins at approximately 24 hours but may take as long as 8 days to appear. Marked tremors, hyperactivity, insomnia, nightmares, and hallucinations may be observed. The onset of the third stage may be at 12–48 hours and is characterized by the appearance of grand mal seizures. Reportedly, 3–5% of untreated patients progress to the third stage.

The fourth and most serious stage of the syndrome is referred to as **delirium tremens** (DT). DT occurs 3–5 days after abstinence and sometimes as late as 10–12 days after cessation. The symptoms are similar to other stages but are more severe. The essential features of delirium are reduced ability to maintain attention or to shift attention appropriately to new external stimuli, and disorganized thinking, as manifested by rambling, irrelevant, or incoherent speech. Vivid hallucinations are common. Physiologic changes such as tachycardia, hyperthermia (elevated body temperature), hyperventilation, sweating, and diarrhea resulting in fluid loss may also be present. There is a 5–15% mortality rate owing to vascular collapse.

Treatment

Benzodiazepines remain the treatment of choice for acute alcohol withdrawal. They target symptoms of anxiety and autonomic hyperactivity and, most important, raise the seizure threshold. They have rapid onset, a moderate duration of action, and possess anticonvulsant properties capable of inducing a state of calm without causing respiratory depression. In patients who have hepatitis, lorazepam is preferable to chlordiazepoxide because it bypasses the liver and thus is less toxic to the liver and less likely to produce toxic drug levels. Nutritional supplementation is provided with thiamine 100 mg orally or intramuscularly daily, multivitamins 1 tablet orally daily, and folate 1 mg orally daily. Other supportive measures, including provision of adequate food and hydration are helpful.

Most cases of alcohol withdrawal are uneventful and may not need interventions with medications. Symptom-triggered individualized treatment has been found to be more efficient than round-the clock coverage with benzodiazepines. This means that detoxification proceeds with treatment targeted on symptoms such as increased blood pressure, increased heart rate, and so on. Table 11–5 summarizes pharmacological treatment options for alcohol withdrawal and dependence.

Alcoholics Anonymous (AA) is a self-help group founded in 1935 that has continued to offer support and help to thousands of patients. AA is a spiritual program that helps its members maintain sobriety by lending support in organized settings. These programs are based on a 12-step model that involves adherence to a series of basic principles. The first of these principles is for the patient to admit to a lack of control over the substance use. A desire to stop drinking, not sobriety, is a requirement. Individuals derive support from meetings and being assigned a partner whom they can contact if the desire to drink become overwhelming. Although AA is not a religious group, alternative self-help groups such as Rational Recovery are available for those who prefer nonspiritual groups. Other support groups for family members of individuals who are dependent on alcohol, such as Al-Anon (for spouses), Alateen (for teenagers and children of alcoholics), and ACA (for adult children of alcoholics), help the family members to avoid enabling behaviors and to care for themselves whether or not a loved one is drinking.

Although abstinence is always the long-term goal, clinicians must provide support and guidance to patients as they progress through the different stages of change, toward the goal of abstinence. This is particularly important for patients who have medical or psychiatric illnesses in addition to being dependent on drugs.

Ted S, aged 42, was brought to the emergency room by the police after his neighbors called 911. He had a long history of alcohol dependence, and his problem was now complicated by the fact that he had AIDS and had difficulty following through with his medical appointments. He usually consumed one pint of vodka a day and often was found incoherent and in an unkempt state in his disheveled apartment. His mother had paid for his treatment in several reputable programs, but Mr. S usually left most programs prematurely.

He was admitted to the detoxification unit, where the goal was to help reduce his alcohol use, so that he would be able to care for himself and get to medical appointments. Although the goal would be abstinence eventually, this goal was not pursued aggressively at first. A more gradual approach worked better with Mr. S, and he was agreeable to going into a residential treatment program after completing his detoxification. Mr. S stayed in the residential program several days before leaving and returned to the

Table 11–5. Pharmacological treatment of alcohol withdrawal and dependence.

Alcohol Withdrawal

Medication	Parameters	Dosages	Effects or Limitations
Benzodiazepines	Systolic blood pressure (SBP) >170 Diastolic blood pressure (DBP) > 100 Pulse > 100 Clinical Institute Withdrawal Assessment (CIWA) > 8		
Chlordiazepoxide		25–100 mg orally every 1–2 hours as needed (if there is no impairment of liver function); maximum daily dose of 600 mg	
Lorazepam		1–2 mg orally every 1–2 hours as needed (if there is impairment of liver function); maximum daily dose of 8 mg	

Alcohol Dependence

Medication	Action	Dosage and Effectiveness	Comments
Disulfiram (Antabuse)	Disulfiram inhibits the enzyme aldehyde dehydrogenase, which is involved in the breakdown of ethanol.	250 mg/day for maintenance; randomized controlled studies have shown mixed results for the drug's efficacy.	Side effects include facial flushing, tachycardia, hypotension, nausea and vomiting, and physical discomfort. Occasionally, chest pain, seizures, liver dysfunction, respiratory depression, depression, cardiac arrhythmias, myocardial infarction, and even death have been reported.
Naltrexone (Revia)	Naltrexone is an opioid antagonist. Alcohol is thought to increase endogenous opioid activity, and activation of opioid receptors may be involved in the reinforcing properties of alcohol	Clinical trials have shown that doses of 50 mg once a day produce lower relapse rates, fewer drinking days, and less alcohol craving.	Naltrexone has long been approved for the treatment of opioid dependence but is rarely used in that capacity.

detoxification unit a few more times. He had decreased his total consumption of alcohol, had some periods of sobriety, and no longer had blackouts, which made it possible for him to follow up with his medical care. Mr. S continued to receive encouragement from his case worker and internist to further decrease his alcohol intake.

Diagnosis. Alcohol dependence (Axis I); AIDS (Axis III).

SEDATIVES, HYPNOTICS, & ANXIOLYTICS

The **sedative-hypnotic-anxiolytic** class of substances includes benzodiazepines, carbamates (eg, glutethimide, meprobamate), barbiturates (ie, secobarbital), and barbiturate-like hypnotics (ie, methaqualone). These substances reduce anxiety but are depressants like alcohol and are susceptible to being abused because of their rapid onset of action.

Biology

The first barbiturate, barbital, was introduced in 1903. Benzodiazepines were introduced in the 1960s and have been used widely because of their relative margin of safety compared to other sedative-hypnotics. They were considered the miracle cure for many ailments in the 1970s, at which time their addictive potential was not recognized, and they continue to be among the most widely prescribed medications in the United States.

The most significant risk factor for abuse of sedative-hypnotics is a current alcohol- or drug-related disorder. Patients who have a history of alcohol- or drug-related disorders are also vulnerable to abusing medications that produce euphoria. Clinicians should be cautious when prescribing medications that have addictive potential, although they should not hold back medications that can provide adequate treatment of acute anxiety.

Clinical Effects

Sedative, hypnotic, or anxiolytic intoxication produces clinically significant maladaptive behavioral changes such as inappropriate sexual or aggressive behavior, mood lability, impaired judgment, or impaired social functioning. One or more of the following signs and symptoms may be present:

- slurred speech
- incoordination
- unsteady gait
- nystagmus
- impairment in attention or memory
- stupor or coma

Sedative, hypnotic, or anxiolytic withdrawal usually occurs after cessation of significant doses of sedative-hypnotics that have been taken over an extended period of time. For example, a dosage of approximately 40 mg/day of diazepam would produce clinically significant withdrawal symptoms, whereas a dosage of 100 mg/day might lead to withdrawal seizures or delirium. Two or more of the following signs and symptoms may be present:

- autonomic hyperactivity
- increased hand tremor
- insomnia
- nausea or vomiting
- transient visual, tactile, or auditory hallucinations
- psychomotor agitation
- anxiety
- grand mal seizures

Treatment

Sedative, hypnotic, or anxiolytic detoxification may be achieved by gradually reducing the substance of abuse itself or by substitution therapy, in which the abused substance is substituted with a cross-tolerant, longer-acting substance that is then withdrawn gradually over a period of time. Table 11–6 illustrates a

phenobarbital substitution protocol that may be used in sedative, hypnotic, or anxiolytic detoxification.

The total daily amount of the phenobarbital equivalent dosage is determined and administered in divided doses, usually every 4 hours, up to 300 mg/24 hours. The patient should be monitored for evidence of intoxication. Once the patient is psychologically stabilized, the dosage may be decreased by 30–60 mg/day and more gradually toward the end of the detoxification process. While a benzodiazepine is being tapered, addition of antiseizure medications such as carbamezepine or valproic acid may be helpful in accomplishing a faster detoxification process.

Patients who are dependent on benzodiazepines may be difficult to treat. They are usually well-educated, very familiar with medical terminology, and possibly involved in the health-care industry. They request treatment for the problem most often when their source of benzodiazepine is lost for some reason, for example, if their physician is relocating or has decided not to prescribe the medication anymore.

Patients should never be maintained on long-term benzodiazepines. These drugs are useful in short-term treatment of anxiety, agitation, and insomnia,

Table 11–6. Phenobarbital substitution protocol for sedative, hypnotic, or anxiolytic detoxification.

Drug of Abuse	Dose Equivalent of 30 mg of Phenobarbital
Barbiturates	
Amobarbital	100
Butobarbital	50
Pentobarbital	100
Secobarbital	100
Other sedative-hypnotics	
Chloral hydrate	500
Ethchlorvynol	350
Glutethimide	30
Meprobamate	400
Methyprylon	300
Benzodiazepines	
Alprazolam	1
Chlordiazepoxide	25
Clonazepam	2
Clorazepate	15
Diazepam	10
Flurazepam	30
Lorazepam	1
Oxazepam	30
Temazepam	30
Triazolam	1

and are used widely in acute inpatient settings for severe agitation, but several other agents are available for treatment of anxiety disorders and sleep disorders in outpatient settings. Physicians should always inform patients that they are at risk for developing dependence on benzodiazepines whenever these substances are used for more than a few weeks.

Juanita N, aged 35, presented to psychiatric emergency services for help with alcohol withdrawal. She usually consumed several glasses of wine daily. She stated that alcohol had been a problem for her and that she had gone through several treatment programs in the past. She mentioned that she was under the care of a psychiatrist who prescribed clonazepam (Klonopin) for treatment of post-traumatic stress disorder (PTSD) and panic disorder. She stated that she was taking up to 12 mg of Klonopin per day for her panic attacks. She was admitted to the inpatient detoxification unit, and the admitting physician started her on 2 mg of Klonopin four times a day, up to a maximum daily dose of 12 mg.

The inpatient attending psychiatrist contacted the treating psychiatrist, who was reluctant to reveal the exact amount of Klonopin prescribed. He was evasive about the treatment and hung up abruptly. When Ms. N was approached with the possibility that Klonopin was a problem, she became angry and stated that she would not agree to any change in her Klonopin regimen. She then signed out against medical advice.

Diagnosis. Benzodiazepine and alcohol dependence, PTSD, panic disorder (Axis I).

STIMULANTS

Amphetamines and cocaine are the most widely used stimulants. Amphetamines and amphetamine congeners compromise a large group of stimulant drugs. They were most prevalent from the 1930s, when they were first synthesized, until the 1970s. Epidemics of intravenous amphetamine use raged in Japan at the time of World War II and in Sweden and the United States through the 1960s and 1970s. With the burgeoning of the cocaine epidemic in America in the 1970s and 1980s, amphetamine use decreased but has made a comeback in the 1990s.

Biology

The most commonly used amphetamines are dextroamphetamine (Dexedrine), methamphetamine (also called Methedrine or speed), and methylphenidate (Ritalin). Ice is a synthetic pure form of methamphetamine that can be either inhaled or injected intravenously. Most of the effects of amphetamines are similar to those of cocaine, except that they lack the local anesthetic property of cocaine. They have a lower risk of producing arrhythmias and seizures, and their psychoactive effects last longer than cocaine.

The so-called **designer amphetamines** are structurally related to the classic amphetamines (such as methamphetamine) and have neurochemical effects on both the dopaminergic and the serotonin systems, unlike the classic amphetamines, which release primarily dopamine from presynaptic nerve terminals. The designer amphetamines include 3,4-methylenedioxymethamphetamine (MDMA), N-ethyl-3,4-methylenedioxyamphetamine (MDEA), 5-methoxy-3,4-methylenedioxyamphetamine (MMDA), and 2,5-dimethoxy-4-methylamphetamine (DOM). Their behavioral effects appear to be a combination of the effects of classic amphetamines and hallucinogens. MDMA, also known as Ecstasy, has been popularized in dance clubs (at so-called raves) and has been associated with a severe adverse effect of hyperthermia. This effect, combined with excessive activity, as in dancing in hot, crowded clubs, can be fatal in some cases.

Methamphetamine use was popular in the 1950s and made a resurgence in the 1990s. It is especially prevalent on the west coast of the United States, especially among young gay men. The drug produces a powerful high, and it is difficult for clinicians to intervene effectively because the user views methamphetamine as a drug that makes one omnipotent. Methamphetamine has been rumored to have aphrodisiac potential, as well as to delay progress of HIV disease, a claim that remains unsubstantiated.

Cocaine is a benzoylmethylecgonine, an ester of benzoic acid and a nitrogen-containing base. It is an alkaloid derived from coca leaves. Historically, natives of Peru, Bolivia, and Columbia chewed the leaves to prevent fatigue and to increase energy. In the nineteenth century, cocaine, the active principle in the coca leaves, was identified and purified by Albert Neimann, a German chemist. It was found to have powerful local anesthetic effects and hence was used in the practice of medicine.

Sigmund Freud wrote about the medical and recreational uses of cocaine, while underestimating its addictive potential. Cocaine was popular in Europe and America until the early 1900s, used widely as a so-called tonic, and was commonly used as an additive in beverages such as Coca-Cola. Cocaine was placed under legal restrictions by the Harrison Act of 1914 and was viewed as having very limited legitimate use in medicine.

The most important therapeutic property of cocaine is its ability to block the initiation or conduction of the nerve impulse following its application. In higher concentrations, cocaine can affect the cardiac action potential, slowing conduction and impairing contractility of the heart, effects possibly contributing to cardiac arrhythmias and sudden death. Cocaine, a sympathomimetic, exerts its clinical actions by blocking the reuptake of norepinephrine, serotonin, and dopamine. In the brain, cocaine acts primarily on the dopamine reuptake system, blocking the dopamine transporter, thus resulting in prolonged concentrations of dopamine in the synapse and stimulation of dopamine receptors. Dopamine release, particularly in the mesolimbic and mesocortical pathways, has been linked to the rewarding effects of cocaine, although other neurotransmitters such as serotonin may be involved.

Clinical Effects

The method of cocaine administration determines how much of the substance is absorbed into the bloodstream as well as how fast it is absorbed:

- Oral: When coca leaves are chewed or cocaine powder is ingested orally, onset of action is in about 1 hour, effects last for several hours, and the drug appears in the blood at low levels.
- Intranasal: When snorted in the powder form, onset is in about 3–5 minutes, with duration of 45–60 minutes, and the drug appears in the blood at moderate levels.
- Intravenous: When injected in the powder form, onset is in 1–2 minutes, with a duration of 10–20 minutes, and the drug appears in the blood at high levels.
- Inhalation: When smoked in the freebase form, onset is in 30 seconds, with a duration of 5–10 minutes, and the drug appears at high blood levels.

The first high is almost always the best high that users recall. Tolerance develops very quickly in all users, whether chronic or infrequent users. The pleasurable effects fade dramatically even before the blood level falls significantly. This phenomenon encourages the user to use high doses in binges, or so-called runs, in a desperate attempt to make the high last. A cocaine binge can last 24 sleepless hours or more, during which time users take several hits per hour before crashing. The crash is marked by depression and exhaustion and may last for several days. This is followed by intense craving, which can last for weeks.

Intoxication with cocaine and amphetamine produces maladaptive behavioral changes such as euphoria, hypervigilance, impaired judgment, or impaired functioning. One or more of the following signs and symptoms may be present:

- tachycardia
- pupillary dilation
- elevated blood pressure
- perspiration
- nausea or vomiting
- weight loss
- psychomotor agitation
- chest pain or cardiac arrhythmias
- confusion
- seizures
- dystonias

- coma
- brief psychotic episodes, anxiety, or depression

Stimulant withdrawal produce dysphoric mood and at least two of the following signs and symptoms:

- fatigue
- vivid, unpleasant dreams
- insomnia or hypersomnia
- increased appetite
- psychomotor retardation or agitation

Treatment

Treatment of stimulant intoxication and withdrawal is symptom specific. The patient may experience increased fatigue (while crashing) and may do well with rest and nutrition. For increased agitation, benzodiazepines such as lorazepam may be helpful. For stimulant-induced psychotic disorder, antipsychotics are indicated.

A variety of medications have been used to treat the biochemical changes that may play a role in relapse to compulsive cocaine use. However, none have proven or consistent efficacy in treating cocaine dependence. Antidepressants have been used because they block re-uptake of biogenic amines and hence may relieve symptoms secondary to cocaine withdrawal. Studies have shown that desipramine and fluoxetine may be helpful. Cocaine can produce or exacerbate seizure activity, and treatment with antiseizure medications such as carbamezepine, which blocks kindling (potentiation of seizure activity), may be clinically useful.

Many stimulant users seek treatment because of legal issues pertaining to prison sentences or child custody. Although these situations can provide powerful motivation, efficacy of treatment is limited. Psychosocial interventions with group and individual therapy are currently the most widely used approaches, although these interventions also have limited success in bringing about long-term abstinence.

Gordon H, aged 25, was brought to the psychiatric emergency room by police after he was seen breaking store windows on a crowded street. Mr. H had numerous brief psychiatric admissions for psychosis not otherwise specified (NOS) and a long criminal record stemming from robbery charges. Mr. H was noted to be paranoid and belligerent. He had loosely formed delusions about being pursued and said that he was trying to "cut off their access" to him by breaking the windows. He admitted to using methamphetamines on a near-daily basis. Urine toxicology confirmed the presence of methamphetamines and trace amounts of marijuana.

Mr. H was admitted to an inpatient psychiatric service where his mental status cleared within 5 days on low doses of antipsychotics. He related well to other patients but was noted to be manipulative with staff members. His family history was remarkable for substance use, but there was no indication of major mood or psychotic disorders.

Mr. H refused placement in a drug rehabilitation program for his methamphetamine use. He had completed a brief program 18 months earlier as part of court-ordered treatment but admitted to returning to methamphetamine use as soon as the program ended. He had been using intravenous methamphetamine since age 18 and downplayed the consequences of his drug use. He was no longer deemed to meet criteria for an involuntary psychiatric hold and was released.

Diagnosis. Methamphetamine use, psychosis secondary to methamphetamine use (Axis I); consider antisocial personality disorder or traits (Axis II).

Discussion. Brief psychotic episodes can result from methamphetamine or other stimulant use. Lack of significant family history for psychotic disorders and rapid clearing of psychotic symptoms with or without antipsychotic medication helps to distinguish these individuals from patients who have schizophrenia. It is possible for chronic heavy methamphetamine users to develop more chronic psychotic symptoms without clearing; therefore, these patients may appear to have schizophrenia.

OPIOIDS

Biology

Opium has been used throughout the world for several centuries. Opium is derived from the opium poppy, which contains approximately 20 opium alkaloids, including morphine. The *DSM-IV* defines the term **opioid** as encompassing **opiates** (any preparation of opium) and opioids (synthetic narcotics such as Demerol). Heroin (diacetylmorphine) is pharmacologically similar to morphine and is the most commonly used opiate among opioid-dependent individuals. A heroin habit can cost several hundred dollars a day, and individuals who become dependent often resort to criminal activities to sustain their habit. **Injection drug users** (IDU) are at high risk for serious illnesses such as AIDS, hepatitis, and tuberculosis.

Clinical Effects

Opioid intoxication produces initial euphoria followed by apathy, dysphoria, psychomotor agitation or retardation, impaired judgment, or impaired social functioning. The characteristic drowsiness is described as being "on the nod." Signs and symptoms include the following:

- pupillary constriction
- drowsiness or coma
- slurred speech
- impairment in attention or memory

Severe intoxication following an opioid overdose can lead to coma, respiratory depression, unconsciousness, gastric hypomotility with ileus (paralyzed bowel), pulmonary edema (fluid collection) from noncardiac causes, or even death. Opioid overdose is a medical emergency and requires immediate attention. Administration of naloxone hydrochloride, an opioid antagonist, can be life-saving and can help reverse cardiorespiratory depression.

Opioid withdrawal occurs after the cessation of heavy and prolonged opioid use. The administration of an opioid antagonist after prolonged use can also produce the withdrawal syndrome. Three or more of the following signs and symptoms may be present:

- dysphoric mood
- nausea or vomiting
- muscle aches
- watery eyes or runny nose
- pupillary dilation, piloerection, or sweating
- diarrhea
- yawning
- fever
- insomnia

Treatment

Short-term substitution therapy is used for opioid detoxification. Methadone, a long-acting opioid agonist with a half-life of 36 hours, is approved by the FDA for narcotic detoxification either for short-term detoxification lasting up to 30 days or for long-term treatment not in excess of 180 days. It is used orally and is cross-tolerant with heroin and morphine. In an inpatient setting, detoxification can be accomplished in 4–7 days, whereas 21-day detoxification is preferred in the outpatient setting in order to minimize patient discomfort. Table 11–7 gives the protocol for methadone detoxification.

Table 11–7. Protocol for methadone detoxification.

1. Ascertain that the patient has definite opioid withdrawal symptoms.
2. Objective withdrawal symptoms such as pupillary dilation are helpful.
3. Ascertain amount of opioid ingestion and frequency of use to establish whether opioid use is prolonged and heavy.
4. Start with methadone 10 mg as needed for withdrawal symptoms for the first 24 hours, with maximum daily dose of 40 mg.
5. After the first 24 hours of (as-needed) prn methadone administration, assess the patient and start on once-a-day dosing, usually 30–40 mg.
6. Dosage may be decreased by 5–10 mg/day as tolerated until total daily dose of 10 mg/day is reached.
7. Reduce to 5 mg/day of methadone for 1–3 days.
8. Observe patient for 48 hours after the last dose of scheduled methadone.

LAAM (L-α-acetyl-methadol), a long-acting congener of methadone, has also been used for detoxification. LAAM has a half-life of 47 hours and is metabolized to two active metabolites: nor-LAAM (which has a half-life of 62 hours) and dinor-LAAM (which has a half-life of 162 hours). The prolonged half-lives of LAAM and its metabolites allow for alternate-day dosing or thrice-weekly dosing, without the problem associated with take-home regimens in methadone maintenance programs.

Clonidine, an α2-adrenergic agonist, is very helpful in targeting symptoms of opioid withdrawal. It acts on the locus coeruleus in the brain, resulting in inhibition of norepinephrine release. It may also be used along with methadone, in controlling symptoms not alleviated with 40 mg/day of methadone. Clonidine is used in doses of 0.1–0.3 mg every 6 hours as needed for opioid withdrawal symptoms. The medication should be stopped temporarily if systolic blood pressure is less than 90, diastolic blood pressure is less than 60, or if pulse is lower than 50. Hydroxyzine, an antihistaminic agent may be used for treatment of anxiety, in doses of 25 mg every 6 hours as needed.

Buprenorphine is a partial agonist of µ-opioid type and is a clinically effective analgesic agent that has an estimated potency 25–40 times that of morphine. Detoxification with buprenorphine is as effective as methadone or clonidine. The dosage is 8 mg/day sublingually, and it is also effective in alternate-day therapy.

Florence P, aged 28, was admitted to the hospital for evaluation and treatment of bacterial endocarditis. She reported using 1 gm of heroin daily, sometimes mixing it with cocaine (called speedballing). She started using heroin at age 15 and had used it daily since age 17. She was drug-free for a total of 2 years while she was in prison. She told the interviewer that currently she was using heroin at least 4 times a day and last used it 12 hours before coming to the clinic. On examination, her pupils were dilated and bowel sounds were increased. Her eyes and nose were runny and she complained of body aches and pain. She also reported feeling depressed and suicidal and was admitted to the psychiatric inpatient unit.

Ms. P was started on methadone per protocol, and she required a total of 40 mg of methadone in the first 24 hours for treatment of withdrawal symptoms. She was given 40 mg of methadone the second morning and observed for somnolence. She stabilized quickly and was no longer feeling hopeless or suicidal. After endocarditis was ruled out by negative blood cultures, she decided to enroll in a residential treatment program and was discharged to the outpatient 21-day methadone detoxification program.

Diagnosis. Opiate dependence, withdrawal (Axis I).

Before starting a patient on methadone, the physician must ascertain whether the patient is dependent on opiates. A urine toxicology screen should be obtained as soon as possible. It is also helpful to define the patient's "drug of choice." Individuals who are dependent on heroin usually use the drug or "fix" several times a day, but polysubstance users may use several drugs sporadically. Heroin may be used occasionally, and for such patients methadone should not be initiated. Methadone has a half-life of 36 hours and builds up gradually in the body. Methadone should be used cautiously in patients who are not opiate dependent (as when methadone is prescribed for control of chronic pain due to cancer) or in patients with impaired liver function due to alcoholism or infection with hepatitis B or C.

HALLUCINOGENS

Biology

Several natural and synthetic hallucinogens have been used by humans. Lysergic acid diethylamide (LSD), the classic synthetic hallucinogen, was synthesized by Albert Hoffman in 1938. The naturally occurring hallucinogens include psilocybin (mushrooms), mescaline (peyote cactus), dimethyltryptamine (DMT), harmine, harmaline, and ibogaine.

Clinical Effects

Hallucinogen intoxication results in maladaptive behavioral changes such as marked anxiety or depression, ideas of reference, fear of losing one's mind, paranoid ideation, impaired judgment, or impaired social functioning during or shortly after hallucinogen use. Perceptual changes such as depersonalization, derealization, illusions, and hallucinations may occur in a state of full wakefulness and alertness. Two or more of the following signs and symptoms may occur:

- pupillary dilation
- tachycardia
- sweating
- palpitations
- blurred vision
- tremors
- incoordination

Hallucinogens also produce EEG changes simulating those of REM-stage sleep, which accounts for the dreamlike quality of the high experienced with these drugs.

There are no clear symptoms of hallucinogen withdrawal, but an individual may experience intense cravings after stopping hallucinogen use.

Treatment

Hallucinogen flashbacks or **hallucinogen persisting perception disorder,** when associated with marked impairment, may be treated with low-dose antipsychotics. Flashbacks are transient recurrences of disturbances in perception that are reminiscent of those experienced during one or more earlier hallucinogen intoxications. They may occur episodically, triggered by various drugs, anxiety, fatigue, or other stressors.

Zeke P, aged 42, was referred for psychiatric evaluation after telling his primary care provider that he had been experiencing vivid visual hallucinations. He reported having used LSD and other hallucinogens heavily 20 years earlier but currently used LSD "rarely, maybe once a year or so." He had been diagnosed as having HIV two years earlier and reported that the hallucinations had become more intense then. He used to experience trailing images, intensified colors, and halos around objects. Now he was also seeing and hearing angels and devils arguing around him. These visual images and auditory hallucinations were intense and troubling to him. At times he reported considering suicide "just to make it stop."

He responded well to a low-dose neuroleptic and experienced a decrease in visual and auditory hallucinations within one week.

Diagnosis. Post-hallucinogen perceptual disorder (Axis I).

PHENCYCLIDINES

Biology

Phencyclidines or phencyclidine-like substances include phencyclidine (PCP, Sernylan) and similarly acting compounds such as ketamine (Ketalar, Ketaject) and the thiophene analogue of phencyclidine (TCP; 1-[1-2-thienyl-cyclohexyl]piperidine). A common contaminant of PCP is 1-piperidinocyclo-hexanecarbonitrile (PCC), a byproduct of illicit synthesis, which on decomposition releases hydrogen cyanide in small amounts. These substances can be taken orally, intravenously, or they can be smoked.

PCP is available under a variety of names such as Hog, Tranq, Angel Dust, and PeaCe Pill. PCP was used originally as an anesthetic in animals, but its exact mechanism of action is unknown. It is cheap and is often used to adulterate other street drugs.

Clinical Effects

Phencyclidine intoxication results in clinically significant maladaptive behavioral changes such as belligerence, assaultiveness, impulsiveness, unpredictability, psychomotor agitation, impaired judgment, or impaired social functioning. Two or more of the following signs and symptoms are present within an hour after PCP ingestion:

- vertical or horizontal nystagmus
- hypertension or tachycardia
- numbness or diminished responsiveness to pain
- ataxia

- dysarthria (difficulty articulating words)
- muscle rigidity
- seizures or coma
- hyperacusis (magnification of sounds)

Involuntary isometric muscle activity can lead to acute rhabdomyolysis (muscle breakdown), myoglobinuria (presence of muscle breakdown products in urine), and renal failure. Clonic movements and muscle rigidity may sometimes precede generalized seizure activity, and status epilepticus (continuous seizure activity with significant chance of death) has been reported. PCP intoxication can lead to death resulting from hyperpyrexia (high body temperature) and other autonomic instability.

Treatment

Treatment of acute PCP intoxication focuses on symptomatic treatment. Benzodiazepines are useful in the treatment of agitation, muscle spasms, and seizures. Antipsychotics may be used for management of psychotic symptoms, although they may lower the seizure threshold and hence should be used cautiously. High-potency antipsychotics are preferred since PCP has some anticholinergic properties, and illegal drugs are often contaminated with belladonna alkaloids.

Jody T, a 21 year-old college student, was admitted to the inpatient psychiatric unit for treatment of psychosis. She was agitated and paranoid and stated that voices were telling her to kill herself and her grandmother.

Ms. T had started smoking PCP at parties and soon was using PCP as often as she could, sometimes 2 or 3 times per day. She dropped out of college a few months earlier. She started hearing voices that told her what to do. She was agitated and was continually mumbling to herself. She appeared disheveled and was unable to care for herself at home. She had last used PCP a few weeks prior to admission. She improved on low-dose neuroleptics and was released to her parents' care. She continued to experience less intense hallucinations intermittently for several weeks.

Diagnosis. Hallucinations secondary to PCP (Axis I).

PCP-induced psychosis may last for a long period of time. PCP, being lipophilic, remains in the body for several weeks. In the case of acute intoxication, antipsychotics should be used cautiously for treatment of agitation, since they lower seizure threshold. Antipsychotics are effective in treatment of PCP-induced psychotic disorder.

INHALANTS

Biology

Inhalants are aliphatic and aromatic hydrocarbons found in substances such as gasoline, glue, paint thinners, and spray paints. Less commonly used are halogenated hydrocarbons (found in cleaners, typewriter correction fluid, and spray-can propellants) and other volatile compounds containing esters, ketones, and glycols. Inhalant use is most common among adolescents, usually in group settings. Inhalants often leave visible external evidence, such as a rash around the nose and mouth, breath odors, and residue on the face.

Clinical Effects

Inhalant intoxication results in clinically significant maladaptive behavioral or psychological changes such as belligerence, assaultiveness, apathy, impaired judgment, or impaired social functioning. Two or more of the following signs and symptoms develop shortly after exposure to volatile inhalants:

- dizziness
- nystagmus
- incoordination
- slurred speech
- unsteady gait
- lethargy
- depressed reflexes
- psychomotor retardation
- tremor
- generalized muscle weakness
- diploplia (double vision)
- stupor or coma
- euphoria

Death from inhalant use may result from central respiratory depression, cardiac arrhythmias, asphyxiation, laryngospasm, or accident. A serious risk is irreversible damage to the lungs (including chemical pneumonitis (inflammation of the lungs) and emphysema), liver, kidney, and other organs from benzene and halogenated hydrocarbons. Permanent neuromuscular and brain damage are possible because inhalants often contain high concentrations of copper, zinc, and heavy metals.

> Thomas J, aged 16, was picked up by the police and brought to the emergency room after he was found wandering half-naked in the snow. He appeared confused and had significant short-term memory impairment. He had difficulty expressing himself, and a strong odor emanated from him. His physician noted a pronounced rash around his mouth. He admitted to sniffing glue daily for a few years. He said that he had started using inhalants with a group of school friends and that his use had escalated quickly. He was currently using inhalants on a daily basis and had dropped out of school. His condition was explained to his parents, who enrolled him in an outpatient day treatment program.
> **Diagnosis.** Inhalant use and intoxication (Axis I).

Treatment

Treatment of inhalant use is neither well-researched nor well-understood. Education about the health risks of inhalants may be helpful for prevention and treatment of inhalant use. Because the majority of users are in their teens and 20s, family therapy may also be of benefit.

CAFFEINE

Caffeine is used by more than 80% of Americans in average doses of a half-gram per day, mostly in coffee. Caffeine is found in coffee, tea, soft drinks, chocolate, over-the-counter stimulant drugs (eg, No-Doze), and various headache medications.

Biology

Caffeine is absorbed rapidly in the gastrointestinal tract and is believed to act as an antagonist at adenosine receptor sites in the central nervous system. Caffeine probably affects adrenergic and dopaminergic neurotransmitter systems to produce clinical effects.

Clinical Effects

Caffeine in low doses leads to heightened concentration, wakefulness, and a feeling of well-being. Larger doses produce anxiety, agitation, insomnia, and restlessness. Physical effects of caffeine intoxication include tremulousness, increased blood pressure and flushing, nausea, and polyurea.

Longer-term caffeine use is associated with tolerance, so that larger doses are required to achieve the same effects. Chronic heavy use of caffeine can also produce symptoms of generalized anxiety disorder, panic disorder, and insomnia. Caffeine may worsen fibromyalgia, peptic ulcer disease, and cardiac arrhythmias. Withdrawal phenomena are often noted when patients go more than 1 day without caffeine. Withdrawal symptoms include headaches, fatigue, and cravings for caffeine.

> Carl M, a 39-year-old attorney, was referred for psychiatric evaluation by his primary care physician. He complained of "heart palpitations" and anxiety that had worsened over the previous 4 months. The onset of his symptoms coincided with his starting a new job at a prestigious law firm. His primary care physician had started him on fluoxetine (Prozac), but Mr. M stopped the medication after 1 week because the medication made him feel "jittery." The physician's forwarded notes indicated that Mr. M drank three cups of coffee per day. His psychiatric history was unremarkable, with no prior history of anxiety or depressive disorders or substance use and a negative family history for psychiatric problems.
> When the psychiatrist asked Mr. M about his caffeine intake, he replied that he had actually reduced his intake of coffee and had switched to

drinking tea when he started his new job. Mr. M said that he knew that tea was much healthier than coffee. He was drinking one to two cups of black tea every hour at work. He also had two chocolate bars in the afternoon and drank one diet soda in the evening.

The psychiatrist estimated that the patient's caffeine intake was almost 2 grams per day. Mr. M was skeptical that reducing his caffeine intake would help but gradually cut back by substituting bottled water for tea and by eliminating soda and chocolate from his diet. At a 3-week follow-up, he was doing well and had no symptoms of anxiety or palpitations.

Diagnosis. Anxiety due to caffeine intoxication; caffeine dependence and intoxication (Axis I).

Treatment

Treatment for caffeine dependence usually is initiated in response to health problems or anxiety and consists of having the patient reduce caffeine intake gradually. Partial substitution of caffeinated beverages with decaffeinated coffee, tea, or soda allows the patient to consume the same quantity of these beverages if they wish.

MARIJUANA

Marijuana is the most frequently used illicit substance in the world, and the third among all potentially addictive substances after cigarette smoking and alcohol. One-third of Americans have tried marijuana, and over 6 million people smoke the drug once a week or more.

Biology

Marijuana is collected from the plant *Cannabis sativa*. The top leaves, flowers, and stems (buds) contain a variety of 400 chemicals. Smoking marijuana in rolled cigarette-like form, a pipe, or a water-filtered apparatus known as a "bong" releases over 2000 compounds, some via pyrolysis (burning). Of these compounds, 60 are of the **cannabinoid** class that are thought to be responsible for marijuana's psychoactive effects. The concentration of psychoactive compounds may vary widely, although plants are bred for increased potency. The best understood of the cannabinoids are Δ-9-tetrahydrocannabinol (THC), its precursor cannabidiol (CBD), and one of its more than 100 breakdown products, cannabinol (CBN). The existence of cannabinoid receptors in the human brain was discovered in 1988. The location of these receptors, primarily found in the cerebellum, cerebral cortex, hippocampus, and substantia nigra, neuroanatomically overlap with the dopaminergic system, implying a possible neurochemical relationship.

Cannabinoids from marijuana may be psychoactive because they are similar to the endogenous compound anandamide, just as heroin is active because the human body has receptor sites for naturally occurring opiate molecules known as endorphins. Effects in the hippocampus and basal ganglia are believed to be responsible for marijuana's effects on short-term memory and coordination, respectively. Cannabinoids appear to affect brain cells via a second messenger system that is activated within the cell when cannabinoids occupy membrane receptor sites. In vitro studies of cannabinoids on cells show general slowing of cellular function and reproduction. This observation correlates with clinical studies showing depressed thinking and decreased energy level, sperm counts, and ovulation in human subjects. Pulmonary problems may be the result of comorbid cigarette smoking rather than marijuana smoke itself.

Metabolism of marijuana takes place via the cytochrome P450 system. Urine toxicology screens may be positive for up to 1 week in light users, although chronic and heavy users may test positive for up to 1 month because of the storage and release of cannabinoids, which are lipophilic, from fat stores.

Marijuana has been used to treat cancer and AIDS patients who experience nausea and cachexia (severe malnutrition). Some patients report that they receive more relief from marijuana cigarettes than THC in pill form. Because marijuana reduces intraocular pressure, it has been used to treat patients who have glaucoma.

Clinical Effects

Effects of marijuana peak within 30 minutes of smoking the drug. Eating hashish (a tar-like residue from the cannabis plant) produces a more gradual, longer lasting but less intense effect. The psychoactive effects of marijuana vary between users. Many people experience giddiness, elevated mood, and enhanced visual and auditory perceptions. Some individuals become more talkative and witty, while others feel more tranquil or tired. Fewer users experience anxiety, panic, paranoia or hypervigilance, or post-intoxication lethargy or depression.

A minority of individuals who use marijuana experience brief but full-blown psychotic symptoms, including auditory and visual hallucinations and delusions. Although psychotic symptoms have been documented in individuals who have preexisting vulnerability to psychotic disorders (eg, schizophrenia, schizoaffective, or borderline personality disorder), the occurrence of psychosis in healthy individuals is considered rare. Physicians should warn patients who use marijuana that decreased coordination, slowed reflexes, and impaired judgment make driving and operating machinery dangerous and inadvisable while under the influence of the drug. Tolerance to marijuana's effects does occur, although withdrawal is unusual and may not exist clinically.

Two aspects of marijuana use are considered controversial. These include the existence of an amotivational syndrome marked by apathy, lethargy, and an inability to initiate or follow through with goal-directed activities. It is also unclear whether marijuana facilitates the use of "harder" drugs. This so-called **gateway hypothesis,** if it truly exists, would likely occur indirectly by exposure of heavier users to people and situations associated with cocaine, heroin, and methamphetamine use.

Treatment

Treatment of marijuana dependence should begin with the elimination of premorbid psychiatric conditions such as depression or anxiety disorders and co-morbid substance use (including use of alcohol). Education and 12-step programs such as Narcotics Anonymous are often effective for motivated users. Some users engage in chronic recreational use of marijuana, and the effects of such use have not been characterized adequately. The use of marijuana for medical purposes is the subject of intense medical and political debate.

NICOTINE & CIGARETTE SMOKING

Approximately 25% of the United States population smokes cigarettes regularly, and 75% of those sampled had tried cigarettes at least once. Cigarette smoking is found at increased rates among patients who have psychiatric disorders, perhaps in part because of the anxiolytic effects associated with smoking. Individuals who drink alcohol or have given up alcohol also smoke cigarettes at high rates. Public health measures to reduce smoking have begun to confront the growing numbers of new smokers who "replace" the ranks of those who either successfully stop smoking or die. Thus antismoking campaigns have focused on preventing experimentation and addiction in teenagers. Snuff, a tobacco product that is placed between the gums and cheek and is chewed, is used by approximately 15% of all tobacco users.

Biology

Nicotine binds to nicotinic receptors in the acetylcholine system, accounting for the subsequent release of catecholamines, epinephrine, and norepinephrine. Possible links to the dopaminergic system may provide insight into high rates of cigarette smoking among patients who have schizophrenia. Pyrolytic byproducts of cigarettes result in dramatic increases in lung cancer, heart disease, stroke, and cancers at other sites (eg, pharynx, bladder, colon). Damage to lung tissue exacerbates chronic obstructive lung disease and causes emphysema. Snuff and cigar smoking are associated with increased pharyngeal cancer.

Clinical Effects

Physiologic nicotine tolerance and dependence develop rapidly. Toxicity and overdose are possible but occur infrequently. Withdrawal phenomena, including irritability, anger, dysphoria, and insomnia, occur within hours of reducing or stopping cigarette intake. The fact that smoking a single cigarette relieves these symptoms rapidly provides powerful reinforcement of smoking and contributes to the high failure rate among individuals trying to stop smoking. Dependence is partially a biological process but is also facilitated by culturally sanctioned stereotypes and advertising.

Treatment

The long-term success rate of smoking cessation programs is approximately 30%. Although many physicians still believe that they can educate or frighten patients into quitting smoking, education alone does not produce effective results. More successful programs combine behavioral techniques and peer support with education. Useful adjunctive measures include hypnotherapy, acupuncture, Nicorette gum, or transdermal nicotine patches to reduce cravings; group therapy; relaxation therapy; and the use of props such as plastic cigarettes. However, a majority of people who stop smoking do so without any treatment.

Poor social support systems (including having family members who smoke) and environmental stress are associated with poor cessation rates. Anxious individuals, or patients who have schizophrenia in particular, often find that nicotine's calming effect makes cessation difficult. Heavy smokers who have histories of depression, dysthymia, or certain troublesome affective states (eg, anxiety, anger, impatience, and other pressured "Type A" behaviors associated with increased cardiac disease) have more difficulty quitting smoking. Depression may also recur in these patients when they stop smoking, further decreasing success rates. Numerous trials have used tricyclic antidepressants, serotonin specific re-uptake inhibitors, and the antianxiolytic buspirone to help depressed patients stop smoking. Buproprion (Wellbutrin) in a sustained release (long-acting) formulation has been shown to help nondepressed patients quit smoking. When used for smoking cessation, buproprion has been marketed as Zyban.

SPECIAL ISSUES & SPECIAL POPULATIONS

HIV & AIDS

Substance abusers are clearly at risk for HIV infection through the obvious route of needle use—if needles are used—and through the less obvious route of impaired judgment consequent to alcohol or drug use with a resulting failure to practice safer sex guidelines. Alcohol use may be the greatest cofactor in the continuing spread of HIV infections.

Some substance users will learn about their positive HIV status while undergoing medical procedures; some will seek out their status on their own.

Substance use may impair an individual's ability to fully understand the meaning of being HIV-positive and hence may interfere with the individual's compliance with medical care. Such limited compliance is almost always secondary to the substance use, not an innate indifference to health needs. Some individuals in recovery may relapse in the period between taking an HIV-antibody test and receiving the results. Helpful interventions include additional clinical visits, extra 12-step meetings, and attempts to expedite the return of the results.

An active abuser's positive HIV status may present an opportunity for treatment intervention. Although there is no evidence that reducing or stopping use will lead to greater longevity, the patient's quality of life will improve, and he or she will be able to make more informed choices about treatment for HIV infections and AIDS.

SUBSTANCE USE AMONG GAY MEN & LESBIANS

The incidence of substance abuse among gay men and lesbians (30%) is much higher than among the general population (10%). Alcohol and amphetamine abuse (including intravenous use, cocaine abuse, and use of designer drugs such as Ecstasy) may be especially prevalent and may play a complicating role in HIV-prevention efforts in the gay community.

Clinical evidence shows that successful treatment interventions include a need for the gay man or lesbian to fully accept his or her sexual orientation, thus dealing with internalized homophobia or self-loathing, which may be an excuse or trigger for relapse. A gay-sensitive or gay-affirmative treatment program may be most effective for intervention and treatment. Younger gay people may be especially sensitive and prone to excessive substance use or outright abuse.

CROSS-CULTURAL ASPECTS OF SUBSTANCE USE

Rates of substance abuse differ among ethnic and cultural minority groups, and some groups are more likely than others to abuse particular drugs. These observations may be related to socioeconomic factors and cultural norms more than to any genetic or biological factors. As with gay men and lesbians, supportive programs sensitive to the cultural and ethnic factors involved—including making counseling and literature available in the user's native language—may work best and offer the best chance for recovery for people of different cultural and ethnic backgrounds.

SUBSTANCE USE AMONG WOMEN

Women abuse substances at rates nearing those of men. The issues for women in society need to be considered in planning for treatment and recovery: limited financial resources, child-rearing concerns, the "hidden" nature of the use or abuse if the patient is homebound, and the possibility of sexual or physical abuse complicating the clinical picture. Providers, clinicians, and treatment programs need to be sensitive to these issues in order to make sobriety and recovery likely. More detailed discussion of these issues appears in Chapter 18.

EMOTIONAL REACTIONS TO PATIENTS

Substance use engenders a strong emotional response across society, perhaps more so in health-care providers. Emotional reactions may include denial on the clinician's part, which can lead the clinician to ignore subtle or obvious signs of substance use. Or the clinician may not inquire about substance use, instead making assumptions as to which patients might use which types of substances based on unconscious stereotypes associated with appearance, gender, ethnicity, or socioeconomic class. For example, a physician might ask about alcohol use in a 58-year-old male patient but omit questions about marijuana, heroin, or cocaine.

Clinicians will also tend to make "stunted" inquiries into a patient's substance use. While clinicians might ask a dozen or more questions about pain, their inventory of follow-up questions beyond "How much alcohol do you drink?" might be minimal. Better training and practice will allow physicians to perform a complete characterization of substance use and its place in the context of the patient's life.

Some patients who initially deny that they use substances but later admit (or it is discovered) that they have a substance use problem explain that they were afraid that if they had revealed their dependency, their physician would have been angry with them, refused to treat them, or would have provided a lower standard of care. These fears are sometimes justified.

Studies have also documented the undertreatment of acute and chronic pain in patients who have substance use histories, in excess of the usual rates of undertreatment. Emotional responses to patients may also cause physicians to unknowingly undertreat or withhold treatment for withdrawal from alcohol or heroin. Physicians who are acting on unconscious feelings of anger may also sabotage potential treatment plans.

Mary A, a 51-year-old woman who had a history of multiple hospital admissions for complications of alcohol dependence, was admitted to the hospital for treatment of pneumonia and malnutrition. The medical team was infuriated at her readmission, her third hospitalization in 6 months. The senior resident finally announced, "This is the last admission that woman is going to have here. Doesn't she realize what she's doing to herself?"

He then led the medical team into Ms. A's room. Ms. A appeared pale and thin, propped up in bed wearing a nasal tube carrying supplemental oxygen. The senior resident stood at the foot of her bed. "Mary," he boomed, "this is going to stop now!" Ms. A nodded wanly.

"I mean it, Mary." The resident continued to speak loudly and sternly. "Your liver and lungs have just about had it. Any more alcohol and they will quit. You'll bleed to death or die of an infection. One drink, that's all it will take. Do you understand?"

Ms. A started to respond, "I know doctor, I'm trying. . . "

The resident cut her off. "Trying won't do it anymore, Mary. You have to stop. This is your last chance before it's too late. We've worked too hard. Do you know how aggravating it is for us to fix you up and then have you come back messed up again?" Ms. A began to cry.

The resident motioned for the team to exit the room. The team members, formerly angry and frustrated, were relieved and upbeat. One resident clapped the intern on the back. "I think we finally got through to her," the chief resident said.

Diagnosis. Alcohol dependence (Axis I), other psychiatric diagnoses possible but not evaluated, see discussion below; pneumonia, malnutrition (Axis III).

Discussion. Of course, the team's interventions made little impact. If anything, their warnings to Ms. A about her precarious health and the implicit threat to abandon her care may have made her so anxious or hopeless that she may have drunk even more after returning to her home.

If the team had performed a more appropriate history and evaluation, they would have asked why Ms. A drank alcohol. (A consulting psychiatrist later learned that Ms. A's heavy alcohol use started 8 years earlier when her husband and son were killed in a car accident. She suffered from depression and anxiety and was socially isolated. Ms. A was ultimately referred to an alcohol treatment program, but only after two years of repeated medical admissions.) Although the hospital had highly trained substance abuse counselors who could evaluate patients and direct them to appropriate treatment programs, the medical team did not bother to call them or even familiarize themselves with the services that the counselors provided. While the team felt better after venting their frustrations, Ms. A had not been helped. Although she sought treatment repeatedly for complications of severe alcohol use, Ms. A was not given contacts for available treatment resources, and her cycle of substance use continued unabated.

Physicians generally do not do well when confronted with limitations of their own power to effect change in a patient's life. They may be frightened by the seemingly out-of-control nature of substance use, so far removed from the ideal of the physician's training and professional ethos. Anxiety about the often repeated self-destructive nature of the patient's substance use, possibly coupled with the high rate of substance use in physicians (upwards of 10% in many studies), may cause physicians to vent unrecognized fear and anger at patients. These feelings must be recognized so that physicians can provide optimal treatment for patients who have substance abuse problems.

LEGAL & ETHICAL ISSUES

Many ethical concerns arise in the treatment of patients who abuse or are dependent on substances. These concerns include issues of confidentiality between patients and physicians, the allocation of resources to patients who are former or current substance users, and the issue of physician control and authority versus patients' rights and freedoms.

Myra G, a 36-year-old woman with a 15-year history of intravenous heroin use, was hospitalized for bacterial endocarditis. Cardiac ultrasound showed that her tricuspid valve was severely eroded from bacterial infection in spite of powerful intravenous antibiotic therapy. The infection was compromising her cardiac function and threatening her life. The cardiac surgery team assigned to Ms. G's case agreed that an operation to replace her damaged valve with a prosthetic valve was necessary to save her life.

The surgery team met with Ms. G the day before the operation. They produced a consent form that they had specially designed for her that day to supplement the standard surgery consent form. They explained that they would perform the valve replacement surgery, but Ms. G would have to agree to enter a drug treatment program and would agree never to use heroin again. If she did return to using heroin or other substances, Ms. G would agree that she would never be eligible to receive another heart valve replacement. Ms. G felt intimidated by the surgery team's strong stance and signed the consent form.

The surgery was successful, and Ms. G made a rapid physical recovery. She entered a drug rehabilitation program and began a methadone maintenance program. Two years later the rehabilitation program was "defunded" in a round of federal and state cutbacks. Ms. G was unable to enter another drug treatment or methadone maintenance program, and despite her motivation and gains over the previous 2 years, she returned to active heroin use.

Ms. G presented 1 year later with a recurrence of heart valve failure. She was hospitalized in serious condition, and again despite antibiotic therapy her prognosis appeared grim. Although heart valve replacement therapy was indicated clinically, the surgery team refused to proceed. They argued that expensive surgery would be "wasted on someone who has proven that they can't be trusted to give up drugs." They also showed the primary medical team and Ms. G a copy of the special consent form that she had signed 3 years earlier.

The case was brought before the hospital ethics committee, where it was pointed out that the surgery team had developed a unique form without the consent of the hospital's policy review committee and that a special standard was being enforced on a small number of patients in a way that violated the principles of fairness and justice. For example, by this reasoning the surgeons should also refuse to perform cardiac surgery on patients who smoked, overate, or otherwise elevated their risk of cardiac disease.

The ethics committee also held that Ms. G's signature on the special consent form was invalid, because she signed it under duress, knowing that if she refused to sign she would not receive the heart valve replacement. As one committee member put it, "You can't consider signing a form 'informed consent' if there's a loaded gun pointed at your head." The surgery team relented, and Ms. G received her second heart valve replacement.

Discussion. The same issue of whether past or current substance use should affect allocation of scarce resources has also emerged in the decision to give liver transplants to selected patients who have alcohol dependence histories.

Studies show that if patients have been abstinent from alcohol for 6 to 8 months prior to transplantation their risk of relapse is considered small, and their prognosis is similar to other liver transplant recipients.

As part of a new hospital policy psychiatric patients were not allowed to smoke on the inpatient unit. They were escorted by the staff as a group to the patio three times a day except when it was raining. The patients were upset, stating that cigarette smoking calmed their nerves and that being deprived of cigarettes was very stressful. They approached the hospital's patient advisory board to lodge a protest against the smoking ban, which they claimed violated their civil rights.

Discussion. The ethics of prohibiting smoking presents a difficult dilemma. Although cigarette smoking is a health hazard, it also provides comfort and pleasure to patients. Proponents argue that psychiatric inpatients should be free to make this decision.

The question of morality and responsibility in substance use has been highlighted by the 1997 decision of the United States Congress not to offer social security disability benefits for substance dependence. Patients with dual diagnoses of substance use and another major psychiatric disorder such as depression, schizophrenia, or anxiety disorders recently were reevaluated for their need to receive benefits. Physicians working in larger health care systems such as public health settings may also be asked to give opinions on public policy pertaining to substance use. This may include controversial topics such as the funding of needle exchange programs.

CONCLUSION

Substance abuse is epidemic in the United States and in many other parts of the world. The issues facing clinicians in the medical care of the substance abuser and in intervening with and treating the substance abuse itself are myriad, complex, challenging, and rewarding. Substance abuse is one of the few medical and psychiatric conditions that can be treated successfully, with great benefits associated with the recovery from the illness: Both quality of life and longevity can be enhanced dramatically.

Each abused substance has its own set of medical results and clinical manifestations, as well as some specific treatment and intervention strategies. Even with such a wide range of abused substances, fairly typical patterns and consequences exist, and successful treatments follow certain patterns and paths.

Recognition of the substance abuse problem is paramount to intervention; working with the patient through the stages of change is essential to effective treatment. The process of abstinence, early sobriety, and recovery depends on the help of the treating clinician, the social network, and 12-step or other recovery-oriented programs. Though substance dependence is never "cured," on-going recovery—remaining clean and sober—provides hope and can reverse the medical and social problems that result from the substance abuse. Recovery is essentially a successful treatment collaboration among the patient, the provider, and the social supports that places a life-long illness in remission.

REFERENCES

Alcoholics Anonymous: *The Big Book.* Alcoholics Anonymous World Services, 1973.

American Psychiatric Association: Practice guidelines for the treatment of patients with substance use disorders: alcohol, cocaine, opioids. Am J Psychiatr 1995;152 (11):1-59(Suppl).

American Psychiatric Association: *Psychiatric Services for Addicted Patients: A Task Force Report of the American Psychiatric Association.* American Psychiatric Press, 1995.

Andreasen NC, Black DW: Alcohol-related disorders. Pages 375–393 in: *Introductory Textbook of Psychiatry,* 2nd ed. American Psychiatric Press, 1995.

Batki SL et al: Fluoxetine for cocaine dependence in methadone maintenance: quantitative plasma and urine cocaine/benzoylecgonine concentrations. J Clin Psychopharmacol 1993;13(4)243.

Benowitz N: Clinical pharmacology and toxicology of cocaine. Pharmacol Toxicol 1993;72:3.

Bohn MJ, Babor TF, Kranzler HR: The Alcohol Use Disorders Identification Test (AUDIT): validation of a screening instrument for use in medical settings. J Stud Alcohol 1995;56:423.

Brady KT, Roberts JM: The pharmacotherapy of dual diagnosis. Psychiatr Ann 1995;25(6):344.

Cabaj RP: Substance abuse in gay men, lesbians, and bisexual individuals. In: Cabaj RP, Stein TS (editors): *Textbook of Homosexuality and Mental Health.* American Psychiatric Press, 1996.

Centers for Disease Control and Prevention: *HIV/AIDS Surveillance Report.* US Department of Health and Human Services, Public Health Service. 1995;7(1).

Chester G, Greely J: Tolerance to the effects of alcohol. Alcohol, Drugs Driving 1992;8(2):93.

DiClemente CC: Motivational interviewing and the stages of change. Pages 191–202 in: *Motivational Interviewing: Preparing People to Change Addictive Behavior.* Guilford, 1991.

Gawin FH et al: Desipramine facilitation of initial cocaine abstinence. Arch Gen Psychiatr 1989;46:117.

Goldstein A: The wild addictions: cocaine and amphetamines. Pages 155–167 in: *Addiction: From Biology to Drug Policy.* Freeman, 1994.

Halikas JA, Kuhn KL, Maddux TL: Reduction of cocaine use among methadone maintenance patients using concurrent carbamezepine. Ann Clin Psychiatr 1990;2:3.

Kaplan HI, Sadock BJ, Grebb JA: *Kaplan and Sadock's Synopsis of Psychiatry,* 7th ed. Williams & Wilkins, 1994.

Landry DW: Immunotherapy for cocaine addiction. Sci Am 1997;Feb:42.

Minkoff K: An integrated treatment model for dual diagnosis of psychosis and addiction. Hosp Commun Psychiatr 1989;40:1031.

Minkoff K: Intervention strategies for people with dual diagnosis. Innov Res 1993;2(4):11.

National Clearinghouse for Alcohol and Drug Information (Services for SAMHMSA): http://www.health.org.pubs.htm

National Household Study on Drug Abuse (NHSDA): ftp://ftp.health.org/ncadi/publications/meth.txt

National Institute of Drug Abuse. http://www.nida.nih.gov/

National Institute of Drug Abuse: *National Household Survey on Drug Abuse Highlights.* US Government Printing Office, 1991.

O'Malley SS et al: Naltrexone and coping skills therapy for alcohol dependence. Arch Gen Psychiatr 1992;49:881.

Rosenthal RN: Comorbidity of psychiatric and substance use disorders. Prim Psychiatr 1995;2(7):42.

Saitz R et al: Individualized treatment for alcohol withdrawal. A randomized double-blind controlled trial. J Am Med Assoc 1994;272(7):519.

Schuckit MA: Alcohol and alcoholism. Pages 2146–2151 in: Wilson G et al (editors): *Harrison's Principles of Internal Medicine,* 12th ed. McGraw-Hill, 1990.

Sorenson JL, Batki SL: Management of the psychosocial sequelae of HIV infection among drug abusers. Pages 788–792 in: Lowinson JK et al (editors): *Substance Abuse: A Comprehensive Textbook,* 2nd ed. Williams & Wilkins, 1992.

Stuppaeck CH et al: Assessment of the alcohol withdrawal syndrome—validity and reliability of the translated and modified clinical institute withdrawal assessment for alcohol scale (CIWA-A). Addiction 1994;89(10):1287.

Tsuang D et al: The effects of substance use disorders on the clinical presentation of anxiety and depression in an outpatient psychiatric clinic. J Clin Psychiatr 1995;56 (12):549.

Volpicelli JR et al: Naltrexone in the treatment of alcohol dependence. Arch Gen Psychiatr 1992;49:876.

Zorumski CF, Isenberg KE: Insights into the structure and function of GABA-benzodiazepine receptors: ion channels and psychiatry. Am J Psychiatr 1991;148:162.

12

Personality Disorders

Amelia J. Wilcox, PhD, James M. Mol, PhD, & David Elkin, MD

Personality disorders differ from other psychiatric disorders in that they are chronic and tend to result in severely impaired relationships. In most psychiatric disorders, patients are upset by their symptoms, which are experienced as foreign and distressing, or **ego-dystonic.** For example, the patient who is depressed is likely to feel sad and tired and may report not feeling like himself or herself. Similarly, someone having a panic attack will usually report feeling overwhelmed by tremendous anxiety. But a hallmark of personality disorders is that they are **ego-syntonic;** that is, from the patient's perspective, nothing is wrong. Rather, something is wrong with the world and others in it, and the patient can do little to change things until other people begin to act differently. Although it is extremely challenging to work with these patients, every physician must be familiar with basic principles of the assessment and management of personality disorders.

Personality disorders create difficulties in interpersonal relationships. The level of dysfunction varies among patients who have these disorders, from a lower-functioning patient who may be unable to sustain work and may require intermittent psychiatric hospitalization, to a higher-functioning individual who may, for example, be relatively well-adapted to much of adult life but may be unable to sustain mature, healthy, and satisfying relationships.

Many of the traits discussed in this chapter are common to healthy individuals. We all may, at times, be mistrustful, avoidant of certain situations, or in search of immediate gratification. But what may be a temporary or situational state in the healthy adult is a fixed and unchanging trait in an individual who has a personality disorder. According to the *DSM-IV,* personality disorders are marked by a "pervasive, maladaptive pattern of behavior that remains stable across time and circumstance." For example, the patient who has paranoid personality disorder is mistrustful regardless of the objective circumstances; the patient who has antisocial personality disorder has poor impulse control and constantly seeks easy and immediate gratification of wishes. These disorders are typically observable in late adolescence or early adulthood, and they continue across the life span. Some of the disorders are preceded by childhood diagnoses, as is the case with antisocial personality disorder, which is preceded by conduct disorder.

Defense mechanisms are the largely unconscious, automatic mental operations that protect individuals from being overwhelmed by anxiety. Sources of anxiety that compel individuals to use these defense mechanisms include internal pressures and impulses, as well as pressures and requirements of the external world. Defense mechanisms are a part of both pathologic and healthy functioning; however, the use of maladaptive defense mechanisms in a rigid and pervasive manner distinguishes individuals who have personality disorders from those who are healthy.

ETIOLOGY

The genesis of personality disorders has been discussed widely. Psychodynamic theories focus on poorly resolved or unresolved developmental tasks as the root of personality disorders. Recent investigations into biological substrates have highlighted heightened limbic system arousal in patients who have these disorders. Although research suggests that genetic factors may play a role in the development of some personality disorders, environment and early childhood experience are considered much more significant causal factors.

Philosophers and scholars have endeavored for centuries to understand the nature, causes, and effects of personality. In the past century, psychotherapeutic treatment failures have led to an increased awareness of the significance of personality and ongoing character traits. The theory and technique of assessing and treating patients who have personality disorders is uniquely linked with the early history of psychoanalysis. Patients who had personality disorders initially appeared to be similar to neurotic patients.

However, these patients not only failed to benefit from analysis, they often became more regressed, disorganized, and less functional. Many also developed extremely intense romantic attachments to their therapists.

At the turn of the twentieth century, Dr. Franz Breuer had been using hypnotherapy to relieve his patient Anna O's psychosomatic symptoms that stemmed from her father's death. Dr. Breuer realized that his patient was developing romantic feelings towards him, to which he was beginning to respond. He abruptly deemed Anna O "cured" and terminated therapy. He was called back to Anna O's house that same night and found her in the throes of hysterical childbirth (psuedocyesis) and yelling, "I'm having Dr. Breuer's baby!" Shaken, the doctor contacted a young neurologist colleague to assume care for Anna O. That neurologist was Sigmund Freud, who undertook a "talking cure" with the patient. Thus Anna O became the first psychotherapy patient and is linked to the founding of the psychoanalytic movement.

After thus being identified, personality-disordered patients were deemed untreatable until the 1920s and 1930s when modifications in therapeutic techniques led to a better understanding of patients' psychopathology and increased successes in treatment. Subsequent advances in theory and practice during the 1970s and 1980s by Kohut, Kernberg, and Masterson considerably improved therapeutic outcomes. They also expanded the notion that personality disorders originate from arrested psychological growth in early childhood resulting from patients' failures to achieve critical developmental goals such as attachment, separation, and individuation with parental figures.

DIAGNOSTIC ASSESSMENT

As recognized by the *DSM-IV,* personality disorders are placed on Axis II. The *DSM-IV* divides the personality disorders into three cluster groups, which are descriptively similar. This division does not imply that the disorders are mutually exclusive, either within or among cluster groups. In fact, patients sometimes demonstrate symptoms of more than one personality disorder. When a patient is characterized as having "traits" of a personality disorder, he or she exhibits features of that personality disorder without meeting all of the criteria for a diagnosis. With a diagnosis of more than one personality disorder, the patient meets the criteria for each of those diagnoses given. When a personality disorder not otherwise specified (NOS) is diagnosed, features of more than one personality disorder are present, without the pa-

tient meeting the full criteria for any one of the disorders. Table 12–1 lists the cluster groups outlined in the *DSM-IV.*

Most people tend to regress under stress, meaning they revert to much less mature ways of thinking and behaving. Thus any patient entering the hospital or facing a serious illness may think, act, and behave in a manner that does not reflect his or her baseline level of functioning. Clinicians should diagnose personality disorders only after obtaining comprehensive historical information, making collateral contacts (ie, contact with other professionals or family members for the purpose of gathering data on the patient's history and function), and maintaining patient contact over time.

CLUSTER A: ECCENTRIC OR ODD

Patients who have cluster A personality disorders have difficulty trusting others. In addition to being suspicious and mistrustful, they tend to interpret the actions of others as deliberately threatening, and they tend to project distorted feelings onto others. Given these tendencies, patients who have these disorders are unlikely to seek treatment themselves.

Paranoid Personality Disorder

Epidemiology. According to the *DSM-IV,* the prevalence of paranoid personality disorder in the general population is 0.5–2.5%. In treatment settings, the prevalence is 2–10% for outpatients and 10–30% for inpatients. There is an increased family incidence of chronic schizophrenia and delusional disorder, persecutory type. This diagnosis is more common in men. It is often preceded in childhood and adolescence by social anxiety and isolation, poor school performance, and oddities of thought and fantasy.

Core Features. The predominant characteristic of paranoid personality disorder is a pervasive mistrust of others. Patients who have this disorder are often consumed by the belief that others are "out to get them," and they appear guarded, suspicious, and

Table 12–1. Personality disorder cluster groups.

Cluster A: "Eccentric or odd"
  Paranoid personality disorder
  Schizoid personality disorder
  Schizotypal personality disorder
Cluster B: "Dramatic, emotional, or erratic"
  Histrionic personality disorder
  Narcissistic personality disorder
  Antisocial personality disorder
  Borderline personality disorder
Cluster C: "Anxious or fearful"
  Avoidant personality disorder
  Dependent personality disorder
  Obsessive-compulsive personality disorder

hypervigilant. They often misperceive others actions as exploitative, anticipate exploitation, and bear grudges for real and imagined exploitation. They tend to be socially isolated and rarely confide in others.

Because these patients struggle with issues of basic trust, they often present in medical settings in a guarded and suspicious manner, denying problems and refusing assistance. They may be reluctant to confide in clinicians because of mistrust of others' motives or of how information shared will be used. This presents particular problems in an inpatient, involuntary setting, when legal decisions require patients to provide information about their mental status. Patients who have paranoid personality disorder are likely to fear being controlled by others, a fear heightened by involuntary contact with the mental health system.

Robert E, a 55-year-old man, was admitted to an inpatient psychiatric unit after exhibiting suicidal ideation. He was placed on an involuntary hold and brought in by ambulance from his office after his wife received a call from him during which he appeared quite upset and said he was "just going to get it over with." Initially Mr. E denied any problems and said to the resident interviewing him, "I don't need to be here or need your help." He appeared most concerned about the rules and regulations surrounding his involuntary hold, asking how long it would last, carefully reviewing his advisement, and angrily taking issue with its wording.

Mr. E remained angry and silent throughout the initial interview, turning his head away and then finally saying to the resident, "There's nothing I want from you. I know what you're trying to do, and I don't want to talk to you now."

The resident asked Mr. E if he could return later to continue the meeting, and they agreed on a time for later that day.

When once again settled into the interview room, Mr. E launched into an angry account of "the bozos" at work who hired a new employee to learn his job duties. With increasing anger and anxiety he reported that he was sure his boss had been planning all along to replace him "with the new jerk," adding, "I'm just waiting for the ax to fall." He described arriving at work that morning to find on his desk a sealed envelope from his boss and told the resident he had not yet opened it, saying, "I just know it's a pink slip."

During a collateral interview with Mr. E's wife, she described her growing awareness over the years that her husband's suspicions were generally inaccurate. She said, "I used to believe him and get worried, too. He'd come home every day and complain his bosses were out to get him. He's always angry about how they do things and thinks he could do better."

"I used to try to reason with him, but that didn't work. Then I tried to joke with him, but you know, he doesn't have a sense of humor." She added, "It's not easy living with someone who thinks there's only one right way to do everything."

During a subsequent couple's session, Mr. E's wife removed an envelope from her purse and said to her husband, "Your boss called last night. He was worried about you and mentioned he'd left a message on your desk thanking you for the help you've given to the new employee."

Diagnosis. Paranoid personality disorder (Axis II).

Discussion. Patients who have paranoid personality disorder may be resentful, envious, and extremely sensitive to power differentials in relationships. They may try to gain control in an interview, for example, by second-guessing the clinician's purpose for questions. It is often helpful to provide these patients with appropriate opportunities for control, for example, by allowing them to pick a mutually convenient time for the interview.

The lack of a sense of humor is characteristic of patients who have this disorder. Their personal relationships are characterized by a cold and aloof stance, a heightened need to be in control, and at times by pathological jealousy and a fear of betrayal.

Patients who have paranoid personality disorder use primitive defenses such as **denial,** which allows the avoidance of uncomfortable, anxiety-provoking thoughts and feelings. In addition, they use **projection,** by which they attribute their unwanted thoughts and feelings to others, resulting in a distorted view of reality.

These patients often struggle with persecutory fantasies, which may be interspersed with fantasies of a more grandiose nature. Often, the conviction that others are out to get them becomes a partial reality. This occurs when their hostile, suspicious, irritable, and controlling behaviors arouse the concerns of those around them. It also may result in poor adjustments to work and relationships.

Patients may appear quite suspicious and difficult to engage in the psychiatric interview. In other medical settings, problems with trust may lead to a decreased ability to confidently work with a physician and may result in difficulty accepting recommendations for care. Physicians should remember that this is a function of the patient's character structure, as this will reduce the likelihood that the apparent lack of trust will be experienced as a personal affront. John Nardo cautions that patients who have paranoid personality disorder may request and require second and third opinions regarding medical decisions.

Associated Disorders. According to the *DSM-IV,* when under stress, patients who have paranoid personality disorder may suffer from very brief psychotic episodes. This disorder may be the precursor to the development of delusional disorder or a schizophrenic disorder. In the diagnostic interview, it is essential to differentiate the patient's persecutory thoughts and fantasies from the psychotic symptoms of a patient who has delusional disorder, persecutory type; major depression with psychotic features; or schizophrenia, paranoid type. Other associated disorders include major depressive disorder, agoraphobia, and obsessive-compulsive disorder. As always, these patients should be assessed for the presence of alcohol and substance abuse. Personality disorders most likely to occur in conjunction with paranoid personality disorder include the other cluster A disorders, as well as narcissistic, avoidant, and borderline personality disorders.

Schizoid Personality Disorder

Epidemiology. Schizoid personality disorder is uncommon in clinical settings. This disorder is slightly more prevalent in men. There may be an increased prevalence of the disorder in relatives of individuals who have schizophrenia or schizotypal personality disorder (see below). Cultural factors may lead to an incorrect diagnosis, for example, when emotional shutting-down occurs in immigrants from other countries or in people who have moved from rural to urban settings.

Core Features. Schizoid personality disorder is characterized by a fundamental inability to form social relationships. As follows, the patient who has schizoid personality disorder almost always chooses solitary activities. In addition, these patients have few or no close relationships and appear indifferent to praise or criticism from others. They are cold, detached, and have a restricted range of emotions. In addition, they have little or no interest in sexual relations with others and take pleasure in few, if any, activities.

Another common feature of this disorder is a poorly defined, or perhaps absent, sense of self. These individuals are disengaged from others because of their detachment from a sense of their own identity. Patients who have schizoid personality disorder deny experiencing strong emotions such as anger or joy, although they may be preoccupied with angry and at times violent fantasies.

Internal fantasy and omnipotence can serve as defenses for the patient who has schizoid personality disorder. The core issues of these individuals have to do with basic trust and attachment.

Malcolm H, aged 23, was a resident of a halfway house for mentally ill young adults. He had lived there for nearly 5 years, longer than any of the other eight residents. During this time he had finished high school by passing the GED examination, had been in stable employment as

an attendant at a local gas station, and had not required psychiatric hospitalization.

Despite Mr. H's history of relatively stable functioning, he had minimal contact, at best, with the other halfway house residents or with others in the community. He maintained no contact with family members. He had never been in a sexual or intimate relationship. When the residents of the halfway house watched television or spent time together, Mr. H could typically be found alone in his room, listening to alternative rock music on his stereo. His only interest was in music, which seemed to provide him with the motivation to work so that he could add to his compact disc collection.

The only times Mr. H interacted with others were during mandatory house meetings, group therapy, and meals. However, these interactions were superficial at best, and Mr. H appeared to be a separate and disinterested observer of those around him. A senior staff person noted that Mr. H seemed mildly interested in developing relationships with two of the staff members. He sought them out (when they were not with other residents) to discuss his latest compact disc purchases and to share lyrics from some of the more poetic and nihilistic of his favorite songs. Sometimes Mr. H also reported to these staff members graphic accounts of sadistic fantasies, usually involving a violent misfortune befalling an irritable gas station customer or images of Mr. H torturing his boss, whom he perceived as being demanding.

Diagnosis. Schizoid personality disorder (Axis II).

Discussion. Intricate fantasies (often angry and violent) may be shared with the few people with whom a schizoid patient has some interest in relating. Although communication of these fantasies may appear significant in their relative depth of disclosure, it is notable that the physician may feel little emotional connection or empathy for the feelings underlying these fantasies or other material presented in these interactions. Even a person well-liked by a schizoid patient will tend to feel that he or she has little knowledge of the patient.

Associated Disorders. Schizoid personality disorder most often co-occurs with schizotypal, paranoid, and avoidant personality disorders. Patients who have these personality disorders exhibit marked interpersonal withdrawal. These disorders can be difficult to distinguish. Table 12–2 identifies the key features of these disorders.

Schizoid personality disorder, like schizophrenia, has features of impaired interpersonal relationships and disordered thinking. However, schizophrenia and other Axis I psychotic disorders are characterized by

Table 12–2. Comparison of schizoid personality disorder and other co-occurring disorders.

	Interpersonal Impairments	Desire to Form Relationships	Cognitive or Perceptual Distortions (eg, magical thinking)	Psychotic Symptoms (eg, delusions, auditory or visual hallucinations)
Schizoid personality disorder	Yes			
Schizotypal personality disorder	Yes		Yes	
Avoidant personality disorder	Yes	Yes		
Schizophrenia	Yes		Yes	Yes

periods of persistent psychotic symptoms (such as delusions or hallucinations). In schizoid personality disorder, psychotic symptoms are rarely present and are usually more transient and less severe than frank delusions or hallucinations. According to the *DSM-IV,* schizoid personality disorder may precede delusional disorder or schizophrenia. Individuals who have schizoid personality disorder may also develop major depressive disorder.

Schizotypal Personality Disorder

Epidemiology. Schizotypal personality disorder occurs in approximately 3% of the general population. Family members of individuals who have schizotypal personality disorder may have an hereditary predisposition to the disorder. They may also be more likely to have schizophrenia or other psychotic disorders, suggesting that this personality disorder is a partial penetrance of the same factors leading to schizophrenia. As Cameron and Rychlak pointed out in 1985, this hereditary factor may be much stronger in schizotypal personality disorder than in schizoid personality disorder. According to the *DSM-IV,* schizotypal personality disorder may be somewhat more prevalent in men.

Core Features. Schizotypal personality disorder is characterized by deficits in social and interpersonal functioning, as well as by cognitive or perceptual distortions and oddities of behavior. These interpersonal, cognitive, and perceptual disturbances begin by early adulthood and must be present in a variety of contexts for diagnostic criteria to be met.

Specifically, individuals who have schizotypal personality disorder have no close relationships outside of their immediate family, and they experience marked social anxiety that does not decrease with familiarity. They are markedly suspicious and paranoid. There may be ideas of reference (not of delusional proportions), odd beliefs or magical thinking, and unusual perceptual experiences. Finally, patients

who have schizotypal personality disorder typically display oddities of speech, inappropriate or constricted affect, and behavior or appearance that is unusual or frankly bizarre.

Schizotypal individuals, like schizoid individuals, have core issues with basic trust and attachment. However, the defenses used by patients who have schizotypal personality disorder differ in that they reflect a greater impairment in reality testing. In addition to defenses of internal fantasy and omnipotence, these patients also use the defenses of denial, projection, and **displacement** (shifting the focus of uncomfortable feelings to less threatening individuals or circumstances).

Cultural factors must be considered before attributing religious or spiritual beliefs or rituals (eg, believing in a sixth sense or in an ability to control health and illness) to magical thinking.

Frank K, a 30-year-old resident of a board-and-care home, was brought to the psychiatric emergency services unit for evaluation after taking into his room all of the sharp knives in the residence, "in case anyone does that again." When questioned about why he was feeling unsafe, he responded with a stilted and convoluted tale that involved other residents of the home attempting to damage items from his "precious collection of grand historical movie stills and memorabilia from the age of giants."

Mr. K was wearing all-black clothing from the 1940s, including a dingy bowler hat and worn leather gloves. He was unemployed and receiving mental health disability and spent all his time alone, cutting out pictures of movie stars from magazines he purchased at antique and novelty shops. During the mental status examination, Mr. K indicated, in obtuse fashion, the belief that he may secretly be related to Clark Gable, stating that when he becomes "very still" he actually becomes the deceased star for "fractions of moments."

At the conclusion of the interview, the staff psychiatrist decided that Mr. K's behavior did not meet the criteria for dangerousness to himself or others, or grave disability. The board-and-care operator, who had brought Mr. K to the emergency room, had stated that the knives had been collected from the patient's room, and Mr. K agreed to notify him if he continued to worry that someone was attempting to destroy his property. Mr. K was sent home with a prescription for a low-dose antipsychotic, and a follow-up appointment was scheduled with his psychiatrist for the next week. Mr. K quietly and stiffly thanked the psychiatrist for her "gracious professionalism and resounding good sense," shook her hand, and formally tipped his hat as he exited the unit.

Diagnosis. Schizotypal personality disorder (Axis II).

Discussion. Often a confusing or vague explanation regarding a problem or concern is indicative of suspiciousness or paranoia. The obfuscation may reflect convoluted thinking, or it may be an attempt to hide a mistrust for the interviewer. Stilted or idiosyncratic speech are examples of oddities of speech frequently found in patients who have schizotypal personality disorder.

The bizarre appearance of these patients may be disorganized, or organized, as in this case. An unusual physical appearance and clothing may give the impression that the person is playing a role and thus wearing a costume for a part in a production or play. Impaired or largely absent interpersonal relationships are central to the schizotypal patient's psychopathology. Magical thinking may appear to be of delusional proportions at times but is generally less severe, less long-standing, and not presented with the same conviction as a delusion.

Associated Disorders. According to the *DSM-IV*, significant psychotic symptoms (eg, hallucinations or delusions) may develop in patients who have schizotypal personality disorder. These symptoms could qualify the patient to receive a diagnosis of brief psychotic disorder, schizophreniform disorder, delusional disorder, or schizophrenia. Many patients who have schizotypal personality disorder may have a history of major depressive disorder or a current coexisting major depressive episode. Schizotypal personality disorder sometimes coexists with schizoid, paranoid, avoidant, or borderline personality disorders. As previously mentioned, schizotypal personality disorder differs from schizoid personality disorder in that there are eccentricities in the schizotypal person's thoughts and behaviors, or oddities in their speech.

CLUSTER B: DRAMATIC, EMOTIONAL, OR ERRATIC

Patients in this cluster group have core difficulties with disorders of self (unstable, unrealistic, poorly defined, or absent senses of their own identity; and poor self-esteem). Other core difficulties include problems with separation from others and guilt or other conflicts regarding sexuality. Treatment is usually sought for problems in relationships and within the community that are the result of these patient's disturbances, rather than the direct symptoms of the personality disorders themselves.

Borderline Personality Disorder

Characteristics of what is now referred to as borderline personality disorder were documented by psychoanalysts in the late 1930s, who began observing patients who were too fragile for classical analytic treatment but were not disturbed enough to warrant a diagnosis of schizophrenia. These patients tended to regress and become disorganized under stress, many severely enough to demonstrate psychotic symptoms. The term **borderline** was adopted because these patients' symptoms were thought to exist at the border between neurosis and psychosis. At this time, borderline personality disorder is recognized not as a state between two levels of functioning, but rather as a habitual level of functioning with specific symptomatology. Patients who have borderline personality disorder are on a continuum. Some function well, others more poorly, with comorbid conditions and a poor prognosis across their life spans.

Epidemiology. The *DSM-IV* states that 2% of the general population, 10% of outpatients in mental health settings, and 20% of psychiatric inpatients meet the criteria for a diagnosis of borderline personality disorder. The diagnosis is approximately five times more common among first-degree biological relatives. Family incidence of mood disorders, substance abuse disorders, and antisocial personality disorder is also increased.

Core Features. The hallmarks of borderline personality disorder include a pervasive instability of affect, impulse control, interpersonal relationships, and identity. In addition, patients frequently engage in suicidal and parasuicidal behavior and other self-injurious acts, such as cutting and burning themselves, potentially dangerous sexual behavior, and substance abuse. Under stress, they may demonstrate transient paranoid ideation or in some cases even brief psychotic episodes or dissociative symptoms.

Borderline patients' experiences are marked by a pervasive internal emptiness and intense fear of abandonment by others. They cannot tolerate ambivalence and commonly use **splitting** as a defense. This defense is part of their tendency to see the world and the people in it as "all good" or "all bad," as it separates competing or conflicting feelings from one an-other so that the individuals can avoid anxiety by feeling only one emotion at a time. These affective states may shift rapidly.

Sheila R, a 34-year-old woman well known to the hospital and carrying a diagnosis of bor-derline personality disorder from her outpatient therapist, was admitted to the surgery service af-ter a below-the-knee amputation necessitated by compartment syndrome (swelling and ischemia of tissues in the extremities) after an apparently inadvertent overdose. A review of Ms. R's prior medical record indicated that she had several re-cent admissions for other "accidental" over-doses. This discovery led to a psychiatric evalu-ation. On initial interview, the student on the psychiatry consultation service observed multi-ple scars and what appeared to be cigarette burns on Ms. R's left arm and thighs.

Later during rounds, the mere mention of Ms. R's name caused eyes to roll as groans filled the room. This puzzled the psychiatry student who had just met Ms. R for the first time. To the stu-dent, Ms. R had seemed sweet, a little helpless, and quite sure that this hospital admission was going to be immensely helpful to her. Ms. R had already accepted the student's referral to the in-house substance abuse service. Also, when the student reviewed Ms. R's chart and spoke with her about her history, she was quite moved by the sad and painful experiences of Ms. R's life. After that first meeting, Ms. R thanked the stu-dent for the time spent with her, commenting on what a "wonderful listener" the student was and what a "good and understanding" physician she would be.

Later that day the student received a call from the nursing staff with complaints that Ms. R had been smoking in her room, had thrown a juice pitcher at her nurse, and had attempted to get out of bed into a wheelchair, claiming "if you're not going to let me smoke in here, I'm going to go outside." She refused a nicotine patch, yelling, "I'm not quitting!" The student arrived at Ms. R's room to find her sobbing loudly in bed. Although Ms. R initially had been glad to see the student, she became angry when the stu-dent told her she could not grant special permis-sion so that Ms. R could smoke in her room. Af-ter a lengthy conversation, Ms. R agreed to a nicotine patch but reportedly only because the student thought "it [was] a good idea." Ms. R further claimed, "I wouldn't do this for anyone else."

Ms. R's two-week acute hospital stay pro-ceeded in much the same way. She alternately praised and derided the primary medical team and nursing staff and occasionally made com-ments about the student's status as "just a stu-dent." This made the student feel both inade-quate and curiously angry and hostile in return. Ms. R wreaked havoc on the medical-surgical floor, and the nursing staff found it increasingly difficult to manage her constant use of the call button. Some staff members began to discuss her as "a manipulative drain on the system," while others viewed her as an unfortunate vic-tim of a difficult life and limited resources. In desperation, a team meeting was called to set clear rules and expectations. The student was surprised at how differently people viewed Ms. R, almost as though different patients were be-ing discussed.

The student continued to see Ms. R daily, with a focus on assessing suicidal ideation and potential for harming herself and preparing her for a transfer to rehabilitation. Ms. R adamantly denied suicidal ideation but refused to discuss her pending transfer from the acute hospital stay, saying only, "that's a long way off," when-ever it was brought up.

On the day of the transfer the student re-ceived a frantic call from the medical social worker, who reported that after a stormy night with the nurses, Ms. R left the unit and was nowhere to be found. The student became anx-ious and upset, and began thinking the worst—that perhaps Ms. R had killed herself or been victimized. Hurrying to the unit, the student found that Ms. R had returned from a two-hour "smoke break" and seemed secretly pleased by the uproar.

When reminded of her transfer, Ms. R ini-tially denied she was due to leave, then angrily refused to go. Finally, when the ambulance at-tendants arrived, she left, commenting that the student had been "absolutely no help at all."

The student felt depleted and questioned whether her involvement in the case had served any purpose. Later that day she felt relief that Ms. R was gone and caught herself making jokes about Ms. R with the intern and medical student on the primary team.

Diagnosis. Borderline personality disorder (Axis II).

Discussion. Parasuicidal behavior or overt suicide attempts are common in patients who have borderline personality disorder. These in-cidents often occur impulsively when the patient is feeling angry or depressed, or after the loss of a relationship. Lower-functioning borderline pa-tients often use self-mutilation as a means of re-lieving anxiety. Some patients may report self-mutilation as an attempt to punish themselves or to "feel alive." They may become dissociative under stress, which is characterized by deper-sonalization and derealization, and when mutilating themselves, may describe themselves as being "out of their body" or unable to feel pain. Some clinicians believe that naturally produced opiates (endorphins) account for some of the perception of diminished pain.

Affective instability and the intense expression of affect are also typical of borderline patients. Some patients will alternate between brief episodes of hypomania and depression in reaction to life events. Borderline patients often feel entitled to special treatment, and the dependency inherent in a hospital admission provides a perfect breeding ground for regression to more infantile behavior.

Another common trait is idealization, which is often followed rapidly by devaluation. Furthermore, clinicians, even the most experienced ones, often have strong and immediate emotional reactions to these patients. These feelings may fluctuate, paralleling or opposing the patient's affective state. Often they include intense anger, inadequacy, self-doubt, and depletion. Strong emotional reactions, both positive and negative, may be best addressed in medical hospital settings by team meetings focused on unifying the approach to patient care. This often involves setting clear limits on the amount and timing of nursing contact and picking one person from the primary team as the representative to the patient regarding ongoing care.

Borderline patients may make a better adjustment to the hospital in semiprivate rooms closer to the nursing station, as this location helps combat the fear that accompanies isolation. When the patient feels more secure, he or she is less likely to make excessive demands on the hospital staff. Abandonment fears are also common among borderline patients, making transfers and hospital discharges difficult to manage. Patients may act out fear of abandonment in a variety of ways, including vehement denial, rage-filled attacks on or devaluation of the perceived abandoner, and at times attacks against the self with the conscious or unconscious intent to avoid the transition at hand.

Clinicians should carefully assess the patient's trauma history when considering a diagnosis of borderline personality disorder, as many features of complex post-traumatic stress disorder overlap with those of borderline personality disorder.

Associated Disorders. Patients who have borderline personality disorder often have other associated Axis I disorders, including mood disorders (eg, cyclothymia and bipolar disorder type II), post-traumatic stress disorder, and substance use disorders. These patients also may be more vulnerable to eating disorders. Lower-functioning patients may be subject to psychotic regression under stress. Additional co-

morbid diagnoses include brief reactive psychosis, cyclothymic disorder, panic disorder, dissociative disorders, and gender identity disorders, particularly in lower-functioning borderline patients. These individuals may struggle with somatoform disorders as well, and borderline personality disorder is commonly associated with other personality disorders. As discussed previously, the incidence of suicide is increased among these patients.

Antisocial Personality Disorder

The diagnosis of this disorder has a long history, at times complicated by the influence of judgmental, overly moralistic, and outright discriminatory thinking. The *DSM-IV* cautions that as socioeconomic and cultural factors often play a role in what is considered appropriate versus antisocial behavior, this diagnosis should be made with caution when the patient is of low socioeconomic status or from an urban environment.

Epidemiology. According to the *DSM-IV,* twin studies indicate that both environmental and genetic factors play a role in the development of antisocial personality disorder. First-degree biological relatives of individuals who have antisocial personality disorder have the highest risk of developing this condition. Interestingly, the risk of developing antisocial personality disorder is greater if the relative with the disorder is a woman. The diagnosis of antisocial personality disorder in the general population is 3% for men and 1% for women. In clinical populations the disorder is estimated at 3–30%, depending on the population studied.

Not surprisingly, antisocial personality disorder has a higher incidence in populations of substance abusers and prison inmates. The risk of developing this disorder is increased if the patient had an onset of conduct disorder before age 10 and a childhood diagnosis of attention-deficit/hyperactivity disorder. Despite the chronicity of antisocial personality disorder, symptoms tend to decrease or remit as age increases, particularly by the fourth decade. This decline may be the result of patients finding more socially sanctioned means of expressing their impulses, a general slowing of energy, or an age-associated decrease in their tendency to act out.

Core Features. The primary feature of antisocial personality disorder is a pervasive pattern of behavior marked by a disregard for prevailing social norms or by the violation of the rights of others. This pattern sometimes includes recurrent illegal behavior, though it is important to stress that every person who engages in illegal acts is not antisocial, nor is involvement in illegal behavior necessary for a diagnosis of antisocial personality disorder.

Patients who have antisocial personality disorder are often irresponsible and deceitful and at times lie, con, or otherwise manipulate or misuse others. Most significantly, these patients lack remorse for their behavior. Other features of antisocial personality disorder include impulsivity or lack of planning, low tolerance for anxiety, inability to delay gratification, irritability and recurrent physical fights or assaults, and a disregard for the safety of self and others.

The principle defense mechanism used is the projection of their own hostility onto the environment, leading to an increased expectation that others will be hostile toward them, and rationalization of their behavior. Although these patients may be superficially facile and charming when things are going their way, they may be resentful, demeaning, and demanding at other times.

Because antisocial personality disorder is perhaps the most difficult of the personality disorders to treat, assessment of the severity of this disorder is essential. In 1975, Otto Kernberg listed negative prognostic signs for severe antisocial psychopathology:

- no personal values
- no awareness of values systems in other people
- no awareness of the interpersonal implications of not having such values systems and the effect of this deficiency on others
- the predominance of generalized ruthlessness toward others, in contrast to the aggressive, impulsive, tumultuous behavior of patients who have borderline personality disorder
- contradictions between stated ethical values and behavior and the toleration of these contradictions without guilt or concern
- no **signal guilt,** by which adults self-correct inappropriate behavior after receiving some clue that they are acting unethically or violating personal or commonly held societal values

According to the *DSM-IV,* patients must be at least 18 years of age and have demonstrated evidence of conduct disorder prior to age 15 in order to meet the diagnostic criteria for antisocial personality disorder. **Conduct disorder** (a diagnosis given only to children or adolescents) is characterized by a pattern of behavior such as aggression toward animals or people, destruction of property, deceitfulness or theft, and serious violations of rules.

The deficiency or absence of conscience is central to antisocial psychopathology. Simply put, although some antisocial people may experience shame when their acts are discovered, they do not experience guilt and feel no compunction to conform to the rules that govern social behavior. These patients commonly complain of feeling bored and, more accurately, may experience a paucity of emotion. Theodore Millon stated that they may be keenly aware of the moods and feelings of others. However, rather than responding to other's emotions in an empathic manner, antisocial patients typically use this awareness to manipulate and take advantage of others. They may relish the pain they cause and find pleasure in their own ability to dominate and control.

Moira V, aged 30, presented at an outpatient clinic for a psychotherapy intake appointment. She relayed a lengthy history of loss and appeared genuinely distraught and tearful throughout the session. The psychiatry resident was moved by her story and impressed by her openness but at the same time felt oddly on guard. Ms. G, with apparent shame, reported a history of shoplifting and passing bad checks for which she had been caught many times and incarcerated in the past. She described a difficult personal history, including a neglectful and abusive childhood and her parents' expectation that she steal food to feed her family.

She also described prior psychotherapy, which she reported ending abruptly when she was accused of stealing property from the clinician's office. When asked if the accusations were true, she replied, "Well, if he was stupid enough to leave money and stuff lying around, he deserved whatever happened."

With only 5 minutes remaining in the session, Ms. V hurriedly reported that she was due in court the next day for her most recent arrest for shoplifting and that she required a letter stating that she was in psychotherapy and successfully addressing the problems which led to her stealing.

Wanting to assist her, the resident felt pressured to provide Ms. V with a letter stating that she had come for an intake appointment but told her he had to discuss doing so with his supervisor. Ms. V pleaded tearfully, "Write the letter now, you can talk with him about it later." Now quite uncomfortable, the resident stood his ground, stating that he would contact her that afternoon.

Later, the clinic secretary reported that she had stepped away from her desk and upon returning several minutes later found Ms. V with clinic letterhead and an envelope in her hand.

Diagnosis. Antisocial personality disorder (Axis II).

Discussion. Patients who have antisocial personality disorder are unlikely to consider the consequences of their actions, change their behavior, or learn from their experiences. Though these patients often create feelings of apprehension, suspicion, or anger in those around them, they are frequently accomplished at deception and the maintenance of a veneer of social appropriateness. Thus they are often able to "take people in." Problems arise when clinicians are unaware of the ways in which they are being deceived. For example, patients who have this disorder may count on the pressure of an ending clinical hour to coerce a clinician into granting inappropriate requests.

Patients who have antisocial personality disorder are unlikely to seek treatment voluntarily for symptoms of this condition. Typically, they come into contact with the mental health system after having been detained, incarcerated, or otherwise required to participate in court-ordered treatment. They may also come into contact with the medical system when their dangerous behavior results in physical injury, for example, an orthopedic injury sustained by a patient who jumped from rooftop to rooftop while fleeing the police. In these cases, indications of depression sometimes appear after incarceration. However, this depression is usually short-lived and is thought to be related both to having been caught and to the patient's inability to discharge intolerable affect in a structured setting such as a jail. The depression may also be accompanied by rage and anxiety. The possibility that the antisocial patient may seek treatment to avoid legal punishment should be considered as well.

Associated Disorders. According to the *DSM-IV*, common comorbid disorders include anxiety disorders, depressive disorders, substance abuse–related disorders, somatization disorder, and disorders of impulse control. Antisocial patients often have additional personality disorders, especially other cluster B disorders.

Narcissistic Personality Disorder

Narcissistic personality disorder is a relatively new diagnostic category, first used in the *DSM-III*. Some clinicians attribute the increased prevalence and significance of this disorder to sociocultural factors such as the rise in self-indulgence and in self-improvement movements popularized after World War II. In 1978, Christopher Lasch wrote a book describing these sociocultural changes, characterizing recent decades as creating "the culture of narcissism."

Although this diagnosis is relatively new, in 1931 Freud described "narcissistic libidinal types" in a manner consistent with the current diagnostic criteria. More recent theorists hold that narcissistic personality disorder has much in common with borderline personality disorder. Despite similarities in the defensive structure of these disorders (both rely heavily on the use of splitting and projection), narcissistic patients' attitudes and manner tend to be quite different from those of borderline patients. While borderline patients' self-perception is inconsistent, narcissists have overly inflated and unrealistic senses of self that often appear impenetrable.

Epidemiology. According to the *DSM-IV*, fewer than 1% of the general population meet the criteria for narcissistic personality disorder. In clinical populations, 2–16% may have this disorder. Significantly, 50–75% of those diagnosed as having narcissistic personality disorder are men. Although narcissistic traits may be especially common in adolescence, these traits do not necessarily indicate that an individual will develop narcissistic personality disorder as an adult. Often individuals who have this disorder encounter unusual difficulties adjusting to physical and other changes associated with aging.

Core Features. The core features of narcissistic personality disorder include a grandiose sense of self-importance and the concomitant desire to associate only with others also perceived as unique or exceptional. Preoccupation with grandiose fantasies and the need for excessive admiration are common. These patients exhibit arrogant and entitled attitudes and behaviors. They lack empathy and use other people to achieve their own ends. They are frequently preoccupied with envious feelings or the belief that others are envious of them.

The core conflict for patients who have narcissistic personality disorder is the fear of depending on others. A grandiose sense of self serves as a defense against an underlying sense of inadequacy and associated desperate reliance on others. When these defenses are not operating well, these patients are particularly vulnerable to damage to their underlying fragile sense of self, becoming susceptible to exaggerated hurts, or **narcissistic injuries.** When feeling these injuries, patients who have narcissistic personality disorder typically react with rage. Common defense mechanisms used by these patients include splitting and projection.

Interpersonally, individuals who have narcissistic personality disorder tend to engage in volatile relationships. Often these relationships begin with a period of intense involvement and idealization of the other, followed by devaluation, and rapid, sometimes explosive, severing of the relationship. Narcissistic people do not take responsibility for relationship difficulties. They lack capacity for empathy and are unable to truly understand the feelings of others.

Patients who have narcissistic personality disorder often elicit extreme emotional reactions from clinicians, ranging from idealization (which mirrors the patient's own grandiose sense of self) to angry devaluation. In the latter case, clinicians feel slights or injuries to their own narcissism when working with these patients.

Fernando L, a 45-year-old man, was brought to the medical emergency room with chest pains that began during a business meeting. Mr. L, a local businessman, insisted that his secretary be allowed to ride in the ambulance on the way to the hospital, and when the emergency medical technician (EMT) suggested that the secretary might follow in her own car, Mr. L became angry over the EMT's "inability to understand the important business" that he needed to finish. When he arrived at the emergency room and was assigned to a medical resident, he refused to speak with her, insisting that he would only be seen by the head of the emergency department.

After being diagnosed with a myocardial infarction, Mr. L was admitted to the hospital. He refused to be seen by students and residents, insisting, "I will only be treated by Dr. A, the head of cardiology. He's widely published and very well-known." Mr. L reduced a nurse to tears when he belittled her for placing him in a semiprivate room. When his roommate complained that he could not use the telephone they shared, Mr. L insisted that his business was "much more important than just chatting on the phone." Mr. L's nurse reminded him of the need to share the telephone and to remain calm because of his vulnerable cardiac status. Mr. L began screaming, "My heart is fine, I'm in excellent shape, and I have more important business than anyone else here!" He also threatened to file a lawsuit against the hospital.

Later Mr. L refused to go for a scheduled cardiac catheter because he was waiting for "an important call." Nursing staff complained that he ordered them around, expected them to take telephone messages, and required them to wait to take blood draws and vital signs. When the head nurse approached Mr. L regarding this behavior, he once again flew into a rage, telephoning the president of the hospital in order to complain about "the disrespectful and shoddy treatment" he was receiving. Later that evening, nursing staff overheard Mr. L berating his wife for her "sloppy attire" when she arrived in the emergency room that afternoon.

Diagnosis. Narcissistic personality disorder (Axis II).

Discussion. Although a strong sense of one's self-importance and worth is valuable and adaptive in many situations, it is the extreme and pervasive presence of these features that distinguishes a person who has narcissistic personality disorder from the healthy individual. Narcissistic people protect themselves against underlying self-doubt by requiring others to share a grandiose and distorted view of their self-importance. As a result, they have few and mostly superficial (or volatile) relationships with others. They have little capacity for mutuality or empathy and are largely unaware of how isolated and egocentric they are.

Often the hospital setting exacerbates these patients' symptoms as they attempt to compensate for feelings of vulnerability associated with the physical or psychological difficulties that led to the hospitalization. This can result in increased grandiosity, demands, and entitlement. At times, it may be necessary to assign only a few individuals to work with these patients. This strategy increases the likelihood that the patient will feel valued and understood by the physician.

Associated Disorders. According to the *DSM-IV*, dysthymic disorder and major depressive disorder

may be associated with narcissistic personality disorder in patients who are struggling with feelings of shame or humiliation. Patients may become more hypomanic when grandiose. Substance abuse–related disorders are a common problem, as is anorexia nervosa. Narcissistic personality disorder is associated with paranoid personality disorder and with all of the cluster B disorders.

Histrionic Personality Disorder

Epidemiology. Approximately 10–15% of mental health outpatients have histrionic personality disorder. Studies suggest a prevalence rate of 2–3% in the general population. Clinicians should review cultural norms regarding emotional expressiveness and sex-role expectations when considering this diagnosis.

Core Features. Core features of histrionic personality disorder include pervasive emotionality and attention seeking. These patients are reliant on others for admiration, are sensitive to the slightest sign of indifference or disinterest, and readily shift their behavior in attempts to sustain others' attention or admiration. When this fails, they easily succumb to feelings of dejection, anxiety, and emptiness.

Histrionic patients are often manipulative in their attempts to gain the attention of others. They are superficially charming and gregarious, in a sense, masters of "cocktail party sociability." Theatrical and dramatic, they draw attention by dress, mannerism, and an often charming, warm, and clever interpersonal style. This is often coupled with overt seductiveness or inappropriate sexuality. Given their superficiality, tendency to maintain multiple targets for affection, and emotional lability, they appear fickle and likely to "change with the wind."

Beneath this lively, dramatic, and engaging style lies an immature, poorly developed self-structure characterized by difficulty experiencing genuine feelings of love and intimacy, limited frustration tolerance, a craving for excitement and change, and a tendency to become easily bored by day-to-day routine.

Contact with medical professionals may be characterized by overt seductiveness and inappropriate overtures for physical contact.

Eleanor N was referred to the psychiatry clinic by her primary doctor, who reported that she had contacted him with multiple vague physical complaints in the past several weeks. When seen in the outpatient clinic, Ms. N complained of feeling "sad and lonely" at the end of a relationship. Though the psychiatrist had a difficult time eliciting details from Ms. N, over the course of two sessions he learned that the recently failed relationship was the latest in a series and that none had lasted more than several months. Ms. N wondered vaguely if there was a pattern. The psychiatrist considered this observation a possible sign of Ms. N's capacity for insight, despite her inability to take the observation further.

At her next appointment, Ms. N arrived looking carefully groomed. She commented on her brightly colored short dress, crossed her legs seductively, and asked the psychiatrist whether he liked how she was dressed. The question made the psychiatrist feel uncomfortable. Ms. N explained that she had gone out with friends after the last session and "met this wonderful man." She continued, "We've seen each other almost every evening this week, and he finds me special and wonderful, too. I think he may be the one." She reported that she would be seeing him soon after the session, adding that she thought they might "spend the night" for the first time that night. She looked momentarily uncomfortable at this prospect. When the psychiatrist asked how she was feeling, she answered breezily and with a bright smile, "Really, just fine!"

Diagnosis. Histrionic personality disorder (Axis II).

Discussion. Millon points to external preoccupation, massive use of repression, and superficial social relationships as factors that contribute to the perpetuation of histrionic patterns of behavior and dependence on others.

The experience of being with histrionic patients is unique. Often entertaining, they may relay stories in a vibrant and theatrical manner that conveys a sense of fun and adventure. Nevertheless, the histrionic use of repression, denial, and dissociation leads to a shallow, impressionistic, and global view of the world; a paucity of internal richness; and a lack of a cohesive inner self. These patients' preferred focus is on the external world and on gaining the approval of others. There is little self-reflection; thus, there is little cohesive inner experience from which to draw.

Histrionic patients tend not to present for psychotherapy unless confronted by some degree of social isolation. Psychotherapy focused on gaining insight into conflicts and inner dynamics is quite possible, though not easily tolerated. Early stages of therapy would likely focus on shoring up the patient's failing defenses and tolerating what is likely to be a strong, idealizing emotional reaction from the patient.

Although histrionic patients have an insatiable need for attention, and often behave in a seductive or even exhibitionistic manner to gain the attention of others, the capacity for mature intimacy on both a physical and emotional level is extremely limited, and their sexual function is often impaired. Given their tendency toward competitiveness, histrionic patients may have few friends of the same sex.

The histrionic-obsessive couple is well-documented in the literature as a common marital dyad. Each individual provides the other something of what is lacking internally. The obsessive person gets access to affect, and the histrionic person, structure and organization. It is not unusual for histrionic female patients to act out infantile fantasies and perceive their partners as all-powerful parental figures.

Associated Disorders. Histrionic personality disorder is associated with increased rates of somatization disorder and conversion disorder. One explanation for this association is the patient's tendency to deny emotional difficulties and express them through physical channels. Patients who have histrionic personality disorder may be more vulnerable to mood disorders, particularly when faced with the prospect of a relationship loss. Common comorbid personality disorders include the other cluster B disorders, as well as dependent personality disorder.

CLUSTER C: ANXIOUS OR FEARFUL

Patients who have cluster C personality disorders share difficulties with self-assertion and self-esteem. In addition, they are uncomfortable with even appropriately modulated expressions of aggression. Social withdrawal, feelings of inadequacy, and hypersensitivity to criticism are also common traits, although the modes of expressing these traits differ greatly from one personality disorder to another.

Avoidant Personality Disorder

Epidemiology. According to the *DSM-IV,* the prevalence of avoidant personality disorder in the general population is 0.5–1.0%. Approximately 10% of patients in outpatient mental health clinics are diagnosed as having this disorder. The *DSM-IV* cautions clinicians regarding the application of this disorder in cultural groups with increased expectation of diffidence, and in the application of this diagnosis to immigrants who may appear avoidant but are struggling with the process of acculturation. Age-appropriate shyness should not be misinterpreted as an indication of avoidant personality disorder in children and adolescents.

Core Features. The core feature of the avoidant personality disorder is a pervasive sense of inadequacy and hypersensitivity to real or imagined rejection, which is manifested in extraordinary social inhibition. Notably, avoidant personality disorder is the only ego-dystonic personality disorder. These patients are distressed by their condition, they long for things to be different, and they see themselves as the cause of their own difficulties.

Avoidant patients' lives often become extremely restricted and isolated in an effort to avoid feared criticism. These patients may associate with few people and then only with those whom they have assured themselves pose little threat of hostility or rejection. Although they may appear as withdrawn and isolated as patients who have schizoid personality disorder, they differ significantly in that they long for attachment to others, as opposed to preferring isolation and detachment.

Susan H, aged 28, made and canceled several appointments before appearing at an outpatient clinic. She complained of anxiety, depression, and "just feeling scared all the time." She appeared shy and distracted in the session and said, "it's always been hard for me to talk."

Ms. H described a 7-year relationship with a man who, by her own description, appeared to have been quite paranoid and emotionally abusive. This relationship ended 2 years earlier. She reported that she lived alone, had contact with her parents and brother, and had one friend with whom she went for an occasional walk, adding, "I guess my best friend is my cat."

She described a history of being an anxious child. She further stated that her parents were and remained "kind of critical." She said, "I was supposed to be the smartest, but nobody could be smarter than Dad." She further reported that although she never talked in school if she could avoid it, she was a good student and graduated from a prestigious university.

Since finishing college, Ms. H had held a series of jobs and described a pattern of poor work adjustment in a competitive and conflict-driven field. She reported "being fired once" several years earlier, which she tearfully described as "devastating." Since then, she claimed she had left several jobs abruptly (once on her lunch hour), "because they were just mean to me, and I knew I would be fired." She had held her present job, reshelving books in a library, for the past 6 months, stating "it's the longest time I've worked anywhere, but it's not very interesting."

Ms. H reported wistfully, "I see other people my age having fun, and I don't know what's wrong with me. I want to have friends and a better life, but I feel like a little kid looking in at a candy store. I want to go in, but I'm afraid someone will tell me I don't belong."

Diagnosis. Avoidant personality disorder (Axis II).

Discussion. Despite evident distress, avoidant patients' fears of rejection may well manifest in difficulty following up with plans to seek psychotherapy. They desire assistance and experience themselves as in need of aid but, as in all other relationships, lack trust and fear rejection and criticism in the psychotherapeutic relationship. Given their very low tolerance level for criticism, what may be experienced as constructive feedback or advice by some individuals is likely to be experienced as harsh, punitive, and horribly rejecting by patients who have avoidant personality disorder.

Avoidant patients are hypervigilant and overly sensitive to irrelevant environmental cues. In addition, they are often flooded with affect, which they attempt to repress. This combination can lead to a distracted and somewhat disorganized thought process. They often express the fear that they will become tearful or otherwise embarrass themselves in public when criticized.

Patients who have avoidant personality disorder fear that they are grossly inadequate and inferior and may carefully review their behaviors for inappropriateness or ineptitude. To others they appear anxious, inhibited, and tense and for this reason may engender the very reactions in others that they fear. These patients often adapt to a level of functioning far below their native abilities. For example, they will often gravitate toward jobs that allow them to work in isolation.

The fear of rejection may be especially problematic in medical settings where time constraints make patient contact brief and to the point. Clinicians are cautioned that these patients will misinterpret the rushed, hurried, and even mildly irritable environment of the clinic and will likely conclude that the physician is hostile toward them.

Associated Disorders. Patients who have avoidant personality disorder may suffer from mood disorders, and somatic complaints are common. Avoidant and dependent personality disorders are often associated, and avoidant personality disorder commonly co-occurs with borderline personality disorder.

Among the most vulnerable to Axis I disorders, patients who have avoidant personality disorder may experience anxiety disorders (including social phobia and panic disorder with agoraphobia). Extremely ruminative thought processes are not unusual in these patients, as they are prone to reviewing interactions for signs of their own inadequacy or the hostility of others. Anxiety disorders, when present, can further inhibit these patients and may lead to complete withdrawal.

Dependent Personality Disorder

Epidemiology. According to the *DSM-IV,* dependent personality disorder is among the most common diagnoses in mental health settings. Cultural factors contributing to sex-role expectations and expectations of increased deference must be considered when evaluating patients from different cultural and ethnic groups.

Core Features. The core feature of dependent

personality disorder is an extraordinary need to be taken care of, which manifests itself in needy, clinging, and submissive behavior. These patients are in search of support and reassurance in all areas of life and have difficulty coming to even simple decisions on their own. They may appear gentle, thoughtful, and generous in nature, but this comes at the cost of denying any strong emotion that may threaten their dependent attachment. These patients have trouble taking initiative, and they express feelings of helplessness when left on their own. They are preoccupied with fears of loss of their caregiver and become frantic to find another caregiver if that relationship comes to an end. Patients who have dependent personality disorder are filled with doubt about their abilities, and although on the surface they may appear positive in outlook, in reality they are quite pessimistic.

The physician is cautioned regarding diagnosis of this personality disorder in patients who are struggling with a serious general medical condition. Increased dependence is common under those circumstances. In order to diagnose dependent personality disorder, the physician must have evidence of dependence that exceeds what might be expected given the patient's medical status, as well as a pervasive pattern of dependent behavior beginning by early adulthood and present across circumstances.

Gordon B, aged 59, had a fever of unknown origin and was medically admitted after complaining to psychiatric emergency services of suicidality with a plan to drown himself. Mr. B reported that his suicidal ideation emerged in response to a growing fear that his sister would ask him to move out of her home.

Mr. B, who completed all but his dissertation for a PhD in chemical engineering, lived with his parents until they died while he was in his mid-40s. He described an abrupt decision at that time to marry a biologist several years his senior, saying, "She thought we should. I wasn't sure, but I was glad not to be alone."

He stated that although he "dabbled" in work and in teaching, he never earned money enough to support himself and his wife, but he said, "I didn't need to. She was very successful. She made all the decisions." Mr. B reported that because he did not work outside the home, he was "obliged to take care of the home and do all the menial and unpleasant tasks, including going under the house where the spiders were to fix the sump pump." He added, "But that was fine, that was the arrangement." The marriage ended by his wife's choice, several years earlier, at which time he made a "temporary but permanent" move to his sister's home.

Mr. B described a several-year decline in function. He said that his ex-wife wanted nothing to do with him, even though he often called to beg her to take him back. Mr. B then asked the psychiatrist to contact a friend of his to let him know that he was in the hospital. Though encouraged to contact the friend himself, Mr. B refused, and the psychiatrist asked his permission to make a collateral call. When interviewed, the friend described Mr. B's growing dependence: "He calls me every day. I started out helping him with his social security disability application, but now he asks for help with everything. He can't even decide what to bring home from the grocery store, it seems."

The nursing staff described Mr. B as "needy" and "expecting a lot of assistance." They reported that he appeared unwilling to initiate tasks without considerable encouragement. While visiting a patient in a nearby bed, the psychiatrist observed Mr. B asking a nurse to change the channel on the TV because he didn't know how and also asking her, "Will you just come talk to me? What do you think I should do about my finances?" When the nurse suggested he could make these decisions without her input, Mr. B became tearful and said, "I can't take care of things myself. I never have."

Diagnosis. Dependent personality disorder (Axis II).

Discussion. Because patients who have dependent personality disorder believe that they are unable to provide for themselves and need to be cared for by others, the threat of loss of the people on whom they depend may precipitate a significant crisis.

These patients are extremely passive and may fear and avoid the development of any competence that may lead to expectations from others that they care for themselves. They allow others to make all decisions, from the simplest to the most complex.

To foster their dependent connections, these patients characteristically assume a "one down" position. They play up their deficits, hide their strengths, and minimize any conflicts that may arise in relationships. These patients often appear naive to others. However, their focus on the good and positive serves as an attempt to avoid confronting difficulties that may threaten their attachment.

Clinicians treating these patients are cautioned that their own emotional reactions may include a tendency to allow inappropriately dependent behavior.

The dependent individual's demands for support and care may be difficult for partners to tolerate and may lead to rejection. When confronted with the loss of a relationship, these patients may be indiscriminate in their search for a new attachment figure. They may go along with things with which they disagree or may put up with extremely noxious or dangerous circumstances, including physical or sexual abuse, in order to avoid the loss of a relationship.

Associated Disorders. According to the *DSM-IV,* patients who have dependent personality disorder may be at an increased risk for mood disorders, anxiety disorders, and adjustment disorders. Common comorbid personality disorders include borderline, histrionic, and avoidant. In children, associated disorders include separation anxiety disorder or chronic physical illnesses.

Obsessive-Compulsive Personality Disorder

Obsessions and compulsions may be present in both obsessive-compulsive personality disorder (OCPD) and in obsessive-compulsive disorder (OCD), an Axis I disorder. **Obsessions** refer to repetitive thoughts, and **compulsions** are defined as repetitive actions.

Obsessive-compulsive symptoms are more extreme and acute in OCD and are experienced as distressing and alien. OCD is often accompanied by prominent rituals or marked repetitive behaviors, in contrast to OCPD. Most patients who have OCPD do not have coexisting OCD.

Epidemiology. According to the *DSM-IV,* OCPD is present in approximately 1% of the general population and in 3–10% of individuals seen in mental health settings. Men are diagnosed with this disorder about twice as often as women.

Core Features. The primary feature of OCPD is a preoccupation with orderliness and perfectionism and the existence of rigid attempts by patients to control others and themselves. There is a marked absence of flexibility, openness, and efficiency that accompanies the former qualities.

Specifically, individuals who have OCPD make perfection a higher priority than actually completing tasks. They lose the point of activities in their preoccupation with details, rules, lists, order, organization, and schedules. They are reluctant to delegate tasks to others, unless those individuals share the same perfectionistic approach. Obsessive-compulsive individuals place work and productivity over friendships and pleasure.

These individuals are also interpersonally rigid and stubborn. They are miserly and stingy, both financially and emotionally, with themselves and others. Finally, they are excessively conscientious and rigid regarding moral and ethical matters.

Core conflicts of individuals who have OCPD revolve around issues of control. Common defense mechanisms include **undoing** and **isolation of affect.** Undoing involves counterbalancing actions or thoughts that remove or minimize the anxiety associated with other thoughts or actions. For example, a patient may state that he is feeling very angry with a family member, then shortly thereafter describe wanting to do something kind for the family member. Isolation of affect involves keeping ideas separate from the feelings typically associated with them. These defenses are used in an attempt to exercise control over thoughts and impulses felt to be unacceptable, as well as to avoid the experience of feeling controlled by others.

Frederick S, a 30-year-old bank manager, was hospitalized after running his car into another car on the freeway. While Mr. S was recovering from a broken pelvis and leg and multiple contusions sustained in the accident, the orthopedic resident requested a psychiatric consultation to address concerns she had about Mr. S's apparent depression and his criticisms that he "deserved this, by God," as well as his repeated complaints of "dirt and germs" in his hospital room.

When the psychiatry resident met Mr. S, she noticed that despite his casts and poor physical condition, he appeared utterly fastidious (clean shaven, extremely well-groomed, and wearing his own pajamas, which appeared starched). His room was equally fastidiously arranged: He was observed stacking and restacking his tidily arranged clothing on the dresser, and his other belongings were aligned in careful order on the desk, above which was a calendar that neatly listed scheduled physical therapy appointments and various medical procedures.

Mr. S said he lived with his parents and had only recently been promoted from bank teller to manager. He described many difficulties in his new position, including his coworker's "sloppiness." He added that he usually does all the work himself, but that "there is never enough time." He described how he had trouble completing projects on time because he checked and rechecked figures before allowing himself to go home, where he usually continued working in his home office.

He continued describing a mostly solitary lifestyle. He occasionally dated women from his church, rarely having a second date because, he claimed, the women had "less than virtuous pasts" and "unclean habits." Mr. S alluded to his injuries being "not completely" accidental, and the psychiatrist learned that several days before the accident he had "picked up a prostitute" and became severely depressed immediately thereafter. He was convinced that he had contracted a sexually transmitted disease and believed the accident and his suspected sexually transmitted disease were "punishments by God."

Mr. S responded well to antidepressant medications and accepted a referral to a private psychologist for outpatient psychotherapy. Several weeks later the psychologist reported that Mr. S was quite guarded but making use of treatment, that he brought long and detailed lists of issues to discuss in therapy, and that he decided to return to his old position as a teller.

Diagnosis. Obsessive-compulsive personality disorder (Axis II); consider major depressive episode (Axis I).

Discussion. Patients who have OCPD display rigidly moralistic thinking that is present in the form of harsh, punitive judgments directed toward themselves or others.

A preoccupation with orderliness, perfectionism, and rigid control may consume all of the patient's time. This focus may be in part adaptive and is often rewarded in contexts that require high performance, such as graduate school or jobs that require great attention to detail. However, this preoccupation typically leads to inefficiency in that the individual loses the point of a given activity by being caught up in the details.

It is essential to ascertain that moral beliefs are not shared by others within specific cultural or religious groups before attributing them to OCPD.

Associated Disorders. According to the *DSM-IV,* associations between OCPD and mood and anxiety disorders may be present. There is considerable overlap between many features of OCPD and Type A personality characteristics, such as competitiveness, aggressiveness, and time urgency. These common features may be present in individuals who are at risk for myocardial infarction.

TREATMENT

Use of Personality Disorder Diagnoses in the Clinical Record

A diagnosis of a personality disorder—especially cluster B disorders such as borderline or antisocial—may be misused by medical teams to justify an unwarranted lower standard of medical care. Any mention of a diagnosis of personality disorder in a patient's record is considered to be a sensitive subject.

In the absence of accurate historical information and a thorough, ongoing clinical assessment, indications of an Axis II diagnosis should be charted in the clinical record as provisional, if at all. As mentioned previously, clinicians should note symptoms of a personality disorder as "personality traits" on Axis II for any individual who does not meet all of the criteria for a given diagnosis. Providing an Axis II diagnosis or provisional diagnosis accompanied by recommen-

dations for intervention may be helpful for several reasons:

- It may help the team unify their approach to caring for the more difficult Axis II patients.
- It may help the team recognize that the observed traits are stable and relatively unchanging and that the patient's response to the hospital admission should not be taken personally.
- It may assist the patient and team in recognizing and preparing for critical junctures in treatment, such as preparation for discharge or receipt of bad medical news.
- It may help the team adjust their approach to a patient who may be unexpectedly sensitive to subtle nuances in individual style, including communication about medical diagnoses and treatment.

In summary, the purpose of diagnosis is to provide the foundation for effective clinical intervention.

Inpatient Medical Settings

When a patient's personality disorder symptoms interfere significantly with his or her ability to participate in care, it is often helpful to contact the hospital's psychiatry consultation service. These difficulties are most likely to occur with patients who have borderline, paranoid, or narcissistic personality disorders.

Whether students are doing rotations on psychiatry services or in other medical specialties, they are likely to be involved in the care of these difficult patients. Useful steps and interventions include the following:

- Seek additional supervision to manage these problematic patients as well as to understand the feelings they arouse in their caregivers.
- Participate in team meetings aimed at predicting and preparing for difficult transitions as well as unifying the approach to patient care.
- Assist staff in the structure of patient contact. This may include having contact with the patient at regular intervals in order to avoid the unintentional reinforcement of dependent and demanding behavior. It may also include assigning particular providers to have direct contact with the patient, to decrease the likelihood of splitting, which may occur when multiple providers are directly involved with the patient.
- Assist staff in providing patients with appropriate opportunities for choice and control.
- Help the staff to respond with clear, nonemotional limits and expectations when behavioral problems arise. Limits are most effective when they are presented to the patient as alternatives. Even when it is not appropriate to comply with a patient's wishes or requests, it is advantageous to present the patient with other options. Behavioral contracts are often a useful tool.

- Predict difficult transitions in advance. This may be helpful with some patients, as it will increase their internal structure and sense of control. However, this approach may be less effective with patients who have paranoid personality disorder, as it may increase their suspiciousness and concern that someone else has control over them.
- Assess and intervene in substance abuse. Substance abuse and dependence are rampant problems in our society, and evaluating and intervening in a substance use disorder is an important component of a successful hospital admission. This includes assessing for drug and alcohol abuse, which may create withdrawal symptoms and lead to difficulties in patient management. It also requires recognizing that in some hospital settings patients may continue using the substance during their admission, endangering their safety and the efficacy of their care. The substance abuse services in the hospital, if available, may be an excellent resource to call upon and are an excellent resource for arranging community follow-up as well.
- Contact mental health professionals involved in the patient's community care. This is only possible if such a person is available and the patient is willing to provide a release of information; however, contact is recommended to learn about recent stressors, the patient's medication history (if any), and approaches to care that may be most helpful. In addition, contact with the provider in the community may minimize the patient's likelihood of splitting (eg, viewing one provider as "all good" while the other is seen as "all bad"), which can occur between inpatient and outpatient providers.

Medications

Contact with psychiatrists in the community and consultation with the in-house psychiatry consultation service may be most helpful in assessing the patient for the appropriateness of a medication trial. Psychiatric medications are considered in the management of some Axis II personality disorders or when a personality disorder coexists with a transient or chronic Axis I mood, psychotic, or anxiety disorder.

Psychotic Symptoms. A psychotic disorder may occur as a separate, ongoing Axis I disorder or transiently in the setting of some personality disorders (eg, in borderline or paranoid personality disorders). A brief period of several weeks to months on a low dose of antipsychotic medication may be useful in intervening in more transient psychotic states. As with all medications, receiving informed consent is important, both for legal and ethical reasons and to discourage the patient from interpreting side effects as a punishment or as carelessness on the physician's part.

Mood Disorder Symptoms. Antidepressant medications may be helpful in treating patients who have dysthymia or major depression co-occurring with a personality disorder. Patients should be observed carefully for side effects, as some antidepressants, most notably some selective serotonin re-uptake inhibitors (SSRIs), may boost vulnerable patients into a hypomanic or manic state (possibly with psychotic features) or otherwise lead to a decrease in functioning. Patients who have borderline personality disorder may be particularly vulnerable to this reaction.

When treating patients who have depressive disorders, suicide risk must be considered. A patient's risk for suicide increases as his or her depressed mood lifts because of the increased energy available to act on impulses. Therefore, the early stages of treatment with antidepressants warrant close follow-up for safety assessment in patients who have an increased risk of suicide. The choice of antidepressant medication must be considered carefully as well. SSRIs may be preferred over tricyclic antidepressants (TCAs), as the chance for a lethal overdose is increased with the TCAs. See Chapter 14 for further discussion on managing suicidal patients.

Mood stabilizers, such as lithium or valproic acid, are used occasionally with patients whose borderline personality disorder is accompanied by lability of mood or cyclothymia.

Anxiety Disorders. Antidepressant medications may be helpful in the treatment of patients who have anxiety disorders and may be preferable to benzodiazepines, given the addictive properties of the latter class of medications. Patients who have cluster C personality disorders are at an increased risk of benzodiazepine addiction, though any patient who takes benzodiazepines over the long-term risks developing tolerance to the medication.

Antidepressant medications may be helpful in treating patients who have OCPD, particularly if prominent ruminations or symptoms of OCD on Axis I are present.

Referrals to the Community

Many of the patients described in cases in this chapter would benefit from community referrals, for example, to substance abuse programs, group therapy programs focusing on parenting concerns or other psychosocial issues, or psychotherapy programs. Making an effective referral—one the patient is likely to follow through with—involves more than simply giving him or her a name and telephone number. The physician should find a way to present the recommendation using the patient's own stated goals and concerns, and to leave sufficient time for the patient to ask questions about the recommendation.

It is useful to have ready access to community referrals. While in medical school and during residency, with rotations that require changes of location and rapid adjustment to each new setting, trainees should contact in-house services such as substance abuse programs, medical social services, and psychiatry consultation services to become familiar and comfortable with these services.

After training, it is strongly recommended that each physician develop a working knowledge of mental health resources in his or her community, including sliding-scale agencies and private practice psychiatrists and psychologists who are interested in working in a collaborative relationship with patients and their referring medical doctors.

EMOTIONAL REACTIONS TO PATIENTS

Patients who have personality disorders are capable of generating significant distress and other emotional reactions in health-care providers. These responses may be especially strong because these patients use primitive defenses that often project problematic emotions onto the people who care for them. The defense mechanism of projective identification results in the clinician taking on the feelings and emotions that originally belonged to the patient. Thus the angry patient who has borderline personality disorder may be relatively calm while the nurses and doctors are left in chaotic disarray, arguing with each other from different viewpoints.

Projective identification and splitting of staff often helps clinicians to understand the patient's subjective experience. Physicians must strive to keep their own feelings in perspective and recognize what is happening with the patient. Otherwise the medical staff will feel increasingly "burned out" and depleted, and the quality of medical care may be undermined. Managing emotional reactions to patients who have personality disorders is also a matter of leadership from the physician, of recognizing emotional responses but not being ruled by them, and of helping others to regain an objective view of their patients. This includes recognizing that patients who are often superficially seen as hostile, dependent, and demanding are struggling with deeper chronic and profound emotional suffering.

LEGAL & ETHICAL ISSUES

Working with patients who may have personality disorders presents numerous legal and ethical issues.

Because personality disorders are generally ego-syntonic, patients may not report critical symptoms and may distort facts and situations to minimize their own contribution to relationship problems. It is therefore critical for clinicians to speak with collateral sources of information (eg, parents, spouses, friends, adult children) to determine the extent of a patient's interpersonal difficulties. Except during emergencies (eg, when a patient is being evaluated for possible suicidal ideation or immediately after a suicide attempt), the patient's permission is required to contact other people in an attempt to learn more about his or her life and functioning.

Case law has largely upheld the confidentiality of patient-therapist privilege and legally prohibits therapists from divulging these accounts to authorities under most conditions. An exception to confidentiality occurs when a patient presents a current or future potential threat of violence to a reasonably identifiable victim. Under these circumstances, even if the patient tries to invoke the principle of confidentiality, therapists must follow the so-called Tarasoff guidelines and warn both the intended victim and the local police of the possible threat.

> Frank L, a 33-year-old patient who had a long history of intravenous heroin use and repeated skin infections, was hospitalized for abscesses and possible endocarditis. Mr. L's history included several jail terms for assault and robbery. Mr. L told the student on the medicine service that he felt that he had been mistreated by the orderlies in the emergency room. He revealed that he was plotting to loiter outside the ER and "sneak up on them and teach them a lesson." Mr. L added that he was telling the student this information "in confidence," adding, "I know that you're not going to betray me."
>
> The student explained that she was part of a team participating in his care and would have to relay his possible threatening fantasies to the resident. A psychiatric consultation was also obtained, although Mr. L was minimally cooperative. Based on his history and his elaborately detailed plans to harm specific individuals, the psychiatrist followed Tarasoff guidelines and called the ER staff and the local police to advise them of the possible threat.
>
> **Diagnosis.** Antisocial personality disorder (Axis II); endocarditis (Axis III).

Patients who have borderline personality disorder often have childhood histories marked by physical and sexual abuse. Clinicians need to determine if the perpetrator (often a parent, family member, or friend) has any current contact with children that might necessitate contact with child protective services, sometimes in direct contradiction to the patient's wishes.

Another question involves whether it is appropriate or advisable to record the diagnosis of a personality disorder in a patient's chart. Making a diagnosis of a personality disorder is often valuable in predicting a patient's behavior, the staff's response to the patient, potential pitfalls in forging a therapeutic alliance, and in defining a treatment plan. Being aware of an Axis II diagnosis may help the medical or psychiatric team avoid floundering unnecessarily for days with difficult interactions with the patient. However, a diagnosis of a personality disorder (especially cluster B disorders) may also be used inappropriately by staff to justify an inferior standard of patient care. Psychiatric disorders also tend to "follow" a patient and are difficult to undo.

Many insurance and managed care companies and health maintenance organizations (HMOs) do not pay for the treatment of personality disorders. These companies state that because personality disorders are chronic conditions that start in early adulthood, they are actually "preexisting conditions" for which they should not be responsible.

> Jennifer A saw Dr. Jones, her primary care physician, for treatment of panic attacks and depression. Ms. A had a history of sexual abuse during childhood and several suicide attempts in her 20s, and she had multiple scars on her forearms from cutting herself. Ms. A's insurance company listed several psychiatric disorders that were exempted for reimbursement, including personality disorders.
>
> Dr. Jones knew that if he referred Ms. A for psychotherapy with a diagnosis of possible borderline personality disorder, her insurance company would not pay for her treatment and that she could not afford consistent alternative care. Dr. Jones therefore listed only Axis I disorders on Ms. A's referral form, ascribing her self-destructive behavior to complex post-traumatic stress disorder. Dr. Jones remained troubled by this decision, wondering whether he was justified in distorting Ms. A's diagnosis to ensure her access to care.
>
> **Discussion.** Readers should be discomforted by Dr. Jones's legal and ethical dilemma. He can no doubt rationalize his decision to omit the diagnosis of borderline personality disorder by insisting that he is trying to provide quality care to his patient, that there is controversy about whether patients with repeated trauma in childhood are erroneously labeled with Axis II diagnoses, and that the insurance company's exemption for personality disorders is itself unethical. However, his actions involve distortion and deception about a patient's diagnosis, which could be legally construed as insurance fraud.

Reiser and Levenson have described a number of inappropriate uses of the personality disorder diagnoses. These include blaming the patient for treatment complications and distorting patients' healthy emotional responses to illness into psychopathology. This may occur when patients refuse recommended treatment.

> A psychiatric consultation was requested for Thomas B, a 51-year-old patient who was refusing dialysis. A review of Mr. B's chart revealed that the medical team had found him to be likable during his initial hospitalization for fatigue and anemia. However, on the day of consultation the medical team's charting changed abruptly to read, "Patient informed that he has chronic renal insufficiency and requires dialysis. Patient refusing dialysis, emotionally labile. Clearly has poor reality testing—likely borderline personality disorder."
>
> However, the psychiatrist interviewed the patient and his medical and nursing teams, and assembled a different story. Apparently the medical team was post-call and very tired, having been awake and working steadily for 30 hours when they met with Mr. B. They told him that he needed surgery to install a shunt for dialysis.
>
> When he anxiously requested more information, the team told him, "We just admitted 12 new patients, and we don't have time to talk with you—the dialysis nurse will stop in later to explain the procedure." Mr. B became panicked and requested a second opinion. The resident and intern were insulted and told Mr. B that this was not how things worked in the hospital and that he needed to sign the consent papers as soon as possible. Mr. B refused, and the psychiatric consultation was requested.
>
> The psychiatrist did not suspect a personality disorder based on the interview with Mr. B and Mr. B's wife and believed that the situation would be resolved if Mr. B and the medical team had a chance to gain perspective on the situation. She allowed Mr. B to share his feelings of frustration and separately allowed the medical team to do the same. She then served as communications "referee" at the next meeting of the team and Mr. B. The meeting went well, with the team spending more time discussing Mr. B's diagnosis, treatment options, and prognosis. Mr. B agreed to dialysis, and there were no further problems during the hospitalization.
>
> **Diagnosis.** Possible adjustment disorder with anxiety due to recent stressor (medical illness) (Axis I); none (Axis II).
>
> **Discussion.** Overdiagnosis of personality disorders in hospitalized and similarly stressed individuals is not unusual. Clinicians who consider any personality disorder diagnosis should remember that these disorders are lifelong rather than situa-

tional and should always confirm diagnostic impressions with collateral information, if available.

CONCLUSION

Personality disorders are frequently encountered in medical and psychiatric practice. It is essential for physicians to develop an understanding of diagnostic and treatment approaches to these disorders. A diagnosis of a personality disorder should be based upon careful and thorough investigation of the patient's baseline state, with information from collateral sources. Overdiagnosis of personality disorders occurs when patients who are emotionally stressed by physical illness and regressed in inpatient medical or psychiatric hospital settings make increasing use of primitive defense mechanisms. Once a personality disorder is accurately diagnosed, it often helps clinicians to predict the patient's reactions to critical events, and assists the medical staff in identifying possible pitfalls in the patient's care.

A treatment plan that includes recommendations on how to interact with the patient on a daily basis is often useful to guide other staff members. Because of the intense nature of the staff's emotional reactions to patients who have personality disorders, clinicians should strive to understand and utilize their own reactions and to provide strong leadership to medical staff to prevent any lowering of standards of care based on negative feelings for the patient. Intense emotional responses must be understood and mastered in order to aid in the detection of personality disorders and to attend to the patient's emotional state.

Clinical formulation of personality disorders has expanded over the past hundred years to encompass a well-researched body of knowledge about different character disorders. However, intriguing puzzles remain to be solved about the origins of personality disorders and personality in general. The relative contributions of genetics and environment—the age-old question of "nature versus nurture"—remain. When does personality first emerge? To what extent do gender and sociocultural factors affect the development of personality? How persistent or malleable are personality traits? It is known for example that many young children are shy and inhibited at age 3 or 4, but by 10 years of age most of these children have outgrown their shyness. A parenting style that provides guidelines for children as if they were not shy has been associated with greatest chance of encouraging more adventurous behavior, alone and interpersonally.

Thus the study of personality traits may yield valuable information and advice to guide parents in raising children to be healthy, resilient, and maximally fulfill their potential. Ultimately, the study of personality raises questions about the nature and meaning of individuality and those precious mental commodities that make each of us unique in spite of our shared genetic and cultural heritage.

REFERENCES

American Psychiatric Association: *Diagnostic and Statistical Manual of Mental Disorders,* 2nd ed, 1968.

American Psychiatric Association: *Diagnostic and Statistical Manual of Mental Disorders,* 3rd ed, 1980.

American Psychiatric Association: *Diagnostic and Statistical Manual of Mental Disorders,* 4th ed, 1994.

Breuer J, Freud S: Studies on hysteria (1893–1895). In: Strachey J (editor): *The Standard Edition of the Complete Psychological Works of Sigmund Freud.* Vol. 11. Hogarth, 1955.

Bychowski G: The problem of latent psychosis. J Am Psychoanal Assoc 1953;4:484.

Cameron N, Rychlak J: *Personality Development and Psychopathology: A Dynamic Approach.* Houghton Mifflin, 1985.

Cleckley H: *The Mask of Sanity.* Mosby, 1941.

Federn P: Principles of psychotherapy in latent schizophrenia. Am J Psychother 1947;1:129.

Freud S: Character and anal eroticism. In: Strachey J (editor): *The Standard Edition of the Complete Psychological Works of Sigmund Freud.* Vol 12. Hogarth, 1958.

Freud S: Libidinal types. In: Strachey J (editor): *The Standard Edition of the Complete Psychological Works of Sigmund Freud.* Vol. 21. Hogarth, 1961.

Hoch A: Constitutional factors in the dementia praecox group. Rev Neurol Psychiatr 1910;8:463.

Internet Mental Health: Borderline Personality Disorder. http://www.mentalhealth.com/dis/p20-pe05.html

Kagan J: *Galen's Prophecy: Temperament in Human Nature.* Basic Books, 1994.

Kernberg O: Structural derivatives of object relationships. Pages 350–384 in: Buckley P (editor): *Essential Papers on Object Relations.* New York University Press, 1986.

Kernberg O: *Borderline Condition and Pathological Narcissism.* Jason Aronson, 1975.

Kraeplin E: *Dementia Praecox and Paraphrenia.* Livingstone, 1919.

Kraeplin E: *Manic-depressive Insanity in Paranoia.* Livingstone, 1921.

Kretschmer E: *Physique and Character.* Kegan Paul, 1925.

Lasch C: *The Culture of Narcissism.* Norton, 1978.

MacKinnon RA, Michels R: *The Psychiatric Interview in Clinical Practice.* Saunders, 1971.

Masterson JF: *The Narcissistic and Borderline Disorders: An Integrated Developmental Approach.* Brunner/Mazel, 1981.

Millon T: *Modern Pyschopathology: A Biosocial Approach to Maladaptive Learning and Functioning.* Saunders, 1969.

Millon T: *Disorders of Personality.* Wiley Interscience, 1981.

Nardo JM: The personality in the medical setting: a psychodynamic understanding. In: *Psychiatry,* Vol. 2. Lippincott, 1989.

Rado S: Schizotypal organization: preliminary report on a clinical study of schizophrenia. Pages 225–236 in: Rado S, Daniels GE (editors): *Changing Concepts of Psychoanalytic Medicine.* Grune & Stratton, 1956.

Rado S: *Adaptational Psychodynamics.* Science House, 1969.

Rapaport D et al: *Diagnostic Psychological Testing.* International Universities Press, 1968.

Reiser D & Levenson H: Abuses of the borderline diagnosis: a clinical problem with teaching opportunities. Am J Psychiatr 1984;141(12):1528.

Siever LJ, Bernstein DP, Silverman JM: Schizotypal personality disorder: a review of its current status. J Pers Disord 1991;5(2):178.

Stone MH: *Abnormalities of Personality.* Norton, 1993.

Vaillant G: The beginning of wisdom is never calling a patient borderline. J Psychother Pract Res 1992;1(2):117.

Eating Disorders

13

Claudia E. Toomey, PhD, & John DiMartini, PhD

Eating disorders form a continuum of severe eating and weight disturbances and underlying psychopathology. A disturbance in the perception of body shape and weight is an essential feature of these disorders. At the most severe end of this continuum is the extreme weight loss characteristic of **anorexia nervosa.** The severe emaciation found in anorexia nervosa may be induced by strict food restriction (**restricting type**); or by either regularly engaging in binge eating followed by purging or purging after eating small amounts of food (**binge-eating/purging type**).

Next on the continuum is **bulimia nervosa,** which is found among individuals of average weight and is characterized by the same chaotic eating pattern found in the binge-eating/purging type of anorexia. In this disorder, periods of restricted food intake are interspersed with episodes during which large amounts of food are ingested. These episodes are followed by self-induced vomiting, laxative or diuretic abuse, fasting, or excessive exercising aimed at counteracting weight gain.

Further along the continuum is **binge-eating disorder,** a new diagnostic category recently listed as provisional in the *DSM-IV*. This disorder is characterized by recurrent episodes of binge eating but without the compensatory behaviors seen in bulimia nervosa. Accordingly, many individuals who have this disorder are of above-average body weight. At the end of the continuum are **eating disorders not otherwise specified (NOS)**, which are disorders that do not meet the full criteria for any specific eating disorder.

Obesity is a general medical condition that has not been consistently shown to be associated with a psychological or behavioral syndrome. However, a subgroup of obese individuals do appear to binge eat and to exhibit the psychological and behavioral characteristics of binge-eating disorder.

Some clinicians may erroneously consider eating disorders to be exotic syndromes whose treatment is best left in the hands of psychiatrists. There are two compelling reasons that argue against this narrow view. First, most patients with eating disorders are secretive about their behavior, and may be especially reluctant to see a mental health professional. General practice physicians and specialists in adolescent medicine, endocrinology, cardiology, gastroenterology, and obstetrics and gynecology thus bear the primary responsibility for the detection and initial referral of patients with eating disorders. Also, the serious medical complications of eating disorders—often extending over many years—are best managed by a multidisciplinary team of physicians who are knowledgeable about these disorders.

INCIDENCE

Women appear to be especially vulnerable to developing eating disorders: they represent 90% of individuals diagnosed as having an eating disorder. The fact that eating disorders are selectively prevalent among women living in industrialized societies—societies in which food is plentiful, where the roles of women are in flux, and where there is an emphasis on thinness as an ideal of female beauty—strongly suggests that sociocultural factors play a significant role in the pathogenesis of these disorders.

Many research studies have indicated that preoccupation with food and weight is surprisingly common in the general female population and that eating disorders have increased over the past 30 years. Distressingly, recent research has also found that restrictive eating, bingeing and purging behavior, and distorted body image problems, once believed to be disorders of adolescence and early adulthood, have been found in many girls as young as age 9. Within clinical populations, eating disorders are still found most commonly among Caucasian females of middle to upper middle class backgrounds. However, ethnic, socioeconomic, and gender demographics appear to have shifted somewhat in recent years.

Bulimia nervosa and binge-eating disorder are more common than is anorexia nervosa. Among adolescent girls and young adult women, the prevalence of bulimia nervosa is believed to be around 1–3%. The prevalence of binge-eating disorder is 0.7–4% in non-patient community samples. These estimates are likely conservative given that these disorders tend to be highly secretive and, as a result, are underreported. Indeed, research suggests that roughly 36% of young adult women exhibit subclinical forms of bulimia nervosa. In comparison, anorexia nervosa is quite rare; prevalence studies indicate a range of 0.5–1.0%. Individuals who have subclinical anorexia (classified as an eating disorder NOS) are encountered more frequently than are those who have full-blown anorexia nervosa.

Little research has been directed at understanding eating disorders among men. Most researchers agree that the ratio of females to males diagnosed as having an eating disorder is 10:1. However, speculation is growing among clinicians treating men that the incidence of eating disorders in men is underreported and that such disorders are surprisingly prevalent among certain subgroups of men. Recent reports suggest that a disproportionate number of gay men have eating disorders. Jockeys, wrestlers, dancers, body builders, entertainers, and other men who are required to lose weight or maintain a physical ideal for their vocational goals are also vulnerable to eating disorders, particularly bulimia nervosa. The manifestations of the disorders are sometimes different for men: Men generally are less interested in a specific ideal weight or clothing size and are more concerned with muscle definition and avoiding body fat.

ETIOLOGY

The etiology of eating disorders remains unclear. Current perspectives propose that biological and psychological factors interact with the sociocultural environment in the development of these disorders.

Biological Factors

Some evidence supports a genetic contribution to the development of eating disorders. First-degree biological relatives of individuals who have anorexia nervosa appear to be at increased risk for the development of the disorder. A significantly higher concordance rate for anorexia nervosa has been found among monozygotic twins than among dizygotic twins. Furthermore, a higher incidence of mood disorders has been found among first-degree biological relatives of individuals who have binge-eating/purging type anorexia nervosa. First-degree biological relatives of individuals who have bulimia nervosa also demonstrate an increased frequency of bulimia nervosa, mood disorders, and substance abuse and dependence.

Psychological Factors

Several theories have been advanced to explain the psychological determinants of eating disorders. Anorexia and bulimia are both characterized by a sig-

nificant disturbance in an individual's self-concept and sense of personal identity. For most individuals who have eating disorders, their experience of self-worth is linked directly to their external appearance and accomplishments. Their preoccupation with body weight and shape and the severe discipline that these individuals exert over their bodies is often a desperate effort to cope with underlying feelings of powerlessness and inadequacy.

Sociocultural Factors

That so many women attempt to control their food intake and body size rather than use some other means of coping is clearly culturally determined. Eating disorders seem to flourish in societies that value thinness, independence, and individual achievement and in societies in which the roles of women are often confusing and conflictual. Many sociocultural perspectives of eating disorders have proposed that these disorders result from efforts to cope with the changing roles of women. Some theorists have postulated that the values of autonomy and individual achievement in industrialized societies conflict with the more relational or interpersonal needs necessary for healthy female development. Women who are psychologically vulnerable, or who may lack the inner resources to establish a sense of connection with others despite the sociocultural environment, may turn to food instead of others in an effort to satisfy their relational needs.

COURSE

Bulimia nervosa usually develops in late adolescence or early adulthood and is often associated with a stressful life event or an effort at dieting. The course of illness can be chronic or intermittent. The long-term outcome is unknown, although several reports suggest that individuals who have bulimia do improve with time and ongoing treatment. The older the individual is at the time of initial clinical intervention, the greater the risk of relapse and, thus, chronicity. This observation suggests that the earlier bulimia is detected and treated, the better the outcome. The mortality rate for bulimia nervosa is unknown, but death, should it occur, often results from dehydration, electrolyte imbalances due to excessive vomiting, or poisoning resulting from the use of purgatives such as ipecac.

The mean age of onset for anorexia nervosa is slightly younger than in bulimia nervosa, with bimodal peaks at ages 14 and 18. As in bulimia, the onset of the disorder tends to be associated with a stressful life event. Some individuals who have anorexia recover after a single episode (49%), while others follow a more chronic (18%) or fluctuating (26%) course. Between 25 and 35% of individuals who have bulimia nervosa once suffered from anorexia. The long-term mortality rate from anorexia is over 10%, usually resulting from starvation, suicide, or electrolyte imbalance. Positive prognostic indicators include early age of onset, good premorbid psychosocial adjustment, less weight loss, and less denial of illness. Poor prognostic indicators include the reverse of the above plus low socioeconomic status and the presence of bulimia, vomiting, or laxative abuse.

MEDICAL COMPLICATIONS IN EATING DISORDERS

Some of the more common medical complications associated with anorexia nervosa are amenorrhea, abdominal pain, increased urination, edema, dehydration, constipation, slow or irregular heart rate, and hypothalamic dysfunction. Laboratory tests may show abnormalities of vasopressin secretion and low estrogen levels. Electrolyte abnormalities can predispose individuals to cardiac conduction abnormalities and are found most commonly among binge-eating/purging anorexics and bulimics but may also be present in restricting anorexics. The most frequent and serious problems leading to cardiac arrest and kidney failure are low potassium, low sodium chloride, and diuretic abuse. In addition, electrolyte imbalances are associated with generalized weakness, confusion, memory and thinking impairment, and emotional lability.

In binge-eating/purging type anorexia and in bulimia nervosa, the use of ipecac and other purgatives can cause irreversible damage to the heart and other muscular tissue. Accordingly, chest pains, skipped heartbeats, and fainting can indicate misuse of purgatives. Enlargement of the parotid glands can give the face a puffy "chipmunk" appearance and is common among those who vomit on a daily basis. Endocrine and gastrointestinal systems abnormalities also occur in bulimia. About 30% of all bulimic women will experience some abnormalities in their menstrual cycle. Peptic ulcers and pancreatitis are potentially life threatening. Some bulimics have been know to ingest up to 15,000 calories in as little as a few hours, leaving the stomach vulnerable to rupture. Gastric rupture is a medical emergency with a mortality rate of more than 80%. Bulimia is often detected by dentists because the acid of regurgitated food causes erosion of tooth enamel or because gum abscesses cause obstruction of the salivary glands.

ANOREXIA NERVOSA

Individuals who have anorexia nervosa have lost 15% of their body weight for what is considered nor-

mal for their age and height. They typically accomplish this weight loss by severely reducing their caloric intake so that they subsist on a highly restrictive diet that includes limited numbers of foods (usually no carbohydrates or fats). Although the term "anorexia" literally means "loss of appetite," few anorexics fully lose their appetite until the disorder is well entrenched. In contrast, they often have to exert extreme self-discipline to override their hunger.

Excessive exercising may also be used to produce weight loss; some individuals exercise incessantly and to the point of sleep deprivation and exhaustion. In addition, some individuals (by some estimates, 50%) will episodically lose control over their food restriction, resulting in bingeing and purging behaviors. Thus, there are two types of anorexia nervosa: restricting and binge-eating/purging. In both types of anorexia nervosa, the individual has an intense fear of gaining weight or of becoming fat, which does not diminish with weight loss and often increases as weight decreases.

Physiologic changes brought about by starvation contribute strongly to the clinical presentation of the disorder. Symptoms include intense preoccupation with food, slowed eating, food hoarding and stealing, binge eating, disturbed sleep, loss of sex drive, reduced concentration and alertness, and social withdrawal.

ANOREXIA NERVOSA: RESTRICTING TYPE

The restricting anorexic's sense of competency and self-worth is tied directly to the extent to which she can control her body weight and shape. She thus feels proud and self-disciplined when weight is lost and unacceptable and a failure when weight is gained. The anorexic does not believe she has a problem and does not consciously experience distress concerning her physical or emotional state.

Kristin D, a 15-year-old high school sophomore from an upper middle class family, was brought to see her pediatrician after having fainted at school. Her father was a successful professional who was frequently away from home on business. Her mother was a homemaker.

Ms. D was resistant to being examined by the doctor, angry at her mother for bringing her, and insistent that nothing was wrong with her. She made little eye contact and appeared lethargic and withdrawn. She was dressed in several layers of clothes even though it was a warm day. Reluctantly she acknowledged that she had been suffering from headaches and insomnia, oftentimes felt cold and lightheaded, experienced regular constipation, and had not had her period for several months. She stated that she exercised regularly and ate a healthy, low fat diet. She insisted that she did not exercise excessively and that she was far from being too thin.

Physical examination revealed that Ms. D weighed 85 pounds and was 5′6″ tall. Her skin had a yellow tint and was dry. She had low blood pressure, and an electrocardiogram (EKG) showed a mild cardiac arrhythmia. Laboratory findings included very low levels of protein and albumin, consistent with malnutrition. A CBC was notable for low hematocrit and hemoglobin, with a microcytic pattern of anemia. Further testing revealed low serum iron concentrations. Based on her clinical presentation and medical status, she was diagnosed as having anorexia nervosa.

Ms. D was angry and defiant when the physician informed her of the severity of her condition and her need for treatment. Her mother was also quite surprised by the diagnosis. She had been aware that Ms. D had been upset and started to diet following a breakup with a boyfriend, but she was unaware of the extent of the weight loss.

According to her mother, Ms. D had always been the "golden child" both within the family and at school. However, in recent months she seemed to be pulling away from her friends and spending more time in her room. She always seemed to be exercising and on the move. She would cook elaborate meals for the family but would rarely eat with them (claiming she had already eaten). When her mother did see her eat, Ms. D seemed to have many rituals around food and eating.

Ms. D and her mother both initially resisted the physician's recommendation that she be hospitalized immediately for medical stabilization and weight restoration. They felt that Ms. D would be able to gain weight on an outpatient basis. Ms. D reluctantly accepted a referral to a psychologist, and therapy on a twice-a-week basis was initiated. However, after 2 weeks of outpatient therapy and regular medical check-ups with her physician, Ms. D continued to lose weight, and she was hospitalized on a pediatric medical unit.

While in the hospital, Ms. D continued to resist the treatment team's effort to improve her nutritional and medical status and was discovered hiding food under her bed, trying to drink large amounts of water prior to being weighed, and secretly exercising in her room late at night.

After a 2-week hospitalization, during which medical stabilization and weight gain were achieved, Ms. D was discharged and received ongoing treatment from a multidisciplinary team consisting of her physician, psychologist, family therapist, and nutritionist.

Diagnosis. Anorexia nervosa, restricting type (Axis I).

ANOREXIA NERVOSA: BINGE-EATING/PURGING TYPE

Several significant features distinguish the binge-eating/purging type of anorexia nervosa from the restrictive type. Many patients who have symptoms of overeating and vomiting associated with anorexia are likely to have been ill for a longer period of time, require more frequent therapeutic contacts, experience a higher degree of emotional distress, and have a poorer prognosis than their restricting counterparts. Bulimic anorexics often begin as restrictors and eventually move into overeating and purging when they are intermittently no longer able to maintain total control over their food intake.

As a group, binge-eating/purging anorexics frequently have more disorganized personal lives and more disturbed family histories, are often more physically ill, and exhibit more psychopathology than restricting anorexics. They are less successful than restricting anorexics at maintaining rigorous control over their behavior and impulses and are vulnerable to disturbances of impulse control such as substance abuse, compulsive shopping, shoplifting, and sexual promiscuity. They are also more prone to suicidal or parasuicidal behavior and to being physically self-injurious (ie, hitting or cutting themselves).

Lisa F, a 35-year-old health professional, sought psychological help because she was feeling overwhelmed and increasingly out of control. She had a tentative manner, was soft-spoken, and was extremely anxious. She was also depressed and suicidal. Three nights before her initial appointment she took a toxic amount of Benadryl. She reported that she did not really want to die: "I just wanted not to wake up . . . I just need all the craziness to stop."

Ms. F was 5′7″ and weighed 80 pounds. She was suffering from extreme binge-purge episodes. Recently she had been vomiting as many as five or six times in succession, typically twice a day, and as many as four or five times a day on especially bad days.

Ms. F's eating disorder began at age 14 and included a combination of bulimic and anorexic symptoms. She began restricting her food intake the summer before she started high school. Eventually severe food restriction was disrupted by periods during which she would "lose control" and binge then purge.

It was not until 10 months into treatment that Ms. F admitted to an addiction to alcohol. She was consuming a minimum of 1 pint of alcohol every night. She reported that the alcohol helped to "numb" her feelings and make it possible for her to fall asleep.

Ms. F's strong feelings of shame prompted her to keep secret both her eating disorder and her substance abuse. Secrecy and shame also dominated her developmental history. From as far back as she could remember, Ms. F was physically abused by her father, a respected physician. Her mother was reportedly powerless and too drunk to protect her from her father. Her memories of sexual abuse, including forced oral copulation, plagued her in her adult life. As was eventually learned in treatment, Ms. F's episodes of repeated vomiting were her attempt to make sure she "gets it all out . . . gets out everything that was never supposed to be swallowed."

Diagnosis. Anorexia nervosa, binge-eating/purging type PTSD (Axis I); alcohol dependence (Axis I); borderline personality disorder (Axis II).

Discussion. This case is complicated by sexual abuse, post-traumatic stress disorder, alcohol abuse, and borderline personality disorder. Ms. F's borderline features manifested themselves in her pervasive instability of mood, interpersonal relationships, and poor self-image that have their roots in her early childhood experiences.

The incidence of sexual abuse among individuals who have eating disorders is believed to be quite high. Accordingly, treating professionals should be attentive to the possibility of a history of sexual abuse in their eating disordered patients.

TREATMENT OF ANOREXIA NERVOSA

The growing role of managed care in medical practice has strongly influenced the manner in which individuals who have eating disorders are treated. Some psychiatric services have established eating disorder protocols; however, many insurance companies no longer cover in-hospital treatment for eating disorders except for brief periods of stabilization and often only when severe medical complications are present. Since primary care physicians are increasingly being placed in the role of gatekeeper, they are often responsible for diagnosing eating disorders as well as determining whether hospitalization is indicated.

Hospitalization

Hospitalization should be considered if the patient exhibits any of the following:

- severe malnutrition (sometimes determined by weight loss below a value set by the treating physician)

- significant medical complications (eg, electrolyte disturbances, hypokalemia, organ damage)
- a persistent cycle of self-induced vomiting or laxative abuse that has not been interrupted effectively by outpatient interventions
- significant suicide risk
- a marked inability for self-care by the patient or her family

A Multidisciplinary Team Approach

When medical complications are not severe enough to require hospitalization, an integrated outpatient program focusing on the individual needs of the patient should be implemented. Typically, an outpatient team will consist of a primary physician who will monitor the patient's medical status, a psychotherapist who will work with the patient on her underlying emotional issues, and a nutritionist who will assist the patient in developing a nutritionally sound meal plan. Sometimes a team will also include a family therapist and psychiatrist when such needs are indicated. Coordination of services and communication among team members is crucial for treatment efficacy.

Pharmacologic treatments of anorexia nervosa are limited. Antidepressants, especially the selective serotonin re-uptake inhibitors such as fluoxetine (Prozac), may be helpful in controlling the binge-purge cycles and in treating associated depression. However, weight gain itself is usually most effective in relieving depression and elevating mood in anorexic patients.

The following case highlights an outpatient multidisciplinary team approach in the treatment of a restricting anorexic. It also illustrates the psychological complexity of eating disorders and some of the difficulties inherent in treating them.

Megan G, aged 24, was referred for a psychological evaluation. Her physician was concerned about Ms. G's low weight and depressive symptoms. Ms. G was 5'6" tall and weighed 95 pounds. She was amenorrheic, and her blood pressure was in the low normal range. Laboratory tests, blood chemistry, and a physical examination revealed no significant medical instability. Ms. G reported that she was having difficulty concentrating and focusing. She had completed her law school studies 3 months earlier and was having problems motivating herself to find a law clerk position or to begin preparing for the bar exam. Ms. G revealed that she was also having trouble sleeping.

Her physician prescribed fluoxetine for depression. Ms. G however was reluctant to take the medication because she was opposed to "taking drugs," did not like the feeling of "not being in control," and objected to having foreign substances in her body. Although Ms. G insisted that she was fine, she agreed to try the medication and took the name and phone number of the psychologist she was to call for an evaluation.

Ms. G arrived for her initial appointment with a great deal of ambivalence. She acknowledged that she had some concerns about finding work and studying for the bar exam, but she was confused about her mother's and doctor's "exaggerated worry" about her weight. She felt that her mother's concern that she was exercising too much was "ridiculous." Ms. G ran 5–6 miles every morning and again most evenings, but she explained that she had been a long-distance runner in high school and had always exercised a lot.

Ms. G became very agitated as she described her interaction with her physician and went to great lengths to describe her dissatisfaction with his approach. She complained about not liking the medication and reported no therapeutic effects. She thought her physician was insensitive, intrusive, and interfering. Ms. G was convinced that the physician had aligned with her mother: "Neither one of them is interested in who I really am." In contrast, she became suddenly complimentary and appreciative of the therapist's demeanor and style.

Upon completion of the evaluation, Ms. G agreed to meet regularly with her physician for medical management and monitoring. Although she was not yet interested in changing her eating behavior, she accepted a referral to a nutritionist to establish a workable meal plan. She also ambivalently accepted the therapist's expressed interest in getting to know her for who she really was and agreed to twice-weekly psychotherapy.

Diagnosis. Anorexia nervosa, restricting type; major depression, single episode (Axis I).

Maintaining the integrity of the treatment team is one of the most significant challenges of the multidisciplinary team approach. Patients will often complain about one professional to another, frequently suggesting that one is being of great assistance while the other is of none. This mechanism is known as **splitting** and is usually experienced by treating professionals as quite manipulative and undermining to the treatment process. Splitting on the part of the anorexic is typically aimed at self-preservation and is usually unconscious and not intentionally malicious or manipulative. Its impact, however, can be quite insidious and destructive and warrants judicious monitoring on the part of all treating professionals.

BULIMIA NERVOSA

Individuals who have bulimia nervosa share many features in common with anorexics who binge and purge, except that they maintain their weight within a normal range. "Bulimia" literally means "ox hunger" and refers to a syndrome wherein individuals experience a powerful urge to consume large amounts of food over a brief period of time (binge eating). They experience these binge urges as being beyond their control and fear that they cannot stop eating voluntarily. The binges end not because the individuals feel satiated, but rather because they experience severe nausea or abdominal pain, are interrupted, fall asleep, or purge. The capacity to identify hunger and satiation is usually impaired as is true for most eating disordered individuals.

Purging behavior most commonly involves self-induced vomiting but may also include laxative or diuretic abuse, severe dieting, or excessive exercising to counter potential weight gain. Two subtypes of bulimia nervosa exist: in the **purging type** the individual regularly engages in self-induced vomiting or the misuse of laxatives, diuretics, or enemas; in the **nonpurging type** the individual uses other compensatory behaviors such as fasting or excessive exercising.

Bulimics often describe feeling depressed (eg, lonely, sad, empty) or anxious before a binge episode. They tend to binge when they are alone, and their behavior is typically a closely guarded secret. They are able to conceal their behavior in large measure because they tend to maintain an average weight and a surface adjustment to work, school, and interpersonal relations. The word "surface" needs to be underscored since, upon closer examination, problems are often prevalent in these areas of their lives as well.

The binges can last from a few minutes to several hours and can occur a few times a week to several times a day. The food consumed during a binge is often easily ingested and high in carbohydrates. During a binge, the bulimic may experience a sense of relief from negative mood states. After the binge, the negative feelings tend to resurface along with strong feelings of self-recrimination and guilt for having lost control. Purging is then used to reinstate a sense of control and reduce feelings of anxiety.

Bulimics also tend to have poor impulse control. Alcoholism, drug abuse, stealing, suicidal gestures and attempts, as well as self-mutilation occur with some frequency. Medical complications in bulimia nervosa can be numerous and severe.

Trisha L was a 17-year-old junior in a college preparatory high school. During the previous year she had been an honor roll student, participated in numerous school activities, and was voted class representative to the student council. Over the past 9 months her grades declined, her interest in school activities diminished, and she increasingly missed curfew. Ms. L's mother complained that her daughter was moody, withdrawn, and openly defiant. Her attempts to reach out to her daughter had been met with aggressive rebuffs.

Ms. L's dentist had discovered advanced erosion of her tooth enamel and questioned Ms. L about her eating and purging behaviors. Ms. L was agitated initially and denied purging; however, as the discussion continued, she became quite tearful and acknowledged that she was inducing vomiting almost every day, sometimes up to four times a day. Her dentist referred her for a complete physical and psychological evaluation.

Ms. L failed to follow through with these recommendations. A month later she was arrested for shoplifting. At this point Ms. L's mother arranged a psychiatric evaluation for her. Findings from the evaluation revealed that Ms. L was of normal weight but quite scared and clinically depressed. She reported feeling overwhelmed and out of control and admitted to self-induced vomiting, laxative abuse, and suicidal ideation.

Medical findings included low blood pressure (secondary to low intravascular volume); low potassium, sodium chloride, and magnesium levels; dysmenorrhea (painful menstruation); edema of the hands and legs; mild inflammation of the pancreas; abrasions on the back of her knuckles on her right hand (caused by self-induced vomiting); and a pasty complexion, yellowish skin, and hair loss associated with chronic protein malnutrition.

Diagnosis. Bulimia nervosa, purging type; major depression, single episode (Axis I).

TREATMENT OF BULIMIA NERVOSA

In severe cases of bulimia nervosa, inpatient intervention may be the only effective means of establishing medical stabilization and disrupting the self-destructive binge-and-purge cycle. Significant suicide risk or an inability to care for oneself are other criteria for hospitalization. However, most individuals who have bulimia nervosa are treated on an outpatient basis. Often the primary care physician is responsible for medical stabilization of the patient as well as initiating the associated psychiatric, psychological, and nutritional consultations. Once again,

communication among team members is crucial for a positive treatment outcome.

Antidepressant medication is effective in the short-term treatment of bulimia nervosa. Studies have found that binge frequency declined by 70% in bulimia nervosa patients treated with amitriptyline (Elavil), and desipramine (Norpramin) produced a 50% decrease in binge frequency. Recently, the FDA approved fluoxetine for the treatment of bulimia nervosa, making it the first drug to be approved for the treatment of this eating disorder. The effective dose for the treatment of bulimia is 60 mg/day, in contrast to the 20 mg/day dosage recommended for the treatment of depression. Length of treatment with antidepressants and the long-term efficacy of psychopharmacologic interventions remains unclear.

SUBCLINICAL EATING DISORDERS

Eating disturbances that do not meet the full criteria for any specific eating disorder are classified in the *DSM-IV* as eating disorders not otherwise specified (NOS). These disorders are quite common and are frequently found among individuals seeking outpatient treatment. According to the *DSM-IV,* examples of eating disorders NOS include the following:

- an individual who meets all the criteria for anorexia nervosa but has regular menses or who, despite having lost a lot of weight, still falls within the normal weight range
- an individual of normal weight who may purge after ingesting only a small amount of food
- someone who will chew and spit out but not swallow large amounts of food
- an individual who meets all the criteria for bulimia nervosa except that the bingeing and purging behaviors occur at a frequency of less than twice a week or with a duration of fewer than 3 months

BINGE-EATING DISORDER

Binge-eating disorder is classified in the *DSM-IV* as an eating disorder NOS and also as a provisional diagnosis in need of further study. Binge-eating disorder is characterized by recurrent episodes of excessive eating that occur at least twice a week for 6 months. These episodes are accompanied by a sense of lack of control or subjective distress. However, unlike in bulimia nervosa, compensatory behaviors such as self-induced vomiting are not used to counteract weight gain. Accordingly, individuals with this disorder are often obese.

Preliminary data suggest that binge-eating disorder is a significant public health problem. Between 2–5% of adult women are believed to have binge-eating disorder. Approximately 30% of individuals seeking treatment for obesity satisfy the current criteria for the disorder. Binge-eating disorder is more common among women, but a proportionally higher percentage of men have binge-eating disorder than any other eating disorder (35%, in comparison to 10% in bulimia nervosa). The disorder typically begins in late adolescence or early adulthood and appears to follow a chronic course.

Individuals who have binge-eating disorder may suffer from feelings of low self-esteem and experience problems at work and in their interpersonal relationships. A high percentage of patients who have binge-eating disorder have a history of some Axis I psychiatric disorder (major depression is most common). Comorbid Axis II disorders (eg, personality disorders) are also prevalent among these individuals. Substance-related problems have also been noted. The role of antidepressants in the treatment of this disorder is unclear, but based on their efficacy in treating bulimia nervosa, they hold some promise.

In contrast to the anorexic and bulimic, binge-eating-disordered patients often have a more receptive and positive relationship with their primary care physicians. The minimization of medical symptoms that characterize the bulimic and anorexic patient is often replaced by a vigilant attention to physical symptoms. The physical symptoms at times can become so prominent that they dwarf everything else in the binge-eating-disordered patient's life. Like bulimics and anorexics, binge eaters experience profound shame associated with their bodies. Binge eaters, however, rarely experience the sense of accomplishment, control, or mastery of their bodies common to both bulimics and anorexics.

EATING DISORDERS & COMORBIDITY

Eating disorders typically are accompanied by other psychiatric problems; however, some of these clinical symptoms may spontaneously resolve once the effects of malnutrition or starvation have been reversed. Restricting anorexics often have a high life-time prevalence of anxiety disorders and cluster C personality disorders—particularly obsessive-compulsive and avoidant personality disorder.

More comorbidity factors are associated with binge-eating/purging type anorexia and bulimia nervosa. Individuals in these two groups experience high rates of mood disorders (eg, major depression, dysthymia), anxiety disorders, substance abuse or dependence disorder, dissociation disorder, and suicide attempts. Cluster B personality disorders—particularly borderline personality disorder—are frequently noted among individuals who have bulimia nervosa. Binge-eating/purging anorexics often exhibit a mixture of cluster B and C character pathology. Comorbid character pathology frequently has a strong negative impact on prognosis.

An estimated 25–30% of individuals who have bulimia nervosa also suffer from borderline personality disorder, making this subgroup especially challenging to treat. These individuals tend to be more polysymptomatic than are nonborderline bulimics, and their prognosis is poorer. They may also have substance abuse problems and numerous other problems of impulse control (eg, promiscuity, suicidality, self-injurious behavior). They may be more inclined to utilize multiple methods of purging, and their emotions can fluctuate rapidly between feelings of rage and depression. Their interpersonal relationships tend to be intense and unstable. A more directive, supportive, and structured therapeutic approach works best with this population group.

Monica R, aged 26, sought therapy for the first time as a result of her self-described "out-of-control behavior." A recent graduate of a top university, she complained of feeling like she was "going out of my mind" and quit her job. In recent months she had experienced deep feelings of depression with strong suicidal urges. Although reportedly not intending to kill herself, she had cut her forearms and thighs with a knife on two occasions. She did not seek medical assistance following these incidents because she feared that she would be hospitalized and thereby exposed to her parents and coworkers.

Ms. R reported suffering from bulimia off and on toward the end of high school and through college. Since that time she had experienced fluctuations in her weight but generally stayed within normal limits and in so doing led "everyone to believe I was cured." She also reported periods in her life during which she drank excessively, took illicit drugs, and was sexually promiscuous.

Ms. R had been hired by a successful computer firm a few months after graduation and had subsequently received a promotion and began supervising a small staff. She felt overwhelmed by this responsibility and traced the onset of her depression to this event. Although she was performing adequately at work, she would come home from work feeling tense and then would binge uncontrollably several times each evening. She would follow each binge by vomiting. She was becoming increasingly exhausted and depressed, distraught by her lack of self-control. She quit her job and sought treatment only after she felt that she could no longer tolerate her behavior.

Upon initial evaluation, Ms. R was found to be an intelligent, attractive woman of normal weight. She was extremely depressed with periodic suicidal ideation and was bingeing and purging two or three times a day. She exhibited little insight into her behavior and had difficulty both identifying and expressing her feelings.

She was the youngest and only girl of an alcoholic mother and a father who was either not present or prone to moments of rage. She denied any sexual or physical abuse but was clearly verbally abused by both parents. She described herself as the good daughter who did well in school and who cared for her mother when she was drunk.

In addition to ongoing individual therapy, Ms. R was referred to her primary care physician for a medical evaluation, given her history of bulimia, substance abuse, and self-mutilating behavior. She was found to be healthy with no medical problems secondary to these behaviors. Because of the severity of her depression, she was also referred for a psychiatric evaluation and was placed on fluoxetine. At 60 mg/day, a reduction in depression as well as bulimic impulses was noted.

After 2 years of therapy and antidepressant medication, Ms. R continued to suffer from depression and bulimia, although with reduced frequency. She experienced one incident of self-cutting but no suicidal ideation.

Diagnosis. Bulimia nervosa, purging type (Axis I); borderline personality disorder (Axis II).

FAMILY DYNAMICS

Family dynamics often play a powerful role in the pathogenesis and perpetuation of an eating disorder. The eating-disordered family member frequently serves an important function in maintaining the status quo within the family system, masking conflicts and problems among other family members (eg, mood or anxiety disorders, marital discord, substance abuse). Denial of the anorexic patient's sometimes highly emaciated state is quite common among family members who may also value thinness and appearance over emotional well-being.

The mothers of anorexics may be overly protective, involved, and enmeshed in their daughters' lives, while the fathers may be withdrawn, uninvolved, or submissive. The families often lack clearly defined interpersonal boundaries and the capacity for effective conflict resolution. For this reason, family therapy is crucial in the treatment of young anorexic girls who must learn to develop a healthy sense of themselves while living within the family system. In contrast, families of bulimics tend to be more disengaged, chaotic, and openly conflictual. There is a higher incidence of substance use and mood disorders among family members of bulimics. The prevalence of sexual abuse also appears to be higher.

EMOTIONAL REACTIONS TO PATIENTS

Patients who have eating disorders can evoke strong emotional reactions from their health-care team. The emaciated physical appearance and the self-destructive behavior of anorexic patients can provoke powerful feelings of fear and anger in medical professionals. The struggle for control that complicates the treatment of many eating-disordered patients can easily destabilize the objective perspective for which physicians strive. The frequent concurrence of borderline personality disorder in this patient population further complicates the treatment plan, as these patients often split health-care professionals into "good" or "bad" categories. Invasive procedures must sometimes be performed against a patient's will and may easily extend to punitive feelings and actions against the patient.

Treating professionals need to be aware of these reactions and seek consultation when appropriate to deal with these feelings. It is often helpful to convene multidisciplinary team meetings to allow the treating team members to vent their feelings and redirect treatment when necessary. Conversely, the seeming "fit" appearance of patients with bulimia nervosa may coincide with treating professionals' own biases that "thin is good" and lead to undertreatment or minimization of the potential severity of the disorder.

The treatment of sexual abuse survivors raises unique countertransference challenges for the treating professionals. Therapists and clinicians are often shocked, horrified, and overwhelmed by descriptions of the abuse. The abuse survivor is generally sensitive to even subtle forms of distancing, and because of the learned tendency to take care of others will often discontinue the disclosure in order to protect and not burden the treating clinician.

LEGAL & ETHICAL ISSUES

Numerous legal and ethical issues arise in the treatment of patients who have eating disorders. As in other psychiatric disorders, involuntary hospitalization may be necessary to treat severely medically ill or overtly suicidal patients. For adolescent patients, the parents' permission must be obtained for involuntary commitment to inpatient psychiatric hospitals and involuntary treatment. For adult patients, psychiatric holds are necessary to detain patients. Medical conservatorship is necessary to perform medical procedures against an adult patient's will. Justification for sometimes invasive procedures such as inserting intravenous lines or nasogastric feeding tubes against the patient's wishes often rests on the ethical principle of physician **beneficence,** the use of authority to protect patients from their own poor judgment and behavior.

The care of a patient who has an eating disorder often involves working actively with the patient's family and raises difficult issues regarding the physician's allegiance to the patient. Working with patients who are minors may present special challenges. When an adolescent patient asks that information be kept confidential from family members, the physician must weigh parental rights to informed consent against the adolescent patient's growing desire for autonomy. When possible, a family therapist should be involved who can act as the family's ally, so that the physician is more free to advocate for the patient. Whenever multiple health-care professionals are involved in a patient's case, it is imperative that a release of information be obtained from the patient or his or her legal guardian.

CONCLUSION

Eating disorders are complex and multi-determined disturbances affecting primarily adolescent girls and young adult women. Primary care physicians play an increasingly crucial role in the detection and treatment of these disorders. Early diagnosis of these disorders contributes significantly to a favorable treatment outcome but is frequently hindered by strong feelings of secrecy, denial, and shame on the part of the patient. Although eating-disordered individuals may resist treatment, a comprehensive, multidisciplinary team approach focusing on the medical, psychological, and nutritional needs of these individuals can significantly enhance treatment efficacy.

REFERENCES

Brownell KD, Foreyt JP (editors): *Handbook of Eating Disorders.* Basic Books, 1986.

Eating Disorders. http://www.mentalhealth.com/dis/p20-et02.html

Fallon P, Katzman MA, Wooley SC (editors): *Feminist Perspectives on Eating Disorders.* Guilford, 1994.

Garner DM, Garfinkel PE (editors): *Handbook of Psychotherapy for Anorexia Nervosa and Bulimia.* Guilford, 1985.

Johnson C (editor): *Psychodynamic Treatment of Anorexia Nervosa and Bulimia.* Guilford, 1991.

Miller JB: *The Development of Women's Sense of Self,* (Work in Progress, Vol. 2). Wellesley College, Stone Center for Developmental Services and Studies, 1984.

Walsh BT, Devlin MJ: The pharmacologic treatment of eating disorders. In: Shaffer D (editor): *Psychiatric Clinics of North America.* Saunders, 1992.

Yager J et al: American Psychiatric Association practice guidelines for eating disorders. Work Group on Eating Disorders. Am J Psychiatr 1993;150(2):20.

Suicide

14

David Elkin, MD, Susan Scheidt, PhD, & Amelia J. Wilcox, PhD

Suicide, in its most basic definition, is the act of intentionally killing oneself. However, suicide obviously has profound implications that this simple definition does not convey. According to Edwin Shneidman, suicide is "the conscious act of self-induced annihilation, best understood as a multidimensional malaise in a needful individual who defines an issue for which the act is perceived as the best solution." Shneidman has also described suicide as "psychache"—the "hurt, anguish, soreness, aching, psychological pain in the psyche, the mind." He posits that suicide takes place when a person experiences this "psychache" as unbearable. Thus suicide can be conceptualized as a way out of a problem that is causing suffering, associated with feelings of despair and hopelessness. Suicide represents a conflict between the will to survive and living with unmanageable stress.

INCIDENCE

According to the 1993 statistics of the National Institute of Mental Health, suicide is the ninth leading cause of death in the United States, accounting for 1.4% of total deaths. The 1993 age-adjusted rate for death from suicide in the United States was 11.3/100,000, accounting for about 30,000 deaths yearly. Generally, the suicide rate has remained constant over the past 90 years, peaking at a rate of 17.4/100,000 in 1932. Estimated rates of suicide attempts have ranged from 8 to 25 attempted suicides to one completion, but precise rates are difficult to determine because of underreporting. Thus, at least 300,000 attempts are made yearly. In the United States, one person commits suicide approximately every 20 minutes, for a total of 75 suicides daily.

Geography

The suicide rate in the United States is at the midpoint of countries that have maintained statistics on suicide. International rates vary. According to the World Health Organization, Hungary has the highest rate of suicide, at about 40/100,000. Scandinavian countries have relatively high rates: 29.2/100,000 in Finland, 21.4/100,000 in Denmark, 18/100,000 in Sweden, and 15.5/100,000 in Norway. The lowest suicide rates are reported in Italy (7.2/100,000), Brazil (5.3/100,000), and Jamaica (0.4/100,000).

Western states have traditionally had higher suicide rates than the national average. In 1992 Nevada had the highest rate (25/100,000), and New Jersey had the lowest (6.5/100,000). San Francisco is the city with the highest suicide rate in the United States: In 1992–1993, the rate was 16.8/100,000, which represented an increase of more than 20% since 1989, possibly associated with the increase in AIDS patients. More people commit suicide at San Francisco's Golden Gate Bridge than at any other site nationwide: Over 1,000 people have jumped since the bridge opened in 1939.

Gender

Men commit suicide four times more often than do women over all ages, accounting for 80% of suicides in the United States. Women are more likely to make suicide attempts. Over 50% of attempts are by women, though the majority of these attempts are not completed. Men are more likely to kill themselves from an attempt because they use more lethal methods—firearms and jumping from bridges or buildings. Women often attempt to kill themselves by overdoses, which are not as likely to result in death. Completed suicide by firearms is the most common method for both men and women, accounting for 61% of all suicides.

Age

Contrary to many beliefs, the suicide rate is not highest in adolescents. The risk of suicide increases with age, with people 75–84 years old having the highest suicide rate of any age group in the United States, at 23.5/100,000. Gender, ethnicity, and age interact, contributing to the highest rate of suicide in elderly white men over the age of 65 (42.7/100,000). By contrast, women over age 65 have a rate of 6.0/100,000; however, the rate for completed suicides in women is highest among those over age 55.

The elderly attempt suicide less often than do younger people, but they are more likely to complete the act. The elderly account for 25% of suicides even though they represent only 10% of the population. Special factors increase the risk of suicide in the elderly, including failing health with impaired physical functioning, changing body image, reduction in available coping strategies, the deaths of loved ones, the ease of culturally sanctioned social withdrawal and isolation, cognitive loss from dementing processes, paranoia that may accompany decreased visual acuity and hearing loss, polypharmacy, and a high incidence of depression and anxiety. Some clinicians have categorized geriatric symptoms under the rubric of "failure to thrive," including impaired physical functioning, malnutrition, depression, and cognitive impairment, although this syndrome by itself is not associated with a higher incidence of suicide in the geriatric population.

Suicide is the third leading cause of death in young people aged 15–24; unintentional injuries and homicide are the top two causes of death. The suicide rate among adolescents has tripled over the past 40 years, to a rate of 13.2/100,000 in 1990. Similar to adult gender distributions, the majority of adolescent suicides (73%) are committed by males, although females make more attempts.

Teenagers may be at particular risk because of the challenges they face: conflicting drives to draw closer to family while pursuing emotional distance; conflict with parents, siblings, peers, and schools; experimentation with substance use; and first romantic relationships. Gay, lesbian, and bisexual teens may be at even greater risk, although precise statistics are unavailable. The past few decades have seen a dramatic rise in rates of adolescent suicide. Numerous factors have been suggested to explain this observation, including increased disruption of family units, availability of guns and drugs, and generalized stress in society affecting its most vulnerable and sensitive members.

Ethnicity

Generally, communities of color have lower rates of suicide than do whites in the United States. As mentioned previously, these differences in suicide rates are especially notable in older adults. Overall, whites are twice as likely to commit suicide as are nonwhites. White males are 1.6 as likely to commit suicide as are black males; 4 times as likely as white females; and 8.2 times as likely as black females. Some Native Americans in certain tribes have rates as high as 44/100,000, especially among male adolescents. The rank order of suicide rates in the United States by incidence within race is as follows (from

highest to lowest): Native Americans, Caucasians, Japanese Americans, Chinese Americans, Hispanics, African Americans, and Filipino Americans. Overall, 70% of all suicides are committed by white males.

In terms of religion, Catholics are less likely to commit suicide than are Protestants or Jews. Although religious communities do not condone suicide, most feel empathy for the individual who commits suicide and provide support and compassion to the individual's family and friends. However, as recently as the 1960s, the Catholic Church considered suicide a public scandal and did not allow those who committed suicide to be buried within the church. In Judaism, a long history of rabbinical practice did not observe mourning for those who committed suicide, considering it to be a moral wrong. Today Jewish leaders consider that most people who kill themselves were having problems coping with life and did not kill themselves out of a "cynical disregard for life." Therefore, all rites of mourning are typically observed.

Marital Status

Marital status also has an effect on suicide rates. The highest rate of suicide is found among individuals who previously were married but were widowed or divorced at the time that they killed themselves. The suicide rate is 24/100,000 among widows and 40/100,000 among divorced women. Among married persons the rate is 11/100,000. Marriage, when reinforced with children, significantly lessens the risk of suicide. Single, never married people are nearly twice as likely to commit suicide as are married individuals.

Socioeconomic & Professional Status

The higher a person's social status, the greater the risk of suicide. The greater the fall in social status, the greater the risk. Work protects against suicide, but certain occupations are associated with a greater risk of suicide. Physicians have been considered to be at the greatest risk among occupational rankings. The suicide rate among physicians is 36/100,0000, three times greater than among the general population. Female physicians have a slightly higher risk than do male physicians and a significantly higher risk than do other women (41/100,000 vs 12/100,000). High levels of stress, easy access to potentially deadly drugs, higher rates of alcohol abuse than average, and reluctance to seek help may contribute to these higher suicide rates. Most physicians who commit suicide had been diagnosed previously as having a mental disorder, usually depression or substance abuse. Psychiatrists are at greatest risk, followed by ophthalmologists and anesthesiologists. Other special populations at risk include musicians, lawyers, police officers, dentists, writers, and insurance agents.

Physical Health

Suicidal behavior is correlated strongly with medical problems. Of all people who commit suicide, 32% have had medical attention within 6 months of their death; this statistic may reflect an attempt to receive attention for depression or other mental disorders. One study showed that 2.44% of primary care patients reported having had **suicidal ideation** (thoughts) during the month before a medical visit. Some studies have shown that the frequency of visits to primary care physicians increase in the months preceding suicide. A national assessment of the risk of suicide among men who had AIDS (analyzing data from 1987–1989) found a rate of 165/100,000, which is 7.4 times higher than the rate among demographically similar men in the general population. It is unknown how new protease-inhibiting medications will affect suicide rates among AIDS patients.

Mental Health

Virtually all mental disorders are associated with a higher risk of suicide, with the exception of mental retardation and dementia. Over 90% of all patients who commit suicide have one or more diagnosed mental disorders at the time of death. (See section entitled "Suicide & Psychiatric Disorders" for a more complete discussion of this subject.)

ETIOLOGY

Psychological Factors

No single psychodynamic formulation or personality structure is associated with suicide. Much can be learned about the psychodynamics of suicidal patients from their fantasies in terms of what they imagine death would achieve, who it would affect, and what the consequences would be. Common themes include revenge, power, control, punishment, atonement, sacrifice, restitution, escape, sleep, social isolation, a desire to be rescued, rebirth, and reunion with the dead. A preoccupation with suicide often can be a way of fighting off intolerable depression and hopelessness. Ambivalence about committing suicide is encountered frequently, as reflected in conflicting thoughts and behaviors.

Clyde J, aged 30, was injured on a loading dock at work when a falling crate crushed his right leg. Physical rehabilitation proceeded slowly with little hope that he would ever regain full function of the limb. Additionally, he was left with chronic pain that medications or surgery did not relieve. Over the next 3 years he developed severe depression with lowered self-esteem and feelings of worthlessness that were accentuated when his wife took a second job to help cover their bills. Mr. J's sex drive also diminished, and he was filled with self-loathing for his body.

Mr. J's anger turned to the worker's compensation insurance company for repeatedly delaying authorization for services such as orthotics for his shoes, a special apparatus for driving with his hands, and surgery that might decrease his pain. He began to experience intense fantasies about committing suicide and having his wife win a lawsuit against the insurance company for wrongful death (his own), which he thought would restore her image of him as "a man who could take care of his family." She would be widowed but wealthy; he would be dead, but his death would restore his sense of honor.

On many days when Mr. J woke filled with anxiety, dread, and anger, he would start his car with the garage door closed. After several minutes wrapped in his fantasies of suicide, he would stop the engine and return to his house, feeling more in control of his life. One day he became dizzy from the exhaust fumes. He was so frightened that he finally revealed his suicidal thoughts and behaviors to his family physician. He was given antidepressant medication and was referred to a support group for depressed patients who have chronic illnesses.

Individuals most likely to act on suicidal feelings may be those who have experienced a **narcissistic injury** (a blow to one's sense of self, such as a job demotion, chronic physical illness, or disfigurement) or the loss of a loved one either through death or a severed relationship, those whose emotions tend to be overwhelming, or those who identify with a family member or friend who has committed suicide.

An 18-year-old woman who was well-loved by family and friends began to use marijuana and cocaine in increasing amounts. She became increasingly depressed and committed suicide by hanging herself in her room, where her mother discovered her body. The mother never seemed to recover fully from the shock of the daughter's suicide and became progressively despondent and socially withdrawn. On the third anniversary of her daughter's death, the mother committed suicide by shooting herself in her daughter's room.

Some people may attempt suicide just as they appear to be recovering from life stresses. This behavior often is seen in patients recovering from depression and may be the result of persistent suicidal ideation combined with an increased energy level.

Biological Factors

Recent studies have examined the neurochemistry of suicide. Suicidal tendencies may be caused by a serotonin deficiency. One study found a decrease in

5HIAA, a metabolite of serotonin, in a group of depressed patients who attempted suicide. Those who attempted suicide by violent means had a lower 5HIAA level in their cerebrospinal fluid (CSF) than did those who were not suicidal or who attempted suicide in a less violent manner.

Genetic Factors

Suicide tends to run in families. A positive family history of suicide is present more often among individuals who have attempted suicide than among those who haven't. In one study, first-degree relatives of suicidal psychiatric patients were 8 times more likely to attempt suicide than were controls. Family members who commit suicide may serve as role models for other members when the option of suicide arises. Other possible genetic factors in suicide may be those involved in the transmission of bipolar disorder, schizophrenia, susceptibility to dependence on alcohol and other substances, and impulsivity, all of which are associated with increased suicide risk.

Richard F, aged 26, had his first psychotic episode after the breakup of a relationship. Since that time, he had multiple episodes of psychosis, as well as episodes of severe depression and mania leading to a diagnosis of schizoaffective disorder. Mr. F was unable to work or maintain stable relationships as a result of continued mood swings and psychotic episodes, some of which were associated with drug use or noncompliance with medication. He made numerous suicide attempts by overdosing on his medication. He also would deliberately drive his motorcycle too fast and crashed it in another suicide attempt.

Two years earlier, Mr. F had discovered his sister's body after she committed suicide. His father had killed himself when Mr. F was a child, and his mother died of a myocardial infarction while he was jogging with her. Mr. F expressed his consistent desire to die, saying, "There's nothing but pain in this life for me, and my family is waiting for me over there to join them."

Social Factors

Social determinants of suicidal behavior were first described by Durkheim. He used the term anomie to describe the profound sense of isolation and alienation from society experienced by many suicidal individuals. More recent studies have focused on socioeconomic variables such as marital status, changes in employment, and ethnic background. These factors are considered later in this chapter.

ELEVEN MYTHS ABOUT SUICIDE

Numerous misconceptions exist about suicide. Physicians must be alert to these inaccurate assumptions so that they can assess and treat patients effectively.

Myth: If you ask someone about suicide, you will either introduce the idea or increase the individual's risk of suicide.
Fact: Often patients will be relieved to disclose these thoughts and to receive assurance that they are not "crazy" for thinking this way. Patients will be even further assured if the information they share can be used to design an intervention to help them.

Myth: People who talk about suicide will not attempt to kill themselves.
Fact: Generally, there are some indications prior to a suicide attempt. An individual may disclose that he or she is contemplating suicide, or there may be hints in the individual's behavior. For example, the individual may give away possessions or clear up financial matters.

Myth: Individuals who commit suicide have made up their mind to die.
Fact: Most people who attempt suicide are in fact ambivalent about dying. They may be very relieved to discuss their suicidal thoughts or to enter into outpatient or inpatient care for treatment of underlying depression, psychosis, or anxiety disorders.

Myth: Everyone who attempts suicide is depressed.
Fact: While this is often the case, suicidal patients may not be depressed but instead may suffer from anxiety, agitation, personality disorders, psychosis, substance use, impulse disorders, or cognitive impairment.

Myth: Suicide is genetic and runs in families.
Fact: An hereditary basis may occur for a variety of psychiatric disorders and plays a role in suicidal behavior; however, suicide is far from a purely biological disorder.

Myth: Suicide is most common in lower socioeconomic groups.
Fact: Suicide crosses all levels of society, and underreporting of instances of suicide is likely to occur in all classes.

Myth: Suicidal patients rarely seek medical help.

Fact: Some studies indicate that more than half of all patients who ultimately attempt suicide have been in contact with a health-care provider in the previous 6 months. Many of these patients will have been seen in the month prior to their attempt. This pattern suggests an openness to getting help, if the physician can either initiate a discussion about the patient's suicidal thoughts or detect the patient's intent if the patient is not forthcoming about his or her state of mind. In addition, because of changes in our society over the past 50 years, patients who formerly might have sought help or solace from friends, family, or religious leaders increasingly turn to physicians in times of physical or spiritual crisis.

Myth: Only medical students planning to specialize in psychiatry need to learn about the assessment and treatment of suicide.

Fact: Patients who have psychiatric problems (including suicide) are more likely to be seen by internists, family practitioners, and other physicians. This trend is the result of the social stigma of mental illness and the low rates at which patients who have these disorders seek help.

Myth: There is no point in asking about suicide because if a patient is serious about killing him or herself, no one will be able to change that individual's mind or make a long-term difference.

Fact: Many suicidal patients welcome help, and effective treatment is available that can reduce the risk of suicide dramatically. This myth can be linked to the preceding false notions about suicide and to the discomfort that many physicians feel regarding mental illness in general and suicide specifically. It may also stem from the emotional responses that health-care providers may have to self-destructive patients, including an overly fatalistic, if not punitive, attitude that may greatly compromise patient care.

Myth: Patients who make "suicide gestures" are just seeking attention and aren't really at risk for suicide.

Fact: Patients who engage in **parasuicidal behavior** (repeated nonlethal suicide attempts) are at high risk for suicide attempts and death in the months and years following any given attempt.

Myth: Severely physically ill or terminally ill patients do not commit suicide.

Fact: Patients who are physically disabled by illness are quite capable of committing suicide. Human motivation and ingenuity is often underestimated, and to many chronically or terminally ill patients, suicide may offer a way for these patients to spare themselves and their family members from prolonged suffering. Even patients who are paraplegic or who are intubated may demonstrate resourcefulness in ending their lives, or they may seek assistance from family members or friends to help them do so.

CLINICAL ASSESSMENT

During clinical assessment, patients suspected of being suicidal should be asked about the following subjects:

- Recent thoughts about suicide. This subject may be broached directly, or more gently, as in a series of questions progressively asking the patient about passive and active thoughts, while simultaneously conveying to the patient that thoughts about suicide are not uncommon. For example, the physician can say to the patient, "It sounds as though your life has been very stressful recently. Sometimes people under stress ask themselves if it wouldn't have been easier if they just weren't here—do you ever find yourself thinking this way?" or "Have you ever had even passing thoughts of suicide?"
- Previous suicide attempts or fantasies about suicide. A history of prior attempts increases the patient's risk of suicide. Physicians should ask about the nature and severity of the previous attempt(s). For example, Was the attempt serious? Did the patient receive medical or psychiatric attention? Did the attempt occur after careful planning or was it more impulsive? Was the patient intoxicated? Did the patient seek out help immediately or was he or she found accidentally? Did the patient receive treatment, such as hospitalization, medication, or outpatient therapy?
- Views about death, including religious beliefs and ideas about an afterlife. Some patients believe that suicide is a religiously proscribed sin and thus is less of an option. Others believe in an afterlife in which they will be reunited with their loved ones, lowering internal barriers to suicidal behavior. These issues can be addressed directly by asking, "What did you think would happen if you had succeeded in ending your life?" or "What do you think happens to people after they die?"
- Presence of symptoms of depression, with special emphasis on anxiety, hopelessness, and exhaustion, which are associated with heightened suicide risk. For example, if a patient states, "I just don't think I can take living like this any more," the physician could ask, "Do you ever feel like you are in danger of just giving up?"
- Plan, intent, and availability of means. The physician must determine how specific the patient's suicidal thoughts have become. A patient may have made aborted attempts recently, for exam-

ple, by placing a dozen pills in his or her mouth and then spitting them out after several minutes.

- Concern for effect on family members. The physician could ask, "What effect do you think your suicide would have on your family?" Patients who feel guilty and believe that their family would be better off without them are at higher risk for suicide attempts.
- Verbalized suicidal ideation to coworkers, friends, or family. One of these individuals may have called the physician to intervene on the patient's behalf.
- Preparation of a will, resignation from a job, or giving away of possessions. Concerned family members or friends can often confirm whether the patient has taken these actions.
- Current or prior life stressors. The physician should ask whether anything has happened recently to increase the patient's stress level? Such stressors include illness, job or relationship loss, financial stress, or the death of a friend or family member.
- Substance use. Substance abuse greatly increases the risk of suicide, by increasing the likelihood of depression and impulsive behavior. The physician should ask the patient about his or her use of alcohol and illicit and prescribed drugs. Physicians should be aware, however, that a significant proportion of patients who use substances will minimize, underestimate, or deny their use.
- Impulsiveness. Does the patient often act impulsively? Is he or she able to make a verbal contract and adhere to it, or is the patient's behavior more unstable? Impulsivity is likely to increase with substance abuse (see above).
- Family history for mental illness, including suicide attempts. Does the patient have any family history of depression, mania, psychosis, substance use, psychiatric hospitalization, and suicide attempts or deaths under suspicious circumstances?
- Support system. Does the patient have a stable group of helpful people to whom he or she can turn? Are these people likely to be understanding, or might they under- or overreact?
- Recent psychiatric treatment. Does the patient have an established, trusting relationship with a psychiatrist, psychologist, or counselor in the community? Can the physician contact the psychiatric treatment provider, and if so, does the provider have a good clinical grasp of the situation?
- Focus on hope. Does the patient retain some hope for relief or improvement? Does he or she have any resources or strengths, such as family or religious beliefs? What inner strength has sustained the patient in the past? This line of questioning also can be used to provide a more uplifting conclusion to an interview, or to shift the patient's focus to building a therapeutic plan.

SUICIDAL BEHAVIORS

Other more indirect suicidal behavior is also very common.

Parasuicidal Behavior

Some patients make multiple suicide attempts but seem particularly ambivalent about these attempts and may exhibit a mixed desire to die as well as to be rescued. These attempts have been termed **parasuicidal behavior,** and they occur most commonly in patients who have borderline personality disorder. Health-care providers often refer to these repeated suicide attempts as "suicide gestures" or "cries for help," but these terms minimize the significantly increased risk of suicide seen in these patients. If a hypothetical cohort were followed through time, beginning with a first ambivalent attempt, one would see a high rate of repeated suicide attempts. Approximately 1% of patients succeed in killing themselves each year, giving a total of 10% dying in one decade. This rate is significantly higher than the rate of completed suicides seen in the general population and underscores the seriousness of the condition and need for treatment.

Indirect Self-Destructive Behavior

Many patients seem to express indirect suicidal behavior through a variety of means, including dangerous lifestyle activities. Some experts would place suicidal behavior on a continuum and consider patients who engage in practices that place themselves at higher risk of death as being "mildly" suicidal. One could consider high-risk sexual behavior, cigarette smoking, overeating, excessive dieting, eating disorders, drug and alcohol use, driving dangerously, or not using seat restraints as partially expressed forms of suicidal impulses.

Alex P, aged 30, was seen in therapy for depression, panic attacks, and self-described "existential angst." Mr. P displayed little sense of care about his body: He was morbidly obese, smoked cigarettes, was noncompliant with medication for diabetes and hypertension, and insisted on walking to work through very dangerous neighborhoods. After 1 year of treatment he had made little progress, except for symptom reduction resulting from treatment with antidepressants.

Mr. P was then noted to have ankle edema and other signs of congestive heart failure, and a mild heart attack was diagnosed. He expressed little concern about his condition, stating, "I always thought my life would be better if a safe were to fall on my head one day." Neither his internist nor his psychiatrist could convince him to take steps to improve his health other than to slightly improve his adherence to prescribed medications.

SUICIDE & PSYCHIATRIC DISORDERS

Ninety percent of patients who attempt suicide have psychiatric illnesses. Accurate evaluation and treatment of these disorders is essential in preventing further suicidal behavior.

Mood Disorders

Unipolar and bipolar disorder (see Chapters 5 and 6) affect about 10% of the United States population. These disorders are correlated strongly with suicide attempts; 15–20% of patients who have mood disorders ultimately kill themselves. A high proportion of these patients are either undiagnosed or undertreated for their disorders. Suicides usually are attempted earlier in the course of illness rather than later. Still, 40% of individuals diagnosed as having depression who attempt suicide give histories of previous attempts when evaluated. Studies suggest that during the first year of depression, comorbid anxiety strongly enhances the risk of suicide. A subjective feeling of hopelessness is correlated with suicide attempts in chronic depressive states.

Historical data suggest that before the advent of mood stabilizers, one in six patients who had bipolar disorder committed suicide. Patients who have bipolar disorder are unlikely to attempt suicide while in a manic episode, except when the mania is complicated by psychotic symptoms. The incidence of suicide attempts rises for patients in **mixed states** (mania with depression and irritability). As in depression, these episodes place patients at high risk of suicide. This risk may be complicated by the tendency of patients to run up large debts or to cause strain in work or social relationships when in manic states. These additional stressors may increase feelings of despair or hopelessness, which subsequently are magnified by depression.

Major depression complicated by psychotic symptoms is associated with severe guilt, paranoia, and social isolation, and a high risk of suicide.

Wendy N, aged 54, became severely depressed after her husband filed for divorce. Her depression deepened, but she refused to consult a psychiatrist, even after friends confronted her with their concern. Ms. N became increasingly socially withdrawn and began to experience psychotic symptoms, including the delusional belief that she was guilty of committing a horrible crime and would spend the rest of her life in jail. She began to hear a voice that offered negative commentary about her life and urged her to "just get it over with." She lapsed into a comatose state after ingesting a bottle of over-the-counter sleeping pills. Her friends found her and called for an ambulance. Ms. N was taken to the hospital and after a medical clearance was transferred to an inpatient psychiatric unit for further treatment.

Schizophrenia & Schizoaffective Disorder

Approximately 10% of patients who have schizophrenia (see Chapter 4) commit suicide. Suicide tends to occur more frequently in patients whose course is deteriorating and in unmarried male patients. Suicide is more common early in the course of schizophrenia, when patients are in adolescence or young adulthood. Substance abuse and depressive symptoms further increase the risk of suicide. The combination of psychosis and mood swings associated with schizoaffective disorder are responsible for the high rate of suicide found in this disorder. The phenomenon of **command hallucinations** (hearing a voice dictating some action, in this case for the patient to kill him or herself) is unusual but should be ruled out in psychotic disorders because it greatly heightens the risk of suicide.

Brian B, aged 24, had been diagnosed as having schizophrenia after a psychotic break 4 years earlier. He responded well when he took the neuroleptic chlorpromazine regularly and had held a job in his uncle's automotive repair garage. However, he tended to be noncompliant with medications and occasionally used cocaine. These behaviors caused frequent episodes of psychosis and resulted in his losing interest in his job.

Mr. B reported that one day after having been off chlorpromazine for almost a week, he saw in his room "a giant flower open up, like a rose." He heard "the voice of God" telling him "to jump out of the window." He leapt out of a three story window, only to land—unscathed—on an embankment. He promptly climbed up the stairs to his room and jumped out of the window again, this time fracturing both legs.

As he lay on the ground, he heard a voice saying, "We love you! We love you!" He was taken to the hospital where his injuries were assessed and treated. As he recovered he told psychiatrists that he believed if he had died God would have given him "a whole universe," adding, "I would be the only one, and I could have anyone there I wanted." His conception of death held many alluring features derived from grandiose delusions that recurred during his psychotic episodes.

Personality Disorders

Individuals who have personality disorders (see Chapter 12) are predisposed to suicidal behavior. The combination of rigid coping styles, impulsivity, and impaired relationships heighten the risk of suicide. Borderline personality disorder (BPD) is characterized by an instability of affect, thought, behavior, interpersonal relationships, and identity. Patients who have BPD sometimes harm themselves by burning or cutting, and multiple suicide attempts are common among this patient population.

Frequently the suicide attempts occur while patients are depressed and angry, often after a disruption or breakup in a significant relationship, and these attempts may be highly manipulative. The suicide rate in patients who have BPD is estimated to be almost 10%. Treatment of the suicidal borderline patient is problematic because of the chronicity of suicidal ideation and attempts, and the psychological regression seen in these patients when they are admitted to psychiatric units for treatment.

Other personality disorders may predispose patients to suicidal thoughts or behavior. In general, personality disorders connote a more "brittle" set of emotional defenses that impair coping with stress or change. The cluster B personality disorders (borderline, narcissistic, antisocial, and histrionic) imply a "dramatic" approach to the world and interpersonal relationships. Patients who have these disorders are more likely to have turbulent relations with other people, marked by conflict and hypersensitivity to feeling rejected or abandoned.

Patients who have narcissistic personality disorder may respond with rage to perceived affronts to their idealized self-image, and this may take the form of self-directed anger. Patients who have antisocial personality disorder often lead chaotic lives marked by legal problems, impulsivity, and substance abuse, all of which are factors that may enhance suicide risk. Patients who have histrionic personality disorder are prone to emotional lability and outbursts that may result in suicide attempts intended to "grab" the attention of people around them.

Anxiety Disorders

Anxiety disorders (see Chapter 7) were not initially thought to be associated with suicide, but studies during the 1980s and 1990s documented a high rate of suicide attempts in patients who have panic disorder and obsessive-compulsive disorder. This relationship may be the result of several factors, including comorbid depression, underlying psychological conflict, social isolation caused by avoidant behavior, and a sense of embarrassment and shame common in patients who have these disorders.

Paolo S, a college student, experienced the onset of panic attacks during his sophomore year. The attacks became increasingly frequent and disrupted his ability to prepare for exams. His family had emigrated from Portugal when he was a teenager, and there was significant pressure on Mr. S to succeed academically in the sciences, while his interests lay in the humanities. Like many people who have panic disorder, Mr. S was too embarrassed to seek help, believing instead that there was something "morally wrong" with him and that he could only bring shame to his family.

Mr. S took an overdose of pills and began to walk out into a nearby bay. He was later found semiconscious on a beach and was admitted to the hospital for treatment of the overdose and hypothermia. He recovered and was transferred to a psychiatric inpatient unit where he participated in individual, group, and family therapy.

Mr. S was able to discuss his desire to change majors and career plans with his family and received education about the medical aspects of panic disorder that relieved his feelings of shame. He returned to school and was doing well without medications at 6-month follow-up.

SUICIDE & SUBSTANCE USE

The use of alcohol and other substances greatly increases the risk of suicide through a variety of mechanisms.

Alcohol

Alcohol has been implicated in 25–50% of all suicide attempts; and up to 15% of alcoholics ultimately commit suicide. Alcohol can serve as a catalyst in suicide attempts in several ways. First, alcohol is used by a high percentage of patients who have affective disorders, and because it is a depressant, long-term use can also result in clinical presentations of major depression. Second, because alcohol also causes disinhibition of thoughts and behavior, some patients will have little or no suicidal ideation when sober but may quickly recover strong suicidal ideation when inebriated. Finally, disinhibition of behavior can lead patients to act on suicidal thoughts. Forty percent of suicidal alcoholics have a history of previous suicide attempts.

Patients who drink are at additional risk for suicide if they are male, if they drink heavily on a daily basis, or if they use other drugs. Many alcohol-dependent patients are socially isolated, and half have experienced a disruption of a significant relationship in the past year.

Gene K, aged 50, was admitted to the hospital after making a suicide attempt in the parking lot. He had a long history of alcohol use and depression. He had dropped out of two rehabilitation programs and continued to drink regularly. On the night he was admitted, Mr. K had been drinking heavily. He told a friend that he was upset about his recent separation from his wife and was going to "end it." He sat in his car in the hospital parking lot and swallowed the contents of a full bottle of acetaminophen. He then walked into the ER and told staff that he had attempted suicide and was able to talk freely about his depression and his intent.

On waking the next morning, Mr. K had no

memory of the overdose and denied any suicidal ideation. He was treated and medically cleared and was permitted to leave the hospital after assuring the staff that he had no further suicidal ideation and intended to pursue treatment for alcohol dependence. He drank alcohol within hours of leaving the hospital and experienced almost immediate resurgence of suicidal ideation. He re-presented to the hospital with a second suicide attempt less than 48 hours after discharge, and was admitted to the in-patient psychiatric unit for treatment.

Other Substance Use

Substance use is a significant cofactor in suicide attempts, either alone or in combination with other psychiatric disorders. The suicide rate in heroin users is 20 times that of the general population and may be higher still if some suicides are misdiagnosed as accidental overdoses. The ease of obtaining a lethal dose of heroin, the experience administering it, and the association of heroin use with impulsivity and personality disorders undoubtedly factors into this elevated rate. Many substances produce feelings of depression, and chronic use of such substances may result in a major depressive episode that may continue after active drug use has stopped. Substance use may also induce states of anxiety or psychosis that increase suicide risk.

David B, a 19-year-old college student, tried LSD for the first time and became psychotic. He was brought to the hospital by police who found him running through campus naked and confused. In the emergency room Mr. B was delusional and believed that he was "stuck in a dream." Unobserved by staff, he proceeded to drink a bottle of hemoccult developer from a nearby shelf because he wanted to "die in the dream," adding, "so I could come back to my own life." Mr. B sustained severe chemical burns to his pharynx and esophagus and was admitted to the gastrointestinal medicine service for treatment.

SUICIDE & MEDICAL ILLNESS

The diagnosis (or mere presence) of medical conditions places patients at higher risk of suicide. Endocrine disorders associated with increased suicide risk include Cushing's syndrome, anorexia nervosa, Klinefelter's syndrome, and porphyria (which can cause mood changes and episodes of psychosis). Peptic ulcer disease and cirrhosis are associated with increased suicide risk, perhaps indirectly through their increased occurrence in patients who have alcohol dependence and abuse. Chronic pain is strongly associated with suicidal behavior.

Vijay D, a 29-year-old man who emigrated from India to the United States to pursue a ca-

reer as an airline pilot, had suffered a severe shoulder injury while working a night job in a department store. Mr. D had been attending aviation school at the time. Even after multiple surgeries, his right arm was useless and he was left with severe chronic pain. He became increasingly depressed as his dream of becoming a pilot became more improbable. He was the youngest of four brothers, all of whom had gone to college and graduate school in the United States and returned to their native land to successful careers and admiration from their family.

Mr. D's wife had divorced him after 5 years of marriage, and he had become withdrawn from all of his friends. He was referred to a psychiatrist after all attempts at rehabilitation and pain control had failed. He was sleeping only 1–2 hours at a time and was anxious and consumed with thoughts about the life he might have had. He had lost all interest in pleasurable activities, including eating, and had gone from a normal weight of 150 to less than 100 pounds. He experienced frequent thoughts of suicide and had already written a letter to his family expressing his shame and regret. He saw death as the only means of diminishing or escaping unbearable emotional pain.

Treatment consisted of the prescription of a selective serotonin re-uptake inhibitor (SSRI) antidepressant, a small dose of an adjuvant tricyclic antidepressant (TCA) for sleep and pain control, and weekly psychotherapy that focused on exploring other career interests and more flexible coping.

Other disorders associated with suicide include central nervous system (CNS) processes such as epilepsy, connective tissue disorders (eg, multiple sclerosis), head injury, cardiovascular accidents (eg, stroke), Huntington's chorea, dementia, and AIDS. Suicide risk is also elevated in patients who have urologic conditions such as benign prostatic hypertrophy (prostate enlargement with age leading to urinary retention) or hemodialysis for kidney failure. Suicide is more common in patients (especially in women) whose medical condition results in a loss of mobility or disfigurement. This increased risk may be secondary in part to adverse effects on the patient's life, such as disrupted relationships and job loss. Medications associated with an increased suicide risk (perhaps partly because of their depressant effects on the CNS) include steroids, reserpine, beta-blockers, and anti-cancer drugs.

Patients who have life-threatening illnesses frequently consider suicide. They often do so as a means of gaining control of a disease process that threatens their autonomy. Many patients do not fear death, but rather the process of dying, including pain or total loss of control. Pain control in patients who have terminal medical illnesses such as cancer is remarkably poor in the United States, partly because of concerns by health-care providers that these patients may become addicted to opiates. In many cases, effective pain relief (which may be augmented by the participation of pain specialists in patient care) is sufficient to reduce suffering and restore hope and a desire to spend remaining time with family.

Ying L, a 49-year-old man who was monolingual in Cantonese, was diagnosed with metastatic liver cancer. His family, who insisted on acting as translators, refused to let the medical team tell Mr. L about the seriousness of his condition. He became extremely anxious, apparently believing that his diagnosis was so terrible that even his doctors were afraid to tell him. He told his daughter that he intended to kill himself, and she rushed home to tell her brother (but did not tell the medical team). Meanwhile, Mr. L committed suicide in his hospital room by stabbing himself in the chest.

Sometimes suicidal behavior is expressed in the form of poor compliance with medication or other medical treatment.

Henry P, a 45-year-old nurse, was treated in the emergency room for acute respiratory distress. Diabetes had been diagnosed 6 years earlier, and Mr. P had responded poorly to the diagnosis. During that time, he had gained over 150 pounds because of overeating. He was poorly compliant with oral medications earlier in the course of his illness and was now erratic in testing his blood sugar or administering insulin. He had been admitted to the hospital several times in the past year with blood sugars over 3–4 times the normal level.

On this admission, congestive heart failure was diagnosed, but Mr. P was adamantly against being placed on a ventilator on a temporary basis until his physical condition could be stabilized. He relented when the head of the emergency room—his former colleague—took charge of the case and personally implored him to accept emergency treatment. He recovered after several days on the ventilator and a 1-week hospital stay.

In spite of post-discharge interventions by friends, his daughters, his ex-wife, and a psychiatrist (who was unable to make a definitive diagnosis), Mr. B continued to engage in high-risk health behavior. He died of a massive heart attack 1 year later.

TREATMENT

Critical first steps in the prevention of suicide involve the physician's ability to identify at-risk patients and take effective steps to reduce the chances that those patients will kill themselves. After identifying an at-risk patient, the physician decides whether that patient needs to be hospitalized in a psychiatric unit. Indications for inpatient admission include the following:

- especially serious suicide attempts involving self-inflicted gunshot or stab wounds, or attempts characterized by little ambivalence
- presence of a major psychiatric disorder such as depression or psychosis
- presence of a personality disorder
- ongoing or recent substance abuse
- impulsivity
- marked agitation
- profound hopelessness
- past suicide behavior
- family history of suicide
- access to means, such as owning a gun or having a large number of pills at home
- corroborative data from other sources such as a spouse, family members, coworkers, or friends

Patients who have poor insight and deny that a suicide attempt was made, or who are entirely centered on how other people or stresses in their life are responsible for the attempt, may be at increased risk of future suicide attempts. Patients who made their suicide attempts in the face of an ongoing acute stressor but display rigid coping styles may require hospital admission to assist in planning alternative responses.

Many suicidal patients see a physician shortly before they act on their thoughts. However, up to two-thirds of psychiatric inpatients who committed suicide after discharge denied suicidal ideation shortly before they died. The treating physician must therefore weigh the overall picture in deciding whether to hospitalize a patient, even one who denies suicidal intention. Sometimes what patients communicate through their behavior is dramatically at odds with what they say. Information from family, friends, or therapists may offer important insights that will raise the physician's level of concern about his or her patients.

Michael L, aged 26, was hospitalized after presenting to the emergency room complaining that he had "taken too much aspirin." He said that he had taken 30 tablets in a 10-hour period for a headache and denied any suicidal intention. He told psychiatric consultants that he had never been depressed. He denied any significant stressors at home or work, stating that his marriage and job at a computer company were "fine." The consulting psychiatrist was on the verge of releasing Mr. L but first wanted to speak to a family member. Mr. L signed a release of information, allowing the psychiatrist to speak to his brother.

The brother revealed a different story: Mr. L's year-old marriage was foundering after he had become romantically involved with one of his coworkers. His wife was staying with his parents, and his work performance had deteriorated to the degree that his employer was considering firing him. Mr. L had complained to his brother about insomnia and profound feelings of hopelessness and despair. When his coworker ended the affair earlier that week, Mr. L called his brother to report feeling suicidal but refused to consider mental health treatment. Feelings of shame and guilt apparently prevented Mr. L from telling the medical staff directly about his distress. He was admitted to the psychiatric unit for treatment and did not protest a continuation of his psychiatric hold.

The physician should always attempt to involve the suicidal patient's family in the treatment plan. Many families are very frightened by suicidal ideation or behavior and welcome education and guidance. However, families commonly deny or minimize the implications of suicidal ideation, sometimes threatening legal action against the psychiatrist for ordering involuntary treatment. This is especially true in families in which insight is limited by substance use, personality disorders, or a shared sense of secrecy and denial.

Psychiatrists were called in to consult when a 17-year-old shot himself in the head. The patient was "fortunate" in that he sustained serious injuries to his face but not to his brain. His parents had separated 6 months earlier. They said that during that time period, their son had undergone a personality change, including social withdrawal, odd affect, and possible auditory hallucinations and delusions. A urine toxicology screen was positive only for alcohol, raising the possibility of depression with psychotic features or more likely, the onset of schizophrenia. The parents appeared to be extremely anxious and upset, displaying inappropriate humor and anger at the nursing staff and downplaying the severity of their son's actions.

The patient's mother expressed the belief that her son was "developing psychic powers," adding, "It runs in my family." The father insisted that his son was "just horsing around." He continued, "He must've been drunk and fooling around, shooting the gun in the air. He just didn't aim straight." When the psychiatrist suggested that the parents might be minimizing their son's suicidal intent, the father exclaimed, "I know all about psychology. I know that denial isn't a river in Egypt!"

Over his parents' strenuous objections, the patient was admitted to the psychiatric unit for continued evaluation.

Families affected by serious problems such as alcoholism or sexual abuse sometimes direct attention to an **identified patient,** a family member who is considered "ill." Attention is thus directed away from family problems. Physicians should be alert for family "secrets" or clues to pathology in the family system of any suicidal patient.

If the patient is released after a short hospital stay, the medical team should encourage the patient to return for outpatient mental health appointments. Even a brief phone call or letter from the hospital several days or weeks after discharge can significantly increase the chances of patient follow-up, and thus can reduce the risk of further suicide attempts.

Many patients who exhibit suicidal ideation can be treated successfully as outpatients. In an era of managed care and dwindling resources in the public sector, stabilization of the suicidal patient on an outpatient basis is becoming increasingly common. Patients who are reliable for showing up for appointments and lack more serious risk factors, such as psychotic symptoms, personality disorders, substance use, or a history of impulsivity, may be good candidates for outpatient therapy.

The physician can ask patients to agree to a verbal or written contract stipulating the actions to be taken should they become acutely suicidal. This contract reminds patients of their ultimate responsibility for their own well-being. If telephone contact between appointments is desired, patients should be encouraged to call whether or not they are doing poorly. This arrangement avoids unwittingly "rewarding" the patient with extra contact for doing worse or having more symptoms.

Care should be exercised in dispensing medications that might be used for a suicide attempt. The LD_{50} (average lethal dose) for TCAs is as low as 750 mg or approximately one week's worth of medication. Potentially lethal medications should be dispensed on a weekly basis. Patients can still stockpile medications at home, but serum levels available for some of the TCAs allow physicians to track compliance. The SSRI antidepressants (fluoxetine, sertraline, and paroxetine) may be preferred for depressed, suicidal patients because they are much less toxic and are less likely to result in death if ingested in large amounts. SSRIs should be started in modest doses and increased gradually because their initial side effects may include restlessness, anxiety, and increased energy, all of which may lead to increased initial suicide risk. All antidepressants are associated with increased suicide risk during the first month of treatment as patients may develop more energy before suicidal ideation diminishes.

ACCIDENTS

Accidents are a relevant concern to physicians for several reasons. First, accidents are extremely frequent, resulting in over 90,000 deaths in the United States annually. Some accidents ultimately are shown to be suicide attempts. Patients may try to make a suicide attempt appear to be accidental to protect family members emotionally or financially (ie, by avoiding circumstances that might void their insurance policies). Other accidents are not overt suicide attempts but appear to be partially determined by stress. The term **psychologically overdetermined** is used to describe events that appear to be strongly linked to psychosocial variables, with or without the patient's conscious awareness. Thus there is a suspicion that patients may unconsciously cause some accidents.

Psychological causes have been implicated in **accident proneness.** While some individuals may be simply unlucky, it has long been observed that a relatively small number of people are involved in a high proportion of industrial and motor vehicle accidents. Studies have indicated that this group of people is not constant, but rather shifts over time with increases or decreases in psychosocial stressors, leading to the concept of **transient accident proneness.** Psychopathology is common in these individuals and includes depression, substance use, masochism, impulsivity, aggressiveness, and paranoid and dependent personality features.

Some repeated accident victims have personal histories that are significant for the early death of a parent. Accidents tend to occur when people are tired, have recently experienced an emotionally distressing event (such as a breakup of a relationship, loss of a job, or receipt of a promotion), especially in the absence of adequate social supports. Thus physicians may also have a role to play in the prevention and evaluation of accidents, by warning at-risk patients to be cautious while driving and working, and by carefully assessing accident victims for psychiatric disorders and possible suicidal intentions.

THE AFTERMATH OF SUICIDE

Families, friends, and physicians may be affected adversely in the wake of suicide. The patient's survivors commonly experience intense feelings of grief, sadness, anxiety, and guilt. Thoughts may take the form of replaying the last contacts with the patient and imagining what could have been done to prevent the patient's death. Anger toward the patient or toward the physician may also be strongly felt. As happens in forms of post-traumatic stress disorder (PTSD), individuals may experience intrusive thoughts and images while awake or nightmares while asleep.

Families that have strong tendencies toward suicide, or physicians who work with high-risk populations (eg, patients who have chronic pain, alcohol and substance abuse, AIDS, or cancer), may have to deal with multiple suicide attempts in a given year. For example, several years ago news was released that three promising AIDS medications had failed to be proven efficacious. In the wake of this news, a rash of suicide attempts occurred among HIV-positive patients.

Family members—or physicians—who have been affected emotionally by a patient's suicide must be able to discuss the event and their reactions with others. Resources include family therapy or referral to mental health professionals or local chapters of organizations such as the National Alliance for the Mentally Ill (a grassroots organization started by family members of patients who have psychiatric disorders).

Although thorough and systematic assessment and treatment of suicidal patients can reduce their risk of suicide, some patients will still attempt suicide, and some will succeed in killing themselves. Physicians should avoid fatalism but should also recognize that they cannot prevent suicide in every case. Occasionally, a patient who attempts suicide may experience a life-altering catharsis after a failed attempt; however, this is the exception and not the rule.

A man who had been depressed for 6 months decided to end his life by jumping off a bridge. Immediately after he let go of the railing, he realized that he had made a mistake and desperately wanted to live. He aimed his feet downward and deliberately made the cleanest entry possible into the water, with his legs and arms straight. He survived the fall and lay in the water dazed but otherwise unhurt. No boats were visible to rescue him, so he swam to shore and called 911. He was brought to the emergency room and treated for hypothermia.

In subsequent meetings with a psychiatrist, the patient explored the feeling that life was precious. He made significant changes in his social and professional life, and volunteered at a suicide prevention service. At 1-year follow-up he retained this perspective and still spoke of "the gift of life" that he was "granted by accident."

EMOTIONAL REACTIONS TO PATIENTS

Suicidal ideation or behavior by patients can evoke extremely strong feelings in health-care providers.

Sometimes these feelings mirror the patient's feelings of ambivalence, self-hatred, or despair. Physicians are trained to be objective in the face of severe illness, but they may still have a difficult time working with people who manifest behavior that is out of control or irrational. This behavior may threaten a physician's irrational ideal of being in control of patients and outcomes. Anxiety, fear, and dread associated with unresolved and powerful existential issues about death may give rise to similar feelings and behavior in physicians. Other powerful feelings include the spectrum of disinterest (ie, a total lack of empathy for patients) to disgust and sadistic rage. These feelings may interfere not only with treatment but also with the detection of suicidal ideation.

A very bright, empathic, and conscientious second-year medical student was assigned to interview a patient in front of a group of other students. He began his interview of the patient, a woman in her mid-20s who was encased in a body cast, by asking "How did this happen?"

The woman replied, "When I was at a party, I fell out of a window." She then smiled oddly and added, "Well, actually, I jumped."

The student became flustered and asked hesitantly, "Um, okay, let's see . . . where were you born?" He proceeded to spend the next hour taking an extremely thorough history—one that was remarkable in that it ended abruptly 1 week before the patient's admission to the hospital. He finished by asking his classmates if they had any questions for the patient.

"Yes!" one of them replied. "You said that you jumped out of a window?!"

The student was shocked and embarrassed that he had not asked about a point that should have been the core issue in the interview. The physical reminder of the body cast had been there all along, and at various points he remembered thinking, "I've got to ask about whether this was a suicide attempt." But these thoughts were transient, and for most of the interview he had forgotten about this issue entirely.

This incident provided the focus for an exciting post-interview discussion, during which the students talked about how discomfort and denial in the interviewer can greatly skew the information gathered in any medical encounter.

Discussion. This case has an interesting postscript. The same student requested a psychiatric consultation 1 year later for a patient on his medical service. The student had been the only person on his medical team to ask about and explore the issue of suicidal inclination with an HIV-positive patient.

The student's assessment of the patient's coping, depression, and potential for self-destructive behavior was so complete that the psychiatrist's consult was almost redundant. The student's perceptiveness and skill may have saved the patient's life. The student remarked, "I always screen my patients for depression and suicidal thoughts. My experience with that patient last year taught me how easy it is to forget something so important!"

Emotional reactions to patients are unavoidable. When properly understood and channeled, countertransference can be a powerful means of understanding patients' emotional experiences. When these strong reactions to patients are not acknowledged, they can lead physicians to be inappropriately controlling, passive, fatalistic, or aloof.

After fielding several difficult consults for suicidal patients, a psychiatrist and a psychiatry resident were called to evaluate a patient on the medicine service who had a recent history of several overdoses on medications. The patient's behavior clearly communicated that he was out of control and remained at high risk for suicide attempts. However, the patient insisted on leaving the hospital, and staff had already wearied of his manipulative behavior and outbursts.

The psychiatrist and resident realized the difficulty posed by admitting a disruptive patient who had borderline personality disorder and seriously considered sending the patient home with outpatient care. They both commented on the hopelessness of the patient's long-term prognosis. Only when discussing the case in rounds did they realize that they were thinking more of the staff than the patient.

Their subsequent discussion generated several interventions that had not been considered, and they transferred the patient to the inpatient psychiatric unit for continued care.

A medical student followed a patient who had chronic back pain and depression in his continuity clinic through his third and fourth years of medical school. The patient killed himself in a carefully premeditated suicide attempt without telling anyone. The medical student was shocked to learn of the patient's death, especially because he had never asked the patient directly about suicidal ideation.

The student began to ask all of his patients about suicidal thoughts. He called for the psychiatry consultation service several times in a single week to involuntarily hospitalize six of his patients whom he worried were at high risk of self-harm. In each case, the patient admitted to having occasional thoughts about suicide. The student was anxious about all of his patients who harbored self-destructive thoughts. Once he discussed his fears about working with suicidal patients, and his guilt about not being aware of the first patient's suicidal intentions, he was able to see that he was overreacting—with the best of intentions—to his patients' actual risk of suicide.

Sometimes the emotions experienced as countertransference are pent up from repeated clinical encounters that leave physicians frustrated and angry. Suicidal patients then serve as the "lightening rods" that catalyze the release of these potentially dangerous feelings. Physicians who are suffering from "burnout" or depression are especially prone to such reactions. The greatest danger comes from countertransference that is acted upon because the physician is unaware of his or her own feelings toward a patient. If a physician communicates disinterest, fear, or disdain to a patient who has attempted suicide, the patient may be less likely to comply with treatment and may be at an increased risk of attempting suicide again.

LEGAL & ETHICAL ISSUES

Most ethical concerns in treating a patient who exhibits suicidal ideation revolve around the physician's right to order an involuntary hospitalization to prevent the patient from committing suicide. A few therapists and philosophers maintain that people should be allowed to behave in whatever manner they want as long as they do not harm others. This is a minority view, however. For the most part, clinicians and legislators agree that, when necessary, suicidal patients should be detained and treated against their will. This view is buttressed by the fact that suicidal patients often are ambivalent, have a wish to be rescued, and may be acting impulsively or out of a transient depressive or psychotic episode.

In most states, if a patient needs to be admitted to a psychiatric unit against his or her will, police or mental health professionals can place the patient on a 72-hour psychiatric hold. A patient can be held for danger to oneself, to others, or for grave disability (inability to provide food, clothing, or shelter) due to a mental condition. A mental health professional can release the patient from a hold if the patient is thought to be sufficiently improved, but a patient cannot legally contest the hold. The hold can be extended for several weeks. The patient—represented by a public defender—then has the legal right to a hearing within several days.

In California, for example, psychiatric holds guarantee that a patient can be hospitalized and evaluated against his or her will. Patients cannot be forced to take medications or be placed in restraints against their will, unless they present an imminent danger to the staff or themselves. If a psychiatrist thinks that a patient would benefit from psychotropic medications but the patient refuses, a separate hearing must be held to determine the patient's capacity to give informed consent and to refuse medication.

Terminally ill patients who have suicidal thoughts and behavior pose a complex legal and ethical dilemma for physicians. Jack Kevorkian's highly publicized physician-assisted suicides have generated (or perhaps revealed) areas of intense conflict in the medical profession and society. Strong disagreement exists over whether it is morally "right" for patients to be able to choose when to end their suffering, and whether physicians have an ethical right to aid them.

For example, what if a terminally ill patient requests increasing doses of pain medication for pain control, and both the patient and the physician realize that increasing the medication is likely to result in death? The Supreme Court's 1997 decision regarding physician-assisted suicide recognized the inadvertent "double effect" of opiate medication to control pain but also to hasten the death of the terminally ill. The court distinguished between the use of medication that accelerated a patient's death as a side effect to achieving pain control and the use of medication solely for the purpose of ending a patient's life. Ethicists would also distinguish between physicians counseling terminally ill, suicidal patients by giving them information about how to end their lives, versus actually prescribing these medications. In the most active physician-assisted model of suicide (currently practiced only in Holland) clinicians may be present as patients take intentional overdoses of prescribed medications.

What are the ethical arguments for and against physician assisted suicide? Proponents hold that physicians should act to ease pain and suffering, and should not abandon these principles by failing to help patients in the process of dying. They contend that modern technology has made an anachronism of a "natural death," and point out that the majority of Americans polled are in favor of assisted suicide of some type. It is notable that Sigmund Freud himself arranged to have his family physician administer an overdose of morphine when his head and neck cancer became overwhelmingly painful and debilitating.

The arguments against suicide are also compelling, however. Opponents of assisted suicide note that many terminally-ill patients experience the desire to die, but only transiently. Those who have more sustained suicidal thoughts are often depressed and suffering significant physical pain, but both of these conditions can be regarded as treatable with antidepressant and pain medication, relaxation techniques, and psychotherapy. Physician condoned or assisted suicide would violate the principle of the "do the least harm," and forever change the social contract in Western medicine on which the patient-physician relationship has been based for two thousand years. The result could be a "slippery slope" on which terminally ill, or even the chronically ill or elderly could be viewed as exhausting health care resources, and be seen as "disposable" by physicians and families. What would be the effect on our society if the value of human life were thereby degraded?

The Supreme Court's decision remands the euthanasia debate to individual states to decide. Because our society and profession remain ambivalent and undecided about these issues, patients may receive varying responses to their requests under the care of different physicians, raising the ethical canons of fairness and justice. For example, in a 1997 survey, half of the physicians working with HIV-positive patients in San Francisco acknowledged that they had prescribed medications that they knew would be used by patients to commit suicide. Oregon is currently the only state where assisted suicide is not illegal, and is serving as a "test case" for this arrangement. But obviously not all terminally ill patients live in areas where they might have access to physicians who would support their choice to end their lives. The only certainty is the continuation of this very difficult debate in medical, legal, philosophical and political circles for many years to come.

are clearly in the domain of mental health professionals. However, primary care and other nonpsychiatric physicians can routinely expect to encounter patients who exhibit suicidal ideation or behavior. Changing gate-keeping roles under managed care will most likely shift even greater responsibility for the management of suicidal patients to primary care health providers. Thus, although psychiatric consultation and referrals may be available, all physicians must be familiar with the basic principles of assessing and managing suicidal patients.

Unfortunately, although most patients are willing to discuss suicidal thoughts, current rates of detection by physicians remains low. Important clinical care principles include screening questions for suicidality, the link between mental illness and suicidality, the benefits and potential risks of psychotropic medication, and triage decision-making to determine the need for inpatient hospitalization versus outpatient management.

Progress continues in research into the biological, psychological, and social causes of suicide. Although advances in the etiology and treatment of suicidality are likely, physicians appear destined to continue to struggle with their own emotional responses to patients who exhibit suicidal thoughts and behavior, and with the difficult question of the ethics of physician-assisted suicide for terminally ill patients.

CONCLUSION

Many physicians and trainees probably consider suicidal thoughts and behaviors as phenomena that

REFERENCES

Abell J: *Information Resources and Inquiries Branch,* OSI, Bethesda, MD, National Institute of Mental Health, NIH, 1996.

American Association of Suicidology: http://www.cyber.psych.org/aas.htm

Appleby L et al: General practitioners and young suicides: a preventive role for primary care. Br J Psychiatr 1996;168:330.

Braun JV et al: Failure to thrive in older persons: a concept derived. Gerontologist 1988;28:809.

Brent DA et al: Alcohol, firearms, and suicide among youth. J Am Med Assoc 1987;257:3369.

Cole TR et al: Risk of suicide among persons with AIDS. J Am Med Assoc 1992;268:2066.

Elliot AJ et al: A profile of medically serious suicide attempts. J Clin Psychiatr 1996;57:567.

Garrison CZ et al: Suicidal behavior in young adolescents. Am J Epidemiol 1991; 133:1005.

Harris EC, Barraclough B: Suicide as an outcome for mental disorders: a meta-analysis. Br J Psychiatr 1997; 170:205.

Klerman GL: Clinical epidemiology of suicide. J Clin Psychiatr 1987;48(Suppl.):33.

Manton KG, Blazer DG, Woodbury MA: Suicide in middle age and later life: sex and race specific life table and cohort analyses. J Gerontol 1987;42:219.

Marcus E: *Why Suicide?* Harper San Francisco, 1996.

Medical Examiner's Office, City and County of San Francisco: Annual Report, 7/1/92–6/30/93.

Mocicki EK et al: Suicide attempts in the Epidemiologic Catchment Area Study. Yale J Biol Med 1988;61:259.

Offson M et al: Suicidal ideation in primary care. J Gen Int Med 1996;11:447.

Sarkisian CA, Lachs MS: "Failure to thrive" in older adults. Ann Int Med 1996;124(12):1072.

Shaffer D: The epidemiology of teen suicide: an examination of risk factors. J Clin Psychiatr 1988;49(9)(Suppl.): 36.

Shneidman E: *Suicide as Psychache.* Aronson, 1993.

Sorenson SB: Suicide among the elderly: issues facing public health. Am J Public Health 1991;81:1109.

Vassilas CA, Morgan HG: General practitioners' contact with victims of suicide. Br Med J 1993;307:300.

15

Psychiatric Aspects of Medical Illness

David Elkin, MD

The study of psychological reactions to medical illness and the psychiatric syndromes encountered in the medically ill has become the subject of intensive investigation during the past several decades. Students and clinicians must be familiar with several important aspects of this area, including the psychological perspective on becoming a patient and common stages of adaptation to physical illness: anxiety, denial, and depression. While these phases may be normal steps toward long-term adaptation, pathological states can also develop in vulnerable patients. Other important issues for clinicians include the challenge of working with dying patients, existential issues faced by patients with life-threatening illness, and various psychiatric aspects of specific medical illnesses such as cancer, cardiac disease, respiratory disease, and chronic pain. Physicians must also be aware of their own emotional reactions to patients whose medical illnesses are affected by psychological factors and must be mindful of the legal and ethical issues that can arise in treating these patients.

PSYCHOLOGICAL ASPECTS OF BECOMING A PATIENT

DEFENSE MECHANISMS AGAINST STRESS

Part of what determines an individual's adaptation to illness is the pattern of defense mechanisms the individual uses to ward off stress. "High-functioning" patients tend to use mature coping styles, with an emphasis on humor, the ability to delay gratification, and altruism (eg, "I can't afford to become frightened when my family is depending on me to be strong"). Less healthy mechanisms include denial, anger, and self-blame.

These styles may leave patients feeling more overwhelmed and prone to social withdrawal and isolation. Other patients will tend to feel more overwhelmed or to be more emotionally dazed, or they will be more likely to "act out" by forgetting to take medication. Anxiety and depression may signal a failure of these defense mechanisms to contain the patient's stress. A patient's stress level also depends on the patient's previous experience or family exposure to serious illness. Coping styles can also be characterized on the basis of the dichotomy between **internal copers,** who tend to make emotional adjustments to life stressors, and **external copers,** who are more likely to attempt to change circumstances in the world around them.

Most individuals **regress** when confronted with life-threatening illness, that is, they use more primitive, often child-like, defense mechanisms when they are ill. Thus some patients who usually function well might suddenly meet some of the criteria for a personality disorder but regain their previous level of functioning after the stressor has passed or they have made a more long-term adaptation. The patient's relationships with others often change as well. Regressed patients often display increased levels of dependency, paranoia, or other aberrant behaviors toward family members or clinicians.

THE SICK ROLE

The sociologist Talcott Parsons coined the term **sick role** to define the special social attributes afforded to those who are ill. Reductions in interpersonal stress brought about by changes in patients' relationships with family, friends, coworkers, and medical staff associated with the sick role are known collectively as **secondary gain** and include regression, increased dependency on others, and temporary relief from personal and professional responsibilities.

Other tasks faced by the patient include adapting to novel circumstances, including pain and discomfort as well as the hospital environment; assigning a sense of meaning to symptoms and suffering; and making difficult decisions. These changes may also be reflected in changing roles within families, such as children assuming more adult responsibilities when a parent is ill.

THE EFFECT OF PERSONALITY ON ADAPTATION TO ILLNESS

Personality is one of the important variables determining the pattern of responses an individual will use to adapt to stress. Personality traits and styles are essential features of all individuals. A patient's style often becomes accentuated as a result of illness-induced stress, affecting the patient's ability to make necessary decisions and affecting how the patient processes information. Thus patients who are more ruminative and obsessive may become mired in specific minor details related to their illness and miss the overall picture. In contrast the patient who is more histrionic is likely to become emotionally overwhelmed by information and be unable to weigh specific facts in making important medical decisions. Clinicians can assist patients in their decision making by helping them to keep their illness and their emotions in perspective. An understanding of how personality styles can affect coping behavior can greatly enhance physicians' effectiveness in providing this guidance.

Because personality traits also determine interpersonal relationships and may intensify under stress, these traits are likely to emerge in dealing with health-care professionals. An anxious patient may become overly dependent on his or her physician. A patient prone to fearfulness and paranoia is likely to mistrust health professionals and to express anger over imagined "dangers" of perceived medical incompetence.

Psychiatric consultation was requested for Helen A, a 45-year-old patient who had renal failure. During Ms. A's second hemodialysis treatment, she was observed holding a stopwatch on the treatment table. When the treatment was completed, she shouted, "You are going to kill me with exposure to dangerous chemicals." Ms. A had timed her treatment and was convinced that the dialysis technician had given her an extra 5 minutes of treatment. Ms. A was not consoled by repeated assurances from several technologists and physicians that all equipment was checked on a daily basis. "Of course you will all cover for each other," she said.

Ms. A had been raised in China and had been 9 years old when her mother sent her to live with her father in a small town at the border of Mexico and the United States. Ms. A struggled to learn English and to be accepted as the only member of her ethnic group in her town. She became extremely guarded, self-reliant, and suspicious and had no close friends or relationships, even with her father. Her paranoia about the dialysis treatment was an exaggeration of underlying personality features.

The psychiatrist suggested that Ms. A should receive extra information about proposed treatments and that care should be taken to involve her as much as possible in her care—even calling out "start" and "stop" to help her perform her confirmatory time checks. The medical staff was asked to view Ms. A's behavior as a sign of emotional distress rather than a personal affront. Ms. A remained suspicious but completed her course of hemodialysis.

Diagnosis. Paranoid personality disorder or traits (Axis II); chronic renal failure (Axis III).

PSYCHOLOGICAL STAGES OF ADAPTATION TO MEDICAL ILLNESS

ANXIETY

Anxiety disorders that occur frequently in medically ill patients include adjustment disorder, panic disorder, generalized anxiety disorder, and post-traumatic stress disorders. In many respects, patients reacting to news of a life-threatening illness can be considered similar to patients who have acute stress disorder (see Chapter 8). These patients are often in shock and experience dissociative phenomena and other symptoms seen commonly in survivors of motor vehicle accidents, natural disasters, and crime. While some anxiety states are transient adaptive stages, other symptoms may persist for weeks, months, or years. Clinicians should bear in mind the intensive subjective experience of anxiety and its effects on information processing in medically ill patients.

Sylvia V, aged 34, was informed by her family physician that her recent symptoms of dizziness, numbness in her right hand, and temporary loss of vision in her left eye were most likely caused by multiple sclerosis (MS). The presumptive diagnosis was based on her symptoms, a family history of MS, and neurological examination showing residual deficits. Her physician went on to explain the plan for a lumbar puncture and an MRI to confirm the diagnosis. He continued to explain in great detail the cellular mechanism for MS, treatment options, and the possibility of a truncated life span with increasing physical infirmity. Ms. V said later, "I went home in a daze. I couldn't concentrate, and I just felt numb. I don't even remember what my doctor told me—I was just too 'out of it.'"

Diagnosis. Acute stress disorder (Axis I); probable multiple sclerosis (Axis III).

This common experience helps provide a guide for physicians who are giving their patients bad news. Patients are often overwhelmed, and clinicians should adjust the amount and nature of information given to conform to a particular patient's emotional state. Physicians often react to a patient's anxiety by overloading the patient with too much information about the diagnosis and treatment in their first meeting. A physician needs to devote a great deal of attention to the patient's level of coping, asking how the patient is doing emotionally, ensuring that the patient has family members or friends who can give support, and offering a brief summary of medical information before discussing a return appointment time to review the plans in detail.

Patients may complain of chronic symptoms of low-level distress that meet criteria for adjustment disorder. Other patients have acute episodes of anxiety that are clinically identical to panic attacks. Treatment of these conditions is similar to that for panic disorder—medications in conjunction with cognitive behavioral or insight-oriented psychotherapy. When these conditions are left untreated, they may be complicated by depression or substance use. Before beginning treatment, clinicians should also exclude a medical cause for these anxiety disorders, such as medications, pulmonary embolus, electrolyte abnormalities, or substance use.

Longer-term anxiety disorders can also result from illness or medical treatment, even after the acute threat of death or disfigurement has passed. Recent studies have revealed a high rate of symptoms consistent with post-traumatic stress disorder following diagnosis and treatment (especially with invasive procedures) for serious illness. Symptoms include anxiety, increased vigilance for danger, and invasive thoughts or images during wakefulness (flashbacks) or sleep (nightmares). Changes in body image have also been reported.

After developing severe shoulder pain, Robert M, aged 33, underwent a complete workup, including an MRI scan. He began to experience claustrophobia after being in the scanner for only 10 minutes, but his calls for help were obscured by noise in the control bay and went unanswered. He was finally released after his pleas for help were detected another 10 minutes later. Mr. M was told to come back the following day to complete the scan. He was unable to do so because of extreme anxiety.

Three months later he was referred for a psychiatric consultation for complaints of severe insomnia. Mr. M reported being wakened "every night" by nightmares about "being sealed in a coffin" and had many intrusive visual memories of the trauma during the day. Mr. M said, "I was always scared of coffins after my parents made me go to an open-casket viewing of my grandfather when I was 5 years old." Treatment consisted of low doses of an SSRI (selective serotonin re-uptake inhibitor) antidepressant and cognitive behavioral therapy, with good results.

Diagnosis. Post-traumatic stress disorder (Axis I).

DENIAL

After the initial phase of outcry and shock passes, patients who have a serious medical illness often enter a period marked by episodes of mild denial. Patients often remark that they find themselves temporarily "forgetting" that they have a life-threatening illness, particularly if there are no current physical reminders of the disorder. Denial appears to be a natural phase in the process of adapting to illness. An analogy has been made between denial and the iris of the human eye, which automatically constricts in bright light and opens later as accommodation takes place. In much the same way, denial seems to help protect the patient from the full psychological impact of illness, allowing time for the patient to adjust and regroup for coping in the longer term. Denial tends to diminish with time and generally is not so complete as to entirely block awareness of a serious disorder. Patients can be assured that this phase is entirely normal.

Denial can be problematic in certain circumstances, including situations in which a patient pervasively avoids of any reminder of illness, thus affecting his or her ability to follow through with medical appointments or to take medications. This is particularly true in such "silent" illnesses as hypertension, where adherence rates are estimated at only 20–30%. Other studies have documented delays in seeking treatment among cardiac patients who deny or minimize chest pain related to their illness.

In unusual cases, denial may take such an extreme form that the patient's efforts to deny or distort information will appear delusional to the outside observer. This is more likely to occur in patients who engage in heavy substance use or in those who have personality disorders and are prone to psychosis or delusions.

Kristen F, aged 38, was admitted to the intensive care unit after presenting to the emergency room for treatment of a "cough." Ms. F was reluctant to allow the physician on call to place his stethoscope on her chest. When she eventually agreed, the doctor was dismayed to see a large visible mass that had partially eroded Ms. F's right anterior chest wall. Ms. F would not answer any questions about the mass and grew visibly agitated and anxious. Her doctor wisely retreated from this line of questioning and told Ms. F that she would need to be admitted to the hospital for treatment of a possible pneumonia.

Ms F lived alone in an apartment. She lived on a small inheritance and did not work or have close friends. She drank alcohol throughout the day. In the hospital, Ms. F accepted antibiotic treatment for her pneumonia but refused to discuss the mass on her chest wall. She was treated for alcohol withdrawal. Her hospital records showed that 7 years earlier she had reluctantly permitted a needle biopsy of a small breast mass. Pathology examination of the biopsy at that time showed the mass to be cancerous, and surgery and chemotherapy were recommended. Ms. F had refused treatment.

On this admission, a chest x-ray revealed that the mass had grown to 18 cm (7 inches) in diameter and had infiltrated Ms. F's lung and caused an obstructive pneumonia. Ms. F refused all other attempts to evaluate or treat her breast cancer. She was discharged to hospice care, still not acknowledging her illness.

Diagnosis. Psychological factors affecting a general medical condition (pathological denial) (Axis I).

The preceding case illustrates several additional points. First, an extreme degree of denial can jeopardize the patient's ability to understand his or her illness and to weigh the risks and benefits of proposed treatments. Thus denial reduces the patient's capacity to give consent and, hence, legal competency. This is often encountered in patients who have just suffered a heart attack and wish to leave the hospital, claiming they are "fine." The best approach to dealing with patients who are using denial is not to confront them or try to challenge their use of denial. Denial is an automatic and unconscious defense mechanism based on repression and dissociation, and efforts to limit its use tend to produce increasing anxiety and may result in a desire to flee from perceived threatening people and situations. Clinicians should approach patients as objectively as possible, being careful not to display anger or frustration. It may be helpful to inquire about the personal meaning of the illness—a history of childhood experiences with illness (particularly catastrophic illness) may offer clues about the nature of the patient's capacity for adaptation over time and which approaches are most likely to be helpful. Contact with other patients with similar illnesses, either one-on-one or in support groups, may offer support as well as educational opportunities that avoids the difficulties sometimes inherent in interactions with authority figures such as physicians. If a patient is extremely anxious and is willing to take benzodi-

azepines, these medications can be beneficial. Antipsychotics may be useful for patients experiencing hallucinations, paranoia, or delusions (especially if the delusions are of shorter duration). "Tincture of time" and a nonjudgmental attitude may produce the best results.

Velma S, aged 63, was brought to the emergency room after fainting in a department store. She was profoundly anemic, apparently because of lower gastrointestinal bleeding. A physical examination showed the source of the bleeding to be a large rectal mass, which a biopsy revealed to be malignant. When Ms. S was informed that she had rectal cancer and needed radiation therapy, she insisted, "It's not cancer, I've had it since I was a child." She insisted that she felt much better and wanted to leave the hospital.

Ms. S's daughter told the medical team that her mother was "eccentric" and "can't be pushed into doing anything that she doesn't think is right for her." The medical team was not confrontational but continued to recommend treatment. On the third hospital day Ms. S remarked, "I have a friend who had cancer." The medical team encouraged her to call the friend.

The next day Ms. S said that her friend had recommended treatment but that she wanted to "go home to take care of some things." She arranged to come back the following week to start radiation therapy. To the surprise of some medical staff members, Ms. S did come the next week and to subsequent treatments.

Diagnosis. Delusional disorder (Axis I); rectal cancer (Axis III).

Clinicians should also be watchful for other major psychiatric disturbances that may be associated with severe forms of denial. Any problems with the processing of information should trigger a cognitive screen for memory problems that might result from a medical cause, such as dementia or delirium. Substance use in general, and alcohol use in particular, can also produce profound memory problems on an acute or chronic basis. Patients who have personality disorders may be prone to using denial to distort information. To handle such situations, clinicians can try to emphasize their own need for thoroughness and to back away from a power struggle over specific treatment issues.

DEPRESSION

Depression in the medically ill is often underrecognized and undertreated by physicians. Many clinicians use their own subjective expectations to predict how patients "should" respond to their illness. Until recently depression in medically ill patients was considered appropriate, particularly in patients facing terminal diagnoses. With this sweeping generalization, many patients never received treatment for depression, dooming them to extreme emotional suffering.

Incidence

The incidence of depression varies greatly in different medical disorders. Depression occurs both in medical disorders with or without central nervous system involvement. In patients who have central neurological disorders such as Parkinson's disease, Alzheimer's dementia, Huntington's disease, and stroke, the rates of depression are 30–50%, and can be as high as 55% in patients who have epilepsy. The location of lesions in the central nervous system (CNS) correlates with the frequency of depression; this correlation is well-documented in patients who have had a CVA (cerebrovascular accident or stroke). In right-handed individuals, strokes on the right side are more likely to produce **neglect** (a neurological syndrome in which patients fail to attend to deficits in physical function such as motor paralysis) and a lack of emotional reactions to resulting physical deficits such as motor paralysis. CVAs on the left side (the dominant side in right-handed people), especially when they occur toward the frontal lobes, tend to produce depression in up to half of all patients.

The incidence of depression is also higher in other medical conditions, including cancer (an average of 25% with considerable variability depending on the site, from 5% in patients who have malignant melanoma to over 50% in patients who have metastatic or terminal illness), diabetes (15–20%), heart disease (20% of post–heart attack patients), and HIV (10–20% of seropositive patients). These rates should perhaps be best compared to those of other medical outpatients, who have depression prevalence rates of 10–30%, which is already much higher than in the general population.

The considerable variation in rates of depression is associated with a number of factors, including the variability in study methods, the site of illness, the effect of the illness on relationships and work function, the amount of physical impairment or disfigurement, and the prognosis. Depression in cancer patients, for example, is most commonly encountered in those who have pancreatic cancer (up to 55%) and head and neck cancers (40%). Pancreatic cancer is believed to secrete neuropeptides that act on the CNS to produce appetite and mood changes, while head and neck cancers often are disfiguring, carry a poor prognosis, and occur in patients who smoke and drink heavily.

The overlap of symptoms of medical illness (fatigue, insomnia, decreased appetite) often complicates the diagnosis of depression. While these neurovegetative signs may be interpreted ambiguously, other subjective features (hopelessness, guilt, and suicidal thoughts) are often more reliable markers of depression.

Etiology

The etiology of depression in medical disorders is still being investigated. Particularly in CNS disorders, depression may be the result of either physical damage to CNS structures and resulting neurotransmitter imbalances, or from the psychological impact of physical disease processes, physical limitations, and anxiety about the prognosis.

Depression clearly produces emotional suffering and can also strongly affect a patient's physical health. Depression is also associated with nonadherence to treatment regimens, longer hospital stays, and significantly higher morbidity and mortality. For example, in studies of patients who had heart disease, depressed patients were 4.5 times more likely to have a myocardial infarction than their nondepressed peers and 2 times as likely to have coronary artery bypass surgery in the next year. Remarkably, 6 months after a heart attack, depression (not other physiologic markers such as cardiac output) was the most important factor in predicting death. At 18 month follow-up, depression was the second most important prognostic indicator. Current studies are attempting to delineate the mechanism by which depression increases the risk of death and morbidity.

> Beatrice B, aged 40, was diagnosed with breast cancer immediately after the birth of her second child. She had several rounds of chemotherapy and was started on benzodiazepines for nausea, but she gradually came to rely on them for sleep and to control daytime anxiety and occasional panic attacks.
>
> The diagnosis of a metastasis to her hip led to an increase in her emotional distress, including severe insomnia, agitation, despair, hopelessness, markedly low self-esteem, anhedonia, and guilt. These problems, in addition to poor concentration associated with medical illness, led to her inability to work. Ms. B found that if she tried to work at home, she would avoid the material she needed to read and find herself unable to concentrate well enough to accomplish anything. At the end of the day she would feel less self-confident and more guilty because she felt she was wasting her company's money and betraying their trust.
>
> Ms. B's earlier image of herself as being a strong, independent person in control of her emotions made it difficult for her to meet with a psychiatrist or to consider antidepressant medications. She was therefore given several hour-long sessions that focused on education about depression and medications, as well as a chance to form an alliance with the psychiatrist. The symbolic meaning of medication and its relation to Ms. B's self-image was a major theme in these discussions. Starting medication was "reframed" as a powerful means of regaining emotional health and functioning more effectively at work and at home.

Because of the presence of symptoms of major depression, anxiety, and panic attacks, Ms. B was started on imipramine, a mildly sedating tricyclic antidepressant (TCA) with a good track record in patients who have panic attacks. She was started on a low dose (25 mg at night) and given several days to acclimate to that dose before it was increased, step-wise, to 100 mg. Benzodiazepines were discontinued gradually.

After 1 month, Ms. B's depressive symptoms began to clear and at 6 weeks had largely subsided. She was still anxious about her illness but was able to taper off of anxiolytics completely. She was also able to return to work and to begin to regain her self-confidence. Her only complaint was a 20-pound weight gain, which she attributed to the imipramine. Group and individual therapy provided much-needed support and an opportunity to work through her fears and concerns. She was tapered off of the imipramine uneventfully after 6 months and promptly lost the weight she had gained.

Ms. B underwent bone marrow transplantation several months later, without medical or psychiatric complications. However, her cancer recurred 1 year after the initial diagnosis. Ms. B began to experience early warning signs of depression, including sadness, crying spells, hopelessness, anxiety, and recurrent thoughts of dying. A meeting with the psychiatrist led to a "wait and see" attitude, particularly since Ms. B was reluctant take antidepressants again. When her symptoms worsened over the next 2 weeks, she returned to the psychiatrist with a desire to start another antidepressant trial, but one that wouldn't make her gain weight. The psychiatrist agreed and prescribed paroxetine, at 10 mg every day, to minimize side effects.

Despite mild insomnia during the first week, Ms. B was able to take a 20 mg dosage after a week, and her symptoms of depression subsided. She experienced her decision to begin antidepressants as a necessary and powerful means of retaining her high level of functioning, of safeguarding her energy level to take care of her family, and of coping in the face of a devastating illness.

Diagnosis. Major depression (Axis I); breast cancer (Axis III).

Differential Diagnosis

Because other medical processes can cause depression, clinicians should attempt to rule out or treat any medical factors that might cause or exacerbate depression. This includes reviewing any medications the patient may be taking, especially corticosteroids, benzodiazepines, H^2 blockers, and hormonal manipulation. When medications cannot be stopped or substituted, dose reductions may be beneficial. Patients should also be screened for substance use, which may

develop or become exacerbated as they attempt to cope with the stress of illness. Patients who are in remission from substance use are prone to relapse as they adjust to the news and impact of medical problems. As stated above, clinicians should attempt to distinguish between depressive features caused by psychiatric disturbance or those symptoms caused by medical illness or treatment.

Treatment of Anxiety & Depression in the Medically Ill

A. Medications. The treatment of patients who have depression and anxiety due to medical illness follows several basic treatment principles previously outlined in Chapters 5 and 7. Medication can be extremely helpful, but clinicians should remember that patients may be biased against diagnosis and treatment of depression because of the stigma of mental illness. Prescribing should take place in the context of a strong therapeutic alliance. Patients require an opportunity to express their concerns about medication, and should receive adequate informed consent about side effects as well as desired responses. While antidepressants may prove helpful in treating depression, they should be viewed as one component of treatment, along with psychotherapy and other modalities. High doses should be avoided when patients are physically ill, particularly in initiating therapy. Side effects should also be considered in selecting a therapeutic agent and potential interactions with other medications should always be researched. Patients who have diarrhea may benefit from the constipation that TCAs can cause. TCAs are also useful as adjunctive pain management medications that can help patients with chronic pain, whether or not depression is present. Unfortunately, the newer antidepressants such as the SSRIs and other novel agents have not shown the same effectiveness for pain control. The use of TCAs in patients who have cardiac conditions is ill-advised, however, due to an increased chance of arrhythmias, decreased intracardiac conduction and increased heart failure.

Low-dose SSRIs generally are used to treat depression in the medically ill because of their favorable side effect profile and clinician and patient familiarity. Dosages may need to be adjusted downward in patients who have impaired renal or hepatic clearance. Because of the delay in onset of antidepressant effects (2–4 weeks with most antidepressants), psychostimulants such as dextroamphetamine or pemoline are sometimes used to treat patients when a faster response is desired. These medications should be tried in the morning and their efficacy can be evaluated several hours later. Their principle side effects include appetite suppression and insomnia if they are given too late in the day.

B. Psychotherapy. While psychotherapy may require referral to a mental health specialist, non-psychiatric physicians are also capable of utilizing basic principles, and may choose to lead or co-lead psychotherapy or educational groups for their patients. Psychotherapy is remarkably effective for treating anxiety and depression in patients who have medical illnesses. Psychotherapy provides a neutral forum in which patients can express their fears without concern for the usual time constraints encountered with other medical specialists. Psychotherapy often involves a more active approach that helps patients to develop and assess alternative coping styles. For example, patients who vacillate between extremes of complete optimism and pessimism may need assistance in developing more realistic expectations. Patients can also learn how to master their more fear-provoking thoughts and explore existential issues that may have been dormant for many years (see below).

The social isolation and pervasive sense of being different that is encountered so often in the medically ill makes group psychotherapy an appealing option. Patients can share their concerns, coping skills, and strategies for optimizing contact with health-care professionals. Some groups also highlight stress reduction by ending each session with a relaxation exercise. These groups are effective in improving the quality of life of patients who have cancer, heart disease, and other medical problems.

Most remarkably, group psychotherapy may also have a positive effect on the course and prognosis of medical illness. In a groundbreaking study by David Speigel in 1989, women who had metastatic breast cancer were randomized to a weekly support group. These women not only coped better with their cancer but lived for over a year longer than those women assigned to the control cohort. This study has been replicated on a larger scale to determine the precise nature of the benefits of group therapy.

Researchers at the University of California, Los Angeles, Medical Center attempted the same approach with patients treated for local malignant melanoma, which has a high rate of recurrence and mortality. In this study the patients were given only six sessions of group therapy. However, this brief form of therapy had remarkably long-lasting effects. At 6-month follow-up, patients in the experimental group had enhanced levels of immune function, including increased activity of killer T-cells that defend against tumors. And although the patients in the group had the same rate of relapse as controls, relapses occurred significantly later, and patients were more likely to survive the recurrence compared to the control group.

CHRONIC PAIN

Pain that continues for more than 6 months is considered chronic. Several important aspects of chronic

pain are relevant to psychiatric providers, including comorbid depression, suicide risk, difficulties in assessment by clinicians, and the need to integrate psychopharmacologic, psychological, and behavioral interventions into treatment plans.

Depression is encountered frequently in patients who have chronic pain. Various studies show comorbid depression in up to 100% of patients with chronic pain syndromes. Not surprisingly, chronic pain is also a significant risk factor for suicide, either alone or in combination with depression.

Given the widespread incidence of acute and chronic pain in medical patients, the availability and efficacy of treatment methods for pain, and the importance of preventing suffering due to pain, one might expect that health-care professionals would excel at accurately assessing pain. Unfortunately this is not the case; health-care workers do not always inquire about pain, and when they do their assessment of a patient's pain is usually an underestimate with little relation to the patient's experience. Most patients who have acute or chronic pain in either outpatient or hospital settings are undertreated for their discomfort. Some patients and their families are more stoic and tolerate high degrees of pain without alerting doctors or nurses, whereas others are not aware that pain is safely treatable.

Among health-care staff, barriers to the appropriate assessment and treatment of both acute and chronic pain include a lack of knowledge about pain pathophysiology, assessment, and management. Patients may be suspected of exaggerating their level of pain, and studies show that physicians and nurses are often inconsistent in their evaluation and rating of pain severity (which often bears little relationship to the patient's reports). Standardized protocols for pain assessment are available, are considered very reliable, and should be used more widely. One of the simplest methods involves asking the patient to rate his or her own pain on a scale of 0 to 10, with 0 indicating no pain and 10 indicating the worst pain the patient has experienced. This question can be posed verbally or using a visual analog scale drawn on a piece of paper.

Treatment principles are also relatively simple. A three-step approach to pharmacologic interventions includes

1. nonsteroidal anti-inflammatory drugs
2. adjunctive psychotropic agents such as low-dose TCAs (desipramine, nortryptiline, and amitryptiline are the most researched) or anticonvulsants such as carbamezapine, gabapentin, or lamotrigine (SSRTs have been shown to be no more effective than placebos)
3. opiate medication for more severe pain

Using fixed doses of long-acting preparations, given at preset intervals around the clock (called a standing dosage), is preferred to using medications on an as-needed (prn) basis. Medications given on a prn basis often result in undertreatment of pain, increase the patient's anxiety level, and may cause tension between the patient and nursing staff. Behavioral techniques to reduce pain, including relaxation therapy and biofeedback, are highly effective in combination with other basic techniques. Primary prevention of pain is also desirable and should be a feature of treatment for medical illness as in the goal of adherence to insulin in diabetes to prevent the onset of peripheral neuropathy. The optimal treatment plan involves a multidisciplinary approach involving personnel from medicine, anesthesiology, neurology, psychiatry, nursing, and pharmacology.

PSYCHIATRIC ASPECTS OF SURGERY

The surgical patient is faced with a number of sources of anxiety. These include concerns about pain, disfigurement, and the disruption of body image; the loss of control during general anesthesia; and fears about death. These concerns may be magnified in patients who have preexisting psychiatric disorders including anxiety and affective disorders, post-traumatic stress disorder, or personality disorders. Patients who have psychotic disorders such as schizophrenia should be evaluated before and after surgery for the early detection of exacerbation of their psychiatric conditions.

Kevin A, aged 24, was admitted to the surgery service after his motorcycle was hit by a passing car. Mr. A's left leg was badly injured, and he required several surgeries for repair of damaged blood vessels. Mr. A had a history of schizophrenia and had been hospitalized several times for psychosis and suicidal thoughts. Psychiatric consultation confirmed that Mr. A was coping relatively well with the stress of illness and continued to be compliant with his antipsychotic medication.

Mr. A was extremely anxious after surgery, and nursing staff noted that he was paranoid and fearful that they would put poison in his IV. He was reluctant to express his concerns but did so at the urging of family members. When he had regained consciousness after the surgery, he misinterpreted stains from presurgical disinfectant on his legs and groin as "chalk marks" the surgeons had drawn on his body, developing the delusion that his doctors were planning to separate parts of his body for use in scientific experiments. Mr. A accepted the explanation of the medical team about the nature of the stains, and his delusions and paranoia did not return during his hospital stay.

Delirium occurs in up to one-third of postsurgical patients. Surgeons, anesthesiologists, and consulting psychiatrists must therefore have a thorough working knowledge of these areas of overlap among their specialties. General anesthesia can also produce temporary depressive states and can delay the onset of alcohol withdrawal by several days. Anesthesiologists need to be informed if patients are taking antipsychotic medications, which may need to be reduced to avoid synergistic interactions with general anesthetic agents.

PSYCHIATRIC ASPECTS OF DISEASE PREVENTION

Physicians should note that psychological factors are involved in major risk factors for premature death, including smoking (addiction to nicotine tends to be more severe in patients who have depression or schizophrenia and is associated with increased risk of cancer, pulmonary and cardiovascular disease), alcoholism, obesity (in which behavioral and mood factors are often overlooked), accidents, and suicide.

The latest advances in medicine have led to the identification of genetic markers that indicate an increased likelihood of developing diseases such as breast and ovarian cancer. However, these markers may lead to stressful awareness and decision-making among patients and their families at risk for disease.

Karen C, a 27-year-old woman, was referred by a genetic risk counselor after her older sister was diagnosed with breast cancer. Ms. C and her younger sister and cousin were tested for the gene that would indicate a 60% lifetime risk of developing either breast or ovarian cancer. Ms. C faced a difficult decision when her blood tests showed her to have the gene. She could elect to have prophylactic bilateral mastectomy and oopherectomy (removal of both ovaries) to greatly reduce her risk of developing cancer. Or she could opt for careful screening with monthly breast exams and annual mammography and abdominal ultrasounds that might detect cancer at an earlier stage. Ms. C had no history of psychiatric disorders but reported feeling "stressed out" trying to decide her best course of action, with anxiety during the day and insomnia at night. Eventually, after much discussion with her physician and family members, she decided to wait two years before having her ovaries surgically removed so that she and her boyfriend could try to conceive a child, and undergo frequent screening for the early detection of breast cancer. Ms. C commented, "The hardest part is having to make decisions based on probabilities, but at least I've come up with a strategy that will give me a chance at becoming a mother and still minimize my risk of developing cancer."

Diagnosis: Adjustment disorder with anxious mood.

EXISTENTIAL ISSUES RELATED TO MEDICAL ILLNESS

Life-threatening illness frequently raises existential questions for patients. These issues include the meaning of life, the nature of death, the dilemma of intimacy with other people, and the conflict between responsibility and the desire for freedom. The possibility of death—which is a part of the challenge of any serious illness, no matter how good the prognosis—tends to bring these issues to the foreground. Patients may report being distracted or "tortured" by profound questions that they have not considered for many years but that are now exceedingly compelling and often poignant. This is illustrated in the following case:

Gregg V, a patient in his mid-40s, had been admitted for treatment of *Pneumocystis carinii* pneumonia, signaling an advance from HIV-positive status to AIDS. His pneumonia responded well to antibiotic therapy, and his physical condition improved during his first week of hospitalization. Psychiatric consultation was requested to evaluate anxiety and possible dementia, as Mr. V had been noted to have memory lapses and difficulty concentrating.

Examination revealed Mr. V to be a pleasant, intelligent man with a sophisticated vocabulary. He formed an easy attachment to the psychiatrist and cooperated fully in the cognitive examination, which revealed slight problems with short-term memory and concentration.

The psychiatrist inquired about Mr. V's background, including his religion, after Mr. V had made numerous veiled or vague references to death and dying. Mr. V was dismissive of these questions; he was, he said, a "lapsed Catholic" and did not believe in an afterlife, saying, "you just quit, and return to nothing." Mr. V was also asked about depression but denied most symptoms except loss of energy, which he attributed to infection with the HIV virus and pneumonia. However, he wanted to know about antidepressants. His friends had mentioned one to him, which he thought was called "Resurrectin."

This word prompted the psychiatrist to

rechallenge Mr. V's assertion that he had abandoned his religious beliefs completely. Mr. V acknowledged that he was very distracted by questions about "what comes after this world" and fears generated by early experiences in church with a minister who often spoke about "hell, and the fate of the damned, the sinners." Mr. V added, "At some level I guess I'm afraid that's where I might end up." He benefited greatly from referral to an AIDS support group for patients with a similar background.

While it is not necessary to find "answers" to these existential questions, clinicians should remember that these issues are often exceedingly important to patients. Some patients seek answers within the framework of organized religion, whereas others do so in a more secular fashion. Some resolution or "coming to terms" with pressing existential issues is often encountered in patients who are in the process of dying and are "taking stock" of their lives as they look back on their life's work and relationships.

Key existential issues may also be encountered in a more hidden form. It is often worthwhile to inquire about patients' dreams, which may contain symbolic references to these issues and may also offer possible solutions.

Psychiatric consultation was requested for Robert J, a 48-year-old man who had diabetes. Mr. J was only partially adherent to his insulin regimen and, as a result, had developed an infection in his foot that required a 2-week course of antibiotics and the possibility of amputation if he did not improve. Mr. J worked in construction and was extremely frightened by the idea of losing his foot. His fear was expressed as anger toward the medical staff and nurses, blaming them for the complications of his illness and accusing them of providing substandard health care.

Mr. J was resistant to psychiatric consultation initially but gradually began to share details of his life. He had been lonely and socially isolated after the death of his wife 10 years earlier. His alcoholic father had verbally and physically abused him as a child, leading to a lifelong distrust of authority figures, including physicians. He related a dream he had in the first week of his hospitalization in which he was working on a platform high above the floor of a desert. The platform tilted suddenly and Mr. J was flung off, not falling only because his foot became caught on the platform. He hung by his foot in midair, terrified, and looked down to see that he would crash directly onto "cactus plants with huge, sharp spikes."

The psychiatrist asked if anyone came up to rescue him. "Oh, no," replied Mr. J. "But finally the crane operator flipped the platform, and I landed on my feet." The psychiatrist, using this metaphor, suggested that even if the medical staff could not "climb up" to help him, Mr. J could direct them to help him from farther away. The psychiatrist also acknowledged the extra difficulty and courage necessary for Mr. J to trust others with his life. Daily sessions in which Mr. J was able to discuss his fear, his depression and dissatisfaction with his life, and the connections these emotions had to his childhood helped him to understand his feelings. He gradually became less anxious and angry toward staff. Ultimately his foot was amputated, and he made a gradual but successful recovery.

NARRATIVE APPROACHES TO MEDICAL CARE

The focus of medical care is often on the patient's recent history of dealing with the current illness. The alternative **narrative approach** borrows from anthropologic concepts and focuses on understanding medical illness from within the context of the patient's entire life and his or her own explanation model for the illness. Rather than assigning meaning based on the average patient's experience, this approach features an emphasis on values derived from the patient's own life experience. This often leads to a fuller picture of both the patient and his or her adaptation to illness. It also reduces physicians' tendencies to categorize patients based on psychopathology.

Psychiatric consultation was requested by the oncology service for Karen M, a 29-year-old woman who refused a lumpectomy for a breast mass. Ms. M had detected the mass on self-examination and came to her doctor for evaluation. A mammogram could not distinguish between a benign mass or malignancy, and Ms. M received a referral to the surgery service. The surgeon was alarmed when she tried to schedule a biopsy and possible lumpectomy and Ms. M refused, telling her, "I'll have to think about this."

Ms. M accepted the psychiatry consultation reluctantly. She appeared slightly anxious but exhibited few psychiatric symptoms. There was no evidence of delusions, and her reality testing appeared intact. Ms. M explained that she did not want to be pressured into surgery, saying, "I know all about breast cancer." In the course of two meetings with the psychiatrist she described her mother's lingering illness and death from breast cancer and her role as her mother's caretaker when Ms. M was 16 years old.

Three months after her mother's death her father married their neighbor, and the family did not mention the mother again. Ms. M felt that she was the only one who kept her mother's memory alive.

She said, "Everyone wants me to rush into surgery so I can forget about it, but I want to talk about it first." The psychiatrist commented, "Maybe you are worried that having surgery quickly will also lessen your mother's memory, after being reminded of her so much." By the next appointment, Ms. M had made the appointment for surgery, which revealed a benign mass. However, Ms. M decided to continue psychotherapy, saying, "This cancer scare made me think about some of the things that I need to change in my life."

EMOTIONAL REACTIONS TO PATIENTS

Physicians are trained to respond objectively to medical illness, but less rational and more emotional reactions often pervade clinicians' experiences. Empathic responses may help the clinician understand the the patient's subjective experience. Some responses are based on the values of modern medicine, which tends to consider illness an aberrant state and death an unacceptable conclusion. By inference, clinicians minimize their anxiety about their limitations as healers by assuming that they have total control over the outcome of each case.

A medical student was assigned to perform a history and physical on Ahmad W, a 68-year-old man who was scheduled to undergo cardiac valve replacement surgery the next morning. Mr. W had signed the consent form for surgery and had been educated about all of the possible complications, including a 10% chance of death. He expressed his fear that he would die during the operation and wondered if he should say goodbye to his family "just in case." The student assured Mr. W that the surgery team was highly experienced and that his chances for a full recovery were excellent. The student even pointed out that his own grandmother had undergone the same surgery at age 75 with a good outcome. Yet Mr. W continued to verbalize his concern.

The next day the student "scrubbed in" for the operation with the surgery team. Although the surgery proceeded smoothly, Mr. W abruptly suffered cardiac arrest in the final stages of the operation. Cardiopulmonary resuscitation was unsuccessful, and Mr. W died. The student wondered if he should have listened to Mr. W's concerns more receptively and realized that he had tried to reassure Mr. W about surgery to lessen his own anxiety about the limitations of medical treatment and the possibilities of failure and death.

Other situations arise in which the technical prowess of medicine is decoupled from the necessary grounding in humanism or an appreciation of the patient as a person. Patients using denial or who are poorly adherent to medication regimens are perceived as frustrating because they do not act "rationally," while physicians who are working with anxious or depressed patients may avoid exploring their patients' emotional states. Clinicians under these circumstances often distance themselves from an empathic stance that would allow them to understand or to help their patients emotionally, concentrating exclusively on the technical aspects of the cases. Unfortunately this behavior is often modeled by attending and resident physicians, and then is emulated by trainees.

Rita T, aged 37, was diagnosed with advanced ovarian cancer with a poor prognosis. The medical team engaged in lengthy discussions about the unusual clinical presentation of the disease, the combinations of chemotherapy and advanced treatments that might be used, and the latest research contributions to understanding the genetics of ovarian cancer. There was no mention of how the diagnosis would affect Ms. T's life or her responsibility as a single parent to three children.

A medical student tried to raise these issues but was told by the resident that "the important thing now is to start her in treatment." The medical student brought to the team's attention a study citing improved survival in cancer patients who receive psychological support, and a pamphlet about local cancer support groups. Again he was told that this information was not a priority. The attending physician led the medical team to Ms. T's bedside and announced the diagnosis, the high likelihood of death within the next year, and the plan to begin chemotherapy immediately. Ms. T sat, stunned, and began to weep openly.

The team stood at Ms. T's bedside, and the attending asked "Do you have any questions?" Ms. T continued to sob and was so distraught that she was unable to respond. After a brief silence, the attending said, "You need to be alone to think about this" and motioned for the team to leave the patient's room.

This distancing probably accounts for some of the instances in which physicians miss or gloss over diagnoses of major depression in medically ill patients. Unfortunately both patients and physicians suffer from a failure to connect in these situations: Patients are left feeling alone and abandoned, while physicians develop technical competence while neglecting their own sense of meaning and purpose as healers. Interestingly, medical students often excel at forging therapeutic alliances with their patients, characterized by good communication and an avid interest in balancing a sense of personal connection with objective information gathering and decision making. Thus the task for medical students and other trainees is not so much to "learn" a bedside manner as it is to further develop these skills rather than sacrificing them in exchange for increased technical expertise.

Issues related to death and dying tend to be emotionally charged for patients and their physicians. Practitioners of Western medicine have an unfortunate tendency to be reductionistic, regarding the human body as a collection of parts that must be tuned or fixed. The language of medicine reflects the manner in which diseases become the enemy (eg, the "war on cancer"). A physician's frustration with his or her inability to completely control life and death may also turn to anger at patients, blaming them for their illnesses. This model is prone to being overly focused on outcomes and neglectful of efforts at prevention that are less dramatic but quite effective. Death is viewed as a "poor outcome," rather than an inevitable part of life. It is not surprising that hospital staff spend considerably less time with patients after they have been found to be terminally ill.

LEGAL & ETHICAL ISSUES

Numerous and complex ethical dilemmas may complicate the treatment of patients whose medical conditions are affected by psychological factors. Severe denial is unusual but can limit a patient's capacity to give informed consent, potentially to the point that the patient will be found legally incompetent to make decisions about his or her medical care. Although the preferred approach is to bide time and provide a supportive environment in the hopes that the patient will become more aware of the medical illness, this is not always possible. Clinicians must then decide whether to obtain surrogate decision-making from family members or the legal system, and whether the physician's prerogative to help the patient outweighs the patient's desire and right to autonomy.

A psychiatric consultation was requested for Albert F, a 54-year-old patient who was attempting to leave the intensive care unit (ICU) against medical advice. Mr. F had been admitted several days earlier for treatment of a dissecting aortic aneurysm.

A review of Mr. F's records and an interview with him revealed that he had been diagnosed with hypertension 2 years earlier. He appeared to be compliant with his high blood pressure medication and had previously presented to the outpatient clinic with blood pressure in the normal range. Several weeks before the hospital admission, Mr. F read an article about the possible dangers of his medication. He stopped the medication that day without attempting to discuss his decision with his physician or the advice nurse. He soon had chest and abdominal pain. He delayed treatment for weeks but ultimately sought medical attention in the emergency room, where his blood pressure was dangerously high and an x-ray showed an ominous ballooning of his aorta.

Mr. F refused surgery to correct the aneurysm, explaining that he was not even certain that he had suffered from hypertension, and despite the x-ray and other evidence, he did not believe that he had a life-threatening aneurysm.

Mr. F appeared to meet the criteria for schizoid personality disorder, having no contact with friends or family members and a suspicious and aloof attitude toward physicians and nurses. Attempts to scare Mr. F with dire predictions about his prognosis without surgery had failed and led to his abrupt decision to leave the hospital. The psychiatrist concurred that Mr. F's use of denial was so extreme as to preclude an ability to understand (or even believe) his diagnosis.

The cardiology team decided that in the absence of Mr. F's capacity to give informed consent, and without available family members, they would seek medical probate conservatorship from the local court to proceed with surgery. However, the team reversed their decision when they realized that Mr. F had passed the acute phase in which surgery had been shown to offer significant chances of improving survival rates and that he would do better if he continued to control his blood pressure with medication. They were concerned that Mr. F might be even less compliant if they forced him to have surgery. It also appeared unlikely that the court would force Mr. F to undergo invasive surgery that carried a 30% mortality rate. Ultimately he was discharged and was encouraged to continue his medication. After discharge he did not return for clinic appointments and was lost to follow-up.

The preceding case illustrates some of the limitations faced by physicians. Even when a patient is clearly not capable of making medical decisions, the proposed intervention may be too invasive or carry too much risk, or both, to proceed over the patient's objections. The other risk to be weighed in such a decision is the potential loss of trust between the patient and the physician, which may greatly hamper efforts to provide crucial ongoing care. Thus clinicians must look beyond the short-term medical crisis and to longer-term goals of adherence and coping within the context of a viable doctor-patient relationship.

A more common dilemma arises in treating patients whose decision-making and behavior related to their medical illness are adversely affected by depression or personality disorders. Clinicians may perceive, for example, that patients are making decisions that are influenced by pessimistic thinking that stems from depression and is not representative of their baseline state.

Susan R, aged 48, was diagnosed with diabetes shortly after her husband died 1 year earlier. Although her compliance with oral hypoglycemic medication had been adequate and her diabetes was under control, she complained of feeling poorly at her regular clinic visit. Her blood sugar was found to be markedly elevated despite continued adherence to medication. Her physician recommended that, given the progression of her diabetes, she start insulin injections.

Ms. R refused to take the prescription. She burst into tears and said that she had decided "not to fight the diabetes." She stated, "If it is my time to die, then it would be better for me to go quickly." Her physician learned that Ms. R, a formerly vivacious and outgoing person, had become extremely isolated in the previous 6 months. She slept poorly, had lost weight, had no interest in her hobbies, and cried frequently. Her daughter noted that Ms. R was no longer spending time with her grandchildren and added, "This isn't like my mother—I think that she's very lonely and depressed."

Ms. R was resistant to trying psychotherapy or antidepressant medication. Ultimately her depression worsened, and her physician and daughter acted together to seek an involuntary inpatient psychiatric hospitalization. Her daughter gave permission for Ms. R to receive insulin injections against her will to manage her diabetes. Ms. R. improved dramatically on an SSRI antidepressant and was discharged from the hospital 3 weeks later, noting that she was relieved that everyone had decided to help her. She said, "I'm so glad to be able to have more time with my grandchildren. Even when I was feeling the worst I still wanted someone to reach out to help me."

Patients who have personality disorders may benefit from behavioral interventions that offer positive incentives for desired health-related behavior. Physicians should be certain that they are acting in an ethical and responsible manner that preserves respect for the patient's autonomy and dignity. Any behavioral plan should satisfy the ethical cannon of justice; that is, decisions to limit care should not be applied uniformly to all patients who exhibit similar behavior. Arbitrary attempts to limit access to care or to "punish" patients who are noncompliant should be suspected as an often unconscious outgrowth of the physician's frustration and often punitive desires to "get back at" the difficult patient.

CONCLUSION

Psychiatric factors in disease prevention and medical illness are poorly integrated into the current practice of medicine. Psychiatric factors have a significant impact on adherence to medications, lifestyle habits that prevent or foster disease, and ultimately the individual patient's response and adaptation to medical illness. Depression and anxiety are all too common complications in the setting of medical illness and, as in other settings, remain woefully underdiagnosed and undertreated. Recent studies suggest that psychological variables that determine how patients adapt and cope with illness can be altered through psychosocial interventions and that such interventions produce not only better psychological coping but may positively influence the course of the medical illness itself. Although Western medicine draws a distinction between "mind" and "body," the body does not, and physicians who neglect psychological components of medical illness place their patients at risk for increased emotional suffering, morbidity, and death. Thus an imperative exists for physicians to gain familiarity with the possible range of responses to illness and to help guide patients toward improved coping with illness.

REFERENCES

Academy of Psychosomatic Medicine: http://www.apm.org/
Bauby J-D: *The Butterfly and the Diving Bell.* Knopf, 1997.
Byock I: *Dying Well: The Prospect for Growth at the End of Life.* Riverhead, 1996
Cain JM, Hammes BJ: Ethics and pain management: respecting patient wishes. J Pain Symptom Manage 1994;9(3):160.
Cassell E: *The Nature of Suffering.* Oxford University Press, 1991.
Cassem EH: Depression and anxiety secondary to medical illness. Psychiatr Clin N Am 1990;13(4):597.
Cassem N: The dying patient. In: Cassem EH, Stern TH, Rosenbaum JF (editors): *Massachusetts General Hospital Handbook of General Hospital Psychiatry,* 4th ed. Mosby Year Book, 1997.
Dreifuss-Kattan E: *Cancer Stories.* Analytic, 1990.
Evans WO: The undertreatment of pain. Indiana Med 1988;81(10):842.
Fawzy I: A critical review of psychosocial interventions in cancer care. Arch Gen Psychiatr 1995;52:100.
Fishman S: *Bomb in the Brain.* Avon, 1988.
Freeman H: Cancer in the socioeconomically disadvantaged. Ca–A Cancer J Clin 1989;39(5):266.
Groopman J: *The Measure of Our Days.* Viking, 1997.

Holland JC, Rowland JH (editors): *Handbook of Psychooncology: Psychological Care of the Patient with Cancer.* Oxford University Press, 1991.
Katon W, Sullivan MD: Depression and chronic medical illness. J Clin Psychiatr 1990;51(6)(Suppl):3.
Kaufman DM: Neurologic aspects of pain. Pages 333–352 in: *Clinical Neurology for Psychiatrists.* 4th ed. Saunders, 1995.
Kleinman A: *The Illness Narratives: Suffering, Healing and the Human Condition.* Basic, 1998.
McCormick TR, Conley BJ: Patients' perspectives on dying and on the care of dying patients. West J Med 1995;163(3):236.
McDaniel JS et al: Depression in patients with cancer. Arch Gen Psychiatr 1995;52:89.
Reiser DE, Rosen DH: *Medicine as a Human Experience.* University Park, 1984.
Rosenbaum EE: *The Doctor* (formerly published as *A Taste of My Own Medicine*). Ivy, 1988.
Shapiro PA, Lidagoster L, Glassman AH: Depression and heart disease. Psychiatr Ann 1997;27(5):347.
Wyszynski AA, Wyszynski B: *A Case Approach to Medical Psychiatric Practice.* American Psychiatric, 1996.
Yalom I: *Existential Psychotherapy.* Basic, 1980.

Psychiatric Aspects of HIV Infection

16

Kristine Yaffe, MD, David Elkin, MD, Francisco Gonzalez, MD, & Sophia Vinogradov, MD

The human immunodeficiency virus (HIV-1) is a relatively small molecular weight RNA retrovirus. Infection may occur through a variety of routes involving an exchange of bodily fluids. Such routes include sexual intercourse and exposure to blood products or needles contaminated with the virus (as occurs in intravenous drug users who share syringes or needles, transfusion recipients, or less commonly by accidental needle-sticks received in medical facilities). The virus then infects human cells, "pirating" their DNA replication mechanisms to produce and release multiple viral copies that go on to infect other cells.

The cells that are particularly targeted by the HIV virus are the T-Helper cells of the immune system. These cells provide the human body's defense against infection; thus, the patient with advanced HIV infection becomes susceptible to opportunistic bacterial and fungal infections (OIs) such as pneumocystic pneumonia, cryptosporidium, and toxoplasmosis. The presence of HIV is determined by an immunologic test for antibodies to HIV known as an ELISA test. A Western-blot test may be even more specific. T-Helper cells are measured by a CD4 count, which is normally over 1000 per cubic millimeter of blood. Declining CD4 counts mark the progress of HIV infection, while measurements of viral load are closely correlated with the rate at which the disease progresses. A term for an intermediate stage of HIV infection, ARC (AIDS-related condition), is no longer used. AIDS is an advanced form of HIV infection, defined by the presence of opportunistic infections, dementia due to the direct effect of HIV infection of the CNS, Kaposi's sarcoma, or a CD4 count of less than 200 (which is generally associated with these other medical diseases).

Psychological and social factors unique to HIV infection lead to stresses that may not be relevant in other illnesses. For example, the history of the HIV epidemic in the United States was marked by a notable lack of news coverage or directed attention by government officials in the early 1980s. Furthermore, in contrast to most other medical illnesses, HIV infection involves stigmatization and frequent marginalization from society, most likely because of the association of the virus in Western countries with homosexual or bisexual activity or IV drug use. Finally, "clustering" of HIV infection in a minority of the populace also makes it likely for HIV-positive individuals to have known other infected individuals who have become ill or died. These factors, as well as advances in care that have led to prolonged survival of HIV-positive patients, have become important considerations in the psychological adaptation of individuals to HIV infection (see Chapter 15 for more detailed consideration of the psychiatric aspects of medical illness).

The care of patients infected with HIV raises complex issues in assessment and patient care. The changing demographics of the AIDS epidemic to younger patients with coexisting problems of substance use, personality disorders, and psychiatric disorders presents challenges in the clinical care of patients. A patient's adaptation to HIV is influenced by the patient's psychological state as well as by diverse social and environmental factors. Depression, anxiety disorders, delirium, and psychosis may result from biological and psychological aspects of HIV infection. HIV-associated dementia exists in both mild and clinically significant forms, requiring prompt assessment and appropriate treatment. Caring for HIV-positive patients may stimulate difficult emotional reactions in medical teams, and physicians must also deal with multiple ethical and legal issues raised by HIV infection.

CHARACTERISTICS OF THE HIV EPIDEMIC

The Centers for Disease Control estimate that as many as 1 million people in the United States are infected with HIV. Since HIV infection was first diagnosed in the early 1980s, over 200,000 people, primarily gay white men, have died from the disease. Between 80,000 and 100,000 new cases of the infection are expected each year, and that rate may increase as HIV-infected patients live longer. While gay white men still constitute the largest group of infected individuals, the incidence of infection is rising among adolescents, intravenous drug users, women, and communities of color. AIDS has become a leading cause of death in adolescents and young adults, especially in urban areas.

Prevention strategies have helped stabilize rates of new infection among gay white men, but individuals who continue to engage in high-risk behaviors may do so for a variety of complex reasons. Social and political factors may play important roles (consider the battles around needle exchange, for example). Some individuals may not have access to information, counseling, or treatment in their language of origin or in terms that are culturally relevant.

Psychiatric morbidity may also play a role in HIV transmission. For example, a patient who has mania, typified by feelings of invulnerability and heightened sexual drive, might engage in increased risk-taking. Or poor reality testing might obscure a psychotic patient's judgment. Alcohol and substance abuse have often been implicated as potential risk factors, but even this relationship is not clear: use of intravenous amphetamines, for instance, is correlated with much higher HIV infection rates than is use of intravenous heroin. While early prevention strategies were aimed at providing information to urban gay white men, perhaps we now need interventions that explore social and interpersonal issues in a variety of cultural and psychosocial settings.

PSYCHIATRIC ASPECTS OF HIV INFECTION

Being tested for HIV infection is an anxiety-laden experience. The process involves evaluating past risk, deciding to seek one's HIV status, tolerating the waiting period before the results are in, and psychologically preparing for a positive or a negative result. Individuals who have a history of psychiatric illness may be at risk for exacerbations during this often stressful time. A careful psychiatric history should include not only a review of past illness and treatments but also

- attention to the motivation for obtaining HIV testing at the current time
- explicit and nonjudgmental discussion of sexual practices and needle use
- discussion of the relationship between at-risk behaviors and psychiatric symptoms and/or substance use

- safer sex guidelines and needle-cleaning techniques
- history of past reactions and coping strategies for stressful situations or trauma
- expected outcome(s) of the HIV test
- a plan of action for both positive and negative results

Clinicians should not assume that a negative result signifies the end of the process. Posttest counseling should focus on strategies to minimize risky behavior. A patient who has bipolar disorder, for example, might engage in impulsive, unprotected sexual encounters while manic or hypomanic, so the clinician might emphasize compliance with mood-stabilizing medications. Exploration of the context in which substance use occurs (eg, at a bar, in the streets, at a crack house) may lead to a fruitful discussion about harm reduction tactics. Amphetamine use, which has been particularly prevalent on the West coast, has been highly correlated with HIV risk. The clinician should help the patient explore ways to stay safe even when using substances and should make sure the patient knows how to use condoms and how to use bleach to sterilize needles.

For patients who test positive, the course of their existing psychiatric condition may be altered: For example, depressed or manic states may intensify in patients who have mood disorders, and substance use may increase among patients who already use alcohol or drugs to manage their stress. Information gleaned from the pretesting session will be invaluable in determining the patient's risk for suicide or decompensation. Posttest counseling for HIV-positive patients should include emotional support as well as a plan for obtaining medical care.

ASYMPTOMATIC HIV INFECTION STAGE

Infection with HIV often precipitates emotions and reactions similar to those seen in other life-threatening chronic illnesses. **Seroconversion,** the point at which the patient becomes HIV positive (assuming the patient is aware of this status) is often accompanied by a range of emotions, including shock, anger, guilt, anxiety, and denial. Clinicians need to help patients with medical questions and other issues. These issues include disclosure of HIV-positive status to friends, family, and employers; feelings of alienation and isolation; decisions about finances and work; and concerns about relationships, changes in body image, and psychological or spiritual crises. The latter often involves consideration of existential issues such as the meaning of life and death, both in a philosophical and a personal sense.

In many cases patients have a diminished capacity to take advantage of resources in the health-care system because of preexisting mood, psychotic, personality, or substance use disorders, or extreme fear or denial. Some patients learn that they are HIV positive after contracting an opportunistic infection, such as pneumocystosis (pneumonia caused by the *Pneumocystis carini* parasite), with an associated low CD4 lymphocyte count. Thus some patients rapidly advance from believing they are HIV negative to having to accept that they have full-blown AIDS.

Adjustment disorder with symptoms of depression, anxiety, or mixed emotional features is the most common diagnosis at this stage, affecting 10–20% of HIV-positive patients. Increased vulnerability to stress may occur in patients who are young, unemployed, have poor social support systems, or who use avoidance as a key coping style, including substance use or other self-destructive mechanisms for short-term escape of anxiety.

New drugs have had a significant impact on this stage. Average life expectancy may be increased significantly by the advent of protease inhibitors and other novel antiretrovirals soon to be released. However, the uncertainty surrounding prognosis and the longer-term impact of the latest generation of medications for treatment of HIV is a source of stress for many patients. A changing expectation about one's life span may produce stress in other less direct ways. For example, some patients in the mid-1990s took advantage of reverse mortgages or early settlement on life insurance policies, or they went into debt based on the assumption that they should be prepared to die within a year or two. With the development of protease inhibitors they found themselves regaining their health but were confronted with the financial burdens they had incurred. Other patients lost their disability status and stipends and needed to find jobs quickly to cover their expenses and debts.

NEUROPSYCHIATRIC DISEASE IN HIV INFECTION & AIDS

Before diagnosing a primary psychiatric disorder in an HIV-positive individual, the clinician must rule out other illnesses (both central nervous system and systemic). It is helpful to know the patient's psychiatric history, level of immune suppression, medical history, and medications taken. Most psychiatric disorders in HIV-positive patients are treatable, but accurate diagnoses must be made based on signs, symptoms, and history.

A complete physical and laboratory workup is essential in the care of any patient who has HIV but is especially critical in HIV-positive patients who have dementia. Most asymptomatic HIV-positive patients have normal central nervous system (CNS) test results. These studies tend to become more abnormal as patients progress to AIDS. Lumbar puncture analysis of cerebrospinal fluid (CSF) often shows pleocytosis and elevated protein levels. Computed tomography (CT) and magnetic resonance imaging (MRI) head scans may show several types of abnormalities, including focal abnormalities from opportunistic infections such as toxoplasmosis, or generalized atrophy and ventricular enlargement.

HIV-ASSOCIATED DEMENTIA

HIV-1-associated cognitive/motor complex is the general diagnostic category for the syndrome manifested in HIV-infected patients with disabling cognitive, motor, and behavioral symptoms that interfere with social and occupational functioning. There are three subtypes:

- **HIV-1-associated dementia complex** (previously termed subacute encephalitis, HIV encephalopathy, and AIDS-related dementia)
- **HIV-1-associated myelopathy** (previously termed HIV encephalopathy)
- **HIV-1-associated minor cognitive/motor disorder** (previously termed HIV-1-associated neurocognitive disorder or HIV-1-associated neurobehavioral abnormalities)

The three syndromes may represent a single entity with a broad spectrum of clinical presentations and severity, or they may signify discrete syndromes. The manifestations of the first two types, which are more severe, are sufficient for a diagnosis of AIDS. They usually occur in combination with other AIDS-defining illness and are usually seen in patients who have low CD4 counts. The third form, which is milder, is not sufficient for an AIDS diagnosis, although it may be present in patients who have AIDS.

Incidence

Studies from the 1980s suggested that a majority of patients who had AIDS would develop dementia, and that many HIV-positive patients in the earlier stages of the illness would have noticeable cognitive problems that would interfere with their daily lives. Newer studies estimate the annual incidence of HIV-associated dementia (HAD) at 7–14%, and many studies show that significant cognitive dysfunction does not occur in patients who have higher CD4 counts.

The most recent research from the National Institute of Mental Health (NIMH) seems to suggest a convergence of these views: 16% of HIV-negative/at-risk men demonstrated mild cognitive impairment, 33% of asymptomatic HIV-positive men showed impairment, and 44% of late-stage AIDS patients had milder or more severe dementia. The criteria used to determine dementia create a threshold that has implications for incidence, since a lower threshold yields greater detection of milder disease. If one looks carefully enough with sensitive measures, subtle or subacute cognitive impairment can be found in many patients; but most early-stage patients have such mild cognitive problems that the findings are not clinically relevant. The problem of dementia tends to be more important in patients who have more advanced HIV disease.

Etiology

Dementia is a well-known complication of HIV, resulting from other CNS pathology or the direct effect of HIV on the human brain. Studies revealed evidence of the HIV virus in 90% of autopsied patients who had dementia, and evidence indicates the HIV virus can invade the CNS early in the course of infection. The virus is rarely detected in neurons, however. Instead, it is found in mononuclear and microglial cells and occasionally in endothelial cells. The virus shows special affinity for macrophages, resulting in inflammation and cell death.

Although brain biopsies are not conducted as a standard diagnostic tool, autopsies have revealed various neuropathic changes, including astrocytic gliosis (inflammation of the cells that help scavenge byproducts of neuronal metabolism and form scar tissue in damaged portions of the CNS), microglial nodules (dense formations in the cells that function as the phagocytes, or scavengers, of the CNS), and vacuolar changes. Multinucleated giant cells derived from macrophages are a hallmark of CNS infection with HIV. Mononuclear cells or astrocytes may be capable of producing cytokines that interfere with neuronal functioning. These cells may generate abnormal neurotransmitter metabolites (such as quinolinic acid) that are neurotoxic. Viral fragments may interfere with neuronal function by docking at critical receptor sites. The result at the end-organ level is diffuse white matter disease and atrophy, which are visible in later stages on head CT or MRI. CSF obtained by lumbar puncture often shows nonspecific findings such as increased protein and white blood cell counts. This is an important area of investigation because neuronal dysfunction may be reversible in the early stages of CNS disease since neurons are not directly invaded by HIV-1.

Clinical Manifestations

At a clinical level, HIV-associated dementia tends to resemble other dementias such as Alzheimer's disease, multi-infarct, and alcohol-related dementias, with disruption of short-term memory, concentration, visuospatial abilities, and abstracting ability, as well as personality and behavior changes. HIV typically produces a subcortical pattern of cognitive dysfunc-

tion similar to dementia from Huntington's chorea, with psychomotor slowing, relative sparing of language, apathy, and gait abnormalities. Although patients who have cortical dementia have difficulty learning items for the test of short-term memory and are likely to make up answers when tested at 5 minutes, patients with HIV show less difficulty learning test items. They tend to have difficulty retrieving these words at 5 minutes, but prompting with hints often leads to recall in patients with mild to moderate dementia. Thus the memory problems of HAD indicate a problem with short-term memory retrieval as opposed to new learning.

HIV-1-associated dementia complex is characterized by disabling cognitive impairment usually accompanied by motor dysfunction, behavioral change, or both. Manifestations include

- poor concentration
- forgetfulness (poor recent memory, particularly rapid decay of acquired information)
- mental slowness
- speech alterations (eg, quieter, slower speech)
- frank confusion (consistent with delirium), which may complicate the clinical presentation
- spatial problems and disorientation
- temporal disorientation
- frontal-executive system problems, including poor conceptual skills, difficulty with sequencing and tracking, or poor mental flexibility
- frontal lobe release signs such as glabellar, palmar-mental, and snout reflexes (neurologic signs elicited on physical examination)
- behavioral changes (eg, apathy, lethargy, loss of sexual drive, diminished emotional responsiveness, social withdrawal, irritability, and increasing inflexibility to change)
- early motor symptoms, including tremors, unsteady gait, and weakness that is greater in upper than lower extremities
- later motor symptoms, including slowed rapid movements, limb incoordination, hyperreflexia (increased deep tendon reflexes), hypertonia (increased motor tone), and peripheral neuropathy (such as diminished perception of pain and temperature in hands and feet)

HIV-1-associated myelopathy refers to the condition in which patients have greater muscular dysfunction than cognitive impairment and includes

- progressive gait disturbance
- lower extremity spasticity
- leg weakness and spasticity (paraparesis)
- extensor-plantar responses (dorsiflexion of the great toe due to upper motor neuron pathology)
- urinary incontinence
- mild cognitive impairment

In the milder form known as HIV-1-associated minor cognitive/motor dysfunction, cognitive impairment can be detected only with detailed neuropsychological testing but may be clinically evident only in the most demanding situations. The bedside mental status examination may be normal, but symptoms include

- inattention and impaired concentration (as evidenced by difficulties with serial sevens, digits backward, and more difficult tests of concentration)
- mild memory loss (low delayed recall relative to immediate recall or low immediate recall relative to peers)
- mild psychomotor slowing
- blunted affect
- normal neurological examination in most cases

Differential Diagnosis

Care should always be taken to rule out treatable causes of dementia. These include infectious diseases of the CNS such as toxoplasmosis, cytomegalovirus (CMV) and neurosyphilis, thyroid disorders, vitamin deficiencies, and medication side effects.

The symptoms of depression may overlap with HAD and should be considered carefully. In some cases patients may have a clinical picture of combined depression and dementia. If no practical separation of the two entities is possible, standard treatment of depression with psychotherapy and antidepressant medication may be warranted. In many cases cognitive ability and other measures of dementia may improve when a patient is started on a therapeutic dose of antidepressant.

Prognosis

Severe HAD primarily affects patients who have low CD4 counts (generally below 200) and is associated with a short life expectancy on the order of 6 months, although these figures have not been updated to include the benefits of antiretroviral agents.

In studies conducted in the late 1980s, as many as one-third of HIV-positive patients had at least a mild degree of dementia. The use of AZT may have protected against dementia by activity against HIV, even in the CSF, along with improving the survival of HIV-positive patients. Because antiretroviral medications do not cross the blood-brain barrier and the HIV virus easily enters the CNS, there is now concern that longer life spans for HIV-positive patients will also be accompanied by a rise in the incidence of HAD.

Treatment

Treatment for HAD consists of following principles:

- Conduct a thorough workup to characterize dementia etiology, if possible.
- Assess and treat for reversible causes of dementia (such as neurosyphilis, medications, endocrine abnormalities).
- Ameliorate associated conditions that complicate dementia such as delirium, depression, substance use, and malnutrition.
- Assess patient's capacity for activities of daily living (ADLs). Home nursing or placement to a structured setting may be necessary for patients who are unable to care for themselves.
- Provide support and education to families. Support and bereavement groups may play a critical role.

Steve C, aged 32, had AIDS and was hospitalized for pneumocystic pneumonia and "failure to thrive." He was extremely malnourished and withdrawn, with impaired memory and concentration problems on cognitive testing. He also wept frequently, ruminated about death, and had many of the key symptoms of major depression. His pneumonia cleared, and the health-care team considered placing him at a hospice. He continued to require help dressing and feeding himself. While he was waiting for placement he was started on an SSRI antidepressant. Within 2 weeks, his mood, memory, and concentration had improved and he began to take a much more active role in his own care. By the time a bed was available at the hospice, he was able to take care of himself at home with part-time help from a visiting nurse in spite of continued mild cognitive deficits.

Diagnosis. Dementia and depression secondary to AIDS (Axis I); AIDS, pneumonia (Axis III).

DEPRESSIVE SYNDROMES

Depressive syndromes that may occur in HIV-positive patients include episodes of major depression, dysthymia (chronic depression), and adjustment disorder. Current studies suggest that the rate of major depression in HIV-positive patients is approximately twice that of healthy controls. Depression is even more likely to occur in hospitalized patients. A past history of depression places the patient at further risk for depression in the course of infection with HIV.

Differential Diagnosis

CNS processes such as toxoplasmosis, cryptococcol meningitis, progressive multifocal leukodystrophy (PML), and lymphoma should be ruled out before proceeding with treatment. Patients with HIV are often on complex medication regimens, some of which can cause depression. Symptoms of dementia may overlap with those of depression, particularly psychomotor slowing that occurs in subcortical patterns of HIV-associated dementia.

The concurrence of any physical illness may complicate the diagnosis of depression because of the overlap of symptoms such as lethargy and fatigue; insomnia; poor concentration; or reduced energy, appetite, and weight. The clinician should therefore rely on the patient's self-reported symptoms and ask specifically about the patient's mood and feelings of sadness, guilt, hopelessness, anhedonia (lack of pleasure in most activities), and suicidal ideation. If suicidal thoughts are present, the clinician should follow up with standard questions about how often these thoughts occur, whether the patient has a plan for suicide, and if there is a personal or family history of suicide attempts. The risk of suicide should not be underestimated in patients with HIV. Among the causes of death in HIV-positive patients, suicide is second only to medical complications of the illness.

Treatment

Just as patients who have chronic illness such as cancer were once considered to have "appropriate depression" in the face of a life-threatening illness, and hence not warranting treatment, there may be a bias against treating depression in HIV-positive patients. However, clinical studies have repeatedly demonstrated that depression is associated with significant suffering, and in medically ill patients depression often reduces adherence to medications, as well as increases mortality through a variety of mechanisms. Depression is also suspected to reduce the effective function of the body's immune system and to jeopardize the patient's physical well-being.

The treatment of depression in HIV-positive patients includes psychotherapy with the possible addition of antidepressant medication if the depression is of moderate or greater severity. Given the difficulty of establishing whether a patient is depressed or dysthymic in the midst of a serious chronic medical illness, clinicians may need to treat patients empirically in the absence of a firm diagnosis. Various forms of psychotherapy are helpful, including individual psychodynamic or cognitive therapy, or group psychotherapy.

HIV-positive patients may be significantly more sensitive to all psychotropic medications and their side effects; thus, certain medications should be avoided and others used cautiously. Tricyclic antidepressants (TCAs) with strong anticholinergic properties such as amitryptiline (Elavil) or clomipramine (Anafranil) should not be used because of the risk of inducing anticholinergic delirium. Suicidal patients can easily use TCAs to overdose.

The SSRI antidepressants are effective in HIV-positive patients but should be started at a low dosage and increased gradually to minimize side effects, which may include agitation, insomnia, nausea, headache, and decreased sex drive. Nausea may be

particularly problematic in HIV-positive patients who are already malnourished.

Psychostimulants have been used to treat depression in medically ill patients, including patients who have HIV. Psychostimulants rapidly alleviate depressive symptoms, sometimes within days, but may suppress the patient's appetite or induce psychosis. All antidepressant medication has the potential to induce manic states in patients who have known or previously undiagnosed bipolar disorder.

> Roberto L, a 35-year-old gay man, had learned he was HIV positive 2 years earlier, soon after the death of a close relative from AIDS prompted him to get tested. Though he had felt quite overwhelmed and depressed at that time, he had not sought treatment. He now presented to an outpatient clinic with symptoms of depression characterized by insomnia, sadness, decreased energy, difficulty concentrating, fleeting suicidal ideation, and guiltiness after breaking up with his lover of 1 year.
>
> He spent many of his waking hours obsessively ruminating about complicated dynamics with his ex-lover, whom he felt was the one person who had really supported and understood him since his HIV-positive status had been discovered. He cried easily and felt overwhelmed and helpless. In the context of psychotherapy and case management services, Mr. L was started on paroxetine, at a half dose of 10 mg in the morning. Because of his acute anxiety and insomnia, he was also prescribed lorazepam (0.5 mg) on an as-needed basis to help manage his feelings during the crisis. His symptoms improved considerably after a few weeks, and the lorazepam was tapered off slowly.
>
> **Diagnosis.** Major depression (Axis I); HIV infection (Axis III).

MANIA

Differential Diagnosis

Symptoms of mania are an unusual presentation in HIV-positive patients. A complete differential diagnosis includes screening for preexisting bipolar disorder, but other causes should be sought. Some medications such as prednisone or isoniazid can induce mania, as can CNS pathologies or cocaine and methamphetamine use. The cytotoxic effects of the HIV virus in the brain seem to be capable of producing mania, as evidenced by the higher than expected rate of mania in HIV-positive patients who lack a past or family history that would place them at risk of primary psychiatric disease.

Treatment

Treatment for manic episodes includes neuroleptics and a mood stabilizer (eg, lithium carbonate, divalproic acid [Depakote], or carbamezepine [Tegretol]). Lithium may be less effective in preventing future episodes of mania than are the anticonvulsants. In patients treated with lithium prior to HIV infection, the clinician should consider changing to one of the anticonvulsants. HIV disease promotes shifts in fluid volume (eg, through diarrhea), which can place patients at greater risk for lithium toxicity. Some physicians have been wary about starting HIV-positive patients on carbamezepine because of the potential side effect of reducing white blood cell counts, but this seems to be more an anecdotal than a proscriptive concern. Patients who have severe mania may also have psychotic symptoms and may require inpatient psychiatric treatment.

Sylvia S, a 22-year-old woman, was admitted to the medicine service with fever of unknown origin and altered mental status in the context of AIDS (her CD4 count was around 100). Chest x-ray revealed a bacterial pneumonia, which was treated to resolution with intravenous antibiotics, but her mental status did not improve. Ms. S suffered from a severely disturbed sleep-wake cycle and insomnia, pressured speech that was tangential and disorganized, and hyperreligiousity in which she believed she was on a divine mission to save the world.

An extensive medical workup was inconclusive: CT and MRI scans were normal, the rapid plasma reagin (RPR) test (for syphilis) was nonreactive, lumbar puncture revealed a mild elevation in protein but was otherwise normal, as were standard chemistries and hematological tests (except for the CD4 count) after treatment for the pneumonia. Low-dose perphenazine (4–8mg) and lorazepam (0.5–1mg) were used on an as-needed basis to help manage her behavioral disturbance. She was transferred to a psychiatric inpatient unit for further stabilization.

History from collateral sources revealed that Ms. S had been using methamphetamines the week prior to her admission but had previously been relatively high functioning and had no formal psychiatric history. There was no psychiatric history in the family. Although her sleep-wake cycle had stabilized (she was no longer sleeping during the day), she was sleeping only 3–4 hours each night. She would often disrobe on the unit and stand gazing at the ceiling, yelling, "I am Jehovah!"

The team decided to start her on valproic acid (250 mg three times daily [TID]), targeting manic symptoms. The dose was increased rapidly to 2500 mg daily in divided doses, with therapeutic blood levels. Ms. S's delusions and disorganized thoughts diminished over the next several weeks, and she began to engage staff in reality-based conversations for the first time.

She was discharged to a residential treatment site for further stabilization.

Diagnosis. Bipolar disorder, manic phase, versus mania secondary to HIV infection or substance use (Axis I); AIDS (Axis III).

ANXIETY DISORDERS

Patients who have HIV are at risk for several different manifestations of anxiety, including episodes of generalized anxiety as well as acute panic attacks. These disorders can occur at any stage of the illness.

Differential Diagnosis

Medical causes for anxiety should always be ruled out, including alcohol withdrawal or medication side effects. Other psychiatric disorders such as depression with prominent symptoms of anxiety should be considered. Early delirium from a medical illness such as pneumonia may have early manifestations of anxiety. The psychological stress of the HIV virus may reactivate old anxiety disorders. Patients are commonly very anxious while awaiting results of an HIV test or determination of viral load and other indicators of the progression of the illness. Later complications such as CMV retinitis that cause progressive blindness may cause considerable emotional distress.

HIV-positive patients are also at risk for post-traumatic stress disorder (PTSD) from invasive medical procedures. Multiple losses of friends to AIDS often produce symptoms of emotional numbing and intrusive phenomena similar to PTSD. Survivor guilt may develop among those who are doing well with their illness or among HIV-negative individuals who have HIV-positive lovers or friends. Some studies suggest high degrees of emotional distress among HIV-negative gay men, resulting from these factors as well as from the general marginalization of gays in society.

Treatment

Treatment for anxiety disorders varies depending on symptomatology. Psychotherapy, treatment of existing substance use disorders, and behavioral prescriptions such as exercise or relaxation techniques are some of the options. Benzodiazepines can be useful in managing acute anxiety with two important caveats. First, in patients who have dementia, benzodiazepines can promote clouded thinking and delirium. Mid-potency neuroleptics, in low doses, are helpful in reducing anxiety in this group of patients. Second, the clinician must carefully monitor drug interactions, especially with some of the protease inhibitors, which can inhibit metabolism of benzodiazepines. Busprione (BuSpar) or low doses of antidepressants are useful for more chronic, generalized anxiety states. Nonactivating antidepressants such as paroxetine (Paxil) and nefazodone (Serzone) are preferred for more acute symptomatology such as panic disorder.

Several months after the death of his partner of 4 years from AIDS, Jeff D decided to have an HIV test for the first time. Though Mr. D had been the victim of physical abuse in the relationship, he idealized his partner after his death. They had often used alcohol and amphetamines together, but Mr. D now resolved to become clean and sober. He had a month's sobriety when he learned he was HIV positive.

Days afterward, his diagnosis was advanced to AIDS on the basis of a CD4 count less than 200 and the diagnosis of Kaposi's sarcoma (KS) lesions on his arms and face. Mr. D also began to experience pain in his chest and developed a cough. A chest CT scan was added to an extensive medical workup. Mr. D presented to his case manager in a crisis characterized by intense fear, insomnia, nightmares, autonomic arousal, depression, and suicidality. He was subsequently hospitalized. Once on the inpatient unit, Mr. D's suicidality resolved and his sleep improved; however, he remained anxious and overwhelmed. His anxiety was exacerbated by news that the CT revealed pulmonary KS.

The staff decided to proceed with a multifaceted treatment plan. Individual staff members met with Mr. D frequently throughout the day to provide education about medical issues, support his sobriety, and help him develop coping strategies. An HIV support group on the unit also provided containment for his anxiety. He was started on buspirone (5 mg TID) and lorazepam (1 mg) as needed for anxiety.

The treatment team organized a conference with Mr. D and his various providers, including his case manager, a residential substance abuse program director, his primary care doctor, a visiting home psychoeducation nurse, and the inpatient team. A comprehensive treatment plan was formulated that provided needed structure and greatly allayed Mr. D's fears. He was discharged to a residential substance abuse treatment facility and began aggressive medical treatments. His anxiety improved considerably, and he maintained his sobriety. Three months later he required an overnight hospitalization for suicidality during which the buspirone was doubled, but overall he continued to do well emotionally and remained sober.

Diagnosis. Adjustment disorder with mixed emotional features (Axis I); AIDS, Kaposi's sarcoma (Axis III).

PSYCHOTIC DISORDER

Psychosis is an uncommon complication of HIV, more often occurring as a manifestation of a preexisting psychiatric disorder such as mania, depression, or schizophrenia but sometimes as a complication of the HIV virus itself.

Differential Diagnosis

CNS pathology, drug use (especially stimulants or hallucinogens), or severe dementia may also be accompanied by hallucinations or delusions. Some of the medications used to treat HIV infection and its complications may cause psychosis. Delirium may mimic psychosis; if the patient has an altered level of consciousness with a waxing and waning quality, delirium should be considered and medical illness excluded. Severely psychotic patients may be extremely disorganized, suicidal, or a danger to others, possibly warranting admission to a psychiatric inpatient unit for observation and treatment.

Treatment

Antipsychotic medications provide effective treatment for psychosis, but care must be taken to avoid medications that have strong anticholinergic side effects and to use lower dosages. Side effects occur much more commonly in HIV-positive individuals than they do in those who are HIV negative. Such effects include extrapyramidal symptoms, akathisia, and neuroleptic malignant syndrome (NMS). NMS is marked by changes in motor rigidity, autonomic nervous system dysfunction, and delirium, and it carries a high mortality rate. Neuroleptics should be discontinued and supportive care initiated if NMS is suspected.

DELIRIUM

Delirium occurs frequently in HIV-positive patients, particularly those patients who already have dementia, are hospitalized, or have advanced disease. CNS disease, systemic illness, and drug use are also risk factors in the HIV-positive patient. Delirium is commonly underdiagnosed and undertreated, particularly when the patient has a so-called quiet (hypoactive) delirium with subtle manifestations. Symptoms include an altered level of consciousness, cognitive dysfunction, hallucinations, and delusions. The onset of delirium is typically abrupt, often occurring within hours or days.

Differential Diagnosis

Delirium is often a consequence of underlying medical illness, and a search for the cause is always the first priority in workup and diagnosis. HIV-positive patients take many medications, and medications can cause delirium, so medication regimens should be simplified as much as possible. Anticholinergic agents in particular can cause delirium in HIV-positive patients.

Treatment

Treatment should be directed to correct the underlying medical condition. Behavioral cues, such as familiar objects from home, can help orient patients. Medication may be used when appropriate (eg, benzodiazepines for delirium caused by alcohol use, and low-dose high-potency antipsychotics for other causes).

SUBSTANCE DEPENDENCE & ABUSE

Substance dependence and abuse conditions may drastically affect many aspects of patient care. Impairment of judgment and impulse control, both common in substance-abusing patients, represent important risk factors for transmission of HIV, and clinicians can help prevention efforts by aggressively treating patients who exhibit these symptoms. Impairment of judgment and impulse control also have a negative effect on medical care in general, especially on adherence to medication, and particularly for complex treatment regimens with antiretroviral medications. Incomplete or flawed adherence to these medications could theoretically hasten the development of treatment-resistant strains of the HIV virus.

The individual response of patients to HIV is varied. In general, patients who have substance use problems cope more poorly with any chronic illness, and the stress of the illness may encourage patients to abandon attempts at sobriety. For many patients, substance use is a strategy utilized to decrease anxiety, and these patients may experience a greater need for drugs or alcohol to manage increased stress. For other patients, HIV-positive status may serve as a "wake-up call" that increases their motivation to cease drug use. Referral to drug and alcohol rehabilitation programs may be most helpful. When substance use is linked to other psychiatric disorders such as depression or anxiety disorders, treatment with psychotherapy and medications may also help with the substance use.

SUICIDE

The risk of suicide in HIV-positive patients has been estimated at 17–36 times greater than that of the general population and much higher than that seen in patients who have other chronic illnesses. These figures are conservative at best, because they are not likely to include some cases of drug overdose or passive suicide brought about by poor self-care. Several factors contribute to this high rate of suicide:

- high incidence of comorbid psychiatric disorders such as depression, personality disorders, and substance use

- lack of support systems available to gay patients (who face both marginalization in society as well as multiple personal losses to AIDS) and patients who use substances
- relative younger age of incidence, which may create less tolerance for progression of the illness
- access to physicians and other resources to obtain large doses of medication used in attempts
- lack of access to mental health services

Because of the high rate of suicide in HIV-positive patients, it is also likely that many patients have friends who have attempted or completed suicide attempts. Finally, as in Huntington's chorea, dementia associated with reduced judgment and impulse control may increase the risk of suicide.

Until several years ago, the progression from HIV-positive status to AIDS was often greeted with a sense of relief by patients. Now that protease inhibitors are available and the spectrum of HIV-related illness is measured on a yardstick of CD4 counts and total viral load, HIV-positive patients have a reason to hope for further advances in treatment, if not a cure. This is also a contrast to 1994, when a transient increase in suicide attempts was seen in HIV-positive patients after news spread that anti-HIV agents that had been promising at the time had failed in intermediate stages of treatment.

Treatment

Treatment for suicidal HIV-positive patients follows the guidelines for other patients at risk of self-harm. A critical point in the assessment of any suicidal patient involves a consideration of whether the individual can be managed as an outpatient or requires inpatient psychiatric hospitalization. When antidepressants are used, SSRIs and other newer antidepressants are preferred to TCAs (for which a week's supply may be a lethal overdose). Frequent outpatient appointments are preferred, and patients should have access to other emergency contacts in case of increased suicidality.

EMOTIONAL REACTIONS TO PATIENTS

Patients with HIV infection may prompt intense emotional reactions from medical providers and trainees. Dreams about HIV patients are common among medical trainees. These responses are shaped both by the individual health-care worker and by the social perception of HIV. Reactions are complicated by the younger age of patients and by conscious or unconscious feelings about sexual orientation or substance use. The presence of comorbid psychiatric conditions such as mood disorders, psychosis, delirium, dementia, personality disorders, or suicidality may further accentuate feelings. Fear of contamination may influence the attitude of providers, particularly given the possibility of contracting HIV by accidental needle-stick. Overidentification with younger patients (experiencing the patients as like oneself) tends to lead to overinvolvement and inappropriately aggressive medical interventions. Underidentification may cause undertreatment and poor alliance due to boredom, distancing, blaming, and anger at patients.

A medical student assigned to the care of a patient with AIDS noted in the patient profound cognitive deficits consistent with dementia. She proposed a workup for the dementia to exclude reversible causes, including toxoplasmosis and other opportunistic infections. The supervising intern refused to endorse the workup, stating, "It's a waste of time and money to try to treat a demented patient." The medical student discussed the case at morning rounds with the chief resident, who told her to proceed. The intern acknowledged that he felt "burned out by all of the AIDS cases."

LEGAL & ETHICAL ISSUES

Myriad complex legal and ethical issues arise in the care of patients who have AIDS. Since the advent of the HIV test, questions about access to testing and confidentiality have pitted public health concerns against matters of civil liberty. Physicians are required to notify state health agencies when a patient has a sexually transmitted disease such as gonorrhea or syphilis, for example, but there are no such reporting requirements for HIV. Some health-care workers have argued for the right to have patients tested against their will in the case of accidental exposure to body fluids. Some physicians have circumvented informed consent and illegally inferred their patients' HIV status indirectly by ordering CD4 counts in patients who refuse HIV testing.

Similarly, a number of issues arise in trying to carry out patients' wishes. In the case of a late-stage patient who has dementia, health-care workers may have to struggle with the question of placing the patient in a nursing home, hospital, or dementia unit, against the patient's will. Physicians may be called upon to evaluate a patient's capacity to give informed consent for medical procedures, do-not-resuscitate orders, or experimental study protocols.

As in other serious chronic illnesses, a significant number of patients will desire direct or indirect help from their physicians in choosing to end their lives. One study showed that over half of the physicians who had treated AIDS patients in a large urban area had assisted a terminally ill patient in dying. At issue is the individual patient's right to choose death versus society's need to uphold values. Physicians are in the middle of this dilemma and must wrestle with how to deal with their own values, the question of how depression or dementia affect a patient's ability to weigh these choices, and the legal and ethical dangers inherent in the physician's role if physician-assisted suicide is permitted.

Even the procedures for conducting scientific investigation and developing pharmaceutical products have been irrevocably and dramatically changed by the profound ethical challenges presented by the epidemic. Double-blind protocols or slow, detailed studies of new drugs have been replaced, in part, by open-label trials and fast-track FDA development. Policy questions about how to allocate limited resources—whether in ongoing HIV-prevention efforts, access to expensive protease inhibitors, or the development of new treatments—are influenced by ethical concerns.

There is no easy or formulaic answer to these extremely complex issues. In the clinical setting, open discussion can be invaluable. Where possible, an ethics team (now routinely available in most hospitals) can facilitate a conference that might involve the patient and family, representatives from various treatment teams, social workers, clergy, or legal counsel.

CONCLUSION

In the early twentieth century syphilis was regarded as the most protean medical illness. The same can now be said of infection by HIV. There are many psychiatric aspects of the HIV infection. Patients with HIV are at risk for psychiatric illness and vice versa. Psychiatric manifestations of HIV should be considered at various stages of infection, including preconversion, asymptomatic HIV infection, and later stages of the disease. Depression, mania, psychosis, substance use, delirium, and dementia may occur during these stages, requiring adequate assessment and treatment. Living with HIV requires an adaptation similar to coping with other chronic illness but with some important distinctions. Understanding medical staff reactions to patients with HIV and the ethical and legal issues posed by HIV are essential components of patient care.

REFERENCES

Bateson MC, Goldberg R: *Thinking AIDS: The Social Response to the Biological Threat.* Addison-Wesley, 1988.

Boccellari A, Zeifert P: Management of neurobehavioral impairment in HIV-1 infection. Psychiatr Clin N Am 1994;17(1):183.

Chesney MA, Folkman S: Psychological impact of HIV disease and implications for intervention. Psychiatr Clin N Am 1994;17(1):163.

Cohen PT, Sande MA, and Volderbing P, eds: The AIDS Knowledge Base. 3rd ed. Lippincott Raven. 1998.

Fee E, Fox R: *AIDS: The Burden of History.* University of California Press, 1988.

Feldman D (editor): *Culture and AIDS.* Praeger, 1990.

Janicak PG: Psychopharmacotherapy in the HIV-infected patient. Psychiatr Ann 1995;25(10):609.

Koenig B, Cooke M: Physician response to a new, lethal and presumably infectious disease: medical resident and the AIDS epidemic in San Francisco. The meaning of AIDS implications for medical science, clinical practice and public health policy. Stud Health Human Values 1989;(1):63.

Melton ST, Kirkwood CK, Ghaemi SN: Pharmacotherapy of HIV dementia. Ann Pharmacother 1997;31:457.

Monette P: *Borrowed Time: An AIDS Memoir.* Avon, 1988.

National Institutes of Health, Office of AIDS Research: http://www.nih.gov/od/oar/

National Library of Medicine HIV/AIDS Resources: http://sis.nlm.nih.gov/aidswww.htm

NIMH Office on AIDS. http://www.nimh.nih.gov/oa/news.htm

Shilts R: *And the Band Played On.* St. Martins, 1987.

Verghese A: *My Own Country: A Doctor's Story of a Town and Its People in an Age of AIDS.* Simon & Schuster, 1994.

Zeghans LS, Coates TJ (editors): Psychiatric manifestations of HIV disease. Psychiatr Clin N Am 1994:17(1).

17

Systems Issues, Groups, and Families

David Elkin, MD

Modern medicine has an impressive record in treating and preventing illness. Remarkable advances have been made over the past half-century, particularly in the area of biomedicine. Unfortunately, the technologically driven, specialized nature of modern health care tends to focus on single organ systems to the exclusion of other important considerations of the patient as a human being or as an individual who is a part of a family or society. In fact many determinants of both physical and emotional health are features of larger levels of organizations: family, workplace, and society.

To become competent in working with families and other groups, physicians must be familiar with some of the basic elements of a systems approach and must understand the fundamental principles of group psychology. This chapter illustrates the application of a systems approach to several different settings: groups in general, families, and medical teams. Cults represent a special case of group dynamics. Physicians need to develop the skills necessary to work in these settings and should be aware of the legal and ethical dilemmas inherent in working with larger groups and systems.

THE THEORETICAL BUILDING BLOCKS OF SYSTEMS THEORY

The terminology and vocabulary particular to medicine reflects a bias toward reductionism and is poorly suited to an understanding of larger systems. A brief review of terms frequently used in systems theory serves as both a lexicon of essential terms as well as a starting point to introduce key theoretical concepts.

A **system** is an aggregate of parts or units that are interconnected and that influence each other. These units may consist of organs, as in the human body; of people, as in a family or other group; or of groups, as in communities or nations. Individual units are joined and mutually influenced by communication. **Communication theory** emphasizes the flow of information between people or organizations.

Distortions and rumors are easily transmitted throughout hospitals and the medical system. This problem is especially relevant in preventing errors in clinical care due to mistakes and miscommunications, and in minimizing distortions. Consider, for example, how an erroneous psychiatric diagnosis (usually of a personality disorder or schizophrenia) can follow a patient from hospital to hospital, thus priming treating clinicians to make observations that confirm the same diagnosis.

Some ideas that have started with just one person endure and spread to shape the behaviors of large groups or nations, becoming driving forces such as religions or political movements. Some sociologists, biologists, and historians have called these ideas **memes.** Memes seem to have a life of their own, propagating through "replication" in individuals in a manner metaphorically similar to viruses that use host cells to generate and spread copies of themselves.

Communications theory also highlights the concept of **feedback.** The most familiar example for students is the process of being evaluated, usually while on clinical rotation and often for a grade. Patients are also often sensitized to receiving feedback from their physicians about their health status or their progress in combating an illness.

Cybernetics is the name given by Norbert Weiner to the science of feedback and control mechanisms, and how systems seek and achieve purposeful change. The thermostat is one of the most familiar cybernetic mechanisms, adjusting room temperature after comparing input information (the actual temperature) to a preset point. The anthropologist Gregory Bateson, who made numerous contributions to the field of communication, also applied some concepts of cybernetics to human behavior. He noted, for example, the similarity of an alcoholic's drinking behavior to the cybernetic processes in a thermostat and observed how mental health professionals try to change these set points.

Bateson, Watzlawick, and others pointed out that professions such as medicine tend to overvalue verbal communication. They stressed the importance of attending to nonverbal communication such as physical mannerisms (ie, body language) and behavior. They also described an important feature of communication: information about the communication itself, which Bateson termed **metacommunication.** Thus verbal and nonverbal messages may be accompanied by metacommunication that instructs the receiver how to interpret these messages. These dual layers of communication are sometimes referred to as **content** and **process.** Content is the explicit information in the message, whereas process refers to the guiding (and often implicit) context for information. It is often helpful for clinicians to attend to both layers of communication in talking with patients, including directly addressing implicit messages and metaphors.

Thus clinicians can intervene and offer interpretations based not only on what a patient says but also on what the patient communicates (a) through nonverbal communication and (b) about the process of communication. Following are some examples:

> A clinician notes that during a psychotherapy session his patient has related several stories from her past that involve betrayal by key figures in her life. The therapist asks the patient if she is indirectly wondering whether she can trust him or if he too will betray her.
>
> A therapist notices that her patient consistently raises difficult, emotionally upsetting issues every week at the very end of his psychotherapy sessions. She points out this observation to the patient, who says, "I guess it feels safer to bring up these issues at the end, instead of earlier in the session when I would have to feel upset or cry in front of you."
>
> Mr. A complains in group psychotherapy that he feels "alone and lonely." Yet he ignores or is dismissive of other patients when they try to offer advice or empathy. The group therapist asks the group members, "Can anyone help Mr. A understand what he is doing in the group that explains why he feels so alone, even when he is with other people?"

Bateson pointed out that the lack of a message could also communicate information. This observation is particularly relevant in medical settings.

> Frank S was worried that tests his physician had performed would confirm his fears that he had cancer. When he asked his physician what

she thought he had, she sought to placate him by telling him, "It's nothing. Let's wait until this next set of test results is ready." But Mr. S inferred that his physician was dodging the question and did not want to reveal that he did indeed have cancer. Thus Mr. S's doctor had sought to put him at ease but instead inadvertently increased his fears.

One of Bateson's most remembered contributions is the concept of the **double bind,** in which a person is offered an impossible choice. The expression "damned if you do, damned if you don't" is the colloquial formulation of this principle. The psychological response to continuous double-bind messages is often frustration, helplessness, or depression. Paranoia may also develop in children raised in this environment.

The basic principles of **ecology** emphasize the interrelationships between all organisms and their environment. The term **boundary** refers to different terms that involve divisions among elements in a system and includes concepts about space, time, and relationships among individuals. Healthy individuals generally demonstrate semipermeable boundaries, which they control depending on the circumstances. Following are some examples of boundaries:

> A 14 year old demonstrates an increasing desire for privacy and places a sign on his bedroom door reading "Occupant only. Knock before entering."
>
> A patient who has a history of sexual abuse requests that her initial physical examination be delayed until a friend arrives to provide emotional support.

Following are examples of **boundary violations:**

> A man in court-ordered psychotherapy for sexually abusing his stepdaughter attempts to ask the medical student performing an initial evaluation for a date (violation of personal boundaries).
>
> A patient consistently arrives 45 minutes late for his psychotherapy sessions but is difficult to dislodge from the office even when his hour is over (violation of time boundaries).
>
> A resident and medical student discuss a patient's case while riding on an elevator that is crowded with staff, patients, and families (violation of confidentiality).

Patients may have an impaired ability to regulate boundaries for a variety of reasons, including a history of sexual, physical, or emotional abuse in childhood; personality disorders; or dementia. These patients often benefit from attention to these issues. For example, physicians can set limits related to times of meetings (eg, by starting and ending appointments promptly) and to personal boundaries (eg, not allowing inappropriate touching or behavior).

George Engel pioneered the concept and application of the **biopsychosocial model.** The key principle of this model is that illness and health are nested in a series of ever-greater hierarchies, from molecules to DNA to cells to organ systems to individual human beings. Beyond the individual patient are families, workplace, and social and cultural groups. Engel and others have cautioned against the reductionist tendencies of biomedicine that attempt to analyze disease in a limited form exclusive of these larger systems issues. For example, it is of limited validity and benefit to discuss the etiology and treatment of a heart attack without considering the patient's psychological state and the effect of the illness on the patient's family and on his or her ability to function at work.

Living creatures are seen as being **interdependent** with each other, and changes in one individual will affect all others through often complex feedback loops. Interdependency is also characterized by an **equilibrium** or set point that represents a stable configuration of forces and populations. These **set points** are usually dynamic, that is, representing the sum of effects from constantly changing variables.

Paula M and her husband were referred to couples psychotherapy after Ms. M visited the emergency room multiple times for treatment of trauma to her face and arms. Ms. M admitted that her husband physically abused her. The cycle of abuse followed a classic pattern in which the couple would relate well to each other for a brief period of time. Mr. M would then experience a mounting sense of disgruntlement and anger toward his wife that would build over several weeks, leading to verbal assaults and threats. Ms. M would protest and threaten to leave Mr. M. Finally, Mr. M would become violent, shoving and hitting Ms. M, who would then consider leaving the abusive relationship. Mr. M would then send her flowers, apologizing profusely for his temper.

Ms. M explained, "My husband would act so romantically, trying to win me back, as if we were on our honeymoon again. He'd promise never to hurt me again and I'd take him back." After this brief "honeymoon phase," the cycle of tension and violence would begin again.

The previous case describes two people adjusting their relationship in order to maintain a certain average interpersonal distance. Although there is considerable vacillation between extremes of either intimacy or nearly breaking apart, usually they are somewhere in between—at the set point of the relationship.

Although systems often enable people to derive greater and more diverse benefits from less individ-

ual effort, sometimes systems don't work appropriately, and a great deal of energy can be expended to achieve very little. This paradox may occur in medical settings when a difficult patient is encountered. In some cases, the staff's initial response may prevent the medical system from functioning properly.

Max B, aged 23, had a long history of intravenous heroin use and was hospitalized for endocarditis, a bacterial infection of the heart valves. Mr. B was described by staff in such terms as spiteful, hostile, rebellious, and impossible. By the end of the first week in the hospital, the nurses were calling hospital police several times a day to confront Mr. B, who was screaming and throwing trays and bed pans, nearly hitting several staff members. The staff considered pressing assault charges if Mr. B's behavior continued.

Mr. B refused to meet with a psychiatrist, but discussion with a social worker led to a presumptive diagnosis of borderline personality disorder. The psychiatrist learned that the interactions with Mr. B started out relatively smoothly in the morning, but later in the day he would become increasingly irritable, making unreasonable demands and insulting the staff. Finally he would become verbally abusive and throw the adult equivalent of a temper tantrum. Security would then be called, and Mr. B's room would be filled with a half-dozen or more staff members and hospital police officers. Several staff members acknowledged that they were avoiding contact with Mr. B during the day as much as possible and that they felt some relief at yelling back at him during confrontations. All of the staff expressed dismay that the confrontations with Mr. B were continuing to escalate. They wondered why he didn't simply respond and settle down.

Discussion. Mr. B's behavior can be explained by considering the situation from a systems perspective. Mr. B was being told to settle into a quiet routine. Since these interactions were unpleasant for the staff, they assumed that Mr. B would comply. But the staff's inadvertent nonverbal communication to the patient was very different. They were in essence presenting Mr. B with a choice: He could be quiet, in which case he would be ignored, or he could "act up" and be rewarded with considerable attention and interaction and a chance to vent some of his fear, frustration, and anger.

Another important insight from the systems perspective is that the staff and the patient are part of the same system. Staff members often attempt to distance themselves from difficult or unlikable patients, who are often viewed as "bad" and completely separate from the staff's behavior. In this case, staff members had been through a stressful year, and some nurses admitted that it was emotionally cathartic to yell back at Mr. B to relieve pent-up feelings of frustration and aggression. Thus a vicious cycle was established, with the staff inadvertently causing the patient's behavior to escalate.

The psychiatrist suggested the following intervention: The staff were offered a series of meetings to discuss and work through their own frustrations separate from their issues of working with Mr. B. They were instructed to establish a regular schedule of checking in with Mr. B, rather than avoiding him, several times each shift. The staff was to praise him when he was behaving acceptably and reward him by spending time with him. If Mr. B did lose control, the staff were encouraged to be emotionally neutral and to keep their interventions brief and to the point. The situation de-escalated rapidly, and Mr. B's behavior was much better controlled. He admitted feeling very frightened by his illness, and the medical staff was able to develop a more empathic and respectful relationship with him.

The same inadvertent effects can be observed in other systems, particularly when complex rules arise in an organization in which administrative functions are uncoupled from the organization's mission.

In the wake of annual cutbacks to the community mental health system, the outpatient mental health clinics in a major metropolitan area lacked the operating budget to supply full benefits to its client base, who lacked health insurance and could not turn elsewhere for help. A decision was made to treat only the most emergent cases, such as patients who had chronic psychotic disorders or recent suicide attempts. Other patients who had less severe psychiatric disorders—including depression or anxiety disorders with suicidal thoughts or plans, or patients who had major psychiatric disorders complicated by substance use, were referred to the psychiatric emergency room.

These patients were then referred back to treatment at the outpatient clinics, where they had already been refused services. Even patients who expressed active suicidal thoughts were told that in order to be eligible for outpatient care, they would have to have a recent history of a suicide attempt. Instead of promoting mental health, the clinics paradoxically encouraged patients to become more ill to qualify for services.

Discussion. The dilemma faced by patients in this case is similar to that of the protagonists of Joseph Heller's book *Catch-22,* whose title immortalized the double-bind inherent in some organizations.

COMPLEXITY & HIERARCHICAL ORGANIZATION

Group and **grid** are two additional properties that help to characterize groups. Each property can be classified as high or low. Group refers to how strongly members identify themselves as part of a particular group. Examples of high group (characterized by a strong sense of feeling that an individual is part of a group) include a soccer team, the crew of a spacecraft, or members of a medical team. These group members typically feel close to each other, with a strong sense of shared objectives and values. Uniforms or other means of identification symbolically stress the sense of group identity and cohesion. Examples of low group include people waiting in line at a bank or walking on a city block. These people tend to feel only a tenuous bond with each other and have only a superficial sense of joint purpose.

Grid is defined as the degree to which leadership is stratified and divided among group members. Military groups or medical teams feature a high degree of grid; that is, there is a strong sense of hierarchy, and group members can readily identify their own roles in the group, the identity of group leaders, and their place in the chain or pyramid of command. The ability to ascend these levels of power is usually tied to evaluation by senior members and is based on preset accomplishments, usually marked by a ceremony (eg, graduation from school or receipt of a diploma). Groups with low grid have little sense of hierarchical structure; power is shared and decisions are made cooperatively.

GROUP PSYCHOLOGY

Systems science contributes to an understanding of some of the complex forms of communication and behavior seen in organizations and groups. But the interpersonal relationships between group members is also a function of human psychology. Social scientists and psychologists studying group psychology after World War II found interactions that appear to result from the complex interplay of conscious and unconscious forces.

How does the psychology of groups differ from individual psychology? Groups tend to be initially more fragile and more prone to regression and the use of primitive defense mechanisms such as paranoia and grandiosity. Beginning group processes often reflect characteristic developmental stages, whether the setting is a psychotherapy group, a newly assembled medical team, or a student volunteer organization. These stages include an early emphasis on boundaries and the definition of who is and who is not a member of the group. Another early group characteristic is **pairing,** in which two members of the group form a meaningful connection that is often symbolic of group unity to other members. A specialized form of pairing is the union of the group to a specific idea or purpose, often with great emotional intensity and unbridled optimism.

Later, fissures may develop between group members, and the group may enter a stage in which members question whether the group can continue or should disband. Even if the group's agenda has been preset or arranged, group members often struggle over the means to completing that agenda. This tension-laden stage is often associated with a strong fantasy that a powerful, idealized leader will intervene to "rescue" the group and can guide the group to its goal and help to lessen the group's tension and anxiety over its identity, purpose, and cohesiveness.

Groups, like individuals, use psychological defense mechanisms to modulate their anxiety levels. However, groups tend to use more primitive defenses, especially when under external stress such as economic restraints and cutbacks. Internal stress may come from tension between group members or from weak leadership. Groups under these circumstances may demonstrate marked paranoia. Leaders sometimes may invoke the threat of an external enemy to strengthen the group's sense of cohesion and their own power.

INFLUENCE OF GROUP DYNAMICS ON INDIVIDUAL & GROUP BEHAVIOR

A complex interplay exists between the members of a group and their contributions to the group's unique makeup. The group both reflects and determines the psychology of the individual members. The near-universal need to belong and be accepted by others provides much of the social glue or cohesiveness in any group.

Certain stereotyped roles tend to recur in groups, including those of the leader, the practical or capable group member, the joker, the so-called rescuer who helps other group members, and the gadfly who seems to enjoy challenging the group's confidence and perceptions. Members of a group often note that they have a similar role from one group to another. Some group members will feel constrained by these roles and feel resentful or frustrated that they are not able to utilize other skills or personal strengths. But the division of roles in a group is also an incredible strength. A group that is coordinated into a cohesive whole can outproduce and outthink a similar number of individuals. At best, group members feel that they are appreciated for their attributes, and for most group members a satisfactory balance develops between being a valued part of the group and retaining their individuality.

An individual's sense of personal identity in a group setting is partially influenced by social forces. In Western cultures, the celebration of individuality is reflected in cultural icons such as the lone cowboy or the rugged protagonist "fighting the system." This imagery is repeated in literature, movies, and advertisements. However, social scientists have demonstrated repeatedly that individuality is greatly constrained and subsumed by group processes.

The psychologist Simon Ash performed experiments that highlighted the influence of peer pressure in group settings. Test subjects were placed in a classroom with other people and given the task of comparing the size of lines and shapes. The other subjects were actually members of the research study, and they gave the same prearranged incorrect answer to each visual test. The test subjects would then usually give in to the pressure not to conflict with the group's consensus by giving the same incorrect response. As they gave erroneous answers over and over, the subjects grew increasingly dejected. Most of the subjects had described themselves at the start of the experiment as strongly individualistic and not afraid of standing up for what they felt was right. The experiment showed that this was not true. Humans are in fact social beings with a strong predisposition and motivation toward cooperation and the avoidance of conflict with the prevailing social group.

Denial in group behavior is not unusual. The "blind spots" in a group's awareness can be magnified by group members' unwillingness to confront glaring errors. The phenomenon of denial in groups, sometimes referred to as **groupthink,** results in a consensus—often outside of the group's conscious awareness—not to acknowledge problems. This phenomenon has been implicated in some of the most famous technological and political disasters of the twentieth century, including the Three Mile Island nuclear plant meltdown, where plant operators repeatedly turned off alarms that warned of an impending meltdown; the decision to launch the space shuttle Challenger under dangerous weather conditions; and the planned invasion of Cuba by United States–sponsored expatriates, which failed disastrously at the Bay of Pigs. In each case dissenting views had been strongly discouraged or were actively silenced. Medical teams are susceptible to the same problem, which may lead to clinical mistakes that are unchecked by other team members.

Ruth T, a 42 year old woman, had a history of bipolar disorder. She had been doing well for ten years with a stable job and solid marriage. She noticed symptoms of a hypomania episode and requested hospitalization while her mood stabilizing medication was being adjusted. On her fifth hospital day, she began to experience bilateral leg weakness. A neurological examination was "equivocal" with no outstanding findings. Two days later Ms. T's leg weakness had progressed to the point that she could no longer walk, and she complained that she was incontinent of urine. She was taken to the medical emergency room where another neurological examination was performed. The neurologist noted slightly decreased tone and patellar (knee) reflexes. However, his impression was that the patient "was probably malingering" based on her "long psych history." The patient was brought back to the psychiatric unit with no medical diagnosis. Based on the suspicion that the patient was "malingering" the staff decided to place the patient on a special behavioral protocol to "encourage her capacity for independence." She was given a form to sign that she was "physically intact" and would be expected to walk and urinate only in the bathroom. The medical student assigned to Ms T's case was struck by the frustration directed at the patient and the unwillingness of her physicians to consider other diagnoses. Ms. T was extremely upset at the medical staff and frightened by her symptoms. She and her husband insisted on a transfer to another hospital. There, clinicians were alarmed by her progressive physical symptoms. An EMG (electromyelogram) demonstrated slowing of electrical impulses in her legs. She was admitted to the medical ward with a diagnosis of Guillain-Barré syndrome, a rapidly progressive neurologic disorder. She required intubation to protect her breathing, and one year after the episode is still plagued by mild leg weakness and parasthesias.

Diagnosis: Bipolar Disorder (Axis I), Guillain-Barré syndrome (Axis III)

Discussion: The case above demonstrates group denial on the part of Ms. T's physicians. Their belief that she was somehow consciously responsible for her symptoms was likely bolstered by her past history of a psychiatric disorder, and possibly by countertransference (their emotional response to Ms. T) of which they may have only been partially aware. Thus numerous highly-trained health care professionals were able to disregard a compelling history and even (admittedly mild) physical symptoms and remain "blind" to an unfolding medical emergency.

INFLUENCE OF GROUP DYNAMICS ON ETHICAL BEHAVIOR

The aftermath of World War II left lingering questions about the nature of power in groups. Psychological testing of Nazi collaborators and officials in Germany showed that rather than being psychopathological "monsters," most of them tested as obsessive men who blindly followed orders. Each gave an account of obeying his superior officer and disavowing his own responsibility for genocide. How much did this reflect human nature in general?

In one of the most famous—or infamous—experiments of the twentieth century, the psychologist Stanley Milgram attempted to determine how far the average person would follow authority and perform immoral acts. Test subjects in Milgram's study were instructed by a supervisor to push buttons to administer electrical shocks of increasing voltage to other participants when they answered questions incorrectly. The other participants were actually Milgram's associates, who gave frequent incorrect answers and pretended to receive shocks by screaming in mock pain and begging the subjects to stop and release them. Most subjects appeared discomforted, telling the supervisor that they would not continue the experiment. The supervisor would repeatedly insist that the subjects must proceed with the experiment. Most subjects insisted that they were not responsible for what happened during and after the experiment, blaming the supervisor for their actions and attempting to absolve themselves of guilt. Two-thirds of the participants continued to administer shocks even though the buttons they pressed were labeled to indicate extreme physical danger and the possibility of death. The study was so stressful that some subjects reported symptoms of post-traumatic stress disorder for years after the experiment.

These results were met with surprise and dismay by behavioral scientists who had predicted before the experiment that only one subject in one thousand would behave in such a fashion. In experiments such as Milgram's and in literature (William Golding's *The Lord of the Flies* is an often-cited example), disquieting observations have been made about human behavior in groups. Recent research has focused on strategies that organizations can use to empower their employees to maintain their values and capacity to make ethical judgments and actions.

This somewhat bleak view of human behavior in groups has been tempered by recent discoveries and hypotheses. More optimistic perspectives on human behavior in groups highlight the roles of empathy and altruism in human interactions. Even the evolutionary tenet of "survival of the fittest" as it applies to individuals (so-called social Darwinism) may reflect Western culture's bias toward individualism and does not take into account the possible evolutionary advantages of altruism and group cooperation. Evolutionary theorists are examining the role of altruism in groups. An example of the potential positive aspects of group cooperation is found in the efficacy of Alcoholics Anonymous (AA), a group started by two men to help themselves and others who had alcohol use problems. Human beings may have some genetic predisposition toward altruism and mutually helpful behavior. Thus the theory of "survival of the fittest" may be substantially modified by a counterbalancing principle, that of "survival of the most socially cooperative to attain the common good."

APPLICATIONS OF SYSTEMS THEORY

FAMILIES

As a specialized group, the family is the most basic, familiar, and enduring social unit. Families are, metaphorically, the cultural equivalent of the DNA double helix, serving as the framework for the transmission of information, cultural and religious values, and language from one generation to the next. The most basic function of the family is to protect and nurture children in a safe environment.

The family also serves as a stable organizational template for the psychological development of all family members, especially children. It is within the family that the child develops his or her personal identity and learns how to relate to others. Key lessons include learning how to relate to authority figures, how to assess interpersonal needs and communicate effectively with others to meet those needs, and how to regulate boundaries. Initially these tasks are centered on the child's relationship with family members, but with time and critical experiences such as school, these lessons begin to apply to the child's relationships with others outside of the family.

Children also learn how to monitor and regulate their own inner drives and tensions, such as how to delay acting impulsively and how to constructively manage and challenge aggressive or sexual feelings. Children also need to learn to regulate personal boundaries and adjust interpersonal distance with others. These developmental tasks vary with each child; therefore, the task of parents is not to nurture their children in a standardized way but to try to evoke each child's identity in a process of mutual discovery. Over time, children achieve a pathway to independence and interdependence, usually leaving home and starting families of their own. Because each family is distinctive in its constituents, developmental challenges, and values, every family can be viewed as a unique social experiment.

Table 17–1. Common developmental challenges faced by families.

Marriage and the formation of the new family
Parents encountering life stressors (eg, job change or promotion, moving)
Childbearing
Infertility
Remarriage
Blended families
Marital discord, infidelity
Divorce
Physical illness
Mental illness
Death and loss

Families are dynamic, evolving groups, and they often face significant developmental challenges. Just as individuals develop adjustment disorders in response to life stressors, families face temporary disruptions in functioning as a result of stress. Table 17–1 summarizes some of the most frequently encountered crises or turning points that force families to grow and change. Like individuals, families use an array of defense mechanisms in a fairly consistent manner that reflect the identity or personality of the family as a whole. Reactions to stressful events may include increased physical complaints that bring one or more family members into contact with the medical system. However, just as individual patients often shun contact with mental health professionals, families as a whole may be reluctant to use psychiatric services.

Families also create coherent narratives, or myths, unchallenged stories or perspectives in which the family distorts its understanding of events or of individual members in order to protect the family from conflict, at the expense of insight and the ability to work through its own problems effectively. A frequently encountered myth is that of the so-called **identified patient** (see Family Psychopathology below), which preserves the belief that the family is healthy, while identifying one family member as being physically or emotionally unwell. Families may preserve these myths unconsciously. Clinicians must be able to identify and help challenge these myths in order to help families grow and develop.

Family Responses to Illness

How families respond to illness depends on a number of variables, including previous experiences, communication skills, interpersonal boundaries, and role flexibility. Physical illness often represents a real and symbolic threat to family unity and cohesiveness. Depending on the integrity and psychological health of the family system, a family may either grow more cohesive and effective or become more chaotic and dysfunctional.

William P, a 48-year-old carpenter, was injured in his workplace and spent a month in the hospital with complications from a herniated lumbar disk. He was in extreme pain after surgery and could not even walk to the bathroom. By the time he returned home, his condition had improved only marginally. Because of his physical impairment, Mr. P's wife set up his living space in a small downstairs guest room. She was initially able to work full-time while caring for Mr. P; however, as the family's economic picture declined, Ms. P was forced to take on a second job. She became very depressed and anxious and had little time for friends.

Their two teenage children had to help Mr. P dress, bathe, and perform other activities of daily living. Within weeks the children had assumed many adult responsibilities in the house, including cooking, cleaning, writing checks to pay bills, and wielding increasing power in decision making. Meanwhile Mr. and Ms. P became increasingly distraught over their situation.

Mr. P was able to return to work after 6 months, and although some aspects of the family's previous configuration of roles was revived, the children maintained some of their increased stature and power, which led to battles with their parents over curfews and homework.

Mental illness has a profound effect on families, but the effect often differs from that of physical illness. Among the differences is a greater sense of shame and embarrassment because of the stigma of mental illness. Emotional disorders and substance use may be cloaked in secrecy or vaguely reclassified as physical ailments. A family's response to mental illness may have a significant effect on the severity and prognosis of the disorder. Chapter 7 cites several examples of how family members may become caught up in helping patients who have anxiety disorders (eg, panic attacks or obsessive-compulsive disorder), inadvertently providing behavioral rewards for these conditions. Physical or psychiatric illness may cause the family to regress as it deals with an older child who might function on a childlike level. Intense and often irrational guilt may complicate the family's response to chronic psychiatric disorders.

James R, aged 23, had his first psychotic episode 3 years earlier and had since required numerous admissions for schizophrenia. He was unable to function independently and moved home at his parents' request. His parents were guided in their actions by a sense of guilt. They felt they had somehow failed their son in his development and, therefore, were responsible for his mental illness. His parents had never discussed with each other their sense of guilt.

The emotional and financial constraints of Mr. R's illness had drained the family. Mr. R's parents were unable to take a vacation because Mr. R would become suicidal whenever they attempted to spend time away from him. Finally, they decided to hospitalize Mr. R on a preventive basis while they went on their first vacation since his illness had started. Mr. R attempted suicide in the hospital by slashing his wrists with a broken mirror. The staff called his parents on the first full day of their vacation, and they flew home immediately.

In a family session at the hospital, Mr. R's parents were strongly encouraged to contact the National Alliance for the Mentally Ill (NAMI), a grassroots organization started by family members of patients who have psychiatric disorders. By attending support groups, Mr. R's parents were able to realize the depth of their frustration and were encouraged to discuss their guilt for the first time. They were able to establish firmer and clearer limits with their son and helped him to take more responsibility for his own well-being. They left on a trip 2 months later, and Mr. R did well staying with a another couple from the NAMI support group.

Family Psychopathology

Psychopathology often occurs in families. Known in popular parlance as **dysfunctional families,** these families exhibit numerous common characteristics. One family member often exhibits overt pathology, such as substance use, a personality disorder, or other major psychopathology. This person is the so-called identified patient and is often considered by other family members to be the cause of the family's difficulties. The identified patient thus serves as a distraction from other major problems within the family.

Boundaries may be poor between family members within the group, with diminished autonomy among individual family members. At an extreme, the most basic boundaries of children may be violated by sexual or physical abuse. One or more family members may act as **enablers,** individuals who attempt to shield or protect the most disturbed family member but in doing so further accentuate or encourage the behavior. Patients are sometimes confounded by the well-intentioned behavior of group or family members who appear anxious to help or rescue people in need. Although the combination of poor boundaries and an exaggeration of altruism and caring can help individuals feel more secure by giving them a sense of purpose, this behavior frequently leads to unintended destructive effects by facilitating, or enabling, the maladaptive behavior of other individuals. Enmeshed individuals may display reluctance to relinquish their roles, even when the negative effects of their efforts are identified.

Frank B met with a psychotherapist, saying that he wanted to help his son. Mr. B, aged 67, was a missionary who had accepted his "dream job" to work in Africa, although he had returned home after several months because he was worried about his son. Mr. B's son Thomas, aged 34, had not worked in many years and was living in his parents' house. He was facing criminal charges for bouncing checks despite living on an income provided by his parents and for failing to report income or pay income tax for 10 years. Although he had the use of his parents' car in their absence, he had failed to send in checks for the car's registration and insurance and for his driver's license renewal, even though his parents had provided money specifically for these costs.

Mr. B suspected that most of Thomas's money was used to purchase crack cocaine. He did not believe that his son would benefit from facing the legal consequences of his actions and gave up his job in Africa, returning home to take care of his son's financial, legal, and tax problems. Mr. B actively lied to creditors, the courts, and family friends to protect his son "from being stigmatized." Because Thomas was not interested in drug treatment programs, Mr. B himself decided to enroll in therapy so that he could "learn" to help him. Mr. B said that he wanted to be a better parent than his own father, an alcoholic, who left the family when Mr. B was 5 years old.

Mr. B was reluctant to talk about himself but exhibited enough symptoms to be diagnosed as having long-standing dysthymia, the possibility of a current episode of major depression, and significant marital difficulties due to his wife's frustration with Mr. B for "coddling" their son. The therapist was unable to convince Mr. B to continue in therapy to deal with his own depression, or to consider couples or family therapy to change his relationship with his son. Mr. B attempted to turn the focus of the final session to the therapist's religious orientation and became focused on ensuring that the therapist had been baptized, stating, "It's important to me that your own soul is saved."

Discussion. Mr. B's behavior is enabling in that his "protection" actually allows his son to avoid accountability and responsibility for his actions, thus inadvertently helping the behavior to continue unchecked. That Mr. B has become enmeshed in his son's life and has lost personal boundaries is evident in his premise for psychotherapy—acting as if his own therapy will directly help his son.

Boundaries between the pathological family and society tend to be overly thick, characterized by impaired social connections and an insistence on guarding family secrets to prevent openness with other parties. Role diffusion and confusion are often encountered, with parents behaving immaturely and children acting in a hyperresponsible manner either by choice or by parental insistence. Communication patterns and defense mechanisms in these families are strikingly rigid.

Families that are marked by psychopathology may either consciously or unknowingly worsen a patient's physical illness. At the most severe end of the spectrum is the patient who has **Munchausen by proxy,** a disorder in which a parent knowingly simulates physical illness in a healthy child (see Chapter 9). Less extreme forms include exacerbation of a real physical illness to meet other goals in the family. Krener and others have noted similarities between this behavior and family characteristics of parents who abuse their children. Thus families may either help or hinder a patient who is coping with or adapting to illness.

In an extreme form, family members may share bizarre or delusional beliefs, as in a **folie á deux** (a shared and often paranoid delusional disorder). However, the psychopathology might be so well hidden that these families still appear superficially healthy. Only on closer examination might clinicians realize the extent of the family dysfunction. Medical crises often overwhelm the family's brittle defenses and expose the disturbed family dynamics.

Susan G, aged 17, weighed 89 pounds when she was admitted to the medical-psychiatric unit. She exhibited severe electrolyte abnormalities secondary to bulimia and laxative abuse. She had never been seen in counseling before despite having a 2-year history of severe depression and one prior suicide attempt at age 13 (by taking her mother's pills). Her family knew about Ms. G's suicide attempt and her 4-year history of an eating disorder but minimized these behaviors and events as "attention-seeking."

Ms. G's family failed to attend most of the scheduled family therapy sessions, although they always had reasonable explanations for having to cancel or miss appointments. Via phone calls and brief interactions, Ms. G's parents made it clear that they regarded her as the problem and did not seriously consider family therapy to be a necessary part of her recovery.

Despite an initially distant and detached attitude toward staff and other patients, Ms. G made significant progress in the hospital. She was started on antidepressants, gained weight, and experienced fewer episodes of bingeing and purging. She began to participate increasingly in the community and group meetings. She bonded well with a third-year medical student, to whom she revealed that she had frequent nightmares and flashbacks related to repeated episodes of sexual abuse. Her father was an alcoholic who began fondling her at age 11 and initiated intercourse at 13. Her mother was extremely emotional and self-centered, covering for her husband's alcoholism and responding to confrontation by her children with rage, beatings, or threats of suicide. As a child, Ms. G's mother had been sexually abused by her own father.

Ms. G was discharged from the hospital after 1 month, and plans were made for outpatient appointments. Child Protective Services (CPS) initiated an investigation, which was dropped when Ms. G refused to back up her earlier account. Her condition deteriorated at home, where her family appeared threatened by her growing sense of independence, confidence, and maturity. They became increasingly critical of her or ignored her concerns and feelings, which she had learned to express more clearly since her hospitalization. They also rebuked her for "getting the family into trouble with the law" and for the cost of the therapy. Sometimes they would refuse to drive her to therapy or "forget" to give her the car.

Ms. G stopped taking the antidepressants as prescribed, and her depression returned. One night she paged the outpatient therapist to report that she had taken an overdose of her antidepressants and her mother's sleeping pills. She was taken to the emergency room and readmitted to the hospital.

TREATMENT ISSUES IN SYSTEMS THEORY

History provides a useful model for intervening with families. In the 18th century so many trees were cut down at one time that an entire river would become choked with trees. The trees then stopped flowing down-river to the mill; this was the origin of the term "logjam." When a logjam occurred a special person was consulted who climbed to the top of a nearby hill to survey the entire river. This person would then select the one "key" log that when removed would break the logjam and release the flow of water.

The physician has an analogous task in attempting to change a larger system, such as a family or a group, that is stuck at a particular developmental stage or dilemma. Micromanaging every aspect of group change is impractical and unrealistic. Clinicians should strive for an understanding of the dynamic forces beyond the identified patient that keep a family system locked in its unhealthy equilibrium. It is then a matter of helping family members make changes that utilize constructive forces within the system to do the remainder of the work.

Isadore S, a 75-year-old grandmother, was admitted to the intensive care unit (ICU) for treatment of congestive heart failure. She improved within 48 hours on fluid and salt restriction, oxygen, diuretics, and digoxin. Ms. S's daughter, son-in-law, and grandchildren visited her many times. The ICU social worker noticed that Ms. S's chart was thick from multiple admissions to the ICU. Each clinical presentation was almost identical, with Ms. S's heart failure clearing rapidly with treatment.

A detailed interview uncovered some important facts in Ms. S's history. She admitted to "getting sloppy" with adherence to her regimen of medications at home. She also acknowledged going off her diet and eating high-salt foods and drinking large amounts of cola. These indiscretions generally occurred 3–4 weeks after her discharge from the hospital. Ms. S admitted to feeling lonely and ignored in her apartment, where she had settled when she became ill 3

years earlier. She had been widowed recently, and her children convinced her to sell her house and move hundreds of miles to be closer to them. "But I never see them," Ms. S complained. "Sure they visit me in the hospital, but when I'm back at my apartment they're always too busy. I call them and they can't be bothered, like I'm an inconvenience in their lives. I don't know anyone in this town, and they insisted I should move here."

A separate interview with Ms. S's daughter and son-in-law revealed that marital tension has increased between them after her move. The family expressed feelings of resentment over Ms. S's demands. They were also concerned that their 13-year-old son had started to experience declining grades and behavioral problems within months of Ms. S's arrival.

Coordination between medicine, psychiatry, and social services led to a number of simple interventions. Ms. S was referred to a senior support group and assigned a visiting nurse to check on her status twice a week. With increased contact with her new peer group, she began to meet new friends and expect less from her family. To Ms. S's surprise, her children and grandchildren began asking her to come to their house more frequently. She was doing well at 1-year follow-up, with a solid social support network and improved relationships with her family. Her congestive heart failure had also stabilized.

Individuals or families in crisis may display inflexible thinking that can impair their adaptation to stress. **Reframing** is a technique that encourages individual patients or family members to change their perspective on a situation or problem. Physicians should consider using language that incorporates the family's or individual's own experience and symbols to make interventions effective and easily understandable.

Octavio L, the father of a depressed 14-year-old girl, did not understand why he needed to have his daughter seen at the outpatient psychiatric clinic after she had attempted suicide. Mr. L, an automobile mechanic, was intelligent but lacked a sophisticated psychological understanding of his daughter's problems. He was frustrated by the psychiatry resident's explanations. Mr. L and the resident found themselves in a heated disagreement in which Mr. L insisted that his daughter "seems fine now."

The third-year medical student working with the resident interrupted the confrontation by empathizing with Mr. L about how difficult it was to raise a child and how hard he was working. She used an analogy about cars to explain the need for ongoing treatment: "Let's say you fixed a car engine. What would you think if the owner said that he wasn't going to come in for any annual tune-ups?"

"He'd be a fool," replied Mr. L. "He'd be facing big trouble—the car might run fine for a while, and then—boom, maybe another major breakdown."

"Well, your daughter's case is like that, too," the student explained. "She just had a major repair job, so she's better, but the outpatient appointments are like tune-ups. She needs them so she keeps doing all right and doesn't need to come back into the hospital."

Mr. L immediately agreed to bring his daughter in for outpatient sessions and thanked the student for explaining why it was important to do so.

Working with extended families and groups under high-stress conditions is a challenge even for experienced mental health professionals. Essential elements of such work include a thorough evaluation of the entire group or system and well-planned interventions that utilize the group's own constructive forces.

Jose R, aged 30, was admitted to the ICU immediately after having a catastrophic subarachnoid hemorrhage. Mr. R had been in excellent health and had recently taken over his father's ministry at a local church. He was placed on life support, including a ventilator because regular breathing had ceased. An EEG showed no significant activity in the cortex, consistent with brain death; he had no chance of recovery beyond a vegetative state. Mr. R's wife was certain that her husband would not choose to be on life support with no hope of regaining a reasonable quality of life and agreed with the physician to disconnect life support.

Meanwhile a large group of almost three dozen relatives, friends, and members of the church congregation had gathered in the ICU. Mr. R's wife and a handful of family members were ready to allow physicians to discontinue all life support measures and allow him to die. Most family members and church members clung to the fervent hope that Mr. R would recover fully. Mr. R's father, distraught at the loss of his son and his faith shaken by the turn of events, drank some hard liquor a family member offered to him and in a drunken state wept, prayed, and cried at his son's bedside. He offered to kill himself to save his son's life. His increasingly distraught state sent members of the congregation into a frenzy. "This is a test of God's will," they said. "If the doctors give up on him, they are turning their back on the Lord. He will be healed after 3 days, if everyone believes and prays and doesn't give up." They were furious that Mr. R's wife had decided to discontinue life support.

The residents and staff in the ICU were overwhelmed by the situation and asked for an urgent psychiatric consultation. The medical residents then left to perform other clinical duties and refused to come back to the ICU. The psychiatric consultants recognized the difficulty inherent in working with over 30 people and asked a colleague to help. He then invited Mr. R's nurse and the head nurse to help plan an intervention with the group in the ICU. When attempts to calm Mr. R's father failed, the psychiatry team called hospital security to escort the intoxicated man to the psychiatric emergency room for observation and evaluation of suicidal ideation. This immediately helped to calm the group. The team of consultants and nurses next divided the large group into more manageable groups of five people each and sought out one member from each group who could consider Mr. R's predicament more objectively. Again, the distress and anxiety among the entire group was diminished.

The psychiatrist then paged the medical residents and insisted on their prompt return to the ICU, citing their essential role in guiding family members through difficult decisions. Mr. R's wife and mother met with the medical residents. While the wife's permission to stop life support was sufficient to proceed, the psychiatric consultants thought that this would endanger her future connection with family members. Mr. R's wife was able to voice her feelings of profound loss and her anger at the family's failure to support her. Gradually, with the support of the medical staff, she was able to make her and her husband's wishes clear to approximately half of the family members.

After allowing family and church members to pray over Mr. R for several hours, and documenting continued signs of brain death, the medical team turned off the ventilator. The family and medical staff joined hands around Mr. R's bed and stayed with him as he died. The psychiatric consultants then held a meeting to allow everyone to share their memories of Mr. R's life and to help them begin to grieve.

Although working with couples and families requires additional training and experience, students and residents can ask for a more active "apprentice" role, for example, working with consulting mental health professionals for experiential training with their own patients. By learning to work with families, trainees can obtain skills that are valuable for practicing medicine in a more holistic fashion.

MEDICAL TEAM LEADERSHIP

In medical school and residency a great deal of time and effort is devoted to the acquisition of clinical knowledge and skills. Remarkably, medical trainees do not receive formal preparation for one of their most important responsibilities, that of leading a team of fellow trainees in patient care. Despite the prevalent image of the physician as a heroic individual who functions autonomously, most medical care is delivered by a multidisciplinary team consisting of medical residents and students, nurses, orderlies, physical and occupational therapists, social workers, and nutritionists. These teams are usually overseen by a medical director and his or her staff, who may in turn report to a hospital or clinic administrator at a university health-care company or county organization.

Social scientists studied leadership and organizations in three high-stress workplaces in which minor accidents could have catastrophic results: a United States aircraft carrier, an electrical company power grid station, and an air traffic control tower at a busy metropolitan airport. The researchers noted that effective operating conditions prevailed at these sites because of a number of factors related to leadership style.

First, there was good communication between members of each organization, with frequent meetings and active solicitation of information by higher levels of management. There was also role flexibility in terms of which individuals at different hierarchical levels of power interchanged work duties. For example, even the captain of the aircraft carrier joined the rest of the crew each day in walking the flight deck to look for dangerous debris. This task and repeated practice drills symbolized the adaptability expected of the crew, including the leaders, and further illustrated that each crew member's sense of importance was always secondary to the mission of the ship itself: maintaining flight capability whenever it was required.

What are the leadership characteristics of the house officer? Leadership tasks for the medical team are similar to those in other groups. Their basic functions include guiding a team of medical students, interns, and residents in delivering the highest quality of care to patients. The team members' roles must be clearly defined to include, for example, how a decision is made, what communication channels are appropriate or inappropriate, and which team member does what work from day to day. Boundaries related to both time management and relationships between team members must be delineated. The emotional responses of the team must be regulated. A leader must help the team to function calmly and objectively when someone is upset or angry, or in emergency situations such as giving CPR to a patient in cardiac arrest, even when the team has not slept for over 24 hours.

The members of the team also require training, evaluation, and feedback about their work. The med-ical team needs to coordinate with other groups, such as consulting physicians, ward clerks, nurses, and social workers. The physician must therefore be able to model good communication skills and respect for others and to understand and facilitate psychological group processes to help team members function both independently and as a cohesive team.

As students and residents move forward in their training they face greater responsibilities and challenges. These challenges will be determined both by the situations the trainees face and by their own experiences in groups that may derive largely from models of authority they have experienced in their own families.

Mary B was a 27-year-old second-year medicine resident. Her team consisted of two interns and two medical students. Dr. B enjoyed the clinical challenges of medicine but found that she had difficulty leading her team. The two interns were constantly bickering and asking her to mediate in their disputes over their workload, or challenging her decisions about how to run team rounds. Dr. B found herself avoiding the interns and spending most of her time teaching the medical students.

Dr. B sought out her attending physician for advice about how to run her team. He said, "You'll have to grab the bull by the horns, and tell them that you are in charge, period." Dr. B halfheartedly attempted to relay this message at the next rounds, but the interns ignored her. Finally she sought out the chief resident, who encouraged Dr. B to develop her own leadership style. Dr. B continued to observe other senior residents and attending physicians, selecting techniques and skills that were more comfortable to her.

Dr. B met with a psychotherapist for six sessions, which helped her to realize a personal connection to her dilemma. As a child, Dr. B was the only girl in her family and constantly felt that her role had been as "the baby" who was inferior to her four older brothers. Gradually she developed more confidence in her own style of leadership and, encouraged by her success, began testing hypotheses about how best to run her team. Her two interns sensed this change and sparred less often with each other. Dr. B gave them leadership experience by having each of them supervise a medical student.

Dr. B was also able to demonstrate her abilities as a teacher and worked with the interns to develop their own teaching skills. Dr. B was pleased to find that she felt much more emotionally secure with her brothers at her family's next reunion. One year later, she was appointed as the chief medical resident and helped to mentor other residents and students in clinical and leadership issues.

Although it is possible to help teach and develop leadership skills, few medical schools or residency training programs make leadership an overt or integrated part of the curriculum. For most medical trainees, authority is learned by example. Students and residents often notice a wide range of leadership styles among their peers and supervisors and choose to emulate these various approaches. It may be years before the same trainees develop their own leadership style. In classes and experiential workshops outside of medical school, interested students can approach the development of their own unique leadership style with increased knowledge and self-awareness.

CULTS & RESTRICTIVE GROUPS

Cults can be viewed as a specialized form of group. The existence of cults has been highlighted over the past two decades by intermittent media coverage. Infrequent but dramatic mass suicides, such as nearly 1000 deaths at the Jonestown massacre in Guyana and the 1997 Heaven's Gate mass suicides in San Diego, have highlighted the often bizarre nature of cult life and the extent to which individuals can be influenced or coerced by group behavior. **Cults,** or **restrictive groups** as they are also termed, exist along a continuum, from the most restrictive groups that deprive members of many individual freedoms, limit contact with the "outside" world, and make heavy monetary demands, to groups that do not subsume as much of their members' time or sense of identity. Youth gangs can also be viewed as a variant of the restrictive group phenomenon. These gangs have rigid codes of conduct that often encourage violence; a hierarchical power system; punishment for leaving the gang; and "uniforms," colors, or tattoos that symbolize group membership. They often provide a strong sense of belonging and identity to otherwise disaffected people in their teens and 20s.

The prevailing public belief is that only morally weak or mentally unbalanced individuals join cults. Research demonstrates that this is not necessarily true and that many people who join restrictive groups are intelligent individuals who are often at difficult transition points in their lives, for example, graduating from college or graduate school, between jobs, or leaving a romantic relationship. Restrictive groups use a variety of recruitment techniques, often cloaking the group's name and purpose at initial stages. Some use sophisticated psychological techniques such as **thought reform** (colloquially known as **brainwashing**) or overt threats to further bind recruits to the group.

Jessica R, a 25-year-old teacher, was laid off from her job because of budget cutbacks. She was crossing the street at a local university when she was approached by two people who invited her to a meeting to discuss the environment. Ms. R was excited by the prospect of meeting new people and the promise of contacts that might lead to employment in a field that had interested her for many years. At the meeting, food was provided and a number of speakers gave impassioned talks about an organization that was working toward world peace.

Ms. R was encouraged to attend more meetings and finally a week-long retreat in a rural area. There, she and other recruits were pressured to attend meetings 20 hours each day. There was no transportation off the grounds except in the group's van, and the closest telephone was said to be over 100 miles away. Ms. R and other recruits were bombarded with talks and increasingly insistent assaults on their values that left them confused and susceptible to suggestions that they needed to "radically change the course" of their lives by committing to the group. Any resistance or ambivalence was reframed as an example of "insecurity and laziness." It was months later before Ms. R learned that she had joined a well-known cult, but by then she had become a local leader in the organization.

For the next 3 years Ms. R's entire life revolved around the group's activities. She gave all of her income to the organization and lived in a group-owned apartment. However, as she rose through the ranks of the organization, she became increasingly aware of abuses of power by group leaders, including financial indiscretions and payment for prostitutes to provide sexual services to top group leaders.

When Ms. R visited her family for the first time since she had joined, she decided not to return to the group. She was subsequently harassed by group members who called her parents' house throughout the day and night. The callers were friendly and seemed concerned initially, imploring Ms. R to return to the group and expressing fears for Ms. R's "moral compass," but soon the callers began making vague threats. Ms. R was convinced that group members were staking-out her parents' house, observing her.

She was seen at a local community mental health organization at her parent's insistence after she developed paranoia, anxiety, and several panic attacks. Ms. R complained of insomnia, symptoms of depression and anxiety, and post-traumatic stress disorder symptoms of hypervigilance and an easy startle response. On evaluation, she was somewhat paranoid and fearful but showed no signs of psychosis.

A phone call made by a group member to Ms. R's psychiatrist labeling Ms. R as "crazy" confirmed her suspicions of being watched. She refused antidepressant medication but accepted referral to a local support group composed of ex-cult members. The group helped Ms. R feel less alienated and more aware of how much of a sense of loss she felt. During one of the group meetings, she said, "I lost some of my best years and really forgot who I was. My self-esteem is so low from being told that I couldn't survive without the group to help me every minute. Now I have to learn to live my life all over again."

Ms. R made a gradual recovery. Her symptoms abated in individual and group therapy, and she later agreed to try antidepressants, with good results. Two years after leaving the group, she became involved in a romantic relationship for the first time since her early 20s and had found a job teaching biology and ecological science at a local high school.

Restrictive group members stay in these groups for varying amounts of time, from brief interactions to involvement across many years. Depression, anxiety, dissociative symptoms, and confusion, including problems with personal identity, are common. Because of the insular or paranoid nature of some of these groups, children of group members are sometimes raised with minimal contact with the "outside" world. These insular groups may be headed by charismatic but sometimes mentally ill individuals. Boundary violations including emotional, physical, and sexual abuse sometimes occur, and physicians should be alert to the presence of post-traumatic stress disorder and other major psychiatric conditions in patients seeking assistance after they have left restrictive groups.

For patients who are considering leaving restrictive groups, support groups composed of ex-group members may play a pivotal role in empowering individuals to leave and assisting in the transition to life outside of the restrictive group. The use of forced and coercive "deprogramming" techniques by non–mental health professional specialists hired by family members is discouraged because of legal considerations: Involuntary detention is viewed by the legal system as kidnapping. Family members may benefit from referrals to mental health professionals or cult experts who can advise them about interacting with members of restrictive group.

EMOTIONAL REACTIONS TO FAMILIES & GROUPS

Physicians receive little training in working with families and often feel overwhelmed by family demands for time, assurance, and guidance. Other emotional reactions may derive from the clinician's own family background. Clinicians have been known to literally flee from families, insisting that they are only responsible to their individual patients. These attitudes and feelings may derive from a lack of training and comfort with family issues or from the clinician's own family experiences. Recognition of these feelings is important to avoid deviation from optimal care and may be best addressed with additional experience supplemented by guidance from consulting mental health professionals.

Work in larger systems often leads to more basic emotional responses, including confusion, disillusion, and depression. Trainees and more senior physicians often speak with frustration about not being able to "fight the system." Many trainees are discouraged to find that power struggles and conflicts are pervasive in the medical system, permeating clinical care and research.

Stephanie M, a third-year medical student, received a year-long fellowship to conduct basic research in a university laboratory. At the end of the year, she was grateful for the experience but dismayed by the interactions she had seen in the laboratory. Jealousy and personality conflicts between researchers consistently prevented cooperation between different groups in the laboratory, resulting in shortages of vitally needed chemicals and equipment. These conflicts drastically interfered with her being able to achieve many of her goals. She told her classmate, "I was naive and thought that the practice of science somehow surmounted the human foibles of the scientists themselves. I didn't realize that scientists are just as human as anyone else. A successful scientist has to be like a politician to succeed, and I'm just not cut out for that kind of infighting."

LEGAL & ETHICAL ISSUES

The traditional doctor-patient relationship and the physician's role as an advocate for individual patients has provided the keystone for ethical decision-making. Although improved skills and experience in working with families are desirable, a shift to engaging with families or working in larger systems of health-care delivery moves physicians away from the doctor-patient relationship and poses many ethical dilemmas.

Dilemmas that arise in working with families include issues regarding confidentiality. For example, to what degree does a minor have a right to confidentiality? To what extent can the physician effectively support a patient's best interests if the physician is shifting the focus of his or her work to advocate for the family's well-being?

Haley N, a 17-year-old high school senior, was referred for outpatient psychotherapy for anxiety in social situations. Ms. N explained that her parents were extremely intrusive in her activities and that they sometimes spied on her when she went out with her friends. Through therapy, Ms. N began to develop increased self-esteem and assertiveness.

Ms. N's mother called the therapist 1 month later to complain that her daughter was becoming too headstrong. Ms. N's parents were also upset that their daughter was now considering applying to colleges that were "unacceptably far away." They were worried that therapy was making Ms. N too independent. They wanted to monitor her therapy, and because Ms. N refused to divulge the content of the sessions, they insisted that the psychotherapist call them after each session to share the details of the therapy hour.

The therapist realized that she was in difficult double bind. Although Ms. N was a minor and her parents were paying for the therapy, the therapist felt that Ms. N's request for additional autonomy was a healthy step in her development and that her parents were attempting to remain enmeshed in their daughter's life. The therapist explained that the parents' request would sabotage Ms. N's therapy by compromising her right to confidentiality, but they insisted on their legal right to be kept fully informed about their daughter's progress. The therapist convened a family conference, which Ms. N and her parents reluctantly attended. The therapist helped the family to agree that Ms. N would not have to divulge details about her therapy and referred the parents to couples therapy to help them work on their own issues.

Physicians-in-Training and the Health-care Team

Trainees who are lower in the power structure in medical teams also face ethical dilemmas when they are instructed to perform tasks that they suspect or know to be counter to the patient's best interests. Intense team pressure may encourage students to act in violation of their own values, or risk poor evaluations or group ostracism.

A medical student started on his first clinical rotation on the surgery service. He received little orientation but was told to shadow one of the interns. The intern instructed the student to insert a foley catheter in the urethra of a patient who was to have surgery in 30 minutes. The patient was very worried about pain and asked the student to insert the catheter after he was anesthetized. The student relayed this request to the intern, who became angry and told the student, "We all have to do things that patients don't want. We don't have

time to hold their hands, and if you want to pass this rotation and be a doctor, you need to buckle down and get to work!"

The student returned to the patient who again asked the student to wait. The student called the second-year resident, who gave the student permission to follow the patient's wishes. The intern was angry that the student had gone over his head. The student called his mentor, a pediatrician in another hospital, who supported the student's decision and encouraged him not to compromise in his ethical judgments.

Discussion. Although such confrontational incidents are encountered infrequently during clinical rotations, these events often have profound effects on a student's sense of professional identity, possibly paving the way for future ethical compromises. These situations are similar to Milgram's experiment (described earlier in this chapter) in which individuals are pitted against their own limitations in defying authority figures. In this case, the student was caught between conflicting drives to do what was best for the patient (adhering to an ethical standard of care) and the desire to fit into the medical team, obtain a satisfactory evaluation, and continue his or her training. Students are encouraged to maintain contact with mentors or advisors who can provide confidential advice when they find themselves in situations that are not easily resolved.

Physicians & Larger Systems

With the dissolution of the era of solo practitioners and fee-for-service payment by third-party insurers, physicians are increasingly working in groups and are often interacting with or employed by health-care maintenance organizations (HMOs) or managed-care companies. Physicians may therefore find themselves with dual and conflictual allegiances to patients and insurance companies. Physicians who take on **capitated contracts** are given a set amount of funding to care for thousands of patients and in essence assume the responsibility of financial insurers. These physicians must set their limitations or caps on specialty services for patients or risk losing their own income.

These changes, and the growing awareness of physician responsibility and culpability for escalating health-care costs, have encouraged physicians to think about economic constraints on medical care. **Bedside rationing,** the practice of limiting costly health care with a low probability of success, is controversial because of the ethical ambiguity inherent in the physician's dual role as an advocate for the individual patients and the group of patients in the health-care system.

A patient with schizophrenia developed renal failure and required renal dialysis; however, he failed to attend his scheduled outpatient dialysis sessions. Instead he presented to the medical emergency room every 4–6 weeks exhibiting nausea and fatigue related to uremia and electrolyte abnormalities. He would then be admitted to the hospital for a brief stay and two or three sessions of dialysis.

The treating medical team presented the case to the hospital ethics committee, arguing that the patient's refusal to participate in outpatient care and subsequent hospitalizations were "too costly to the system." The team proposed to stop offering dialysis to Mr. M on either an outpatient or inpatient basis. He would be offered palliative care to keep him comfortable during his next admission, in which he would be expected to die within several weeks.

Some members of the ethics committee indicated that such a decision was tantamount to permitting the patient to die, since he could not survive without dialysis. Others were concerned that the team's decision would establish a precedent that could lead to the denial of care for other difficult patients, creating a de facto policy.

It was ultimately pointed out that the patient's medical bills from regular monthly hospitalizations were probably not much more than for dialysis 3 times per week; therefore, there was no economic reason to withdraw care. The medical team explored their frustration with the case and realized that their own emotional reactions to the patient had led them to use a flawed economic premise as justification for abandoning their duty to advocate for the patient's needs. They were encouraged to continue offering the patient ongoing care and otherwise to accept the patient's health behavior.

CONCLUSION

Traditional medical training gives physicians a sense of assurance and competence in managing individual patients. But physicians often are not equipped with the skills or experience needed to work confidently with families and larger groups. It is not sufficient to merely cure a disease; physicians must approach health care from a more holistic, systems-oriented perspective. Fortunately, training is available, but many trainees need to actively advocate for education in these areas or seek experience outside of the curricula of traditional residency programs.

If physicians do partially shift their focus from the individual patient to larger social groups, they will need to establish new guidelines to function effectively and ethically in these areas. Facilitating community health through public health activities; developing programs for families; and tackling social issues such as teen pregnancy, substance use, and violence are a few of the challenges that they may face.

However, the systems approach that features the physician in a role of a "human ecologist" or an expert in group, family, and social interactions and their effects on health and illness, is an appealing and powerful model that offers to surmount the limitations of the current focus on individual patients and expand the role of the clinician in the community.

REFERENCES

Bateson G: *Steps to an Ecology of Mind.* Ballantine, 1972.

Conway F, Siegelman J: *Snapping: America's Epidemic of Sudden Personality Change.* 2nd ed. Stillpoint, 1995.

Feudtner C, Christakis DA, Christakis NA: Do clinical clerks suffer ethical erosion?: Students perceptions of their ethical environment and personal development. Acad Med 1994;69(8):670.

Finkel J: Physician countertransference: impact on patients, treatment team and adaptation to illness. In: Finkel J (editor): *Consultation-Liaison Psychiatry.* Grune & Stratton, 1983.

Gardner H (in collaboration with Laskin E): *Leading Minds: An Anatomy of Leadership.* Basic, 1995.

Goleman D: *Vital Lies, Simple Truths.* Simon & Schuster, 1985.

Greenblatt M: The use and abuse of power in the administration of systems. Psychiatr Ann 1986;16(11)650.

Halperin DA: Psychiatric perspectives on cult affiliation. Psychiatr Ann 1990;20(4):204.

Hughes P, Brecht G: *Vicious Circles and Infinity: An Anthology of Paradoxes.* Penguin, 1980.

Krener P, Adelman R: Parent salvage and parent sabotage in the care of chronically ill children. Am J Dev Childhood. 1988;124:945.

Luepnitz DA: *The Family Interpreted.* Basic, 1988.

Principles of Systems and Cybernetics: http://pcs.pmc1. vub.ac.be/CYBERSPIN.html

Raven B: A taxonomy of power in human relations. Psychiatr Ann 1986;16(11):633.

Shur R: *Countertransference Enactment: How Institutions and Therapists Actualize Primitive Internal Worlds.* Aronson, 1994.

Singer MT, Halich J: *Cults in our Midst.* Jossey-Bass, 1996.

Stein H: *American Medicine as Culture,* Westview, 1990.

Tannen E: *Why Things Bite Back.* Vintage, 1997.

Tolbert WR: *The Power of Balance.* Sage, 1991.

Watzlavick P: *Change: Problem Formation and Problem Solution.* Norton, 1988.

Yalom I: *The Theory and Practice of Group Psychotherapy.* 4th ed. Basic, 1995.

18

Women's Issues in Mental Health

Sudha Prathikanti, MD

Historically, psychological theories based on men's life experiences have determined the clinical standards for mental health assessment and treatment. Because such male-biased models are used, the psychological features of female development frequently have been labeled as immature, passive, or pathologic. Until recently, research in psychiatry did not consider gender differences, and investigators often included in their studies only male subjects—or a disproportionately high number of male subjects. This bias has resulted in very limited knowledge of how gender may influence the etiology and presentation of major psychiatric disorders, the patient's response to psychotropic medications, and the efficacy of various treatment modalities.

A growing body of psychiatric literature now addresses topics relevant to women's experiences. These topics include early psychological development and the establishment of female gender identity, the impact of reproductive function on women's psychological health, gender differences in psychiatric diagnoses and treatment response, and the effects of violence against women.

GENDER IDENTITY & PERSONALITY DEVELOPMENT

Despite changes brought about by the feminist movement, women in most cultures around the world continue to be the primary caretakers of young children; men remain significantly less involved in early child-rearing. This arrangement has far-reaching effects on the personality development of young children and the acquisition of gender identity and gender role constructs.

Gender identity refers to the internalized sense of maleness or femaleness and the knowledge of one's biological sex, including associated psychological attributes. Core gender identity appears to be well established by approximately 18 months of age. Once established, it does not appear to be reversible; however, as a child gets older, his or her gender identity continues to evolve and become more multifaceted.

Gender role refers to the expectations, attitudes, and behaviors considered to be appropriate for each gender in a particular culture. Enormous cultural variations exist in the roles and expectations of men and women; not all cultures value the same traits or see traits as gender specific in the same ways. Furthermore, an individual can have a clear gender identity as male or female but still experience conflict regarding specific gender role behavior.

When the mother (or an adult female) is the primary caretaker of infants, she becomes the identification figure in early childhood for both boys and girls. In this context where a primary male attachment figure is lacking, a little boy's principle way of attaining male gender identity will hinge on (a) achieving an emotional distance and separation from the mother and (b) reinforcing his difference from the mother via rigid adherence to masculine gender roles. As the boy grows up, he struggles against "too much" emotional intimacy with his mother, since an affective re-merger with her would be tantamount to losing his sense of self as a male. To preserve his hard-won masculine identity he becomes vigilant—both consciously and unconsciously—in defining and maintaining strong emotional boundaries. While this may facilitate his ability to be objective in interpersonal decisions, it may also lead to later difficulties with intimacy and with acknowledgment of healthy dependency needs.

As a little girl grows up, she does not have to disavow her primary affective tie with her mother; instead, she develops her sense of self as a girl in the context of an ongoing and intimate bond with her mother. Without needing to break off this bond at an early age, she learns a great deal about nurturance, empathy, and emotional responsiveness to others and often experiences her deepest sense of self-affirmation while in relationships with others. Although the girl may excel in activities and decisions requiring cooperation and accommodation to others' needs, she may have difficulty expressing anger and autonomy, both of which may seem to threaten the integrity of her relationships.

Thus, in a context in which women are the primary caretakers of young children, the acquisition of gender identity leads boys and girls to different psychological strengths as well as to different areas of struggle. Yet, historically, the outcomes of the male developmental process have been considered the hallmarks of psychological maturity for both men and women. Women's tendency to organize their life choices around connections to and concern for others often has been labeled as arising from "masochism," "excessive dependency," or "lack of a strong superego." Women's psychological strengths have been persistently denied or devalued in favor of increased separation, autonomy, and the capacity to make decisions based on abstract principles instead of empathy. As clinicians integrate the recent literature on women's psychology into patient care, they may develop more compassion and respect for women patients, empowering women to make choices more consonant with their values and life experiences.

Ms. T was a 26-year-old married woman who came regularly to her primary care physician for diabetic care. She had two children, both under age 5, and she worked as a housekeeper. During Ms. T's previous clinic visit, she was noted to be quite depressed, exhibiting neurovegetative signs of depression such as insomnia and fatigue. Ms. T's elderly parents had moved in with her recently because of their poor health, and they had been criticizing her child-rearing methods as well as the "filthy condition" of her house.

Ms. T was tearful and overwhelmed during her clinic visit, saying, "Nothing has changed after all these years. My parents are still so harsh and demanding." Yet, she said that she felt responsible for her parents and believed it was her duty to care for them. Although he agreed to share his home with his in-laws, Ms. T's husband had not been able to offer Ms. T much emotional support.

The primary care physician prescribed an antidepressant for Ms. T. Six weeks later, her sleep and energy had improved, but she remained quite tearful and depressed as she recounted her parents' continued harshness and humiliating comments toward her. Her physician felt frustrated and impatient as he listened to Ms. T's story, and he tried unsuccessfully to convince her to find another place for her parents to live.

Later, the physician discussed the case with a consulting psychiatrist and voiced the opinion that Ms. T seemed to be "masochistic" and needed to become "more independent of her parents." The psychiatrist saw the situation differently: Ms. T greatly valued her role as a caring individual; her identity was deeply tied to family relationships that had failed to provide the empathic support of which she herself seemed capable. Rather than having her sever any existing family relationships—an action that would profoundly disrupt her basic sense of self-identity—she would more likely benefit from the creation of new relationships that could offer some of the emotional closeness and reciprocity lacking in her interactions with her parents and her husband.

The primary care physician was advised to continue treating Ms. T's depression with the antidepressant but also to refer her to a neighborhood women's support group as well as to some parenting classes. Ms. T's husband declined to undergo couple's counseling but agreed to watch the children one night each week so that Ms. T could attend her support group. Two months later, Ms. T reported feeling much better. Her parents continued to be critical, but she felt less sensitive to their comments because her parenting class instructor had told her she was a good mother. She had made new friends at the class as well as at the support group, and these women listened sympathetically to her difficulties with her parents while admiring her decision to care for them. After discussing her situation in the support group, Ms. T arranged for her parents to visit a close relative in another town for a few weeks so that she could spend some time with her husband and children.

REPRODUCTIVE FUNCTION & WOMEN'S PSYCHOLOGICAL HEALTH

DEVELOPMENTAL TASKS OF NORMAL PREGNANCY

In classical psychoanalytic theory, a woman's wish to have a child arises from her disappointed recognition that she does not have a penis; she therefore substitutes her wish for a penis with a wish for a baby, and by giving birth, she comes to terms with her "castrated" self-image as a female. Subsequent theorists have rigorously challenged the notion that penis envy is the ultimate source of a woman's wish to give birth. Some of these theorists suggest that the wish for motherhood is an inherent biological drive, while others view the wish as a positive affective identification with what is essentially and uniquely female—the capacity to conceive and give birth. In either case, pregnancy offers women an important opportunity to re-approach and re-work core identity issues related to being female. As a woman prepares to become a mother, pregnancy can also revive unresolved conflicts regarding the parenting she received in her own childhood. Depending on how a woman faces these developmental tasks, pregnancy can be the catalyst for deepening her psychological growth and insight.

In the first trimester, during which pregnancy is usually diagnosed, a woman faces the task of acknowledging this physiologic reality and making an appropriate decision about whether to continue with the pregnancy. Cultural expectations about motherhood as well as the woman's financial situation, religious beliefs, and her relationship with the baby's father will all have a major impact on her initial response. Even when the pregnancy has been planned, the woman may vacillate between intense fear, ambivalence, and elation or excitement as her wish to become a parent moves toward reality. The relationship she had with her own mother will significantly affect her trust in her ability to "carry off" pregnancy and motherhood. If the pregnancy is unwanted or unanticipated, emotional vacillation may be pronounced as the woman confronts the decision of whether to have an abortion. Carr (1993) notes that "pregnancy alters the course of a woman's life irreversibly; once having been pregnant, there is no return to a prepregnant psychology. Even in women who choose induced abortion, [pregnancy] confirms the essential femaleness of her biology."

In the second trimester, as the pregnancy becomes more visible, the woman faces the task of assimilating an altered body image. On one hand, her pregnant abdomen may underscore her fertility and increase her pleasure in her female gender identity. On the other hand, her body may no longer feel like her own, and its increasing girth and other physiologic changes may lead to a sense of resentment, loss, or being out of control as she compares herself to her prepregnant state. It is also during the second trimester, as fetal movement is first experienced, that the woman's emotional bond with the baby often intensifies; this increased maternal-fetal attachment can result in a somewhat passive, inward-focused demeanor on the woman's part. The woman's growing attachment to the baby and the knowledge that she is bringing a new life into being will often help the woman to resolve the ambivalent feelings she may have about her altered body image.

In the third trimester, as the physical toll of the pregnancy becomes more pronounced, the woman often experiences increased fatigue, discomfort, and impatience for the pregnancy to end. At the same time, she may dread the pain associated with labor and delivery and become increasingly anxious about possible fetal abnormalities. Concerns about her own parenting capacities may become heightened, and she may grieve the changes to preexisting relationships that the birth will likely bring. In contrast to the transient ambivalence toward the fetus often seen in the first trimester, emotional rejection of the fetus in the third trimester is often a warning sign of later attachment difficulties with the newborn.

Ms. M, a 34-year-old single woman, presented to the emergency room complaining of back pain. She was thin and mildly disheveled and was dressed in a loose-fitting sweater and skirt. The physician who examined her was surprised to note that Ms. M appeared to be in the third trimester of pregnancy. Her gestational state was confirmed with a urine HCG (human chorionic gonadotropin) test.

When asked why she didn't initially report her pregnancy to the triage nurse, Ms. M replied nonchalantly, "It didn't seem related to my back pain." She had not obtained any prenatal care, and when asked about her due date, she replied, "Next month, I think." Ms. M chatted easily with the hospital staff, but her conversation was notable for the lack of any references to her baby. In a more detailed interview with a consulting psychiatrist, Ms. M exhibited no evidence of psychosis or cognitive impairment.

Ms. M reported that the pregnancy was the result of a brief and very disappointing romantic affair with a man who had subsequently left town. She said that she initially considered an abortion but "didn't have the money for it" and then decided to "just go ahead and have the baby." She said she would keep the baby, but she had made no plans for the baby's arrival and had continued to work long hours at a physically demanding job as a waitress.

After being discharged from the ER with a prescription for a muscle relaxant, Ms. M failed to keep an intake appointment at the obstetrics clinic. Three weeks later, she presented to the hospital in active labor and eventually delivered a healthy baby girl. After the birth, Ms. M did not ask to hold the infant or to visit her in the newborn nursery. She seemed more concerned with obtaining permission for a cigarette break. The obstetrics team asked for a psychiatric assessment of Ms. M's parenting capacity, and the psychiatrist found that Ms. M was having marked attachment difficulties to the newborn. The psychiatrist notified Child Protective Services, and after an extensive interview, Ms. M decided to put the baby up for adoption.

PSYCHOTROPIC MEDICATION DURING PREGNANCY

In addition to the developmental challenges brought on by pregnancy, some women must also contend with serious preexisting or new psychiatric disturbances during this period. The incidence of severe mental disorders such as major depression or psychosis do not increase during pregnancy; however, when psychosis, major depression, mania, or debilitating anxiety disorders do occur in a pregnant woman, these conditions must be treated rapidly and effectively. If the pregnant woman is not treated with appropriate medications for these disorders (while attempting to minimize adverse effects on the fetus), she and the baby might be at risk for the following:

- refusal of prenatal care
- poor nutrition
- attempts at premature self-delivery
- precipitous delivery (when the patient delivers her baby suddenly and possibly under dangerous circumstances)
- fetal abuse or neonaticide

Ms. C, a 30-year-old homeless woman who had a history of schizoaffective disorder, presented with a dead infant at the county hospital on Christmas Eve. She had not taken any psychiatric medications for more than 2 years. She had recently moved to a large urban area and had lived for 2 days in a low-rent hotel. She said she delivered the baby in the hotel bathroom, explaining, "I had to go to the toilet, and when I looked down, he just popped out. I didn't even know I was pregnant."

She reported that the infant was alive at birth and that she cut the umbilical cord with a plastic knife she had saved from a fast food restaurant. She didn't come to the hospital immediately, she said, "because even though there was blood all over, it was a miracle . . . my baby boy was born on Christmas Eve. . . the room was filled with white light when he was born . . . God told me this was a special gift to me, and I didn't want to share it with anyone." She fell asleep soon after the delivery, and when she woke up several hours later, the baby had apparently died of respiratory distress.

Diagnosis. Schizoaffective disorder (Axis I).

Teratogenic effects (birth defects caused by medication) are limited to the first 10 weeks of gestation, when organ development takes place; therefore, most clinicians try to avoid administering psychotropic agents during this period—except in the most extreme cases of psychosis or suicidality. Psychotropic drugs appear to be safer in the second and third

trimester, although many clinicians prescribe lower dosages throughout pregnancy and discontinue the medication 2 weeks before delivery to minimize toxicity and withdrawal in the newborn.

In general, high-potency neuroleptics and tricyclic antidepressants (TCAs) appear to be relatively safe throughout pregnancy. Preliminary data on fluoxetine also seems to indicate relative safety in the first trimester. Because of conflicting data on possible cleft lip/cleft palate abnormalities with use of benzodiazepines in early gestation, most clinicians avoid prescribing these agents in the first trimester. Mood stabilizers such as lithium, valproate (valproic acid), and carbamezepine have been associated with definite teratogenic effects when used in the first trimester: Cardiovascular anomalies are seen frequently with lithium, valproate is associated with neural tube defects, and carbamezepine with craniofacial abnormalities.

POSTPARTUM PSYCHIATRIC DISORDERS

Physicians have long recognized that women are at higher risk for mental disturbance in the year after childbirth. Comparing antenatum and postpartum rates of admission to a psychiatric hospital, Kendell (1987) demonstrated a six-fold increase in psychiatric admissions in the first month postpartum and a nearly four-fold increase within the first 3 months postpartum. More than half of women requiring psychiatric hospitalization after delivery have no history of previous psychiatric illness. Affective disorders are the most commonly diagnosed disturbance, ranging from postpartum "blues" to major depression and postpartum psychosis.

The medical literature reflects controversy regarding the reasons for women's increased psychiatric vulnerability after childbirth. Enormous physiologic change occurs during labor and after delivery, and several authors have suggested that the increase in psychiatric disorders may be related to the fluid, electrolyte, and hormonal shifts that occur during this period. For example, plasma corticosteroids and beta-endorphins are elevated dramatically during labor and then fall rapidly within a few hours of childbirth.

In the first 3 days after delivery, progesterone and estriol levels are reduced drastically, while prolactin levels remain elevated. Several days after delivery, there is usually a significant weight loss, accompanied by an increase in sodium excretion and a decrease in calcium excretion. Other physiologic changes such as postpartum levels of tryptophan, cyclic AMP, and platelet monoamine oxidase (MAO) also may be linked to the development of affective disorders. However, a direct correlation between these biological factors and the onset of specific psychiatric disorders has not been established. Psychosocial factors such as poor family and social support, conflict with the baby's father, breast-feeding and child-care responsibilities, fears about parenting, financial strains, and change in employment status may exacerbate biologically induced stress.

Postpartum Psychosis

Postpartum psychosis is a rare but usually severe form of psychosis with an incidence of 0.1–0.4%. The risk of psychosis is increased up to 1 year after delivery. The most significant etiologic factor for postpartum psychosis appears to be a genetic predisposition to bipolar disorder. Although the differential diagnosis for postpartum psychosis includes schizophrenia, depression with psychotic features, and substance use, the most common cause of psychosis after delivery is mania.

A. Signs & Symptoms. Symptoms develop with an extremely rapid onset, such that the woman can move from reality-based cognition to full-blown psychosis within 48 hours. There is a small but significant risk of infanticide or suicide. The mother frequently develops bizarre delusions involving the infant or herself; she may also experience visual or auditory hallucinations—including command hallucinations to harm the baby or herself. The following signs and symptoms may also be present:

- marked emotional lability
- depressed or elated mood
- confusion
- a tendency to be easily distracted
- insomnia

B. Treatment. Treatment involves separating the woman from her infant until symptoms are controlled with an antipsychotic and a mood stabilizer.

C. Recurrence. There is a 50% chance that postpartum psychosis will recur during future pregnancies, so the woman must be advised strongly to seek psychiatric care before becoming pregnant again.

Kimberly S, aged 27, was brought by her husband to the hospital. She was in an agitated state, having jumped into a nearby river that day. She explained that she was trying to cover herself with mud in order to "get rid of all the prejudice in the world." She was preoccupied with sin and redemption and was convinced that the second coming of Christ was at hand. Her husband explained that he and Ms. S had married a year and a half ago and that they were eager to start a family. She became pregnant within a few months of their wedding. After normal vaginal delivery of a healthy girl, Ms. S breast fed her daughter for about 9 months before weaning the infant.

Around this time, her behavior changed markedly. She became restless and highly energetic, for example, buying and wrapping all her Christmas gifts 4 months in advance. She had difficulty sleeping for more than 2 or 3 hours, and she would get up in the middle of the night to switch on all the lights and turn on all the water faucets in the house because she felt that water and light had a cleansing effect. She denied substance use and a urine toxicology drug screen was negative.

Ms. S's obstetrician requested a psychiatric evaluation of her patient, believing that Ms. S displayed symptoms of postpartum psychosis. The psychiatrist concurred and noted the presence of symptoms suggestive of mania, including grandiosity and reduced need for sleep. Ms. S's family history was remarkable for both a maternal uncle and grandfather who had bipolar disorder. The psychiatrist recommended that Ms. S start on an outpatient course of valproate (a mood stabilizer) and antipsychotic medication. She improved after a few weeks and eventually discontinued the medication. However, she and her husband were not counseled about the risk of recurrent psychotic episodes with future pregnancies.

Eighteen months later, she became pregnant again. Her prenatal course and delivery were once again unremarkable, and she gave birth to a healthy baby boy. About 6 months later, Ms. S's husband noted that she seemed socially withdrawn and internally preoccupied, often lying awake in bed for several hours during the day. He attributed this behavior to the "stress of motherhood" and was not concerned about a recurrent psychotic episode since she was acting so differently from her previous manic presentation.

One day, the husband returned from work and discovered that his wife had drowned their infant son. She had been experiencing recurrent delusions regarding her spiritual mission to prepare the world for the second coming of Christ and had been spending hours in bed praying for her husband's redemption. She had begun to believe that there might be "something evil" about her son and that "he might be like Lucifer after his fall from grace." She was convinced that her son's redeemed soul would cause his body to rise from the dead.

Diagnosis. Bipolar disorder (Axis I).

Postpartum Depression

Postpartum depression is a more common psychiatric disturbance. Its incidence is estimated at 20%; however, many cases go undetected because mothers are ashamed to admit feelings of depression during the supposedly joyful period after giving birth. The disorder is more common after first births. Onset of depression can occur gradually from 4 weeks to 1 year after delivery, and the highest rates of new cases occur in the third and ninth months after delivery. The mother is frequently unable to cope with the demands of child care and becomes withdrawn and unresponsive to her infant's needs. Risk of suicide is rare, but the infant is at high risk for inadequate parenting. Etiologic factors include personal or family history of major depression, psychosocial stressors, and ambivalence about pregnancy.

A. Signs & Symptoms. The following signs and symptoms may be present:

- changes in sleep, energy, appetite, and libido
- tearfulness
- despondency
- feelings of inadequacy

B. Treatment. Treatment generally consists of an outpatient course of antidepressant medication combined with increased social support and psychotherapy. If the depression is severe, the patient may be hospitalized.

C. Recurrence. Recurrence in a future pregnancy depends on the severity of the depression and the degree of psychosocial stressors.

Lisa L, aged 19, was accompanied by an aunt to her obstetrician's office. The aunt voiced concern that Ms. L had become depressed and was "just not herself recently." Ms. L reluctantly agreed to discuss her problems. She told the doctor that she had been feeling stressed since her discovery that she was pregnant. She had been in a stable relationship with the baby's father, a young auto salesperson, when they discovered the unplanned pregnancy.

Despite limited financial resources, the couple decided to carry the pregnancy to term because of their religious beliefs against abortion. The boyfriend increased his work hours to earn more money for child-related expenses. After a healthy infant was born, the young woman's aunt moved in temporarily with Ms. L and her boyfriend so that she could assist with child care.

The aunt was planning to leave after 2 months with the couple, but she hesitated because of her concern for the young mother. She said Ms. L appeared to be getting increasingly tired and irritable during the day and slept for more than 10 hours every night. She had no appetite and was 5 pounds below her prepregnancy weight. She would forget the baby's feeding times and became annoyed when reminded; she misplaced medication that the pediatrician prescribed for the infant's ear infection, and the aunt had to ask the pediatrician to call in another prescription.

Lately, the aunt had taken over more of the infant's care, in response to Ms. L tearful statement: "I'm not a good mother." The aunt accompanied Ms. L and the infant to their next clinic visit, and she reported her concerns to the pediatrician. Ms. L was sent to her primary care physician, who correctly diagnosed her with postpartum depression and started her on an antidepressant. The aunt was advised to continue living with Ms. L for a few more weeks, and the boyfriend was encouraged to cut back on his work hours for the time being.

After 6 weeks, Ms. L's symptoms of depression had improved significantly. She admitted that she felt anxious and overwhelmed with her new role as a mother, and she appreciated the increased support from her aunt and boyfriend.

Diagnosis. Postpartum depression (Axis I).

Postpartum Blues

Postpartum blues represents an extremely common syndrome of postpartum affective lability characterized by mood swings. The syndrome has an incidence of 50% and has no etiologic links to major psychiatric disorders. Typically, symptoms appear within 10 days after delivery, and peak symptoms occur between the third and the seventh day after delivery. No major risks to mother or infant are associated with this syndrome.

A. Signs & Symptoms. The following symptoms may be present:

- crying spells
- tiredness
- physical discomfort
- insomnia
- anxiety

B. Treatment. Since the syndrome resolves spontaneously within 2 weeks of delivery, treatment consists only of reassurance and increased social support.

C. Recurrence. The syndrome is likely to recur in future pregnancies, but mothers can be reassured in advance that this is a self-limiting and fairly benign condition.

PREGNANCY LOSS

Any prenatal or neonatal loss of a desired pregnancy has emotional effects, whether the loss results from spontaneous abortion, ectopic pregnancy, partial fetal loss in a multiple pregnancy, or sudden infant death syndrome (SIDS). However, third trimester pregnancy loss or the death of an infant tends to have a more devastating emotional impact.

Bereavement usually involves several stages: Initial shock and denial are followed by guilt, anger, and despair, often associated with agonizing preoccupation with the lost child. Women frequently report feeling "empty," with a debilitating loss of self-worth and an undermined sense of female identity. They may experience marked envy and resentment toward more reproductively "successful" women friends and relatives, avoiding all contact with these individuals even if it means the loss of their support and caring. Rage toward medical caregivers is also a common response to the pregnancy loss.

For many mothers, the grief reaction can last 6–9 months following loss of the infant. However, there is no consensus among mental health experts regarding the duration of "normal" bereavement; the length of time required to work through the stages of grief and to accept the loss can vary tremendously among women. Psychological studies show that the mother's grief reaction tends to be longer and more intense than the father's. The intensity of the initial grief reaction does not appear to be a predictor for the overall duration of the bereavement.

Pathological or **complicated grief reaction** is a somewhat ambiguous term that refers to a derailment in the normal mourning process; it is characterized by persistent deterioration in physical, mental, or social functioning beyond the norms generally seen in an individual's cultural group. The manifestations of pathological grief following pregnancy loss can include chronic, absent, or distorted grief. When present, distorted grief can appear as furious hostility, aimless hyperactivity, or obsessive wishing for the return of the lost child. One consistent predictor for a complicated grief reaction is the perceived lack of support and concern from medical caregivers.

Other factors involved in complicated grief reaction may include a poor marital relationship, preexisting medical and psychological problems, fertility problems, lack of any living children, advanced gestational age at the time of fetal loss, and ambivalence toward the pregnancy. Couples experiencing pregnancy loss are advised to wait at least 6 months before attempting to have another child; conception within 6 months of a previous fetal loss tends to complicate the bereavement process, increase anxiety in the next pregnancy, and distort the mother's attachment to the next child.

In women choosing to terminate their pregnancies with induced abortion, no psychiatric pathologies or specific patterns of psychological response have been described. Women who are at risk for psychiatric illness following induced abortion are mainly those with prior psychiatric illness, those pressured or coerced into undergoing the abortion, those markedly ambivalent about the decision, and those lacking social supports.

Ms. G, a 40-year-old paralegal assistant, was involved in a somewhat volatile relationship with a man for about 1 year. Soon after a very difficult and protracted breakup, which she resisted to the end, Ms. G discovered that she was pregnant. She contacted her ex-boyfriend, hoping that they would get back together after he learned of her pregnancy. To her disappointment and anger, he merely offered to help pay for an abortion. She refused his help and sought pregnancy counseling at a local health clinic.

Despite several weeks of counseling, Ms. G remained torn about whether to have an abortion. Aware of her "biological clock," she feared that if she terminated the pregnancy, she might not have another chance at motherhood. Yet, she did not feel that she could handle either the emotional or financial obligations of being a single parent. Finally, at 18 weeks gestation, she decided to have an abortion.

Ms. G was lying on the treatment table at the abortion clinic when she suddenly sat up on the table and demanded that the physician stop the procedure. The physician tried to explain to Ms. G that the abortion procedure was too far along for the fetus to be viable. Ms. G began to wail and scream, and tried to get up. To prevent serious medical complications, the physician sedated Ms. G and completed the abortion while she was sedated.

After the sedation wore off, Ms. G was furious with the clinic staff. She accused them of "murdering" her baby, and she refused to accept any responsibility for her ambivalence regarding the abortion. She was referred to the outpatient psychiatric clinic, where she was evaluated for the pregnancy loss.

After several weeks in psychotherapy, she remained unable to accept the loss or to acknowledge the fetus' importance as a symbolic tie to her ex-boyfriend. She obsessed about the lost child and expressed rage at the boyfriend, the staff at the abortion clinic, and the psychiatrist. She eventually lost her job because she was unable to concentrate at work as she mentally planned the details of a "huge lawsuit" against the abortion clinic. Because the psychiatrist did not support Ms. G's plans to sue the clinic, Ms. G left treatment abruptly.

Diagnosis. Pathological grief reaction (Axis I); consider personality disorder (cluster B) based on long history of interpersonal difficulties (predating pregnancy) and externalized rage and responsibility.

INFERTILITY

Infertility is defined as the failure to conceive despite 1 year or more of unprotected intercourse. Between 10 and 15% of couples in the United States may be affected by infertility. Although male reproductive dysfunction partly or wholly contributes to 40–50% of infertility cases, women may be made to feel that the problem is primarily theirs because of societal biases that may also be present in physicians' attitudes.

Among infertile couples, women are significantly more distressed than men about the failure to conceive; for example, 57% of these women thought that infertility was the worst thing they had ever faced in their lives, while only 12% of men felt this way. In another study, 40% of infertile women reported psychological distress of clinical severity compared to only 13% of their male counterparts. Depression appears to be the most common psychiatric disorder in response to infertility, although chronic anxiety with secondary sexual dysfunctions such as impotence, inability to achieve orgasm, and loss of libido may also develop.

Treatment options for infertility have increased with the advent of new reproductive technologies such as in vitro fertilization, gamete intrafallopian transfer, and ovum donation; however, the expense involved in such high-tech treatments is prohibitive for most infertile couples. With success rates of only 15–20%, many couples pursuing these expensive and medically demanding treatments may ultimately experience an even greater sense of anger, disappointment, and loss about their infertility. In these situations, the clinician must help the couple to decide when "enough is enough" and must provide adequate emotional support throughout the infertility evaluation and treatment. According to Downey (1993), the goal in treating infertile couples is "not to achieve pregnancy at any cost, but to assist in resolving their infertility crisis and becoming able to move on in their lives. This may mean having a birth child, adopting a child, or (discovering) a child-free way of life in which a couple's creativity and urge to contribute to the next generation can find expression."

PREMENSTRUAL SYNDROME

Intense controversy exists about the significance of psychological and somatic symptoms that occur regularly during the luteal phase of the menstrual cycle. This possible medical disorder has been studied under the names of **premenstrual syndrome** (PMS), **late luteal phase dysphoric disorder** (LLPDD), or more recently, **premenstrual dysphoric disorder** (PMDD). The principle psychological symptoms consist of markedly depressed mood, heightened anxiety, mood swings, and decreased interest in normal activities. Physical symptoms may include depressive symptoms including changes in sleep, energy, and appetite, as well as headaches, breast tenderness, and sensations of bloating or weight gain. Symptoms occur in the late luteal phase and are absent in the week following menses.

Prospective studies of premenstrual symptoms suggest a rate of LLPDD of 3–5% in women of reproductive age. However, it is unclear what, if any, biological factors are involved in this phenomenon. Numerous studies have shown no consistent abnormalities in peripheral hormone levels of women reporting PMS.

Other studies have linked PMS symptoms to dys-

function in circadian rhythm and serotonin metabolism. Asking whether the disorder is more of a sociological phenomenon than a physiologic entity, some investigators have hypothesized that the physical discomfort, tearfulness, irritability, and anxiety linked to the imminent onset of menses may represent women's internalized response to the societal devaluation of femaleness and the stigmatization of menstruation. Several studies show that women report more negative symptoms when led to believe that they are premenstrual than when they are persuaded that they are not. Regardless of etiology, studies do indicate that fluoxetine and alprazolam may be effective in relieving symptoms of LLPDD.

MENOPAUSE

Since 1900, the average life expectancy of women in the United States has risen from 50 to 80 years. The average age of **menopause**—the cessation of menses—has remained relatively constant at about 51 years, which means that the number of postmenopausal women in the United States has increased dramatically during the past century. At one time, the cessation of menses, and the corresponding hormonal shifts, were thought to lead to a distinctive affective disorder called **involutional melancholia.** Recent studies have dismissed the hypothesis of involutional melancholia as a specific, hormonally induced depression, and this nomenclature is no longer used in the psychiatric literature. However, the question remains as to whether women are at higher risk for developing depression perimenopausally than at other periods in their lives.

Although several epidemiologic studies have failed to demonstrate an increased incidence of depressive disorders in the general population of menopausal women, 65% of menopausal women who seek medical consultation for their symptoms have varying degrees of depression. The most common reason for perimenopausal women to be referred to a psychiatrist is for evaluation of depressive symptoms.

In menopausal women, the appearance of depression—as well as other affective symptoms such as irritability and mood instability—appears to be culturally mediated to a great extent. The psychological impact of menopause is influenced strongly by the cultural importance attached to procreation, fertility, aging, and female roles. In cultures in which women receive increased status and privilege once they reach menopause, affective symptoms are minimal, whereas women in youth-oriented Western cultures experience more serious symptoms. Authors from different countries have also noted that the higher the education and socioeconomic status of the woman, the less pronounced any emotional symptoms will be at menopause.

Psychosocial stressors that may contribute to depression around the age of menopause include decline in physical health, onset of illness or disability in the spouse, departure of children from the household, necessity of caring for elderly parents, and changes in employment and financial status. In nondepressed menopausal women, conventional estrogen replacement therapy appears to have a mood-enhancing effect; however, in women with menopausal mood disturbance, conventional dosages of exogenous estrogen do not alleviate affective symptoms.

During a clinic visit for a routine PAP smear, Anne K, a 50-year-old postmenopausal woman began to cry and told her gynecologist that she felt "useless and old." She described the onset of these symptoms as "2 months after the accident that ruined my life." Eighteen months earlier, she had been hit by a speeding car as she was crossing the street, and her left hip and knee were badly broken. She had undergone several surgeries as well as extensive physical rehabilitation, and she was able to slowly and rather painfully walk on her own again. Ms. K lived with her husband and two college-age children. She was a homemaker, and before the accident, she had been an active participant in her church and in local volunteer groups.

Despite continued encouragement from her family and large community of friends, Ms. K often refused to leave her house. She was physically able to drive, but she insisted that her husband or her children drive her on errands. Before the accident, she had encouraged her daughter to apply for a prestigious out-of-state college program but now wanted her to attend a rather mediocre local university.

After an evaluation with a consulting psychiatrist, Ms. K was started on a serotonin re-uptake inhibitor, targeting her depressive symptoms as well as obsessive ruminations and possible agoraphobia. She was also referred for individual psychotherapy and a support group for menopausal women. In therapy, she admitted that the accident made her realize how physically and emotionally vulnerable she was. She had always been the "family caretaker," but she became afraid that if she were the one requiring assistance, the family would see her as a burden. She unconsciously began acting as the helpless dependent person she feared she might be perceived as being, "just waiting in fear for my husband and kids to tell me that they were sick of me."

In her support group, Ms. K also realized that the accident had heightened the worries about aging and attractiveness she had started to feel around the time of her menopause. She began to discuss with her family the emotional impact of growing older, and they responded with empathy and reassurance.

Six months later, Ms. K's grooming had improved dramatically, and she had bought several new outfits that accentuated her height and slender build. She was pleased and excited that her daughter had been accepted into the out-of-state college program. She was also involved with her church Christmas pageant and drove herself to the planning meetings.

Diagnosis. Major depression (Axis I).

GENDER DIFFERENCES IN PSYCHIATRIC DISORDERS & TREATMENT RESPONSE

SCHIZOPHRENIA

Undifferentiated schizophrenia has a higher incidence in men than in women, whereas paranoid and schizoaffective disorders have a higher incidence in women than in men (see Chapters 4 and 12). Etiologically, prenatal viral infection seems to play a significant role in the onset of schizophrenia for women but not for men. Women who have schizophrenia have a significantly later age of onset than men, resulting in a much better premorbid history for women. For example, women schizophrenics are more likely to be married and to be more developmentally mature than men. Women also have better premorbid social functioning and school achievement.

Women who have schizophrenia exhibit more affective symptoms, paranoia, and auditory hallucinations, while males tend to have more so-called **negative symptoms** such as flat affect, social withdrawal, and loss of will. Women tend to have better treatment outcomes, as measured by fewer hospitalizations, shorter hospital stays, fewer symptoms during remission, and better social adjustment. Limited evidence suggests that young women seem to require lower doses of antipsychotics than do young men and that young women have more complete symptom response than do their male counterparts.

Male children of schizophrenic women exhibit lower birth weights, lower IQs, more neurobehavioral deficits, more aggression, and more schizoid/schizotypal traits than do female children.

MOOD DISORDERS

Epidemiologic data show higher lifetime prevalence rates of unipolar depression in women, as compared to men (see Chapter 5). Overall prevalence rates for bipolar disorder are not increased for women, but the rapid-cycling subtype appears to be more common among women (see Chapter 6). Gender differences in affective symptoms, course of illness, and response to treatment are quite limited. Women appear to respond to MAO inhibitors better than do men, while men respond better to TCAs.

ANXIETY DISORDERS

Prevalence rates for post-traumatic stress disorder (PTSD), generalized anxiety disorder, simple phobias, social phobia, and panic disorder with and without agoraphobia are significantly higher in women, as compared to men (see Chapter 7). For PTSD and agoraphobia, the course of illness is longer for women. Obsessive-compulsive disorder (OCD) is equally prevalent in men and women, but women have later age of onset, less severe illness, and tend to exhibit compulsive hair pulling (trichotillomania) and compulsive washing, while men tend to engage in checking rituals. For women more than men, depression and eating disorders are commonly found in conjunction with OCD. Limited data suggest that in cases of panic disorder with depression, men may respond more favorably to TCAs than do women.

SOMATOFORM DISORDERS

In Western countries, disorders such as irritable bowel syndrome, chronic fatigue syndrome, fibromyalgia syndrome, and chronic pelvic pain are more prevalent in women than in men; in other countries, irritable bowel syndrome is diagnosed more frequently in men (see Chapter 9). Because the prevalence rates for somatoform disorders are derived from treatment samples and not from community samples, higher rates might represent increased help-seeking behavior. Women with somatoform disorders frequently have an undetected history of sexual and/or physical abuse.

EATING DISORDERS

In Western countries, anorexia nervosa and bulimia nervosa occur almost exclusively in women and adolescent girls (see Chapter 13). The prevalence of eating disorders in other countries appears to be much lower overall, although it has not been studied as extensively. The few men who do develop eating disorders appear to experience psychological conflicts similar to those experienced by women, including those related to autonomy, dependence, body image, and sexuality.

WOMEN & CHEMICAL DEPENDENCY

Chemical dependency refers to the compulsive use of one or more psychoactive substance with resulting impairment of physical health, emotional health, social functioning, occupational functioning, or intimate relationships (see Chapter 11). Compared to the data on men, far less is known about the etiology, clinical course, and effective treatment of chemical dependency in women. Women appear to be stigmatized more heavily for drug dependency than are men, which encourages women to minimize or dismiss their drug dependence as a mere coping strategy for dealing with a "real" problem such as family violence, poverty, or interpersonal loss. Women impaired by chemical dependency often first seek help from social service agencies for family or child-related stresses, rather than seeking the help of physicians.

IDENTIFYING HIGH-RISK GROUPS

Clinicians should be alert to the possibility of chemical dependency when treating women from the following high-risk groups: incest survivors, battered women, members of genetically vulnerable families, partners of male substance abusers, and women with chronic pain. Lesbians, women in the military, and inner-city women also appear to have a higher risk for alcohol and drug dependence.

Women with underlying chemical dependency are more likely to experience episodes of anorexia, bulimia, or agoraphobia between periods of substance use than are women who don't use substances. Chemically dependent women are more likely than their male counterparts to carry a concurrent psychiatric diagnosis, especially of major depression. Furthermore, women with chemical dependency often exhibit the following psychosocial features:

- They tend to have a more traditional and rigid view of appropriate female behavior and are acutely aware of their failure to live up to it.
- They believe they are "worse" than chemically dependent men, and the men they know agree with this conclusion; these women lack hope about their lives and feel more guilty and responsible for their circumstances.
- They are far more likely than their male counterparts to be romantically attached to another addict; drug dependency is more likely to become established in the man and then transferred to his female partner, rather than vice versa. Also, while women are likely to remain involved with

substance-dependent men, men often end their relationships with substance-dependent women.

- They are less involved in criminal activity; therefore, they are also less likely to be assigned to court-mandated treatment programs.
- They tend to have less education, make less money, be less likely to have health insurance, and have fewer life options than male substance abusers.

TREATMENT OF CHEMICAL DEPENDENCY IN WOMEN

Successful treatment of chemical dependency in women must take into account the above psychosocial features. For example, the highly confrontational techniques used successfully with male addicts to overcome denial often are counterproductive with women; women addicts are more likely to experience pointed confrontations as further proof of their worthlessness and will drop out of treatment. Thus, clinicians working with women addicts may need to spend more time establishing a treatment alliance by praising them for seeking help before re-labeling their symptoms as addiction related.

Most drug rehabilitation programs emphasize severance of ties with drug-using peers as a major step toward recovery; however, this recommendation can be more difficult for women to follow since they are more likely than men to be living with intimate partners who are also chemically dependent.

To prevent women from leaving treatment because they find rehabilitation programs so enormously disruptive to their interpersonal relationships, care providers might make more efforts to engage intimate partners in the recovery process. In addition, pregnant women and those with young children frequently cannot follow the structure of a standard program of drug rehabilitation; programs that provide on-site child care or that show more flexibility in accommodating pregnancy and child care might be more successful in keeping women in treatment.

Finally, some investigators have argued that women with chemical dependencies should participate only in same-gender therapy groups because clinicians have observed that women sometimes show less improvement than men in mixed-gender groups. Researchers have hypothesized that men are more expressive in mixed-gender groups and that women provide the nurturing support; the net result is that men improve but women do not. Clearly, more treatment outcome research with chemically dependent women is needed to test the validity of these clinical observations.

Alcohol

Alcohol dependence in women is associated with a phenomenon called **telescoping**—that is, accelerated

development of cardiovascular, gastrointestinal, and liver disease when compared to men consuming equivalent amounts of alcohol. Because equivalent alcohol consumption is associated with more severe disease in women, the cut-off level for defining hazardous drinking should be lower for women than for men. When gender-adjusted cut-off levels are used to define hazardous drinking, rates of heavy drinking in men and women are about the same (10%); without gender-adjusted cut-off levels, the incidence of heavy drinking would appear erroneously to be twice as high among men.

For women, the average age of onset for alcohol dependence is 4–8 years later than for men. Women tend to have shorter drinking histories before seeking help. Women alcoholics typically consume less alcohol than do men and drink less frequently and less continuously, with fewer binges. They experience fewer blackouts and fewer episodes of delirium tremens (DTs). They are arrested less frequently for drunk driving. Despite shorter drinking histories than men and less overall consumption of alcohol, the telescoping phenomenon results in women getting just as sick as men at about the same time of life or even earlier. Alcoholic women tend to use prescribed psychoactive drugs more frequently than do male alcoholics.

Prescription Drugs

Psychoactive drugs such as anxiolytics and sedatives are prescribed for women under age 65 more often than they are for men. Women account for 61% of emergency room visits involving sedative-hypnotics; for antidepressant-related emergencies, women account for 64% of the visits. The finding of disproportionate prescribing of psychoactive drugs to women holds up even when adjustments are made for the fact that, overall, women use medical services more and receive more prescription drugs than do men.

The increased dispensing of psychotropic drugs to women may reflect the fact that they have higher lifetime prevalence rates of anxiety and depressive disorders. However, Gomberg & Nirenberg (1995) suggest that because of sex stereotyping and gender bias, physicians may also tend to see female patients as "more anxious, more neurotic, and more emotional than male patients and thus prescribe more psychotropic drugs for women." Physicians must carefully weigh the benefits of controlled use of sedatives and tranquilizers against the risk of drug abuse and dependence. Elderly women experiencing high levels of emotional distress and chronic somatic problems are at highest risk for physician-induced psychotropic drug abuse and dependence. When prescribing lipid-soluble drugs such as diazepam and oxazepam, physicians must consider that higher body-fat levels in women will lead to longer half-lives for these psychoactive agents.

Ms. R, aged 64, visited her internist regularly for management of hypertension. During her last clinic visit, she reported insomnia and restlessness at night and that her thoughts frequently focused on her recently deceased husband. Her appetite, energy, and concentration were at baseline, and she denied any suicidal thoughts or loss of interest in normal activities. She had no history of drug or alcohol abuse. Her internist prescribed a low dose of lorazepam to be taken at bedtime for the next few weeks. Ms. R doubled the dose one night when she was having a particularly difficult time sleeping and continued to take this double dose thereafter. Her physician had authorized a refill, and she renewed the prescription 2 weeks later.

By her next clinic visit, Ms. R had run out of lorazepam. She reported to the physician that she was experiencing increased anxiety, palpitations, and had to urinate more frequently since finishing her medication. Her sleep was by this time quite disturbed, and she reported having vivid, frightening dreams. Her internist restarted the lorazepam, but this time he emphasized to Ms. R that she was on an "addictive" medication from which she needed to be carefully weaned. He outlined a plan to taper off the lorazepam over the next 4 weeks, by which time the medication was successfully discontinued.

Diagnosis. Benzodiazepine dependence (Axis I).

Discussion: While Ms. R's symptoms cleared once benzodiazepines were tapered, patients with sleep disorders should always be screened for mood disorders.

Illegal Drugs

According to the 1992 National Institute on Drug Abuse cross-sectional survey of drug use, 4% of all women reported illicit drug use in the previous month, compared to 7% of all men. For girls and women, intimate male partners are a primary route for being introduced to illicit drugs; continued use of illicit drugs appears to be influenced heavily by social factors such as weekend gatherings and partner's use patterns. For boys and men, initiation into illicit drug use is almost always via male peers; continued use appears more related to availability and the physiologic "high" associated with use.

Among adolescents aged 17 and under, incidence of illicit drug use is slightly higher for girls than for boys, probably reflecting the fact that girls typically date older boys, thereby getting an earlier introduction to illicit drugs. From age 18 and on, however, women have consistently lower rates of marijuana, cocaine, and heroin use than do men. The highest illicit drug use rates were among young adults aged 18–25; 10% of women in this age group reported illicit use within the past month, versus 17% of their male counterparts.

Obviously, the use of illegal drugs carries the potential for criminal penalties, adding to the psychosocial problems already faced by women addicted to these substances. For low-income women, chemical dependence on illegal drugs may involve more participation in prostitution and drug trafficking than does dependence on alcohol and prescription drugs.

VIOLENCE AGAINST WOMEN

Women and girls are the primary victims of rape, incest, and domestic violence. According to Stewart & Robinson (1995), most states define **rape** as "nonconsensual sexual penetration obtained by physical force, by threat of bodily harm, or when the victim is incapable of giving consent due to mental illness, mental retardation or intoxication." When the perpetrator is a family member, rape and other forms of sexual violation may be referred to as **incest. Domestic violence** is a pattern of assaultive and coercive behaviors—including physical, sexual, and psychological attacks—that adults or adolescents use against their intimate partners.

Until the 1970s, when the feminist movement in the United States initiated widespread public education campaigns about these forms of violence, most health-care providers thought their occurrence was relatively rare. When victims did report rape or domestic violence, health-care providers commonly believed that the women had consciously or unconsciously provoked the assault in some way. Fortunately, such attitudes are changing, and medical providers are becoming more sensitized to the chilling frequency of violence against women and its profoundly damaging psychological effects. A visit to the emergency room or the gynecologist's office will often be the first or only contact that abuse survivors make with the medical system; therefore, appropriate diagnosis and treatment in these settings is particularly crucial.

INCIDENCE

In reviewing incidence statistics, one must bear in mind that episodes of incest, sexual assault, and domestic violence are frequently underreported. The reasons for underreporting can include shame, fear of retaliation from the perpetrator, fear of being disbelieved, lack of information about how to get help, social stigmatization, and distrust of the criminal justice system.

For women in the United States, estimates on the lifetime prevalence of completed rape range from 6% to 26%. Using the latter figure, this means that as many as one of four women will be the victim of a completed rape at some time in her life. According to one study, 21% of female rape victims were assaulted by strangers, 39% by acquaintances, 17% by men they were dating, and 24% by their husbands. Contrary to popular belief, date rape and marital rape were more likely to lead to physical injury than stranger rape.

Prevalence studies show that 12% of adolescent girls will experience some form of intrafamilial or extrafamilial sexual abuse by the age of 17. Girls are sexually abused by men 92% of the time and by lone women (usually the mothers) 6% of the time. Less than 20% of cases involve unknown offenders.

Prevalence data on domestic violence indicate that 20–30% of women in the United States will be physically assaulted by an intimate partner or ex-partner at some time in their lives. The level of injury resulting from domestic violence is severe and escalates over time; in one study of battered women presenting to a metropolitan emergency room, 28% of the women required hospital admission and 13% required major medical treatment. A staggering 42% of murdered women are killed by their intimate male partners; the risk of being killed is greater in interracial relationships and increases with a widening age difference between the two individuals. Women are more likely to be killed, raped, or physically assaulted by a past or current male partner than by anyone else.

ETIOLOGY

Sociological Theories

A number of authors have noted that rape, incest, and domestic assault occur along a wider continuum of violence against women; at many points along this continuum, men's domination and control of women is socially sanctioned. For example, pornography, sexist jokes in the workplace, and demeaning media portrayals of women are viewed by some as culturally acceptable ways to intimidate and dominate women.

The difficulty experienced by many rape survivors in prosecuting their assailants is thought by some to reflect society's collusion in having men maintain power and control over women. Legislators and criminal justice personnel may view "marital rape" as an oxymoron because they might believe that a husband has the right to demand sexual intercourse from his wife. In this framework, when men rape and assault women, they are essentially extending and elaborating the basic abuse that some say is routinely perpetrated on women to keep them in a devalued and inferior position. Some authors argue that rape and domestic violence cannot be eliminated effectively until the complex social structures maintaining gender inequality are dismantled and more power and social status are accorded to women.

Modeling Theories

Numerous studies suggest an intergenerational transmission of violence in which both perpetrators and victims come from family backgrounds in which violence was part of their daily lives. According to these studies, boys who routinely witness their father's violent behavior learn to solve disputes or frustration by physical force, later abusing their own children or their intimate partners. Girls who witness family violence in their childhood learn to tolerate high levels of violence in their adult partnerships. In an extensively researched review article on battered women, Hotaling & Sugarman (1986) found that the only consistent risk factor for becoming a victim of marital violence was witnessing parental violence as a child. From these data, many authors conclude that violence against women will not stop until children are raised in environments in which disputes are resolved without resorting to intimidation and physical force.

Biological Theories

Recent biological research suggests that exposure to major psychic trauma sets into motion a complex series of neuroendocrine changes; these changes lead to altered physiologic functioning that places the individual at higher risk for repeated victimization. For example, individuals who have been exposed to severe trauma seem to have excessive central nervous system adrenergic activity. This excessive activity appears to suppress endogenous opioid production, and the traumatized individual may subsequently develop chronic **hyperalgesia** (increased pain perception).

Exposure to a new stressor that is a reminder of the original stress appears to produce a temporary analgesia that is blocked by the opiate antagonist medication naloxone. Thus re-exposure to trauma might transiently re-stimulate endogenous opioid production, which will later be suppressed again by hyperarousal of the central sympathetic system. For example, a traumatized woman with hyperalgesia might engage in self-mutilation to experience a temporary abatement of pain due to a surge in endogenous opioids; once the self-mutilation stops, excess central adrenergic firing will suppress opioid production, and the woman will experience a painful opioid withdrawal. This process might explain in part the "addiction to trauma" that many victimized individuals seem to display.

PSYCHOLOGICAL EFFECTS OF VIOLENCE

The consequences of violence against women can be divided into short-term and long-term effects. Short-term psychological effects lasting a few days after an assault include emotional numbness, social withdrawal, and denial of the trauma; there may also be hypervigilance about safety, as well as recurrent and intrusive recollections, dreams, and flashbacks of the traumatic incident. Behavioral patterns in the immediate aftermath of trauma are characterized typically by either very calm, controlled, and subdued actions, or by intense expressions of anxiety, confusion, helplessness, and crying.

Long-term psychological effects include difficulties in forming and maintaining intimate relationships; a pervasive sense of vulnerability; and chronic feelings of fear, despair, and worthlessness. Long-term behavioral effects include self-mutilation, substance abuse, aggression, suicide attempts, sexual dysfunction, eating disorders, and increased visits to physicians and clinics. The risk of long-term effects is particularly high after childhood sexual abuse, repeated sexual abuse, and sexual assaults aggravated by extreme violence.

A wide spectrum of psychiatric diagnoses is found in women surviving violence. PTSD is probably the most common diagnostic entity among victims of incest, rape, and domestic violence (see Chapter 8). In addition to PTSD, major depression, drug and alcohol abuse, and obsessive-compulsive disorder are significantly correlated with a sexual assault history. Dissociative disorders and borderline personality disorder are particularly common in women with histories of repeated childhood incest. Survivors of domestic violence exhibit more somatic symptoms, substance abuse, suicidal thinking, and suicide attempts than do women from nonviolent homes; in addition, these women are more likely to act out their aggression verbally and physically against nonfamily members. Many women with somatization disorder, conversion disorder, and chronic pelvic pain have an undiagnosed history of sexual and/or physical abuse.

Ms. C, aged 28, was referred by the gynecology clinic for psychiatric evaluation. She reported severe pain during menses since early adolescence, and had decided that the only solution was a hysterectomy. She had requested this procedure several times throughout her 20s but was told each time that she should wait until she was older.

Ms. C was remarkably sensitive to any pain in the pelvic region, so much so that it was impossible for the gynecologist to perform a speculum examination; one pelvic examination had been performed under general anesthesia prior to surgical exploration of the abdomen, and subsequent assessments of Ms. C's reproductive tract were made through pelvic ultrasound. No physical etiology for her pain symptoms could be determined. The gynecologist was extremely reluctant to perform a hysterectomy when there was no clear medical indication and the patient was a young woman with no children.

When the gynecologist asked Ms. C how she would feel about the loss of childbearing potential, she replied that she had never had sexual relationships and while she was interested in being a foster parent, she did not want to have biological children "because that would mean having sex."

In the evaluation with the consulting psychiatrist, Ms. C reluctantly described being sodomized repeatedly at a daycare center she attended for 3 years as a preschooler. She did not report the abuse to anyone at the time. She told her mother when she was 12, but her mother advised her that it was "too late" to do anything and that she should try to forget the abuse. Ms. C was remarkably calm as she recounted this history; she was convinced that her childhood abuse had nothing to do with her pelvic pain or her abstinence from sexual relationships, saying, "[the abuser] didn't touch my sexual parts at all . . . it was only my bottom."

The psychiatrist recommended that Ms. C undergo a course of outpatient psychotherapy to address the possibility that her pelvic pain symptoms might subside as the psychological issues surrounding her abuse were finally addressed. If she continued to experience significant pain symptoms despite good progress in psychotherapy, then the issue of elective hysterectomy might be considered. However, when this proposal was made to Ms. C, she chose not to undergo therapy; she expressed frustration with the medical team and stated that she would have to find another doctor who would perform the hysterectomy "without all this fuss."

Diagnosis. Pain disorder (Axis I).

Discussion: Patients such as Ms. C may generate strong emotional responses among their health care providers. Chapter 9 discusses these reactions, and possible strategies for successful interactions with patients who are diagnosed with a somatoform disorder.

EVALUATION & TREATMENT OF VIOLENCE SURVIVORS

Emergency Management

When a woman first presents to the emergency room after assault or abuse, the following issues should be addressed by the medical providers:

- immediate physical safety from the assailant
- diagnosis and treatment of physical injuries
- careful documentation of all injuries for later help in legal proceedings
- current psychological symptoms and the availability of social supports
- crisis counseling with education about the likely psychological effects of the trauma
- referrals for emergency housing, social service agencies, and police intervention
- mandatory reporting of the assault as per state law (abuse to minors must always be reported, but state regulations vary regarding the reporting of domestic violence to adults)

The victim's personality structure and level of functioning prior to the assault will be important factors in formulating a psychiatric diagnosis and treatment plan; however, these factors often cannot be assessed accurately at the time of presentation and must be deferred to follow-up visits when shock from the acute stress has abated.

Longer-Term Interventions

Several longitudinal studies have shown that violence survivors rarely escape psychological damage. The sooner the victim receives appropriate interventions for psychological symptoms and comorbid psychiatric diagnoses, the more likely she will achieve a reasonable recovery without protracted impairment in her functioning. Yet, in the immediate aftermath of trauma, many women go through a period of pseudo-adjustment in which they deny symptoms and avoid medications or psychotherapy.

Psychodynamic psychotherapy, cognitive-behavioral therapy, pharmacotherapy, and self-help organizations have been successful in helping women to recover from sexual and physical trauma. For a given woman, the optimal treatment modality—as well as the psychological outcome—will depend on many factors, including her preexisting character strengths and defenses, her beliefs about why she should seek help, her attitude toward mental health providers, her financial resources, her social supports, and the level of distress she is experiencing. When psychotherapy is pursued, the following therapeutic features are essential for a good outcome:

- empathy, recognition, and validation regarding the helplessness experienced by the survivor
- assistance that enables the survivor to make cognitive and affective sense of the trauma she has undergone
- understanding and facilitation of the survivor's need to regain a sense of empowerment

EMOTIONAL REACTIONS TO VICTIMS OF VIOLENCE

Clinicians should recognize their own countertransference reactions that could impede the survivor's recovery or even cause her to abandon treatment. These reactions include overidentification with the victim, development of an incapacitating sense of anxiety or outrage, voyeuristic curiosity resulting in inappropriately intrusive questions, impatience with a victim's decision to remain in an abusive situation, and insistence that an adult victim report the assault to police despite her choice not to do so. In addition, clinicians may sometimes be so unconsciously disturbed by the survivor's story that their countertransference reaction will be to minimize or deny the traumatic etiology of the patient's symptoms, focusing instead on achieving immediate and concrete solutions for these symptoms.

Ms. T was a 24-year-old refugee from an Eastern European country ravaged by war. She presented to the outpatient psychiatric clinic with complaints of nightmares, insomnia, hypervigilance, and sudden outbursts of anger at the most minor provocation. She and her sister were living together in a small apartment, struggling to learn English and find employment.

Before leaving her homeland, Ms. T had suffered several brutal physical and sexual assaults as well as the loss of her parents. Her sister accompanied her to the clinic and reported that Ms. T had recently talked about how "pointless" life was and how there was "too much hate" inside her for anything to change for the better; she had become increasingly isolated from others and spent most of her time playing cards by herself.

The young psychiatrist evaluating Ms. T felt anxious as she wrote down the history; she noted that the patient's hair color was strikingly similar to her own. She correctly assessed that Ms. T's clinical presentation was consistent with PTSD, and she prescribed an antidepressant as well as a sedative for nighttime. However, she did not inquire into the details of the war trauma endured by this young woman; nor did she ask about Ms. T's current feelings of pointlessness and hate, or whether Ms. T might be considering suicide as a way to end her suffering.

Instead, she counseled Ms. T to be strong and to think about how much political reform might occur in her homeland over the next few years. She also advised Ms. T to exercise more during the day and to listen to soothing music during the evening so that she would be more likely to get a good night's sleep.

Discussion. The anxiety and helplessness aroused by Ms. T's story, as well as the psychiatrist's possible overidentification with the young woman, rendered the clinician incapable of discussing and addressing the traumatic etiology of the presenting symptoms. These feelings also jeopardized the patient's clinical care as the psychiatrist avoided an important assessment of the patient's suicidal inclination.

LEGAL AND ETHICAL ISSUES

Effective medical and psychiatric care of women patients includes a sensitivity to the legal and ethical issues surrounding reproductive choice, the evaluation of parenting capacity, and the reporting of sexual and physical violence.

For many decades, women's rights to control fertility and birth have been debated with great fervor in medical and lay communities. From Margaret Sanger's public health efforts to make birth control safe and accessible in the early 20th century to landmark Supreme Court legislation involving the right to abortion, to the ongoing discourse about in vitro fertilization techniques and surrogate mothering, women's reproductive choice has been at the center of considerable legal and ethical controversy. While most physicians support the principle of patient autonomy, these same physicians may experience conflict about honoring a woman's reproductive decision because they may feel a strong pull to consider the fetus as the primary "patient." The conflicts of medical providers may be particularly heightened when the patient is a woman with significant psychological disturbance. In some cases, women are placed on long-term psychiatric conservatorship, or even given jail sentences, to ensure the safety of the fetus by preventing pregnant women from using drugs or being non-adherent to their prescribed psychotropic medication. In other cases, women may be misperceived as being incapable of rational reproductive decisions, and in extreme cases, this may lead to involuntary sterilization or undue pressure to either terminate a pregnancy or to continue the pregnancy according to the value system of the treating physician. These principles are illustrated in the following case.

Lisa F., a 32-year-old woman, had a history of schizophrenia since age 19. She had been stable on antipsychotic medication since then, with a job as an administrative assistant and a marriage to her high school boyfriend. She and her husband had been trying to conceive for almost five years. Ms. F and her husband were overjoyed when she did become pregnant. However, her psychiatrist had serious reservations about her decision, believing that any child would have an unacceptably high risk of developing a psychiatric disorder. The psychiatrist informed Ms. F that if she did not have an abortion that he would not continue to prescribe her antipsychotic medication. Ms. F was extremely upset but refused to terminate the pregnancy. She felt too dejected and mistrustful to find another psychiatrist. After taking the last of her medication, she became psychotic for the first time in over a decade, with paranoia and delusions that people were planning to take her baby away from her. She began to hear a voice telling her to kill herself to protect herself and the baby. She jumped from a two-story building but survived, and was hospitalized for the treatment of several fractures in her lower extremities. Ultrasound examination showed the fetus to be healthy and apparently unaffected. The consulting psychiatrist worked to establish a therapeutic alliance, and Ms. F ultimately agreed to restart her antipsy-

chotics. The original psychiatrist was informed of Ms. F's decompensation but insisted that he was justified in trying to force Ms. F to "confront reality" and have an abortion. Ms. F was discharged with an appointment with a new psychiatrist who was comfortable with her decision to become a mother. Ms. F and the hospital consultant filed complaints about her original psychiatrist with the state board of medicine.

Discussion: The case above illustrates some of the pitfalls faced by women with psychiatric disorders who decide to bear children. There are clear dangers of medical providers taking advantage of their power in the doctor–patient relationship to force decisions based upon their own value system of what is "right" for their patients. Issues arising in cases involving reproduction are often emotionally charged and may lead health care providers to act unethically and illegally, overriding the rights of women patients.

When children are born to a woman with severe psychological problems or chemical dependence, most states require Child Protective Services to ascertain whether the infant will have a safe parenting environment with the mother. As a part of its investigation, CPS will generally request a psychiatric evaluation of the new mother to determine whether or not she possesses adequate parenting skills. The psychiatrist must keep the health and safety of the infant at the forefront, but he or she must also keep at bay any preexisting judgments about who would constitute an "unfit mother." For example, contrary to the perception of many physicians, women with schizophrenia or on methadone maintenance may be highly motivated to become good parents, and with sufficient social supports, they can often succeed.

As advanced reproductive technologies such as GIFT (Gamete Intrafallopian Transfer) and embryo transplants become more common, physicians increasingly will have to confront their own biases regarding the suitability of candidates for these procedures. For example, while few people question the appropriateness of a man in his sixties fathering a child, many object strongly to a woman of a similar age becoming pregnant via new fertility techniques. In addition, the cost of the new reproductive technologies is prohibitive to many women, and questions have been raised about whether insurance companies and government-sponsored health plans should cover such procedures so that more infertile women might have a chance to conceive. With rapid advances in the field of reproductive medicine, ethical considerations become more complex but also more essential.

In another important legal and ethical arena, the care of women patients often involves the mandatory reporting of sexual and physical violence. Under state law, medical providers must report cases of suspected child abuse to local child protection agencies, and many states also require physicians to report spousal abuse to appropriate law-enforcement authorities. In some cases, physicians may be ambivalent about these legal guidelines. The reader is referred to chapter 8 for a further discussion of this issue.

The role of the psychiatrist in the ethical and legal dilemmas described above is clearly a difficult one. The psychiatrist is most likely to be seen as the most experienced and skillful judge of parenting capacity, as well as the health professional best able to assess the impact of stressful events on the patient. The conflict between being an advocate for the patient versus an agent of society may produce tension in cases involving notification of CPS or local authorities for child neglect and abuse or domestic violence, respectively. Careful attention to emotional responses to patients that deflect from rational consideration of emotionally charged issues by health care professionals is essential.

tive events throughout a woman's life cycle, the existence of gender differences in the presentation of major psychiatric syndromes, and the acute and chronic effects of violence against women.

However, in the process of consolidating a database on the "mental health of women," we must examine sex differences without dichotomizing gender, perpetuating stereotypes, and oversimplifying treatment approaches. In evaluating the etiology and therapeutic implications of any gender difference, we should remain attentive to the influences of a sociopolitical context where women have significantly less privilege and status than men. Only with such a careful approach can we ultimately offer compassionate and competent care to our women patients.

CONCLUSION

The psychiatric community is becoming more sensitized to the treatment needs of women patients. In the past two decades, there has been more research on and clinical attention given to female psychological development, the emotional impact of reproduc-

REFERENCES

Ageton SS: *Facts About Sexual Assault: A Research Report for Adults Who Work with Teenagers.* National Center for the Prevention and Control of Rape. DHHS Publ. No. (ADM) 85-1398, 1985.

American Medical Association Council on Scientific Affairs: Violence against women. JAMA 1992;267:3184.

American Medical Association guidelines on domestic violence. http://www.ama-assn.org/public/releases/assault/fv-guide.htm

Anderson E, Hamburger S, Liu J, et al: Characteristics of menopausal women seeking assistance. Am J Obstet Gynecol 1987;156:428.

Berrios DC, Grady D: Domestic violence: risk factors and outcomes. West J Med 1991;155:133.

Blumenthal SJ: Psychiatric consequences of abortion: overview of research findings. Pages 17–37 in Stotland NL (editor): *Psychiatric Aspects of Abortion.* American Psychiatric, 1991.

Brownmiller S: *Against Our Will: Men, Women and Rape.* Simon & Schuster, 1975.

Carr M: Normal and medically complicated pregnancies. Pages 15–35 in: Stewart D, Stotland N (editors): *Psycho-*

logical Aspects of Women's Health Care. American Psychiatric, 1993.

Downey J: Infertility and the new reproductive technologies. Pages 193–206 in: Stewart D, Stotland N (editors): *Psychological Aspects of Women's Health Care.* American Psychiatric, 1993.

Frieze IH, Browne A: Violence in marriage. Pages 163–218 in Ohlin L, Tonry M (editors): *Family Violence: Crime and Justice: A Review of Research.* University of Chicago Press, 1989.

Gitlin M, Pasnau R: Psychiatric syndromes linked to reproductive function in women: a review of current knowledge. Am J Psychiatr 1989;146(11)1413.

Gomberg ES: Women and substance abuse. In: Seeman M (editor): *Gender and Psychopathology.* American Psychiatric, 1995.

Gomberg ES, Nirenberg TD (editors): *Women and Substance Abuse.* Ablex, 1993.

Hamilton J: Emotional consequences of victimization and discrimination in special populations of women. Psychiatr Clin N Am 1989;12(1):35.

Hamilton J, Gallant S, Lloyd C: Evidence for a menstrual-linked artifact in determining rates of depression. J Nerv Ment Dis 1989;1779:359.

Harrison WM, Endicott J, Nee J: Treatment of premenstrual dysphoria with alprazolam: a controlled study. Arch Gen Psychiatr 1990;47:270.

Hart B: Battered women and the criminal justice system. Am Behav Sci 1992;36(5):624.

Hotaling GT, Sugarman DB: An analysis of risk markers in husband to wife violence: the current state of knowledge. Violence Victims 1986;1:101.

Jack DC: *Silencing the Self: Women and Depression.* Harper Collins, 1991.

Jensvold MF, Reed K, Jarrett DB, et al: Menstrual cycle-related depressive symptoms treated with variable antidepressant dosage. J Women's Health 1992;1:109.

Kendell R, Chalmers J, Platz C: Epidemiology of puerperal psychoses. Br J Psychiatr 1987;150:662.

Keye WR, Deneris A, Wilson T, et al: Psychosexual responses to infertility differences between infertile men and women. Fertil Steril 1981;36:426.

Kilpatrick DG, Best CL, Saunders BE, et al: Rape in marriage and in dating relationships. Ann NY Acad Sci 1988;528:335.

Koss M: Hidden rape: sexual aggression and victimization in a national sample of students in higher education. Pages 3–25 in Burgess A (editor): *Rape and Sexual Assault.* Garland, 1988.

Leidig MW: The continuum of violence against women: psychological and physical consequences. J Am Coll Health 1992;40:149.

Lerner H: *Women in Therapy.* Harper & Row, 1988.

Margolin G, Sibner LG, Gleberman L: Wife battering. Pages 89–117 in Van Hasselt VB, Morrison RL, Bellack AS, et al (editors): *Handbook of Family Violence.* Plenum, 1988.

McEwan KL, Costello CG, Taylor PG: Adjustment to infertility. J Abnormal Psychol 1987;96:108.

Mercy JA, Saltzman LE: Fatal violence among spouses in the U.S. 1976–1985. Am J Public Health 1989; 79:595.

Rose D: Sexual assault, domestic violence, and incest. Pages 447–483 in: Stewart D, Stotland N (editors): *Psychological Aspects of Women's Health Care.* American Psychiatric, 1993.

Seeman M (editor): *Gender and Psychopathology.* American Psychiatric, 1995.

Sherwin B: Menopause: myths and realities. Pages 227–248 in: Stewart D, Stotland N (editors): *Psychological Aspects of Women's Health Care.* American Psychiatric, 1993.

Steiner M: Postpartum psychiatric disorders. Can J Psychiatr 1990;35:89.

Stewart D, Robinson G: Violence against women. Pages 261–282 in: Oldham JM, Ribe M (editors): *Review of Psychiatry.* Vol 14. American Psychiatric, 1995.

Straus MA: The marriage license as a hitting license: evidence from popular culture, law and social science. Pages 39–50 in Straus MA, Hotaling GT (editors): *The Social Causes of Husband-Wife Violence.* University of Minneapolis Press, 1980.

Unger K: Chemical dependency in women. West J Med, 1988;149:746.

Cross-cultural Issues in Psychiatry

19

David Elkin, MD, Elizabeth Lee, MD, Arthur Sorrell, MD, JoEllen Brainin-Rodriguez, MD, Heather Clague, MPH, & Robert Harvey, MD

Cultural factors play a key role in determining patterns of thought, the modulation and expression of emotions, and modes of communication and behavior in both healthy and mentally ill individuals. The fields of sociology and medical and psychological anthropology have contributed greatly to our understanding of how cultural factors influence health, illness, and medical care. Recognition of the relevance of cultural factors in psychiatric assessment, diagnosis, and treatment has led to the emergence of a subspecialty called **cultural psychiatry.** This chapter introduces the principles of providing culturally sensitive care to an increasingly diverse patient population.

At the time of the 1990 census, ethnic groups including African Americans, Latinos, Asian Americans, and Native Americans comprised over 25% of the United States population, and this percentage is growing rapidly. Between 1980 and 1990 the growth rate of the Asian-American population was 65% and that of Latinos was 44%. Today's medical practitioners can expect to work with patients from a variety of ethnic backgrounds, and thus must become proficient at providing culturally sensitive care.

Culture is defined traditionally as the shared patterns of belief, feeling, and knowledge that guide a social group's behavior. Culture incorporates social relationships, religion and spirituality, technology, and economic values. These shared values, orientations, and beliefs extend to views about the body, the self, illness, and treatment.

A more sophisticated conceptualization defines culture as emerging from everyday patterns of daily activity, including communication patterns and the routines and rituals of community life. Culture reflects patterns of social relations through shared symbolism, language, aesthetics, and other core values. The locus of culture thus becomes the communal self or body, which is highlighted in the form of families, work settings, and whole communities.

Cultural identity attempts to explore the meaning of cultural background from an individual's perspec-

tive or world view. Although a physician may make assumptions about a patient's behavior, thoughts, and values based on the patient's ethnic group, the patient's cultural identity will tend to vary greatly depending on the patient's degree of acculturation, socioeconomic class, and immigration experience, as well as whether he or she has experienced discrimination or stereotyping in the host country. Some people identify closely with their ethnic group; others, especially second- or third-generation émigrés who have acculturated or made assimilation into the host culture a priority, may view themselves as being only minimally affected by their ethnic origins.

Culture is a powerful lens through which perceptions are filtered. This subjective experience becomes a set of values and beliefs that are so ingrained that they are taken for granted. Most people, from Western city dwellers to tribal peoples, tend to accept that their world view is correct and valid. From this viewpoint, other cultural groups are seen as having values and behaviors that appear interesting, exotic, frightening, or disturbing. Approaches to understanding other cultures are often fraught with misunderstandings, oversimplifications, and stereotypes. It is crucial to consider some of these erroneous but pervasive assumptions to better appreciate the task of considering cultural differences.

Cultural psychiatry derives its knowledge base, theoretical conceptualizations, and methodologies from several related fields, including

- psychological anthropology, which uses psychological theories to interpret relationships among elements of society and culture
- comparative psychiatry, which uses epidemiologic and clinical studies to describe and analyze cross-cultural variation in the incidence of psychiatric symptoms and syndromes
- medical anthropology, which elucidates cross-cultural variations in physical and psychiatric illness by examining social constructs of illness, healing, and caretaking roles

Areas of investigation include the relationship of cultural and contextual factors to specific psychiatric disorders; the relationship of psychiatric disorders to universals of human behavior and existence; comparative studies of diagnostic criteria; so-called culture-specific syndromes; and the effect of race, ethnicity, and culture on psychotherapy and pharmacologic treatment. Cross-cultural issues may also affect the clinician's emotional reactions to patients and may raise legal and ethical issues as well.

CULTURAL COMPETENCE

In the process of interacting with and describing a culture that is different from our own, there is a tendency to stereotype the other culture, emphasizing the differences from our own culture in a narrow or rigid perspective. On the other hand, we may also ignore the other culture's uniqueness, adopting an ethnocentric stance by underemphasizing fundamental differences in values, beliefs, and perspectives.

Cultural competence refers to a set of congruent behaviors, attitudes, and policies that come together in an individual and enable that individual to work effectively in cross-cultural situations. Individuals working together in a culturally sensitive system of care acknowledge and incorporate the importance of the cultural background of both the patient and the clinician. There is a consistent, informed approach to assessing cross-cultural relations, noting dynamics that result from cultural and other differences. In this approach, clinicians work to continuously expand their cultural knowledge and adapt their services to meet the culturally unique or diverse needs of their patients.

The adoption of either extreme of cultural bias often occurs unconsciously and can affect the entire spectrum of health care. Access to and utilization of health-care resources, and the diagnosis and recognition of physical and mental illness can be affected. Follow-up care and treatment may be compromised, as evidenced by patients who do not return for appointments or who have poor adherence to prescribed medication or other treatment regimens. Ethnic minorities in the United States have disproportionately poorer access to mental health–care services and underutilize these services even when they are available. Evidence indicates that both misdiagnosis and subsequent dropout from treatment occur more frequently in minority populations.

Cultural competence includes awareness about differences between the culture and values of the clinician and the patient, and a willingness to incorporate

that awareness into strategies for interviewing and treatment interventions with the objective of maintaining the highest standards of patient care. It also involves learning about the patient's cultural background and models of illness and health, as well as an exploration of the clinician's own cultural identity and attitude toward patients. Just as sensitivity and accuracy in detecting physical examination findings are skills that can be acquired with practice and refinement through experience, sensitivity to the nuances of culture and their effects on health care also can be learned and developed.

ASSESSING PATIENTS FROM A CROSS-CULTURAL PERSPECTIVE

In a cross-cultural assessment, general guidelines apply for obtaining a history of present illness, reviewing symptoms, conducting the mental status examination, and completing appropriate physical and laboratory evaluations. Table 19–1 delineates items requiring special consideration during such an assessment. A comprehensive assessment may require several interviews, and more time must be allowed if language interpreters are needed.

The issue of confidentiality must be explained to the patient and his or her family if the concept is new to them. Clinicians may also have to explain why they are asking psychosocial questions when the patient and family may assume the problem is medical. The patient and family should be asked about any treatments they have tried already—although many folk or religious treatments or rituals may be calming and not harmful, the patient or his or her family may be hesitant to reveal them unless asked to do so.

Assessment. It is often easiest on the patient if the clinician begins with open-ended questions related to physical well-being, for example, sleep, appetite, and energy. As a dialogue becomes established, the clinician can then move on to topics such

Table 19–1. Items to consider when conducting a cross-cultural assessment.

Ethnicity
Race
Country of origin
Language
Acculturation
Gender
Age
Migration history
Religious and spiritual beliefs
Socioeconomic class and education

as memory and concentration, irritability, worries and fears, and tearfulness. As trust and rapport develop further, the interview can shift to more personal inquiries regarding productivity and personal, family (including intergenerational issues), and social problems. Potentially upsetting issues (eg, regarding legal status, traumatic incidents, or financial issues) should be approached in a sensitive manner toward the end of the interview.

Migration History. The patient's personal and family history of migration is significant and should be ascertained. For example, what were the conditions under which the move was made? Was the move voluntary or was it involuntary, due to oppression or catastrophe? What was the attitude of the receiving country? Until recently America was considered to be a "melting pot." This stereotype is now being challenged, and the long history of America's exclusionary actions (particularly preventing non-European immigration) is becoming more widely known. The difference between the patient's pre- and postmigration lifestyle, social class, and occupation are all helpful in understanding the patient's current situation.

Language. As always, it helps to know something of the culture in question, including language distinctions. For example, the English language has more than the average number of terms for anxiety; Thai and Laotian have more expressions for sadness and loss. It is vital to remember that the patient and family may be relying on language skills based only on elementary or secondary school language courses. This level of communication may not be representative of the patient's life abilities. Bilingual clinicians should be cautious of using secondary school or collegiate language skills in interpreting patient responses.

Also, nonverbal cultural patterns can be critical when interpreting the mental status examination. For example, many cultures shun direct eye contact when speaking with authority figures, and downcast eyes may be a mark of respect rather than one of shame or depression, as they are in European-American cultural groups.

Mental Status Examination. Culture can thus greatly affect the findings on many aspects of the mental status examination. The cognitive examination can be affected drastically by culture. For example, a refugee patient from rural Southeast Asia would not be expected to know present or past American presidents, much less the political structure of the United States. Emigrants from rural areas of non-Western nations may lack the educational background to perform mathematics tests, and increased anxiety in the interview process may further impair cognitive testing. Proverb interpretation is very much dependent on the patient's cultural background.

A psychiatric evaluation was requested for a 65-year-old Salvadoran woman who had lived in the United States for over 15 years. She received regular medical attention for hypertension, which was under good control with medication, and for mild osteoarthritis. She lived alone and functioned independently in terms of activities of daily living (ADLs). She had episodic contact with children and grandchildren. Her English was good enough for her to communicate with her internist about medical issues, but she was described by the referring family practice doctor as "somewhat concrete and literal." He wondered if her difficulty with abstract concepts indicated the beginning of a dementing process.

The interview was conducted in Spanish and revealed that the patient had a very full and appropriate range of humor and a deep fund of knowledge—she made several literary allusions and referred to current events. No attention or memory deficits were observed, and the referring physician, who knew enough Spanish to follow most of the interview, commented, "She was a completely different person!"

Diagnosis. None (Axis I); hypertension, osteoarthritis (Axis III).

Somatization is thought to be particularly common in patients from non-Western cultures and from rural parts of the United States. This may reflect traditional beliefs in which certain emotions belong to various organ systems, and emotional disturbance is attributed to harmonic imbalances in the body. Clinicians can become frustrated when patients focus exclusively on somatic complaints and ignore emotional connections. In this situation, it can be helpful to recall the universality of these connections in the etymological roots of English expressions, for example, "having heart" as a synonym for courage and compassion, "spleen" as the medieval seat for anger, and the terms "sanguine" or "phlegmatic" personality (from the words for blood and phlegm, respectively).

SPECIAL CONSIDERATIONS FOR IMMIGRANT POPULATIONS

Acculturation is the degree to which one can function effectively and easily in the host country. This differs from **assimilation,** a process marked by individuals maintaining progressively less of a social and cultural identity separate from the host environment. Examples of assimilation include the original European immigrants to the United States from England and Germany, individuals who typically identify themselves as "just plain Americans." A very general assumption is that it takes three generations to become thoroughly assimilated. This may not apply when racial differences are involved, as physical appearance may elicit biased projections from the majority culture.

Before the 1970s, the goal of many immigrants

was assimilation. Children were encouraged to adapt quickly and completely to the American lifestyle and to American English. More recent cohorts of immigrants have adopted a different orientation, becoming **bicultural,** that is, equally comfortable with both the culture of origin and the new culture. Some individuals may deliberately choose not to assimilate, which may evoke strong reactions from host-country service providers as, for example, has been the case for the orthodox Jewish community and the Amish in the United States. Both groups are viewed by many people as odd, anachronistic, and "out of step" with Western society's mainstream values. Others may have less of an opportunity for assimilation even if they desire to become part of the host culture because of gender roles, age, or racism. The process of acculturation is a complex one and depends on the individual's age at migration, his or her communication proficiency, degrees of similarity and difference between the two cultures, and social and historical factors unique to the individual's situation. Stress may occur with the degree of **role strain,** or **role conflict,** felt at any point in time. Role strain or conflict refers to a sudden change in the individual's expected place and functioning in the family or community forced by external circumstances. In medical settings, family members may be thrust into roles they are not ready to accept. For example, young children may be called upon to act as interpreters for older family members.

Stressors in the Refugee Experience

Clinicians should be aware of the many stressors inherent in the refugee experience. These stressors include grief over multiple losses. Some of these losses may be financial, such as property, businesses, investments, and money. Important interpersonal relationships are often lost by forced separation. Individuals who leave their home culture may also grieve for the loss of their cultural milieu: the sound of their own language being spoken, familiar sights of their own landscape and architecture. Social isolation often results from disruption of old social connections and from the loss of protection provided by the old community against stressors.

Outsiders often underestimate the difficulties inherent in forging new connections among fellow refugees. Immigrants often lose their established social role and position and are frequently unable to use previously acquired skills, such as professional degrees, without retraining. There may be significant contrast between expectations about a host country and the reality of life there; and many refugees are unprepared for racism, cultural prejudices, and scapegoating (blaming for social and economic problems) by their new country's inhabitants. Adjustments to modernized host countries, or the contrast of urban life for rural refugees, may produce **culture shock.** Trauma may occur during various phases of the emigration process or after arrival in a new country.

Aroon U, a 30-year-old East Indian man who was born in Uganda, recalled his emigration to Britain when he was 10 years old. The ruling Amin government had embarked on a campaign to push out "foreigners," even those families that had lived in Uganda for several generations. Mr. U remembered little of these events; he only knew that his father had suddenly lost his business and that his parents were frightened. He explained, "But they wouldn't tell us what was happening, probably to protect us. We were all afraid of what might happen next."

Mr. U remembered his parents taking the family to the airport, a modern structure that he said, "terrified us—we had never seen a building larger than a two-story wood and mud home before." The sight of thousands of panicked people in the airport, hostile soldiers, and modern technology was overwhelming. "My parents had to carry my brother and me on the escalator. We were terrified by it." The trip to London was long and the plane crowded. Mr. U said that when they arrived, he and his brother "were in shock. We had never seen a city so large. Everyone thought we would love it. Instead, we cowered whenever a bus came by, and we couldn't go outside because of the crowds."

Mr. U went on to describe feelings of dissociation and anxiety. He and his brother gradually became more used to their surroundings, but he said, "We never felt like we belonged, even though our English was pretty good." They were beaten up at school by a group of older students who taunted them with racial epithets. At age 26 he emigrated to a city in the United States that had a sizable East Indian–American community, but he noted, "I still am homesick for my childhood home in Africa. I often dream of the village where I grew up."

Psychological & Psychopathologic Responses to the Refugee Process

Because of the severe psychosocial stressors noted above and the loss of previously learned coping strategies, many emigrants experience overt psychiatric disorders, including major depressive episodes, dysthymia, or panic disorder. Depression and anxiety are the most common, sometimes lasting for years. Dissociative symptoms may complicate anxiety and depressive disorders. Exposure to traumatic events before, during, and after emigration may result in post-traumatic stress disorder, which may persist because of ongoing psychosocial stressors and lack of access to or awareness of mental health services. Refugees should be screened for insomnia, nightmares, flashbacks, phobias, and signs of avoidance or increased arousal.

Head trauma may have occurred during emigration, with lasting neurologic and cognitive deficits.

Clinicians should be particularly sensitive to the presence of dementia or delirium from medical illness. Many parts of the world do not have high health-care standards; therefore, malnutrition, encephalitis, meningitis, and other infections may have left residual damage that can affect an individual's mental status. Decreased access to standardized education can delay a diagnosis of mental retardation or learning problems. Illiteracy may complicate performance on the cognitive examination.

Physical preoccupations occur frequently, based on culturally sanctioned health beliefs and patterns of communication about feelings that utilize somatic metaphors and symbols. Thus somatoform disorders are often encountered in refugee populations. Substance use, reactive psychosis, paranoia, and occasionally sociopathic behavior are less common psychiatric complications in the face of the severe stresses of emigration.

A family's coping ability may be highly strained by emigration. Marriages may fail in the face of overwhelming stresses and the breakdown of social buffers. Intergenerational conflicts may occur as the generation gap is widened by the pressures of acculturation. The younger generation and women may adapt more easily as they are more likely to welcome the narrowed generation- and gender-based power differentials and increased opportunities for individuation in Western countries. Conflicts between the old culture and the new will flare up throughout the life cycle of each individual with each major life event, highlighting differences between the previous way of life and current circumstance.

Profound conflict may also arise as family members acculturate at different rates and act discordantly to family expectations. Some of the most poignant examples occur among elderly immigrants, who may be socially isolated and dependent on their families for the self-esteem and respect that would have been expected in the old country. However, as the younger generation adapts more quickly to America's youth-oriented value system, this respect and consideration is attenuated considerably. Films such as *Avalon, Dim Sum, The Joy Luck Club,* and *Bajai at the Beach* illustrate the extent to which some of these misunderstandings between generations can exist in different ethnic groups.

LANGUAGE & INTERPRETERS

The most obvious case in which cross-cultural issues may pose a problem is presented by the patient who cannot communicate well, or at all, in English. Such patients will require a translator or interpreter. Ideally, a professional interpreter will be available. Short of that, hospitals and clinics may have a roster of personnel who are bilingual and can be "borrowed" from their departments—which may be related only indirectly to the medical field. Some short-comings may be associated with using this type of interpreter:

- They may be under time pressure to get back to their regular duties (and this impatience may be transmitted to the patient).
- They may lack training in the nuances of psychiatric interviewing.
- They may lack professional distance and dispassion.

An X-ray technician was asked to help interpret for the interview with a monolingual patient brought in for radiation treatment for lung cancer. Throughout the interview, the technician kept glancing nervously at the clock. When the patient did not appear to respond succinctly to questions, the technician began to pressure the patient with a rising tone of voice. When asked what was happening, the interpreter complained that the patient was uncooperative. The patient was later found to be delirious.

Informal interpreters may be dealing with their own acculturation status. They may unconsciously try to shape or distort the interviewer's line of questioning to minimize or heighten cultural differences. If somewhat more acculturated than the patient, an interpreter may try to give advice to the patient (or physician). For example, in the case of suicidal ideation, an informal interpreter may berate a patient for contemplating suicide. Such interpreters may also be less familiar with issues of confidentiality—an important consideration if the community's minority culture is closely knit.

These same pitfalls apply to family members who tend to volunteer (and are often the most readily available resource). Family members have their own needs and expectations for the patient's behavior. They may be the most likely to mistranslate in both directions and partly withhold or distort the patient's responses. Issues of confidentiality can create enormous obstacles. Because of the language differential, the interviewer is at a distinct loss with regard to these hidden agendas. These agendas might include family members trying to protect a patient by preventing doctors from informing the patient of a terminal illness, or attempting to keep the secret of domestic violence within the family.

The best interpreters are those who understand the patient's cultural background and are also well acculturated to the mainstream culture, that is, bicultural. Even with experienced interpreters, it is important to confer with them before interviewing the patient, so that they understand issues related to confidentiality, the purpose of the task at hand, and the means of achieving it (eg, in a mental status examination, the importance of translating or describing the flow of non sequiturs or tangential associations). A general rule when using an interpreter is to at least double the amount of time anticipated for a normal interview. Translation can be broken down into three major types:

- summary translation (best at the outset to obtain a history of present illness or a social history)
- word-for-word translation (the most time-consuming type, used when translating instructions or procedures)
- cultural broker (when the interpreter provides cultural interpretation and explanations in addition to the transmission of direct communication)

Clinicians should also remember that interpreting services add another layer to possible miscommunication and also increase the structure of the interview at the possible cost of valuable information about the patient's spontaneous thought processes. Especially for psychiatric problems, many nuances can be lost.

Carlos C, a 25-year-old Mexican man, had been incarcerated and was awaiting possible deportation when the jail staff noted he was agitated, talking to himself, and seemed paranoid. He spoke very little English. Through an interpreter, he denied suicidal ideation but appeared to have some persecutory ideas about the Mafia. There was no evidence of loose associations or other symptoms of a formal thought disorder, although his grooming and hygiene were fairly disorganized. The psychiatrist was asked to evaluate Mr. C to determine whether his ideas about the Mafia placing a "curse" on him were related to psychosis or some culturally congruent belief in the occult and experiences with organized criminal groups.

Mr. C was interviewed in Spanish and revealed very elaborate persecutory delusions that included the Mafia monitoring him through the window blinds and sending him messages telepathically. There was no account for his current belief of his being cursed, although Mr. C had been involved with small-scale drug smuggling several years earlier and may have been in contact with organized crime figures at that time. He denied current substance use, and his toxicology screen was negative.

By arranging to interview Mr. C in his primary language, the clinician allowed him to express his thought processes in much richer detail, revealing elaborate delusions, auditory hallucinations, loose associations, and ideas of reference. Treatment with antipsychotic medication led to improvement over the next week.

Diagnosis. Psychosis NOS; consider schizophrenia, paranoid type, or schizophreniform disorder (Axis I).

Interpreters are generally best at facilitating open-ended questions, obtaining basic demographic information, and reporting the patient's physical symptoms. They are not as good when it comes to obtaining a detailed social history or gathering information about family problems, sexual dysfunction, hallucinations or delusions, and suicide.

Because the interpreter is the only one who understands both languages, he or she could potentially lead or misrepresent the interview. In addition, if the interpreter is of the same ethnic background as the patient, he or she may be seen as being more powerful than the doctor, as being a compatriot who has successfully acculturated into and is working with the mainstream medical profession. To maintain control of the interview, the clinician should use as many nonverbal cues as possible:

- Arrange seating so that all parties can readily see one another.
- Make sure the interpreter is not physically dominant.
- Always address the patient directly as "you," rather than asking the interpreter to ask the patient about the matter at hand.
- Maintain as much eye contact with the patient as possible.

A resident in internal medicine requested a psychiatric evaluation for her patient, Lily W, a 60-year-old Chinese-American woman in the outpatient clinic. The interpreter was friendly and professional, and he proceeded to translate the psychiatrist's questions about depressive symptoms. Ms. W endorsed most symptoms of major depression including insomnia; weight loss; feelings of guilt and worthlessness; and loss of energy, pleasure, and appetite. She also revealed a preoccupation with death and dying.

The psychiatrist logically wondered whether Ms. W had active ideas about suicide and proceeded to ask this question. The interpreter refused to ask the question. The psychiatrist started to explain why it was important to assess suicidal thoughts, but the interpreter said, "I cannot ask that—it would be insulting. Everyone knows Chinese ladies do not think about such things."

Eventually a nurse was located who spoke Cantonese. She asked the patient about suicide, and the interpreter was shocked when Ms. W said she had thought about suicide a great deal and had a plan to take an overdose of her medications. When Ms. W was able to contract not to harm herself, she was referred to a local mental health clinic specializing in the care of Asian patients.

The preceding case illustrates that clinicians need to attend both to their own interactions and responses to patients as well as to those of interpreters. It is important to attend to "blind spots" that make particular types of inquiries difficult or mask important areas of clinical concern. While these complex interactions may seem daunting at first, clinicians should be encouraged by the concept that working with interpreters is a skill that can be mastered with patience and experience.

MODELS OF ILLNESS, DISEASE, HEALING, & HEALTH

The patient's and the clinician's definitions of mental health and disease have a profound effect on every stage of the patient's illness. The combined interaction of these definitions will determine the patient's motivation for seeking care, the urgency with which they seek it, the type of care provider sought, the nature of the diagnosis and treatment the provider offers, the extent to which the patient chooses to adhere to treatment recommendations, and finally, the efficacy of the healing process.

The **narrative approach** and the **explanatory model** are two useful anthropologic concepts that are helpful in understanding the influence of culture on the patient's experience of medical or psychiatric illness. The narrative approach to understanding illness emphasizes the patient's understanding of his or her illness within the context of the individual's life experience. The explanatory model focuses on the meaning of the illness to the patient, and how the patient accounts for the illness, including its occurrence at this point in his or her life. The patient's understanding of the illness' etiology is also shaped by the prevailing understanding of his or her cultural group.

THE CULTURE OF WESTERN MEDICINE

The basis of a cross-cultural focus in medicine presumes that clinicians are attempting to understand the differences between two distinct cultural systems. Traditionally this has led to a focus on the patient's ethnic background, with the assumption that the clinician's scientific training in medicine somehow surmounts cultural biases through an objective perspective of illness, disease, and human behavior. But this assumption disregards the clinician's own values and perspectives, and presumes that Western medicine is somehow value-free and objective. Explanatory models of illness and of the roles and rights of patients and healers are important aspects of any society and reflect strongly held cultural beliefs. These beliefs are

instilled in a concentrated manner during medical school and residency training but are broadly acknowledged throughout the United States. Television shows such as *ER* and *Chicago Hope,* for example, appeal to a broad audience in part because they depict human drama unfolding in hospital settings. Viewers do not have to be physicians to understand the context of these shows; the rules and the conflicts that guide the stories are familiar to most Americans.

What are the values of the Western, or Anglo-American, medical tradition? Social scientists have attempted to characterize American medicine from an anthropologic viewpoint as a "culture within a culture." Thus medicine is seen to have its own values, language, and implicit viewpoint.

Western medicine has become firmly set on the foundation of biomedicine. The past 150 years have seen dramatic successes of the biological model of disease, including the invention of the microscope; the discovery of the germ theory and medications such as antibiotics, neuroleptics, and antidepressants; and the discovery of DNA as life's unique molecular building block. Western models of illness tend to rest on physical explanations: For example, heart disease is caused by blockages in the coronary arteries; cancer is the result of errors in DNA-guided cellular replication; and depression is caused by an imbalance of neurotransmitters in the CNS. Biological factors are viewed as more important than psychological and social considerations.

Many medical students find that although they are taught about behavioral science in preclinical classes, when they enter clinical rotations they are expected to give brief accounts, if any, of the psychological and social aspects of the patient's life. Thus the "social history" section of the patient evaluation is set aside in a separate category, and students are sometimes told by their preceptors to restrict their comments in this entire category to the patient's cigarette smoking habits and source of income.

The role of the physician in the doctor-patient relationship has changed in the latter half of the twentieth century, from an authority figure who gives orders to patients to that of a highly trained and informed partner who educates and guides patients in making rational choices. An implicit assumption is the Western conception of the individual who is self-sufficient and, in an idealized state, is capable and desirous of independent decision making.

Critiques of biomedicine focus on the small role given to psychological, social, and spiritual issues in understanding health and illness. The specialization in research and medical training leads to a focus on organs rather than the whole person, and the patient's role in his or her social setting—family, workplace, and community—is ignored. Stripping away social factors from disease processes also limits discussion of social problems. For example, a patient who is fired after a corporate merger and is in despair over his or her financial predicament might be diagnosed as having major depression. This objective classification quashes discussion of the effect of changes in the workplace on mental health. Biases also exist toward patients complying with aggressive treatment, "fighting" terminal illness, and excluding the possibility of complementary psychological or alternative aids to healing. Clinicians should be mindful of their own cultural biases, some of which stem from the values inherent in modern biomedicine.

UNDERSTANDING HEALTH & ILLNESS IN DIFFERENT CULTURES

The task of eliciting a patient's explanatory model for his or her illness is an essential part of any interview but is especially important in a cross-cultural setting. Placing the patient's symptomatology into the context of his or her social and cultural background and beliefs is not simply a matter of expressing appropriate curiosity, adopting a holistic view toward the patient, or practicing sensitive bedside manners. It is also a matter of being diagnostically complete. The absence of this approach can lead to gross misunderstanding or confusion about a patient's condition, with often serious consequences.

Given two divergent explanatory models, the clinician must determine which aspects of each model to use in creating a treatment plan. Ideally, the process would be one in which the patient comes to see that the clinician understands his or her explanatory model, after which the clinician infuses that model with his or her own conceptualizations without invalidating the patient's model or attempting to convert the patient. In reality, the construction of an appropriate hybrid model may accomplish the goal of clinical efficacy but may be ethically problematic to create.

A nephrologist requested an urgent psychiatric consultation in order to place his patient, Ryan F, on a psychiatric hold for "suicidal behavior." Mr. F, a 26-year-old Chinese-American man, had been coming to dialysis three times each week for several years after developing chronic renal failure. Mr. F had become interested in his cultural roots and had started acupuncture treatment for his kidney disease. Mr. F informed the nephrologist that his acupuncturist expected him to make a complete recovery through treatment with acupuncture and Chinese herbs, and that he would no longer be coming to the renal clinic for dialysis. The nephrologist was unable to convince Mr. F that he would become very ill and most likely die within weeks if he followed this plan. The nephrologist then called for a psychiatric consultation.

On examination Mr. F did not display signs of any mental disorder, such as depressive or psychotic symptoms. He appeared enthusiastic about the possibility of being "cured" from his disease, in contrast to the chronic disease model offered by Western medicine. He was reluctant to consider what he would do if he did not improve on his acupuncturist's treatment regimen but indicated that he would be disappointed and would probably restart dialysis. The psychiatrist concluded that Mr. F was able to make rational decisions regarding his health care.

Adherence to a treatment plan is also affected by different cultural belief systems concerning medicine and mental illness and by expectations about the behavior the clinician should exhibit. Attitudes toward psychiatry and mental illness in particular are loaded issues for patients and family members of all cultures, including in the United States. People fear being labeled as "crazy" or as a "mental case." Furthermore, many cultures do not differentiate illness into psychiatric and nonpsychiatric categories, and patients may not understand the presence of a separate physician whose function is to evaluate and treat stress-related conditions.

Outward compliance with physicians is often encountered in working with patients from non-Western cultures. Superficial respect and fear may disguise deeply held distrust of the medical process. Patients should be encouraged to voice their own explanatory model of their illness. When this model is explained, the astute clinician can then compare it with her or his own in order to detect conflicts for the purposes of preventing clinical miscommunication, inappropriate help seeking, non-adherence to treatment, and patient and clinician frustration.

Ronald H, aged 62, had emigrated recently from Jamaica to the United States. His initial physical screening examination was remarkable for one abnormality, a mild enlargement of the prostate. The medicine resident explained to Mr. H that he would need an appointment with urology for a needle biopsy of the prostate, saying, "It will be performed transrectally, but it's an outpatient procedure, it's not a big deal."

Mr. H indicated that he understood but failed to show up at the appointment and did not come to a second rescheduled appointment. The medicine resident asked for a psychiatric evaluation of Mr. H, saying to the psychiatrist, "I'll be curious to see what you think. I'm guessing dementia or an underlying psychosis, maybe schizophrenia."

During the interview, Mr. H was observed to be pleasant, if somewhat anxious. The medicine resident was somewhat gruff as he explained, "Mr. H, you've missed two appointments. I'm making a third appointment for a biopsy, but you have to be sure to go!" Mr. H nodded unenthusiastically. The psychiatrist asked if Mr. H understood why the biopsy was necessary. Mr. H indicated he did not, despite the medical resident's previous explanations. However, there was no indication of short-term memory loss or any other cognitive dysfunction on mental status testing, nor any signs of psychosis.

It became clear that Mr. H had never seen a physician before arriving in the United States and literally had no reference for what was expected of him. He had been shocked on his first visit when the resident performed a rectal examination. He said, "I don't understand how doctors work. Maybe they experiment on you. Who knows? But I am not going to have someone stick any needles in me when I'm not sick."

Cultural norms can also directly affect the patient's context and expectations for interactions in the doctor-patient relationship.

Ivana L, a 46-year-old woman, was admitted to the hospital for complications of metastatic breast cancer. Ms. L had emigrated from the Ukraine 5 years earlier. Psychiatric consultation was requested to assist in determining whether Ms. L was capable of giving informed consent. Ms. L referred to her illness as a "cold" and would become agitated when staff used the word "cancer." She also became agitated when the surgery team attempted to review the informed consent form with her. This included informing her about the various risks of infection, paralysis, or death from the planned operation. Ms. L covered her ears and angrily demanded that the team leave the room.

An interpreter who was also from the former Soviet Union explained that in the patient's country of origin, Ms. L's case would be handled much differently. The term "cancer" was never used. Additionally physicians practiced in a much more autocratic or paternalistic manner, telling patients what they planned to do but not leaving the treatment plan open to patient input. Ms. L was agitated in part because she was confused by the American doctor's approach.

It is important to emphasize again that within the United States variations exist in individuals' understandings of different forms of physical and psychiatric illness.

Cassie R, a third-generation American woman of European descent, believed that her depression was biologically based and refused psychotherapy. She did agree to take a selective serotonin re-uptake inhibitor (SSRI) antidepressant and was pleased with her increased mood and energy level. Her primary care provider and her family encouraged her to start psychotherapy, but she said, "I don't need therapy. My doctor says depression is like diabetes, and taking Prozac is the same as needing insulin. That's the only treatment that I need."

Cultural variations in responses to illness have also been observed in how well patients from different ethnic backgrounds are able to tolerate pain (see Chapter 15 for a discussion of chronic pain). The pain experience is the sum of the patient's response to noxious stimuli as mediated by internal psychology, the immediate environment, and the general cultural context. A patient may express pain quite differently in the physician's office than he or she would at home with a family member from whom there are different expectations. Cultures differ widely in pain expectancy and pain acceptance. For example, in the United States there is great expectancy of pain for women during childbirth but generally low acceptance of pain for the same stressor in other cultures. Understanding the cultural and psychological context of patients' experiences can aid in avoiding over- or underprescribing analgesics.

CULTURE & PSYCHIATRIC DIAGNOSIS

The *DSM-IV* contains a guide to assessing the impact of culture, including the patient's cultural identity based upon migration history and ethnic identity. This includes the patient's explanatory models for his or her illness and the cultural norms of help-seeking behavior. Cultural factors related to the patient's development, as well as psychosocial stressors and supports, are used to characterize the patient's level of functioning. The cultural differences between the clinician and the patient should be described in terms of transference and countertransference. The psychiatric diagnosis should be expressed both in Western terms and in the diagnostic categories of the patient's own culture, with an exploration of how the patient's ethnicity might affect the differential diagnosis and treatment plan.

Psychiatry is the one specialty in medicine where the unique experience of the individual is critical for fully understanding and formulating an effective treatment plan for any specific disorder. Most psychiatric disorders will manifest in terms of some behavioral disturbance. Especially when mental health treatment is associated with stigma, patients or their families may wait until dysfunction is extreme before presenting to a medical setting. In any society, only a certain amount of divergence from the standards of acceptable behavior will be tolerated before an individual is labeled deviant.

On the island nation of Singapore, there are very few inpatient psychiatric beds. Most individuals who have mental disorders are treated at home or are sequestered by their families to prevent others from finding out about their illness. If someone has a condition severe enough to warrant psychiatric hospitalization, extreme care is taken to keep the disorder a secret after discharge. In a program similar in method to the United States's Witness Protection Program, a patient is discharged to a new home in a different part of the island. The stigma of mental illness is so great that the patient and his or her family are issued new names, identification cards, and driver's licenses to prevent anyone from learning about the psychiatric disorder or its treatment.

Each culture has its own belief system about the underlying cause of the behavioral aberration. Asians often believe that mental health is a matter of self-discipline and willpower. They may exhort a depressed family member to "snap out of it" or to "stop thinking negative thoughts." Conversely, there may not be any sense of personal responsibility if the underlying belief is that of spirit possession or of an ill-wisher having put a hex on the patient. Most cultures have a common-sense approach to what we would call adjustment disorders, where clear identifiable stressors lead to distress and dysfunction. Oftentimes, however, such problems are treated in a nonmedical arena, so that being questioned about a social history in a medical setting may be experienced as unexpected and intrusive.

The clinician who assesses patients for possible psychiatric disorders is actually defining what constitutes normal versus aberrant behavior. As clinicians learn about different cultures, they should beware of efforts to "normalize" symptoms or to oversimplify their observations and conclusions about patients' symptoms.

Mr. and Mrs. K brought their 16-year-old daughter, May, to her pediatrician. They complained that May had become "unmanageable." They reported that she was talking back to them and to Mrs. K's mother, staying out with boys until very late at night, and experimenting with alcohol. May's behavior might have appeared marginally age-appropriate to a Western observer such as the pediatrician. However, her family considered her behavior to be markedly aberrant by the standards of their own culture, in which adolescents were compliant and respectful of their parents' wishes.

In fact, a child psychiatrist noted that May had two aunts who had bipolar disorder, and on mental status examination, May had accelerated speech and thoughts. May herself noted a diminished need for sleep, increased activity and spending, and two occasions of hearing voices talking to her. She was diagnosed as having bipolar disorder and started on mood stabilizers. Her symptoms cleared rapidly, and she returned to her normal mental state.

Her parents continued to complain about May being "too independent," a reflection of family issues that were more enduring than May's diagnosis.

Diagnosis. Bipolar affective disorder, mania with psychotic features (Axis I).

The medical anthropologist Kleinman has argued that current psychiatric understanding is attached to a model of mental illness that he termed **pathogenicity/pathoplasticity,** in which the form of the disease is determined by biology, while cultural factors primarily shape the content of the disorder. The **category fallacy,** as he calls it, assumes that the categories of mental illness developed by Western psychiatrists and codified in the *DSM-IV* and its international counterpart, the *ICD-10,* represent the true (biological) form of mental illness, untainted by cultural content. The search for the universality of mental illness deteriorates into an effort to justify these Western categories rather than to achieve an understanding of illness as experienced by individuals in different cultures. Thus Kleinman criticizes cross-cultural research for overemphasizing the similarities of mental illness across cultures while underplaying differences, and for repeatedly applying the same disease checklists to clinical populations that are most likely to demonstrate these similarities. Kleinman argues for a more inclusive descriptive approach that attempts to approach symptoms and behavior with fewer preconceived notions of what constitutes mental illness in other cultures.

Fabrega portrays this struggle between competing viewpoints of universalism and relativism. Universal understandings of mental illness seek scientific knowledge that is founded on biomedical principles and that provides an understanding of the etiology of mental illness, leading to treatment and possible elimination of disease. Relativism, on the other hand, seeks descriptions through successive filters of cultural factors that determine the manifestation and course of mental and physical illnesses with less focus on biological factors. Both approaches have inherent weaknesses. Biological theories have undeniable relevance, yet clinicians cannot, to borrow Wittgenstein's metaphor, simply peel away cultural factors to find the universal biological core of any illness. Perhaps a more sophisticated perspective that avoids this dichotomy would view psychiatric—and medical—illness as a dynamic interplay of biology and culture, each influencing the other, shaping the etiology, epidemiology, presentation, and treatment of mental illness.

CULTURE & PSYCHIATRIC TREATMENT

PSYCHOTHERAPY & CROSS-CULTURAL ISSUES

Ethnicity plays an important role in interactions between patients and their clinicians and in patients' perceptions about the health-care system. Transference takes on unique characteristics depending on the patient's experiences but is also greatly influenced by the cultural overlaps or differences between the patient and physician. When the patient and the physician share the same cultural background, the patient's emotional responses may vary. A patient who is less acculturated than his or her clinician sometimes idealizes the clinician and his or her professional status. Alternatively, the patient may feel that the clinician is a "traitor" for becoming part of the medical establishment, as if the culture of medicine has replaced the clinician's own cultural heritage. The patient may also vacillate between these two views.

When the physician is from a different ethnic background, the patient may be overtly mistrustful, suspicious, or hostile. A positive response is also possible: The patient may be friendly and overly compliant or respectful. Some patients will deny any difference between the two cultural groups or at least will deny the impact of any difference.

Physicians need to be alert for signs of these emotional responses in their patients' words or behaviors. The success or failure of psychotherapy and other medical encounters may depend on the clinician's awareness of these issues as well as how these issues are brought to the patient's attention.

Alex M, a Vietnam veteran who complained of depression and severe flashbacks and nightmares, was admitted to the inpatient psychiatric unit at a university-affiliated Veterans Administration hospital. Mr. M was assigned to work with a Vietnamese-American medical student who had emigrated from Vietnam to the United States at age 11. Mr. M was extremely angered by the ethnic identity of the student chosen to work with him, saying, "I'll be damned if I lay my life on the line so I can trust it to you." He demanded a different trainee.

The student also felt anxious about working with Mr. M, who seemed too hostile to form a therapeutic alliance and also reminded the student of the tumultuous war-torn era in his country's history. The attending psychiatrist held firm in the assignment, saying to the patient and the student, "You will have to find a way to work together."

Gradually Mr. M allowed the student to take a history, complete a physical examination, and begin to tend to his medical needs. Over the next several weeks Mr. M increasingly confided in the student about his depression and symptoms of post-traumatic stress disorder. His condition improved dramatically.

At discharge, Mr. M said, "I can't believe it, that I trusted someone I once considered 'the enemy,' and that they could help me so much!" Indeed, the student and the attending physician wondered if the student's ethnic identity, though such an impediment to therapy initially, had served as a catalyst for Mr. M's rapid progress in treatment. Mr. M's feelings of hostility for "the enemy" and fear brought his emotions closer to the surface, and the transcendence of ethnic identity to feeling helped by "another human being" helped restore his level of trust and hope.

Patients may need an orientation to the basic principles of doctor-patient confidentiality that are critically important in any health-care setting.

Mary R, a 28-year-old Filipino woman, was referred by her family practitioner to the neurology dementia clinic for "memory problems." The medical student evaluating Ms. R found her to have mild problems with short-term memory and concentration. Although Ms. R denied feeling depressed, the student was struck by Ms. R's depressed demeanor, psychomotor slowing, quiet voice, and monosyllabic answers to questions.

When the student asked Ms. R how things were at home, she burst into tears. With gradual coaxing, she explained that her husband was always "very angry" with her because she had emigrated from the Philippines 4 years before him, and he suspected that she had had an affair before they met. Her husband had progressed from being verbally abusive to shoving and punching her. Ms. R had contemplated suicide but had not told anyone about her predicament. Her physician also treated her husband, and Ms. R assumed that anything that she told her doctor would be relayed directly to her husband. Ms. R was reluctant to accept a referral to a psychiatrist but finally did so when the medical student reframed her problem as a "common medical problem" and explained the principles of confidentiality.

Therapeutic interactions also depend on a common frame of reference for where problems arise and how they can be conceptualized and treated. Some of these basic assumptions are so overlearned that they are virtually taken for granted. For example, the Western conception of the self is of the self-sufficient individual. The idealized state of psychological health is of a person who functions independently and is competent at mobilizing resources (eg, people or material goods) efficiently. Thus the Western tradition upholds the ideals of self-sufficiency, self-dependence and independence, and similar values that have important correlates in health-care settings, such as confidentiality, informed consent, and autonomy. In many other cultures, however, the individual is defined in relation to other family or community members. The emphasis in these cultures is on the individual's healthy functioning within the larger setting. Family psychotherapy is often a critically important component of working with patients from such cultures.

Care should also be taken to be familiar with cultural issues before beginning therapy to map out potential areas of conflict or difficulty.

The Refugee Health Clinic at a community hospital decided to start a group to treat posttraumatic stress disorder in Bosnian refugees. Patients were interviewed for the group and invited to come to the first session. As soon as patients arrived for the session a fist-fight broke out between Muslim and Christian refugees who had been on opposite sides of the conflict in their home country.

Clinicians should also try to anticipate how the patient's experiences and use of metaphors might affect therapeutic interventions.

A 24-year-old Vietnamese-American woman sought treatment for anxiety related to traumatic experiences in her country. The therapist recommended relaxation exercises to help the patient relax. The therapist suggested that the patient visualize a beach (the therapist's own conception of a relaxing scene). The patient became extremely anxious and tearful and explained that her traumatic experiences had occurred at a refugee camp located on a beach in Southeast Asia.

PSYCHOPHARMACOLOGY & CROSS-CULTURAL ISSUES

Culture can significantly affect the use of psychopharmacologic agents in several significant ways. As described earlier, a patient's culture can influence his or her understanding of mental illness and hence adherence to prescribed medication. Furthermore, interethnic variation in the metabolism of psychotropic medication must also be considered. Although reports of such variation were first noted in the 1960s, only within the past decade have these phenomena been studied scientifically.

Therapeutic responses and side effects may vary by as much as a factor of 40. Differences in metabolism of drugs within the same ethnic group may be based on genetically determined levels of liver enzymes. For example, glucose-6-phosphate dehydrogenase deficiencies exist in some African Americans and Asian Americans, and there are so-called fast and slow metabolizers for acetylation in Asians and Caucasians.

Polymorphic genes determine levels for these and other enzymes that determine the rate of breakdown of medications in the body. In the liver, the cytochrome P450 system determines the metabolism of many drugs. Specifically, CYP2D6 determines the metabolism of many SSRIs, tricyclic antidepressants (TCAs), and antipsychotics; and CYP2C19 affects metabolism of tertiary TCAs and benzodiazepines. Other factors that vary within and between ethnic groups and affect pharmacokinetics include average percentages of body fat, conjugation, and variation in the concentration and shape of drug-binding plasma proteins that transport psychoactive medications. The effects of ethnicity on diet, cigarette smoking, alcohol intake, and the use of herbal preparations exert environmental influences on the activity of enzymes that metabolize psychiatric medications. Researchers are hopeful that specific tests will be developed in the next decade that will allow clinicians to prescribe individually tailored regimens of psychotropic medications based upon blood tests and a more extensive knowledge of drug metabolism.

Recent studies have also documented differences in prescribing practices when the clinician and patient are from different ethnic groups. African Americans are more likely to be diagnosed by non-African-American physicians as having schizophrenia, and they are more likely to be placed on antipsychotic medication regardless of diagnosis. Antipsychotics are also more likely to be prescribed to African Americans in higher doses and in longer-lasting intramuscular preparations.

RELIGIOUS & SPIRITUAL ISSUES

Religion and spirituality are important variables that may greatly modify an individual's values within his or her cultural group and that, as a result, may affect the individual's approach to illness. Although many people have an active belief in God, most physicians and mental health professionals do not integrate religion and spirituality into their work with medical and psychiatric patients. The uses of religion and spirituality range from adaptive to maladaptive and can have a constructive or destructive effect on health and adaptation to illness. The *DSM-IV* includes a diagnostic category for individuals experiencing a religious or spiritual crisis.

Table 19–2. Distinguishing characteristics between religious beliefs and pathological delusions.

Religious Belief	Religious Delusion
Relationship to the community	
Participation and unity with community	Isolation, distancing, exclusion
Requires trust, shared conviction, communal consensus	Built from mistrust, paranoia, idiosyncratic formulation
Product of tradition and history—answers common human needs and shared communal concerns	Created by individual in response to inner need
Use of symbols/ability to participate in transitional realm	
Symbols as representation of transcendent	Real and imminent
Shared reference	Self-referential, idiosyncratic
Ritual and practice deepen life experience	Practices and compulsions limit experience and may harm self or others
Transitional space	Collapse of transitional space
Level of integration and maturity	
Sign of integration	Sign of fragility/fragmentation
Increase in meaning and fulfillment	Increase in distress and suffering
Fits into developmental stage	May involve regression of development
Moderated by ego system	Uncontrollable affect, thoughts, behavior
Effects on social and vocational function	
Enhances function	Impairs function

Patients vary in their religious practices, from privately held beliefs to frequent participation in organized activities. Serious medical illness often results in at least a transient crisis that involves questions along spiritual dimensions: the meaning of life, the nature of life and death, or the question of fate or control of life's course by a supernatural being. Religious and spiritual issues also feature prominently in many psychiatric disorders. The content of psychotic symptoms in mania and schizophrenia, or medically based delusions from temporal lobe epilepsy, frequently involve religious or spiritual dimensions.

Fred A, aged 42, was admitted to the inpatient psychiatric unit after police placed him on a psychiatric hold. Mr. A had been meditating on a public beach for 6 days without food or water and appeared extremely agitated and paranoid. When police approached him, he told them to stay back, saying, "I am the universe. If you touch me, you will disturb galaxies." Mr. A was malnourished and required supplemental vitamins and nutrition to stabilize his medical condition. His toxicology screen was consistent with recent marijuana use.

Mr. A was accompanied by a female friend who identified herself as a "girlfriend and disciple." She explained that Mr. A lived in a nearby park and studied "his own form of religion and metaphysics" that involved intensive meditation and fasting. He had a history of several other admissions for brief psychotic episodes that cleared within several days on antipsychotics.

Mr. A was started on low doses of antipsychotics, and his delusions resolved gradually. Within days his hostility and disorganized thought processes had also resolved. The student assigned to work with Mr. A was impressed by his level of intelligence and knowledge of philosophy. However, she noted that Mr. A regarded himself somewhat narcissistically as having "the key to life." He also refused to acknowledge the possibly permanent muscle weakness in his legs that was likely the result of severe vitamin deficiency.

Mr. A had quit his graduate program in physics and worked briefly in engineering jobs before embarking on a bohemian life path. He had only one friend and had broken off all contact with family members. He lived on his girlfriend's income and was unwilling to investigate his behavior as anything but "the sacred way." He also refused outpatient psychotherapy, saying, "I'll be fine, I just need to meditate for 4 days at a time."

Diagnosis. Psychosis NOS (Axis I); possible personality disorder with schizoidal and narcissistic features (Axis II); malnutrition (Axis III).

Discussion. Table 19–2 compares healthy religious beliefs to pathologic delusions. While this division is somewhat arbitrary and is best thought of on a continuum between healthy and psychopathology, Mr. A's spiritual beliefs and practices are clearly maladaptive in a number of areas: idiosyncratic, facilitating self-inflicted physical and psychological damage, and incompatible with normal social and vocational functioning.

In summary, because religion and spirituality are important components of cultural identity, and because these issues are often activated by the threat of serious physical or psychiatric illness, clinicians should consider the patient's religion and spiritual beliefs and practices when making their assessment.

CULTURE-BOUND SYNDROMES

Culture-bound syndromes usually combine anxiety and depression with behavioral components. One example is the Latino **nervios,** which can encompass a wide range of *DSM-IV* disorders across the anxious-depressive spectrum. A similar syndrome is known in China as **neurasthenia** and is included as a diagnostic category in the *ICD-10.* This diagnosis was also used by Charcot and Freud to describe a combination of anxiety and depressive features with fatigue and weakness in upper-middle-class young women at the beginning of the twentieth century. Although not included in the *DSM-IV,* analogous syndromes, such as **falling out** or **nervous breakdown,** exist in American folklore.

Other culture-bound syndromes are more pronounced in the behavioral components. **Amok** (which has made its way into vernacular English) is defined as a dissociative episode mainly affecting men, accompanied by violent outbursts and repeated automatic behaviors. **Koro** is a phenomenon described in Japan and China, seen exclusively in males, characterized by extreme anxiety, fear, and a near delusional belief that the penis is receding into the abdomen. The *DSM-IV* recognizes that these syndromes do not fit clearly into any one psychiatric disorder and provides a glossary of such culture-bound syndromes and associated condition.

Culture-bound syndromes are often considered highly exotic, unlike any disorders encountered in Western cultures. However, many syndromes of health-related behavior are found primarily in Western cultures, such as eating disorders, the construct of Type A behavior, and the use of surgery to alter body image such as breast augmentation. Although these conditions are not classified formally as culture-bound syndromes in the *DSM-IV,* they may constitute the Western equivalent of the same phenomenon.

EMOTIONAL REACTIONS TO PATIENTS

Physicians' emotional responses that are affected by cross-cultural issues can be divided broadly into reactions that occur when the physician and patient are of the same cultural background (**intraethnic countertransference**) and when the two are of different cultures (**interethnic countertransference**).

Intraethnic responses to patients may be generally positive or negative in emotional tone. A clinician may welcome contact with a patient from the same ethnic background, particularly if the clinician has been feeling isolated or alienated—feelings that are common among health-care trainees, especially when they are from an underrepresented ethnic group. The clinician may rapidly come to consider such a patient as "family," which is not undesirable as long as the patient is not uncomfortable with this relationship and the feelings do not interfere with the clinician's judgment. However, overidentification with the patient may lead the clinician to feel angry or alienated from the rest of the health-care team.

Clinicians may also feel guilty for enduring less or acculturating more than their patients. More negative emotional responses are also possible, including a form of self-loathing based on ethnicity that has been termed **auto-racism.** For example, a physician from an underrepresented ethnic group may regard a less acculturated or educated patient with disdain or scorn, possibly as a result of the unrecognized fear that the clinician's own acculturated status is revealed as vulnerable.

Interethnic reactions may run the spectrum of positive feelings of fascination and admiration for another cultural group, to negative feelings of emotional distancing, ambivalence, disdain, fear, and hatred. Another possible response is for the clinician to fail to recognize or deny the cultural differences between himself or herself and the patient. Even a positive response can result in stereotyping, such as the belief that all members of an ethnic group are emotionally stable, geared toward education, and other commendable traits. Negative stereotypes and reactions to patients also abound. As always, the clinician's goal should not be to suppress or silence these feelings and thoughts but rather to be aware of them and to ensure they do not interfere with accurate assessment and treatment.

Stephanie J, a 25-year-old Caucasian medical student, had majored in anthropology as a college undergraduate and regarded herself as "completely unprejudiced." However, she noticed that she was very uncomfortable with one of her patients, Howard M, a 33-year-old African-American businessman who had been hospitalized for a manic episode. Ms. J was worried that Mr. M might become assaultive even after his psychiatric symptoms subsided.

Ms. J was able to discuss some of her feelings and fears with the resident and connected her apprehension to growing up in an all-white neighborhood and to her parents' fears of people from different ethnic groups. Ms. J discovered that being able to discuss her feelings allowed her to work more easily with Mr. M. She decided to write her final paper on cross-cultural barriers to communication to continue to expand her knowledge and explore her own previously unrecognized beliefs.

Students may also struggle to deal with a patient's racism or other difficult responses based on ethnic background.

David F, a 28-year-old medical student, was assigned to work with Joy A, a 54-year-old woman who was being treated for breast cancer. Mr. F formed a close attachment to Ms. A, until one day while discussing her living situation she described her Jewish landlord in stereotyped, racist terms. Mr. F, who was Jewish, felt betrayed by his own mix of empathy and anger toward Ms. A. He told her that he was Jewish and was dismayed when Ms. A responded, "Really? Well, I guess that explains why you want to become a doctor."

Alfonse E, a third-year student at a metropolitan medical school, was scheduled to do his surgery rotation at a rural hospital several hundred miles away. Mr. E enjoyed his rotation but commented to a classmate that the experience "was like going to a foreign country—I was the only African-American man most of these white people had ever seen." He recounted that visitors to the psychiatric unit appeared frightened about the topic of mental illness and asked him where the ward for "nervous people" was located.

He also related how he had worked closely with one patient who was recovering from cardiac surgery. Mr. E noted that during the week after surgery, the patient was increasingly alert but also seemed puzzled by his presence. Finally the patient asked him, "Aren't you working awfully hard for an orderly?" When Mr. E explained that he was the medical student caring for her, she said, with a tone of shock in her voice, "*You're* my doctor?"

A medical team on morning rounds visited Mina A, a 34-year-old East Indian woman who was hospitalized for ovarian cancer. The attending physician joined the team and, to the embarrassment of the residents and students, attempted to interview Ms. A in Spanish. The senior resident tactfully interrupted to inform the attending that the patient did not speak Spanish but, while somewhat shy, did speak excellent English.

LEGAL & ETHICAL ISSUES

Legal and ethical issues frequently arise when psychiatric or medical treatment is provided across cultures. These issues may come up when a patient's cultural symbols and metaphors are used to increase adherence to treatment regimens or when a terminal illness is diagnosed. Cultural factors may have a powerful effect on how a physician upholds or balances the principles of autonomy, informed consent, beneficence, and justice.

Victor W, a 41-year-old Vietnamese-American man, was being treated on the psychiatric inpatient unit for bipolar affective disorder with psychotic features, including hallucinations and paranoia. Mr. W refused to take the prescribed antipsychotic medication. He explained that he was suffering from an imbalance of "hot" and "cold."

The psychiatrist, who had also emigrated from Vietnam, told Mr. W that the antipsychotic medication would restore his balance of "hot" and "cold." With this understanding the patient began to take the medication, and his psychotic symptoms resolved within several days. The psychiatrist explained that he felt he had acted ethically, since he was able to "bridge" the cultures of American medical practice and Vietnamese beliefs.

A Caucasian medical student on the team wondered if it would be ethical if she used the same explanation to make a patient in a similar situation believe in an intervention, even if she did not come from the same cultural background.

A major cross-cultural conflict could arise in a medical setting when a patient is diagnosed with a terminal illness. American culture and medicine values highly an individual's right to informed consent and individual determination. This value is not always shared by other cultures, where the family or group as an entity is far more important than the individual. Family members may confuse if not overtly try to obstruct the physician's attempt to deal openly with the patient, if these cultural differences are not acknowledged and respected.

Conflict may occur in a case where family members are upset by the need for involuntary commitment, or where surgery or other major treatment decisions must be made without the patient's consent. Patients and families who have emigrated to the United States may be accustomed to physicians in their own country of origin acting in different ways. Patients who are not accustomed to contact with health-care providers may view physicians as authority figures, resulting in a large imbalance of power. Physicians may be tempted to use their enhanced power to unduly influence a patient's decision making.

A medical team sought an ethics consultation for Weng Z, a 72-year-old man who was admitted to the hospital for evaluation of hemoptysis (coughing up blood) and weight loss. Sputum analysis and a chest X-ray revealed widespread lung cancer that carried a poor prognosis even with chemotherapy. Mr. Z's daughter asked the physicians not to tell her father that he had cancer.

She explained that her father had come from China 6 months earlier and that doctors in China would not inform a patient of a terminal illness. Mr. Z gave an indication of his wishes when he told the medical team through a translator, "If this is serious I will need to go home to China to be with the rest of my family." He gave no other intimation of wanting to know his diagnosis. The medical team was struggling with the decision to follow standard procedures in the United States and inform the patient of his diagnosis and limited options, or follow his daughter's description of medical practice in China and not tell Mr. Z. Neither option appeared satisfactory.

The ethics committee advocated a third option: Mr. Z should be told that he had an illness that was serious enough to warrant returning to China without giving him a specific diagnosis. Mr. Z's daughter also found this option acceptable. Mr. Z appeared grave as he received this message from the medical team. He thanked them and made plans to return immediately to China.

Ethical issues that emerge when working across cultural groups encompass a number of potentially problematic areas. Anthropologic studies of the culture of American medicine have also yielded critical reviews of bioethics and its place in medicine. Kleinman, Faberge, Good, Koenig, and others have noted biases within Western bioethics that arise from an emphasis on high technology, on the conception of the individual patient split off from family or community, and on power relationships implicit in the model of the doctor-patient relationship.

CONCLUSION

Because of the increasingly diverse ethnic makeup of the United States, and the cultural differences that exist nationwide between people of various ethnic groups, physicians need to be familiar with theoretical and practical considerations of how culture affects the presentation and treatment of psychiatric disorders. Ethnicity has emerged as a difficult, potentially divisive, and keenly important issue. Ultimately, proficiency in cross-cultural issues should be a celebration of the diversity of human experience and beliefs and should raise the hopes of bridging the distance between individuals. Cultural competence can be acquired as a clinical skill, although many trainees may have to advocate for such training to be added to their current curricula.

Cross-cultural issues in psychiatry should encompass much more than a comparison of illness frequency and clinical presentations in different geographical locations. Instead, cross-cultural issues raise complex questions and appreciation for the key role of culture in shaping health-related behavior and emotional and psychological development. The acquisition of awareness and skill in cross-cultural issues is consistent with the objectives of physicians to be able to work with as diverse a range of patients as possible; to be able to assess critically the values, biases, and perspectives of the Western tradition of biomedicine; and to further the goals of the physician's lifelong quest for self-knowledge and personal exploration.

REFERENCES

Alarcon RD: Cultural psychiatry. Psychiatr Clin N Am 1995;18(3).

Al-Issa I (editor): *Culture and Psychopathology.* University Park, 1982.

Al-Issa I, Tousignant M (editors): *Ethnicity, Immigration and Psychopathology.* Plenum, 1997.

Bateson MC: *Peripheral Visions.* Harper Collins, 1994.

Comas-Diaz L, Green B (editors): *Women of Color.* Guilford, 1994.

Comas-Diaz L, Griffith EH: *Clinical Guidelines in Cross-Cultural Mental Health.* Wiley, 1988.

Desjarlais R et al: *World Mental Health: Problems and Priorities in Low-Income Countries.* Oxford University Press, 1997.

Gaw A (editor): *Culture, Ethnicity and Mental Illness.* American Psychiatric, 1993.

Good BJ: *Medicine, Rationality, and Experience: An Anthropologic Perspective.* Cambridge University Press, 1996.

Kleinman A: *Rethinking Psychiatry.* Free, 1988.

Kleinman A: *Writings at the Margin.* University of California Press, 1997.

Koenig B, Gates-Williams J: Understanding cultural difference in caring for dying patients. West J Med 1995; 163:244.

Lin K-M, Poland RE, Nakasaki G: *Psychopharmacology and Psychobiology of Ethnicity.* American Psychiatric, 1993.

McGoldrick M, Pearce JK, Giordano J: *Ethnicity and Family Therapy.* Guilford, 1982.

Saba GW, Karrer B, Hardy KV (editors): *Minorities and Family Therapy.* Haworth, 1990.

Sargent C, Johnson T: *Medical Anthropology.* Praeger, 1996.

Smith PB, Bond MH: *Social Psychology Across Cultures.* Allyn & Bacon, 1994.

Transcultural Psychiatry (McGill University): http://www.mcgill.ca/Psychiatry/TPRR.html

Tsuang MT et al: *Textbook in Psychiatric Epidemiology.* Wiley, 1995.

Twemlow SW: DSM-IV from a cross-cultural perspective. Psychiatr Ann 1995;25(1):46.

20

Psychiatric Issues in the Homeless

Kyra Minninger, MD, & David Elkin, MD

Mental illness is quite prevalent among the homeless population, although the estimates vary. Some studies have shown that as many as 97% of the homeless have psychiatric disorders, but these studies were carried out in settings such as psychiatric emergency rooms and in clinics where the rate of psychiatric illness would be predictably higher than that of the homeless population in general. More reliable studies conducted through the National Institute of Mental Health estimate that one-quarter to one-third of the homeless population is severally chronically mentally ill, although other studies place the rate at 50% or higher. If substance abuse and other psychiatric disorders such as personality and anxiety disorders are included, the estimates of psychiatric illness among the homeless are much higher.

The homeless mentally ill represent a heterogeneous population in terms of medical and psychiatric diagnoses, level of functioning, previous psychiatric treatment, and prior living situations. These patients may be categorized in terms of their homeless situation. **Street people** often have schizophrenia, substance abuse disorders, or both, and they frequently have a history of psychiatric hospitalizations and medical problems. The **episodic homeless** are usually younger; are more likely to have a personality, mood, or substance abuse disorder; and tend to use mental health services sporadically. The **situationally homeless** are typically without housing because of an event or series of events—such as loss of a job—rather than a psychiatric disorder but may be prone to depression or anxiety disorders as a consequence of their situation.

The homeless have special needs and often have difficulty getting access to mental health services. Such services for the homeless are in short supply because of reductions in public health budgets. Practical problems, such as lack of transportation, and difficulties organizing thoughts and behavior because of a mental illness itself further reduce the likelihood that homeless mentally ill patients will use existing facilities. Effective treatment must be tailored to the needs of this challenging population and includes helping patients arrange for basic needs such as housing and food, drop-in services, and outreach contact.

Many factors contribute to the high prevalence of mental illness among the homeless. The discovery in the 1950s of chlorpromazine, the first antipsychotic medication, led physicians, public health officials, and politicians to release hundreds of thousands of severely mentally ill patients from long-term psychiatric facilities. These patients were expected to receive ongoing care at outpatient mental health centers. However, many patients fared poorly after discharge to the community. Many were too disorganized to seek outpatient care, and outpatient clinics were drastically underfunded and unable to provide care for those patients who did request psychiatric services.

Over the past 15 years, marked social, political, and economic changes have contributed to the dramatic increase in homelessness in general, as well as homelessness among those with mental illness. A decline in the availability of low-income housing, shifting patterns in industrial employment opportunities, deficiencies in the educational system, reductions in social welfare programs, and changing patterns of family relationships contributed to this increase.

People who have mental illness are particularly affected by these changes because of their symptoms, disabilities, lack of resources, and dependence on others. In addition they are susceptible to stigma, neglect, and victimization. Consequently, the severely mentally ill are especially vulnerable and at high risk of homelessness. One study found that homeless people who have mental illness identified their economic and social problems rather than symptoms of mental illness as the principle reasons for their homelessness.

MENTAL HEALTH PROBLEMS AMONG THE HOMELESS

The stereotype of the mentally ill homeless person is of someone who has a severe chronic illness such as schizophrenia. However, most mentally ill homeless people have other mental illnesses such as depression, phobias, and anxiety or personality disorders. The high prevalence of mental disorders and substance abuse disorders is not surprising given that these illnesses likely contribute to an individual's becoming and sometimes remaining homeless.

Combinations of psychiatric disorders are predictably high in the homeless population, since symptoms of one disorder may worsen symptoms of another. For instance, alcohol is a depressant and may cause or exacerbate depressive symptoms, and depression itself may lead to increased alcohol use. Coping with a mental illness is far more difficult in the context of ongoing substance abuse.

Table 20–1 shows the prevalence of psychiatric disorders among homeless patients in a study conducted by Breakey in 1989. This study included 298 men and 230 women who were selected randomly from more than 20 sampling sites serving homeless adults in the Baltimore, Maryland, area (eg, missions, shelters, and the jail). A subsample of 203 subjects randomly selected from the baseline survey underwent psychiatric and physical examinations. The results were striking in that a little over 90% of men and almost 80% of women had psychiatric disorders that were either active or in remission.

Table 20–1. Prevalence of psychiatric disorders in the homeless.

	Men, % (n = 125)	Women, % (n = 78)
Axis I disorders	91.2	79.5
Schizophrenia	42.0	48.7
Bipolar disorders	12.1	17.1
Major depression (unipolar)	11.3	15.8
Dementia	3.3	0
Others	8.0	7.8
Substance use disorders (current and in remission)	75.4	38.2
Alcohol	68.1	31.6
Other drugs	22.4	16.7
No Axis I disorders	8.8	20.5
Axis II (personality disorders)	46.5	45.3

SCHIZOPHRENIA

The worldwide prevalence of schizophrenia is 1–1.5%, but up to one-half of homeless people have schizophrenia. Schizophrenia is a chronic disease that waxes and wanes and is characterized by episodes of psychosis (see Chapter 4). Typically a patient has disorganized thoughts, may experience auditory or visual hallucinations, and may be quite paranoid. Patients' symptoms can vary dramatically: One schizophrenic person may be talkative, exhibit bizarre behavior, and wear odd or inappropriate clothes; another may be mute, withdrawn, immobilized, and immaculately groomed.

Although schizophrenia exists in all cultures and socioeconomic groups, it seems to be more prevalent in the lower socioeconomic groups. The **downward drift hypothesis** holds that affected persons either move into a lower socioeconomic group or fail to rise out of a low socioeconomic group because of their illness. The **social causation hypotheses** postulates that the increased stresses experienced by members of low socioeconomic groups contribute to the development of schizophrenia.

Mr. L, aged 23, was seen in the homeless clinic for a skin infection on his ankle. His clothes were ragged, he had no socks, and he indicated that he had been walking most of the day. He was obviously intelligent, displaying a sophisticated vocabulary and asking astute questions about antibiotic therapy. But when the medical student evaluating Mr. L asked where he usually spent the night, Mr. L became anxious and suspicious.

"Are you in on it?" Mr. L demanded. The student asked Mr. L what he meant.

"You know what I'm talking about, don't you. I can read your thoughts," Mr. L replied.

The student assured Mr. L that he did not know what he was referring to and asked him to explain. Mr. L calmed down and explained that since he was 7 years old, he'd "known about something that the government wants to keep hidden." He described a complex delusional scheme involving Marilyn Monroe, President Kennedy's assassination, global warming, and the North American Free Trade Agreement. He said that he had been the intended victim of several assassination attempts, but he'd "stayed one step ahead of 'them.'" This explained the patient's constant walking during the day and his reluctance to sleep in shelters at night. "I have to keep moving, so they can't get a bead on me," he added.

He was also convinced that "The Company" had placed an electronic transmitter in his head several years earlier. "That's how they can track me and know what I'm thinking. I can even hear them talking about me sometimes, but they don't know that the transmitter is a receiver, too, so I can hear what they're planning."

As an adolescent, Mr. L's parents had taken him to see a psychiatrist, who prescribed high doses of thiothixine, an antipsychotic. Mr. L reported that the medication "made me dopey, I couldn't think straight—there's no way I could defend myself in that kind of state." After high school, he tried college but left after 2 months. His parents helped him apply for disability benefits, which provided income for housing and food, but Mr. L spent 6 months riding Amtrak trains up and down the west coast, stopping only occasionally to call his parents to warn them that they were in "mortal danger" for being associated with him.

Mr. L's disability income ended when he refused to go for his renewal examination. "They have computers in that building, and they're only there for one reason—to download all of the information this thing in my head is storing." Thus in spite of the availability of psychiatric help, and a monthly income that would have provided shelter and food, Mr. L was too paranoid to use these services.

Another student remembered seeing the same patient presenting in the surgery clinic earlier that year asking for brain surgery to "help get this transmitter from my brain." The student encouraged Mr. L to follow-up at the nearby mental health clinic. Although Mr. L was too paranoid to agree to go, he said, "I'll come back here to talk to you, if you want—I think that I can trust you."

This case illustrates how difficult it is for patients who have schizophrenia to benefit from the services that are available to them. However, contact with an open-minded and patient interviewer in a homeless clinic may foster trust and help build a better bridge to these services.

Schizophrenia & Comorbid Disorders

Patients who have schizophrenia are likely to suffer from depression as well. About 50% of patients who have schizophrenia attempt suicide at some time. Male and female patients are equally likely to commit suicide, and 10–15% will succeed in killing themselves. Several risk factors are associated with suicide among patients who have schizophrenia: depressive symptoms, young age, high levels of functioning (eg, college education) before developing psychotic symptoms, recent discharge from the hospital, unemployment, social isolation, and living alone. Approximately 30–50% of patients who have schizophrenia abuse or are dependent on alcohol, 15–25% use cannabis, and 5–10% use cocaine. Sub-

stance use typically exacerbates underlying psychotic symptoms.

Treatment of Schizophrenia Among the Homeless

Individual psychosocial interventions are as important as medications in treating homeless patients who have severe psychiatric disturbances such as schizophrenia. Clinicians should offer services that the patient will value. A homeless patient may be more concerned about eating than anything else, so that assistance in finding free meals may be of great value. Some patients may have had negative experiences in the past and may not trust doctors. Schizophrenia itself often causes paranoia and suspiciousness, which may be directed at the clinician as well as at the entire medical establishment.

Patients should be encouraged to take or at least consider taking antipsychotic medications. They may be more likely to take medications if clinicians explain how these medications can decrease anxiety, improve sleep, and help to organize thoughts in addition to decreasing paranoia, grandiosity, and auditory and visual hallucinations. Although antipsychotics are effective in decreasing psychotic symptoms, the rate of noncompliance is high among schizophrenic patients. (See Chapter 4 for a detailed discussion of the treatment options available for patients who have schizophrenia.)

DEPRESSION

Depression is common among the homeless. As mentioned earlier, depressive symptoms are likely to be exacerbated by the state of homelessness, and depression itself may contribute to an individual becoming and remaining homeless. Depression occurs most often in people who have no close relationships, or who are divorced or separated. Given the high prevalence of depression among the homeless population, clinicians must consider depression in the differential diagnosis. Depression is often missed because clinicians do not ask appropriate screening questions. In some cases, depressive symptoms are viewed as a normal reaction to the stress of being homeless, and the opportunity to assess for a preexisting or more severe depression is precluded.

Depression & Comorbid Disorders

Sometimes people use drugs and alcohol to mask a depression. Although a patient may believe that substance abuse helps him or her cope with symptoms of depression, drug use interferes with the individual's ability to find more constructive ways to face problems and also exacerbates the underlying symptoms.

Mr. D, an African-American man in his early 30s, presented at a medical student–run homeless clinic for treatment of an abscess in his mouth. He asked for codeine to relieve the pain until he could see a dentist. Physical examination showed that he had several cracked or missing teeth and inflamed gums. The medical student examining Mr. D was struck by his intelligence and poised demeanor, although he also noticed that Mr. D's shoulders slumped when he was told that the clinic did not dispense opioid pain relievers. The student said to Mr. D, "It must be pretty hard out there, and it looks like you've been in pain for a while." This empathic comment seemed to help Mr. D feel understood, and he began to talk about how difficult it was to live in shelters or in the neighborhood park.

Mr. D had made other appointments for dental and medical care but had not followed through. When the student asked why, Mr. D explained that he was usually out "scoring some crack—I know it's sick, but I'm weak, I just find myself going after it every time I have any money." Mr. D did freelance art work but had never saved enough money to pay for rent and a deposit on an apartment. He felt too ashamed to ask his parents or sister for help. He expressed self-loathing in his response, stating, "Why would anyone waste their money helping a crack-head like me—it's a hopeless situation, you know." He exhibited many symptoms of depression and described part of the allure of crack as "the best way I know to make those feelings go away, at least for a while."

Mr. D described a 10-month period of sobriety he had 2 years earlier, while he participated in a research protocol using fluoxetine to help with cravings for cocaine. He already had the phone contacts for a drug rehabilitation program but said, "I've had the numbers for a while, but there's a long wait. I keep losing my initiative to go." He was urged to contact the local mental health clinic for follow-up, including an evaluation for antidepressants and therapy, and to become involved in Narcotics Anonymous meetings to help keep his focus on entering a rehab program.

By the end of the interview, Mr. D felt more optimistic about his chances of ending his cycle of drug use and homelessness. "This really helped to put things into perspective," he said of his appointment at the homeless clinic. "I think I will follow through this time." However, a follow-up call to the mental health clinic 2 weeks later revealed that Mr. D had not made an appointment to be evaluated.

Treatment of Depression Among the Homeless

The choice of treatment depends on the etiology of the depressive symptoms. If there is significant ongoing substance abuse, then the recommendation may be for substance abuse treatment and further evaluation of mood symptoms after a period of sobriety has been reached. Antidepressant treatment should be considered for patients experiencing significant distress and difficulty functioning because of mood disturbances. In working with the homeless population, clinicians often encounter barriers to treatment, and it may be difficult to find appropriate psychiatric services, especially if a patient is without resources and unable to keep regularly scheduled appointments.

SUBSTANCE ABUSE

The most prevalent disorders among the homeless are those associated with substance use. According to Breakey's study, the rate of substance abuse was extremely high among the homeless: 69% of the men and 38% of the women were diagnosed as probable or definite alcoholics. The prevalence of other substance use disorders was also substantial, though much lower than for alcohol use, and there was little difference between the sexes. There were high rates of comorbidity for mental illness and substance abuse, as well as physical disorders. Of men who had active or remitted alcohol use disorders, 38% also had a major mental illness; of the women, 32% also had a major mental illness.

SUICIDE

Each year 30,000 deaths are attributable to suicide, and there are probably ten times as many suicide attempts. These statistics do not take into account chronic self-destructive behaviors such as suspicious accident-proneness, alcoholism, cigarette smoking, and poor compliance with treatment regimens for medical illness.

The homeless are at greater risk for suicide than the general population because of a variety of factors. Work is generally protective against suicide, whereas a fall in socioeconomic status (especially prominent declines among the homeless) increases suicide risk. The homeless have higher rates of mental illness and substance use than the general population, factors strongly correlated with suicide risk. The risk of suicide among heroin users is 20 times greater than that of the general public. Failure of relationships and marriages also increases the suicide risk. Other risk factors for suicide frequently encountered in homeless populations include medical illness; histories of legal problems; impulsive behavior; and estrangement from family, poor social support, and feelings of alienation from society.

Although precise statistics regarding suicide among the homeless are unavailable, homeless patients should be screened carefully for suicidal thoughts and behaviors. Access to a lethal amount of drugs, intravenous drug use, antisocial or borderline personality disorders, chaotic life styles, impulsiveness, hopelessness, depression and other severe mental illnesses, and intoxication are all risk factors that should be considered in assessing suicide risk among homeless patients. When patients cannot be stabilized on an outpatient basis, inpatient psychiatric hospitalization may be clinically indicated.

PHYSICAL HEALTH PROBLEMS

The prevalence of physical health problems is high among the homeless. Common health problems include respiratory tract disease, including tuberculosis; peripheral vascular disease; dermatologic problems; infectious disease, including sexually transmitted disease; and trauma. Mortality rates are higher among the homeless, in part because of their increased exposure to environmental toxins and other hazards of street life such as trauma, poor nutrition, poor personal hygiene, and increased risk of infectious disease through crowding and debilitation. People who have schizophrenia have a higher mortality rate from accidents and natural causes than do the general population, and homeless patients who have schizophrenia may be at even higher risk. Studies have shown that up to 80% of homeless patients who have schizophrenia also have significant concurrent medical conditions and that up to 50% of those conditions may be undiagnosed.

TREATMENT ISSUES AMONG THE HOMELESS

The treatment of mental disorders in the homeless requires a comprehensive plan addressing the social problems that compound and cause mental illness. Medications used to treat psychiatric disorders may be helpful, but a purely psychopharmacologic plan is likely to fail because of poor compliance, substance use, a lack of follow-up care, and the destabilizing effect of homelessness on the illness itself. Other treatment options that may help ameliorate both mental illness and homelessness include:

- Social services that can help patients find housing (such as local shelters) or food. Patients can also be assisted in applying for services for which they qualify, including social security disability funding, Medicaid (a health plan for indigent patients), and food stamps.
- Existing public health outpatient clinics, which, though usually underfunded, offer services such

as psychiatric appointments that may help patients break the cycle of mental illness and homelessness. Military veterans can be directed to programs run by the Veteran's Administration.

- Substance abuse programs, which can help patients to reduce or eliminate drug and alcohol problems. These programs have been cut back because of reduced public health budgets, and waiting lists of 2 months or longer are common. Some programs require interested patients to check in by phone or in person to continue to reserve their place. Meanwhile, patients can be encouraged to make use of groups such as Alcoholics Anonymous (AA) that have daily meetings free of charge. The social support offered by groups such as AA is often of great value to homeless people who struggle with dependency on drugs and alcohol and with feelings of alienation.
- Other innovative programs have been created in recent years to help the homeless. Mobile assistance programs take psychiatrists and social workers to the streets, delivering mental health services to homeless patients "in the field." Several medical schools have developed free medical clinics in conjunction with homeless shelters that allow medical students to gain supervised clinical experience while providing much-needed medical and psychiatric services. Although the scope of these clinics is limited, the contact with homeless patients can serve as a bridge to better access and follow-up with existing clinics. Other programs use case managers who perform outreach work, providing homeless patients with comprehensive assistance in obtaining available medical, psychiatric, and social services, and offering encouragement and help signing up for services such as substance use programs and housing.

BARRIERS TO MENTAL HEALTH CARE FOR THE HOMELESS

The same mental illnesses that require care may interfere with a patient's ability to reach help that exists. For example, patients who have schizophrenia may be paranoid and, as a result, fearful and suspicious of health-care facilities. Psychosis, dementia, or substance use may be accompanied by declines in judgment and insight so severe that patients do not realize that they need help. Mental illnesses also lead to disorganization and an inability to plan or execute simple tasks, such as calling or walking in for an appointment. Depression and substance use may keep patients from seeking assistance by removing hope that life can be better.

Many external barriers also prevent the homeless from receiving adequate mental health care:

- Lack of health insurance.
- Lack of money to buy medication or to provide for basic needs such as food or shelter.
- Lack of transportation as a result of poverty or an inability to walk long distances (eg, from foot infections, weakness from hunger, or inadequate clothing).
- Lack of social supports such as family and friends, which are essential for mental health in all individuals.
- Lack of means of receiving communications (eg, a telephone or mailbox).
- Poor quality of services. Fewer outpatient clinics are available, and these clinics may offer care only to more critically ill patients, for example, those who are suicidal or psychotic. Patients who have milder conditions such as depression may be turned away.
- Inadequate commitment from society to ameliorate homelessness and the social problems that foster homelessness, especially poverty.

EMOTIONAL REACTIONS TO PATIENTS

Clinicians' emotional reactions to a homeless patient may be related mostly to the patient's homeless state or to particular illnesses. For instance, clinicians may experience strong feelings of fear about being without adequate resources. Or they may feel guilty, spoiled, or undeserving about having a place to sleep, a home, a car, and other belongings as well as relationships and an education.

Countertransference may also arise in clinicians working with patients who have particular mental disorders. For instance, clinicians may feel angry and frustrated at patients who continue to abuse alcohol despite their efforts to encourage sobriety. They may also have feelings of anger at a patient's denial or minimization of his or her drug dependence; they may experience self-doubt, a lack of self-confidence, or feelings of helplessness resulting from their inability to stop a patient from using drugs; or they may feel hatred toward a patient who may be manipulative. In working with patients who have severe chronic mental illnesses such as schizophrenia, clinicians may experience feelings of confusion, fear, anger, or anxiety. An understanding of these feelings can help clinicians work most effectively with this population.

CROSS-CULTURAL ISSUES

People from different ethnic groups are affected differently by socioeconomic pressures. Numerous studies have documented that disproportionately high numbers of African Americans and Latinos are homeless. Racial and cultural issues affect treatment as well. For example, although the incidence of depression does not vary by race, clinicians tend to underdiagnose mood disorders and overdiagnose schizophrenia in patients who have racial or cultural backgrounds different from their own. Studies have shown that Caucasian clinicians especially tend to underdiagnose mood disorders and overdiagnose schizophrenia in African-American and Latino patients. Cultural factors may affect patients' perceptions of their own illness, their beliefs about what causes and cures mental illness, and their faith in Western treatments.

LEGAL & ETHICAL ISSUES

Involuntary hospitalization is the most common legal issue related to providing medical care for the homeless. Individuals can be hospitalized against their will and placed on a legal hold in most states for up to several days for an initial evaluation period. Patients can be hospitalized involuntarily in three situations: if they are a danger to themselves, if they are a danger to others, or if they are unable to care for themselves, that is, if they are "gravely disabled."

The question of what it means to be able to care for oneself is complex, and at the most basic level focuses on one's ability to obtain food, clothing, and shelter. Many homeless people are able to provide for themselves by living in shelters, in protected tents, or under freeways; they know where to find free food and clothing at churches or community organizations; and they may beg for money or have some financial assistance from the state to buy needed items.

Homeless people who are not able to care for themselves may become hypothermic sleeping on the streets, they may become malnourished and exhibit signs of starvation, or they may develop medical complications such as sunburn or frostbite. At times it can be difficult to determine whether a homeless person is able to care for him or herself, and whether hospitalization is needed. The decision should be thought through carefully since the consequences of not hospitalizing someone can be serious and even life threatening, yet taking away someone's freedom unnecessarily is a violation of an individual's right to make basic life decisions.

The care of homeless patients, who frequently lack health insurance, has become increasingly difficult as funding for health care shrinks. In the past, public health hospitals and clinics that provided medical and psychiatric services were able to recoup some of their costs from state and federal funding, and by charging all patients greater fees. Third-party insurance payers were thus "recruited" to help defer the costs of patients who lacked insurance. Cost-cutting by health maintenance organizations and managed care companies has led to a growing reluctance by these organizations to assume the same responsibility for patients who lack insurance. Reductions in federal and state spending have led to a scarcity of available public money to cover these costs.

Meanwhile, managed care companies—sometimes run on a for-profit basis—are poised to assume management of public health hospitals and clinics. While proponents argue that health-care costs must be contained, critics fear that financial incentives will lead to widespread cutting of services and denial of care, leaving the most vulnerable patients—those who lack insurance or political clout—likely to receive far less medical care than is available now. Because psychiatric services frequently are reduced even more than

are most other types of medical care, homeless patients who have severe mental illness are likely to become even more marginalized. Physicians may find themselves in the difficult position of being told by health-care administrators to deny services to homeless patients—which in turn results in greater chances for disease progression or death due to illness or exposure—or risk losing their jobs.

CONCLUSION

Although the homeless themselves have much in common, each patient is unique in his or her treatment needs. The homeless are disadvantaged in many ways that impede their receiving needed treatment, and they typically underutilize or inappropriately utilize health services. These problems may result from the effects of mental illness itself, which can interfere with one's ability to recognize and acknowledge the presence of a mental illness, affect one's motivation or desire for treatment, and hinder one's ability to negotiate for services in a very complicated system.

REFERENCES

Breakey WR et al: Health and mental health problems of homeless men and women in Baltimore. JAMA 1989; 262:1352.

Cohen CI: Down and out in New York and London: a cross-national comparison of homelessness. Hospital Commun Psychiatr 1994;45:769.

Cohen CI, Thompson KS: Homeless mentally ill or mentally ill homeless? Am J Psychiatr 1992;149:816.

Herman D et al: Self-assessed need for mental health services among homeless adults. Hospital Commun Psychiatr 1994;119(44):1181.

Jecker NS: Caring for socially undesirable patients. Cambridge Q Healthcare Ethics 1996;5:500.

Kaplan H, Sadock B (editors): *Kaplan and Sadock's Synopsis of Psychiatry,* 7th edition. Williams & Wilkins. 1994.

National Resource Center on Homelessness and Mental Illness: http://www.prainc.com/nrc

Susser E et al: Psychiatric problems in homeless men. Arch Gen Psychiatr 1989;46:845.

Index

NOTE: Page numbers in bold face type indicate a major discussion. A *t* following a page number indicates tabular material and an *f* following a page number indicates a figure. Drugs are listed under their generic names. When a drug trade name is listed, the reader is referred to the generic name.